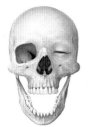

# WinkingSkull.com *PLUS*

## <u>Your</u> study aid for must-know anatomy

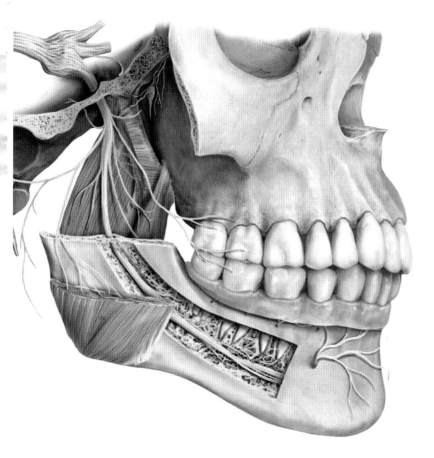

## Register for WinkingSkull.com *PLUS* – master human anatomy with this uniquely interactive online learning tool.

Use the access code below to register for **WinkingSkull.com** *PLUS* to view over 560 full-color illustrations and radiographs from Thieme's bestselling anatomy and radiology publications. After studying this invaluable image bank, quiz yourself on key body structures, including head and neck anatomy. Get your score instantly to check your own progress or to compare with other users' results.

**WinkingSkull.com** *PLUS* has everything you need to prepare for your dental Boards, including:

- 100 full-color dental anatomy images
- More than 460 general anatomy full-color illustrations and radiographs
- An extensive section on head and neck anatomy covering everything from the bones of the head to the neurovasculature of the skull and face
- Intuitive design that simplifies navigation
- "Labels-on, labels off" function that makes studying easy and fun
- Timed self-tests–with instant results
- Exclusive clinical material, including MRIs and CT scans

**Simply visit WinkingSkull.com and follow these instructions to get started today.**

**If you do not already have a** free WinkingSkull.com account, visit www.winkingskull.com, click on 'Register Now,' and complete the registration form. Enter the scratch-off code below.

**If you already have a WinkingSkull.com account,** go to the "My Account" page and click on the "Enter WinkingSkull PLUS Access Code" link. Enter the scratch-off code below.

*This book cannot be returned if the access code panel is scratched off.*

**System requirements for optimal use of WinkingSkull.com PLUS:** **

|  | **WINDOWS** | **MAC** |
|---|---|---|
| **Recommended Browser(s)** | Windows XP or Vista | MAC OS X 10.4.8 or higher |
| **Silverlight Plug-in** | Microsoft Silverlight*<br><br>* *After registering, follow the prompts to download Silverlight, a free plug-in required for use on the study and test pages* | |
| **Recommended for optimal usage experience** | Monitor resolutions:<br><br>• A display capable of reading millions of colors<br>• Normal (4:3) 1024 x 786 or higher | |

** *While you may find that WinkingSkull.com works with some older systems, we recommend the above as minimum requirements for using the capabilities of the site.*

# Head and Neck Anatomy for Dental Medicine

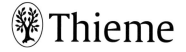

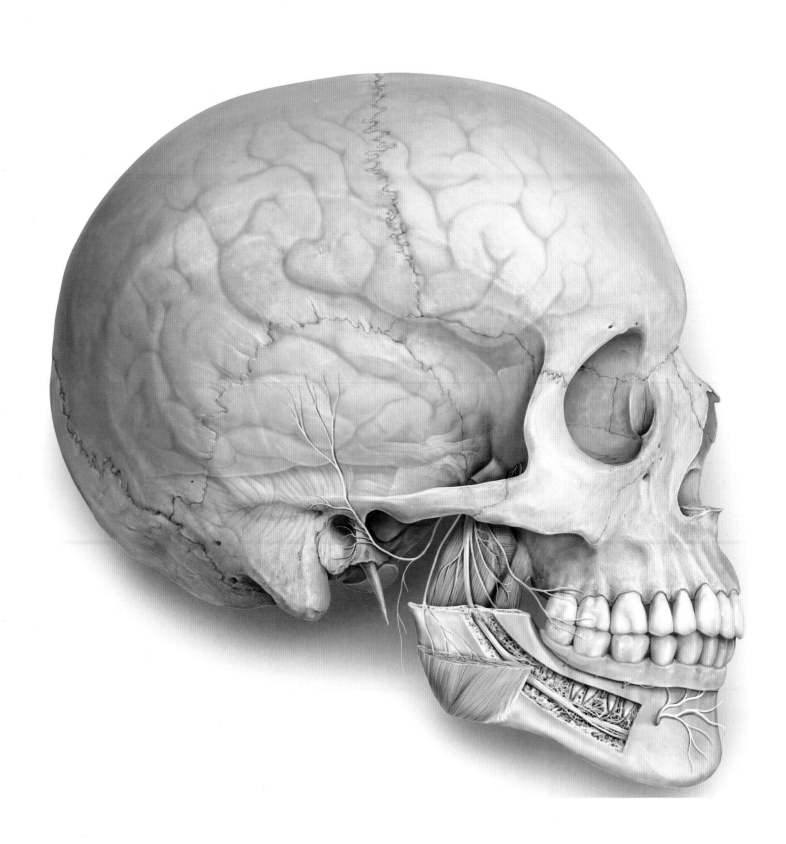

# Head and Neck Anatomy for Dental Medicine

**Edited by**

Eric W. Baker

**Based on the work of**

Michael Schuenke
Erik Schulte
Udo Schumacher

**Illustrations by**

Markus Voll
Karl Wesker

Thieme

New York · Stuttgart

Thieme Medical Publishers, Inc.
333 Seventh Avenue
New York, New York 10001

Based on the work of Michael Schuenke, MD, PhD, Erik Schulte, MD, and
Udo Schumacher, MD

Eric W. Baker, MA, MPhil
Educational Coordinator and Director of Human Gross Anatomy
Department of Basic Science and Craniofacial Biology
New York University College of Dentistry
New York, New York 10010

Michael Schuenke, MD, PhD
Institute of Anatomy
Christian Albrecht University Kiel
Olshausenstrasse 40
D-24098 Kiel

Erik Schulte, MD
Department of Anatomy and Cell Biology
Johannes Gutenberg University
Saarstrasse 19-21
D-55099 Mainz

Udo Schumacher, MD, FRCPath, CBiol, FIBiol, DSc
Institute of Anatomy II: Experimental Morphology
Center for Experimental Medicine
University Medical Center Hamburg-Eppendorf
Martinistrasse 52
D-20246 Hamburg

**Library of Congress Cataloging-in-Publication Data**

Head and neck anatomy for dental medicine / edited by Eric W. Baker ;
based on the work of Michael Schuenke, Erik Schulte, Udo Schumacher ;
illustrations by Markus Voll, Karl Wesker.
        p. ; cm.
    Includes bibliographical references and index.
    ISBN 978-1-60406-209-0 (softcover : alk. paper)    1. Head—Anatomy—
Atlases.    2. Neck—Anatomy—Atlases.    I. Baker, Eric W. (Eric William),
1961–    II. Schünke, Michael.    III. Schulte, Erik. IV. Schumacher, Udo.
    [DNLM: 1. Head—anatomy & histology—Atlases. 2. Dentistry—
Atlases.    3. Neck—anatomy & histology—Atlases.    WE 17 H432 2010]
    QM535.H43 2010
    611'.910223–dc22
                                                            2009041592

*Developmental Editor:* Bridget N. Queenan and Julie O'Meara
*Editorial Director, Educational Products:* Cathrin Weinstein, MD, and
Anne T. Vinnicombe
*Associate Manager, Book Production:* Adelaide Elsie Starbecker
*International Production Director:* Andreas Schabert
*Director of Sales:* Ross Lumpkin
*Vice President, International Marketing and Sales:* Cornelia Schulze
*Chief Financial Officer:* James W. Mitos
*President:* Brian D. Scanlan
*Illustrators:* Markus Voll and Karl Wesker
*Compositor:* MPS Content Services, A Macmillan Company
*Printer:* Leo Paper Products Ltd.

**Important note:** Medical knowledge is ever-changing. As new research
and clinical experience broaden our knowledge, changes in treatment
and drug therapy may be required. The authors and editors of the material herein have consulted sources believed to be reliable in their efforts
to provide information that is complete and in accord with the stand-
ards accepted at the time of publication. However, in view of the pos-
sibility of human error by the authors, editors, or publisher of the work
herein or changes in medical knowledge, neither the authors, editors,
nor publisher, nor any other party who has been involved in the preparation of this work, warrants that the information contained herein is in
every respect accurate or complete, and they are not responsible for any
errors or omissions or for the results obtained from use of such information. Readers are encouraged to confirm the information contained
herein with other sources. For example, readers are advised to check the
product information sheet included in the package of each drug they
plan to administer to be certain that the information contained in this
publication is accurate and that changes have not been made in the rec-
ommended dose or in the contraindications for administration. This rec-
ommendation is of particular importance in connection with new or
infrequently used drugs.

ISBN 978-1-60406-209-0

# Dedication

To my wonderful wife, Amy Curran Baker, and my awe-inspiring daughters, Phoebe and Claire.

# Contents

# Regions of the Head

# Neck

# Neuroanatomy

# Sectional Anatomy

# Appendix

# Preface

I was amazed and impressed with the extraordinary detail, accuracy, and beauty of the material that was created for the three-volume *THIEME Atlas of Anatomy* by authors Michael Schuenke, Erik Schulte, and Udo Schumacher and artists Markus Voll and Karl Wesker. I felt that these atlases and their pedagogical concepts were a significant addition to anatomical education. I was delighted to be invited to use this exceptional material as the cornerstone of an effort to create an atlas that specifically focuses on the structures of the head and neck as they are taught to students of dental medicine.

Starting from the extensive coverage of these structures distributed across the three volumes of *THIEME Atlas of Anatomy*, I have organized, revised, and added new material to create *Head and Neck Anatomy for Dental Medicine*, a learning atlas for the first-year students of dental medicine taking a gross anatomy course. Because of the exceptional quality artwork and explanatory information concerning the structures of the head and the neck, it can also serve as a reference for practitioners of dental medicine and for students and practitioners in the more general field of dentistry (dental hygiene, dental assistants, etc.) and/or any field dealing primarily with the head and neck (ENT, speech pathology, ophthalmology, etc.).

Some key features of this atlas are as follows:

Organized in a user-friendly format in which each two-page spread is a self-contained guide to a specific topic.

Intuitively arranged to facilitate learning. Coverage of each region begins by discussing the bones and joints and then adds the muscles, the vasculature, and the nerves. This information is then integrated in the topographic neurovascular anatomy coverage that follows.

Features large, full-color, highly detailed artwork with clear and thorough labeling and descriptive captions, plus numerous schematics to elucidate concepts and tables to summarize key information for review and reference.

Includes a full chapter devoted to sectional anatomy with radiographic images to demonstrate anatomy as seen in the clinical setting.

The study of head and neck anatomy is challenging due to the intricacies of the structures involved, but this atlas manages to convey detailed anatomical information in a way that is both thorough and efficient, making for a very effective study tool.

I would like to thank Susana Tejada, class of 2010, Boston University School of Dental Medicine, and the group of dedicated anatomy instructors who provided feedback to Thieme as they were developing the concept for this atlas: Dr. Norman F. Capra, Department of Neural and Pain Sciences, University of Maryland Dental School, Baltimore, Maryland; Dr. Bob Hutchins, Associate Professor, Department of Biomedical Sciences, Baylor College of Dentistry, Dallas, Texas; Dr. Brian R. MacPherson, Professor and Vice-Chair, Department of Anatomy and Neurobiology, University of Kentucky, Lexington, Kentucky; and Dr. Nicholas Peter Piesco, Associate Professor, Department of Oral Medicine, University of Pittsburgh, Pittsburgh, Pennsylvania.

I would like to thank my colleagues at New York University who assisted me in this endeavor: Professor Terry Harrison, Department of Anthropology, for fostering my interests in comparative anatomy and instilling an appreciation for detail and accuracy in anatomical description; Dr. Richard Cotty for his keen eye in looking over the sectional anatomy in this atlas; Dr. Phyllis Slott, Dr. Elena Cunningham, Dr. Avelin Malyango, and Dr. Johanna Warshaw for assistance in all things anatomy related, including countless discussions on all aspects of current anatomical education and the need for a detailed head and neck anatomy atlas. Finally, I would like to thank Dr. Inder Singh for mentoring me as an anatomist and serving as an inspirational anatomy professor.

I would like to thank my colleagues at Thieme Publishers who so professionally facilitated this effort. I wish to thank Cathrin Weinstein, MD, Editorial Director, Educational Products, for inviting me to create this atlas. I extend very special thanks and appreciation to Bridget Queenan, Developmental Editor, who edited and developed the manuscript with an outstanding talent for visualization and intuitive flow of information. I am also very grateful to her for catching many details along the way while always patiently responding to requests for artwork and labeling changes. Thanks to Julie O'Meara, Developmental Editor, for joining the team in the correction phase. She graciously reminded me of deadlines, while always being available to work with me on proofs and to troubleshoot problems. Finally, thanks to Elsie Starbecker, Associate Manager, Book Production, who with great care and speed produced this atlas with its over 900 illustrations. Their hard work has made *Head and Neck Anatomy for Dental Medicine* a reality.

Eric W. Baker
New York, New York

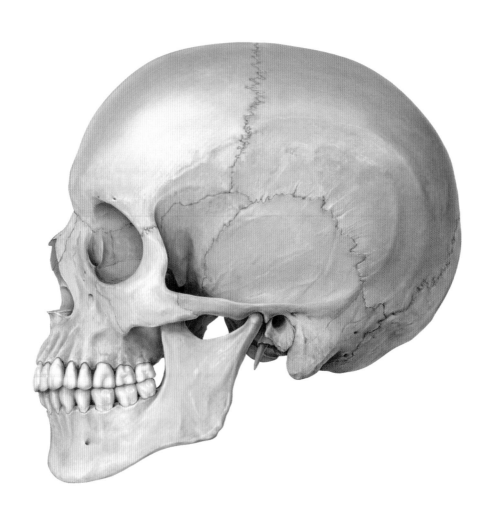

# Head

# Development of the Cranial Bones

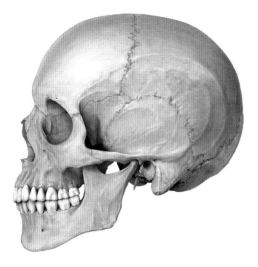

*Fig. 1.1* **Bones of the skull**
Left lateral view. The skull forms a bony capsule that encloses the brain and viscera of the head. The bones of the skull are divided into two parts. The viscerocranium (orange), the facial skeleton, is formed primarily from the pharyngeal (branchial) arches (see p. 61). The neurocranium (gray), the cranial vault, is the bony capsule enclosing the brain. It is divided into two parts based on ossification (see **Fig. 1.2**). The *cartilaginous* neurocranium undergoes endochondral ossification to form the base of the skull. The *membranous* neurocranium undergoes intramembranous ossification.

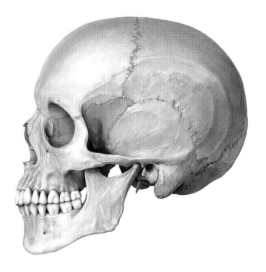

*Fig. 1.2* **Ossification of the cranial bones**
Left lateral view. The bones of the skull develop either directly or indirectly from mesenchymal connective tissue. The bones of the desmocranium (gray) develop directly via intramembranous ossification of mesenchymal connective tissue. The bones of the chondrocranium (blue) develop indirectly via endochondral ossification of hyaline cartilage. *Note:* The skull base is formed exclusively by the chondrocranium. Elements formed via intramembranous and endochondral ossification may fuse to form a single bone (e.g., the elements of the occipital, temporal, and sphenoid bones contributing to the skull base are cartilaginous, while the rest of the bone is membranous).

| *Table 1.1* **Development of the skull** | | | | | | |
|---|---|---|---|---|---|---|
| The bones of the skull can be understood using three major criteria: embryonic origins, location in the skull, and type of ossification. The majority of the viscerocranium (facial skeleton) is derived from the pharyngeal (branchial) arches (see p. 61). The neurocranium (cranial vault) is divided into membranous and cartilaginous parts based on ossification. The cartilaginous neurocranium (endochondral ossification) forms the skull base. | | | | | | |

| Embryonic origins | | Cranium | | Ossification | | Adult bone |
|---|---|---|---|---|---|---|
| | | V | N | I | E | |
| Paraxial mesoderm | | | Nm | I | | Occipital bone (upper portion) |
| | | | Nc | | E | Occipital bone (lower portion) |
| | | | Nm | I | | Parietal bone |
| | | | Nm | | E | Temporal bone (petrous part) |
| | | | Nm | | E | Temporal bone (mastoid process) |
| Neural crest | | | Nm | I | | Temporal bone (squamous part) |
| | | | Nm | I | | Frontal bone |
| | | | Nc | | E | Sphenoid bone |
| | | V | | I | | Sphenoid bone (pterygoid process) |
| | | V | | | E | Ethmoid bone |
| | | | Nc | | E | Ethmoid bone (cribriform plate) |
| Neural crest, pharyngeal (branchial) arches | 1st branchial arch, maxillary process | V | | I | | Maxilla |
| | | V | | I | | Nasal bone |
| | | V | | I | | Lacrimal bone |
| | | V | | I | | Vomer |
| | | V | | I | | Palatine bone |
| | | V | | I | | Zygomatic bone |
| | | V | | I | | Temporal bone (tympanic part) |
| | | V | | | E | Inferior nasal turbinate |
| | 1st branchial arch, mandibular process | V | | I | | Mandible |
| | | V | | | E | Malleus |
| | | V | | | E | Incus |
| | 2nd branchial arch | V | | | E | Stapes |
| | | V | | | E | Temporal bone (styloid process) |
| | | V | | | E | Hyoid bone (superior part, lesser cornu) |
| | 3rd branchial arch | V | | | E | Hyoid bone (inferior part, greater cornu) |

V = viscerocranium; N = neurocranium; Nm = neurocranium (membranous); Nc = neurocranium (cartilaginous); I = intramembranous; E = endochondral.
*Note:* Tubular (long) bones undergo endochondral ossification. The clavicle is the only exception. Congenital defects of intramembranous ossification therefore affect both the skull and clavicle (cleidocranial dysostosis).

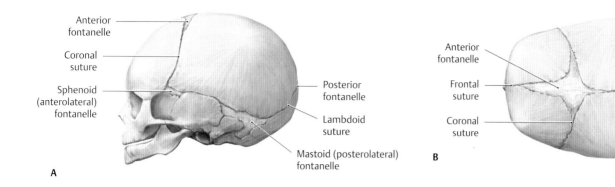

**Fig. 1.3 Cranial sutures (craniosynostoses) and fontanelles**
**A** Left lateral view of neonatal skull.
**B** Superior view of neonatal skull.
The flat cranial bones grow as the brain expands; thus the sutures between them remain open after birth. In the neonate, there are six areas (fontanelles) between the still-growing cranial bones that are occupied by unossified fibrous membrane. The posterior fontanelle provides a reference point for describing the position of the fetal head during childbirth. The anterior fontanelle provides access for drawing cerebrospinal fluid (CSF) samples in infants (e.g., in suspected meningitis).

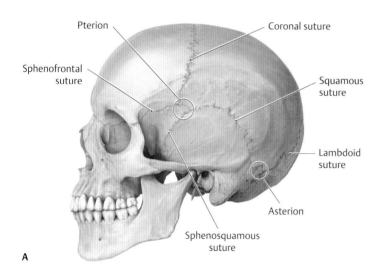
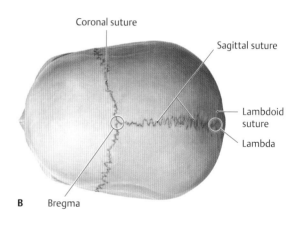

**Fig. 1.4 Sutures in the adult skull**
**A** Left lateral view.
**B** Superior view.
Synostosis (the fusion of the cranial bones along the sutures) occurs during adulthood. Although the exact times of closure vary, the order (sagittal, coronal, lambdoid) does not. Closure of each fontanelle yields a particular junction (see **Table 1.2**). Premature closure of the cranial sutures produces characteristic deformities (see **Fig. 1.14**, p. 9).

| Fontanelle | Age at closure | Suture | Age at ossification |
|---|---|---|---|
| 1 Posterior fontanelle | 2–3 months (lambda) | Frontal suture | Childhood |
| 2 Sphenoid (anterolateral) fontanelles | 6 months (pterion) | Sagittal suture | 20–30 years old |
| 2 Mastoid fontanelles | 18 months (asterion) | Coronal suture | 30–40 years old |
| 1 Anterior fontanelle | 36 months (bregma) | Lambdoid suture | 40–50 years old |

**Table 1.2 Closure of sutures and fontanelles**

# Skull: Lateral View

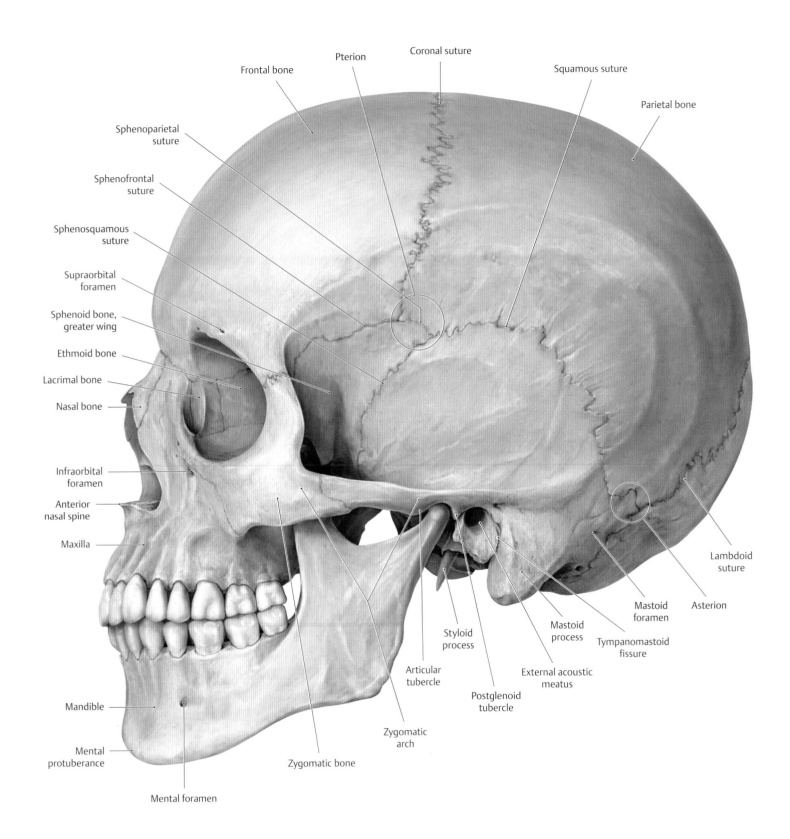

**Fig. 1.5 Lateral view of the skull (cranium)**
Left lateral view. This view displays the greatest number of cranial bones (indicated by different colors in **Fig. 1.6**). The individual bones and their salient features are described in the pages that follow. The teeth are described on pp. 180–189.

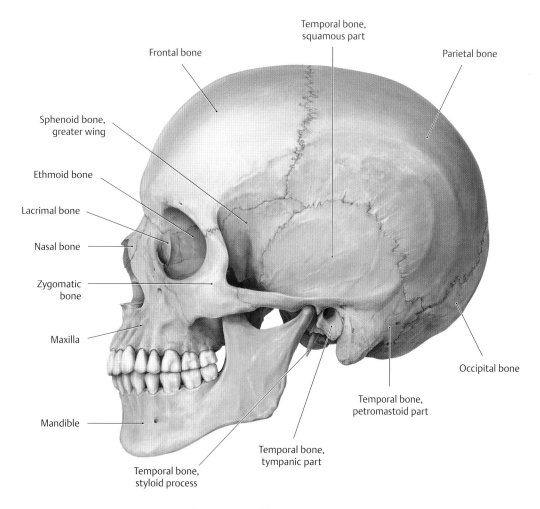

**Fig. 1.6 Cranial bones: overview**
Left lateral view.

Labels on figure:
- Temporal bone, squamous part
- Frontal bone
- Parietal bone
- Sphenoid bone, greater wing
- Ethmoid bone
- Lacrimal bone
- Nasal bone
- Zygomatic bone
- Maxilla
- Mandible
- Temporal bone, styloid process
- Temporal bone, tympanic part
- Temporal bone, petromastoid part
- Occipital bone

| *Table 1.3* **Bones of the skull** | | | |
|---|---|---|---|
| The cranial bones are shown within the skull and some are also shown individually (see referenced pages; boldface page numbers are for bones shown individually). | | | |

| Bone | Page | Bone | Page |
|---|---|---|---|
| Frontal bone | 5, 7, 9, 11, 14, 108, 142 | Temporal bone:<br>• Squamous part<br>• Petrous part<br>• Tympanic part<br>• Styloid part | 5, 7, 9, 12, 14, **18**, **19** |
| Nasal bone | 5, 7, 11, 108, 142 | Occipital bone | 5, 9, 11, 12, 14, **20** |
| Lacrimal bone | 5, 108, 142 | Parietal bone | 5, 7, 9, 11, 12, 14 |
| Ethmoid bone | 5, 7, 14, **21**, 108, 142, 190 | Sphenoid bone:<br>• Greater wing<br>• Lesser wing<br>• Pterygoid process | 5, 7, 9, 14, **16**, **17**, 108, 142, 190 |
| Maxilla | 5, 7, 9, 12, 108, 142, 190 | Vomer | 9, 12, 142, 190 |
| Palatine bone | 9, 12, 108, 142, 190 | Inferior nasal concha | 7, 12, 142, 190 |
| Zygomatic bone | 5, 7, 12, 108 | Hyoid bone | **23** |
| Mandible | 5, 7, 9, **22** | | |

# Skull: Anterior View

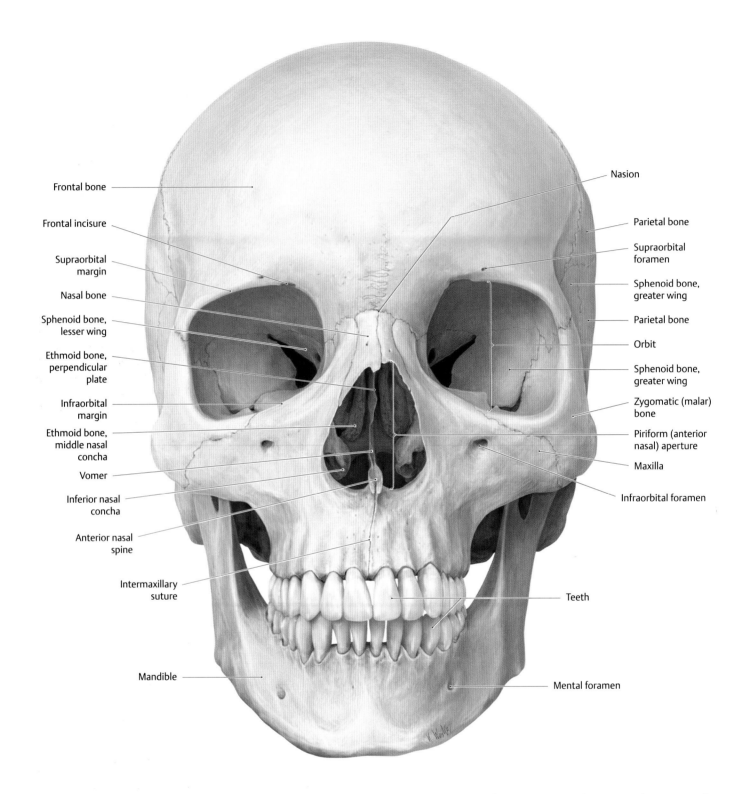

Frontal bone

Frontal incisure

Supraorbital margin

Nasal bone

Sphenoid bone, lesser wing

Ethmoid bone, perpendicular plate

Infraorbital margin

Ethmoid bone, middle nasal concha

Vomer

Inferior nasal concha

Anterior nasal spine

Intermaxillary suture

Mandible

Nasion

Parietal bone

Supraorbital foramen

Sphenoid bone, greater wing

Parietal bone

Orbit

Sphenoid bone, greater wing

Zygomatic (malar) bone

Piriform (anterior nasal) aperture

Maxilla

Infraorbital foramen

Teeth

Mental foramen

***Fig. 1.7 Anterior view of the skull***
The boundaries of the facial skeleton (viscerocranium) can be clearly appreciated in this view (the individual bones are shown in **Fig. 1.8**). The bony margins of the anterior nasal aperture mark the start of the respiratory tract in the skull. The nasal cavity, like the orbits, contains a sensory organ (the olfactory mucosa). The *paranasal sinuses* are shown schematically in **Fig. 1.9**. The anterior view of the skull also displays the three clinically important openings through which sensory nerves pass to supply the face: the supraorbital foramen, infraorbital foramen, and mental foramen.

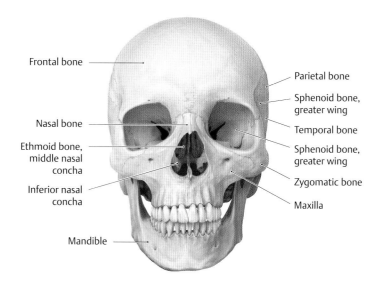

**Fig. 1.8 Cranial bones, anterior view**

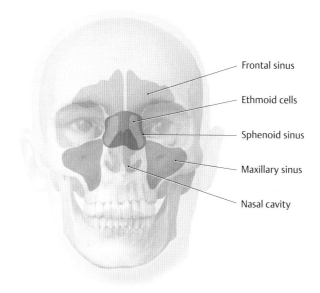

**Fig. 1.9 Paranasal sinuses**

Anterior view. Some of the bones of the facial skeleton are pneuma tized; that is, they contain air-filled cavities that reduce the total weight of the bone. These cavities, called the paranasal sinuses, communicate with the nasal cavity and, like it, are lined by ciliated respiratory epithelium. Inflammations of the paranasal sinuses (sinusitis) and associated complaints are very common. Because some of the pain of sinusitis is projected to the skin overlying the sinuses, it is helpful to know the projections of the sinuses onto the surface of the skull.

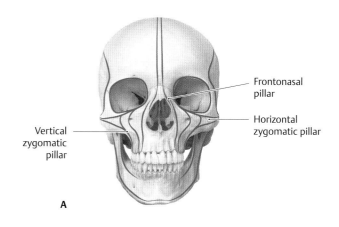

A

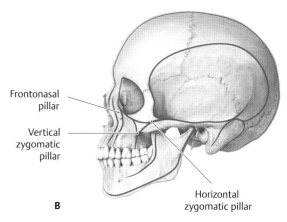

B

**Fig. 1.10 Principal lines of force (blue) in the facial skeleton**

**A** Anterior view. **B** Lateral view. The pneumatized paranasal sinuses (**Fig. 1.9**) have a mechanical counterpart in the thickened bony "pillars" of the facial skeleton, which partially bound the sinuses. These pillars develop along the principal lines of force in response to local mechanical stresses (e.g., masticatory pressures). In visual terms, the framelike construction of the facial skeleton may be likened to that of a frame house: the paranasal sinuses represent the rooms, and the pillars (placed along major lines of force) represent the supporting columns.

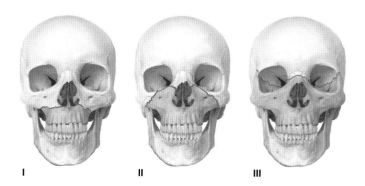

I    II    III

**Fig. 1.11 Le Fort classification of midfacial fractures**

The framelike construction of the facial skeleton leads to characteristic patterns of fracture lines in the midfacial region (Le Fort I, II, and III).

**Le Fort I:** This fracture line runs across the maxilla and above the hard palate. The maxilla is separated from the upper facial skeleton, disrupting the integrity of the maxillary sinus (*low transverse fracture*).

**Le Fort II:** The fracture line passes across the nasal root, ethmoid bone, maxilla, and zygomatic bone, creating a *pyramid fracture* that disrupts the integrity of the orbit.

**Le Fort III:** The facial skeleton is separated from the base of the skull. The main fracture line passes through the orbits, and the fracture may additionally involve the ethmoid bones, frontal sinuses, sphenoid sinuses, and zygomatic bones.

# ull: Posterior View & Cranial Sutures

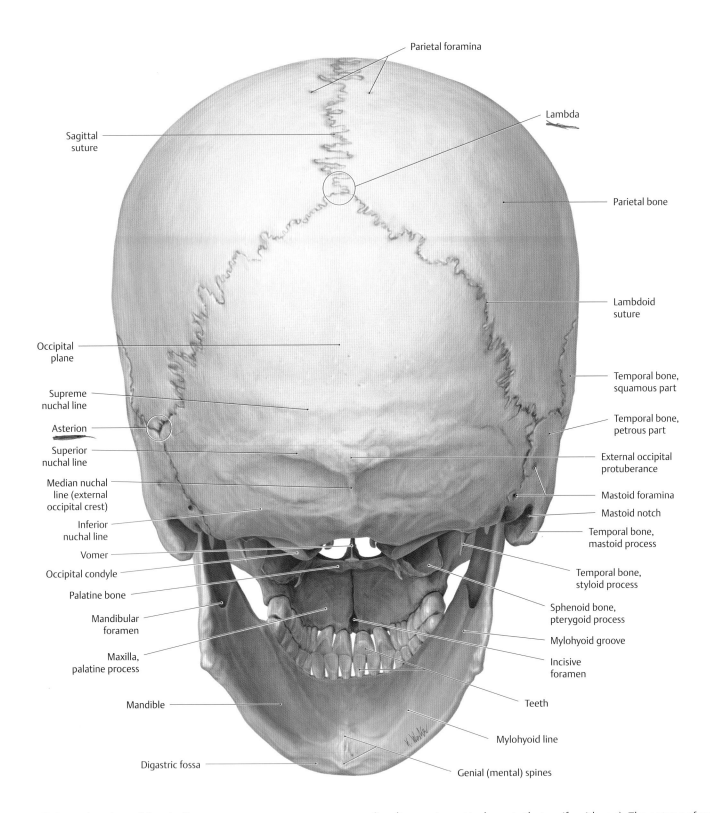

Parietal foramina

Lambda

Sagittal suture

Parietal bone

Lambdoid suture

Temporal bone, squamous part

Occipital plane

Temporal bone, petrous part

Supreme nuchal line

External occipital protuberance

Asterion

Superior nuchal line

Mastoid foramina

Mastoid notch

Median nuchal line (external occipital crest)

Temporal bone, mastoid process

Inferior nuchal line

Vomer

Temporal bone, styloid process

Occipital condyle

Sphenoid bone, pterygoid process

Palatine bone

Mandibular foramen

Mylohyoid groove

Incisive foramen

Maxilla, palatine process

Mandible

Teeth

Mylohyoid line

Digastric fossa

Genial (mental) spines

**Fig. 1.12 Posterior view of the skull**

The occipital bone, which is dominant in this view, articulates with the parietal bones, to which it is connected by the lambdoid suture. Wormian (sutural) bones are isolated bone plates often found in the lambdoid suture. The cranial sutures are a special type of syndesmosis (i.e., ligamentous attachments that ossify with age). The outer surface of the occipital bone is contoured by muscular origins and insertions: the inferior, superior, median, and supreme nuchal lines.

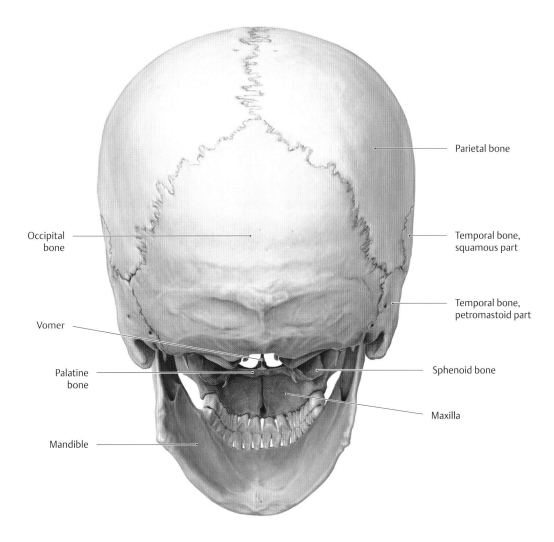

**Fig. 1.13 Posterior view of the cranial bones**

Labels on figure:
- Parietal bone
- Temporal bone, squamous part
- Temporal bone, petromastoid part
- Occipital bone
- Vomer
- Palatine bone
- Mandible
- Sphenoid bone
- Maxilla

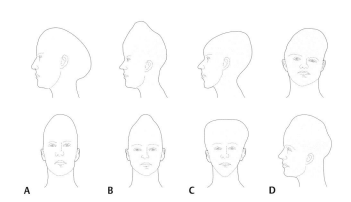

A   B   C   D

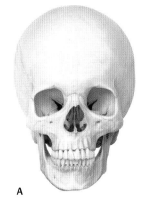

A

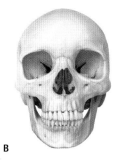

B

**Fig. 1.14 Premature closure of cranial sutures**

The premature closure of a cranial suture (craniosynostosis) may lead to characteristic cranial deformities:

A  Sagittal suture: scaphocephaly (long, narrow skull).
B  Coronal suture: oxycephaly (pointed skull).
C  Frontal suture: trigonocephaly (triangular skull).
D  Asymmetrical suture closure, usually involving the coronal suture: plagiocephaly (asymmetric skull).

**Fig. 1.15 Hydrocephalus and microcephaly**

A  **Hydrocephalus:** When the brain becomes dilated due to CSF accumulation *before* the cranial sutures ossify, the neurocranium will expand, whereas the facial skeleton remains unchanged.
B  **Microcephaly:** Premature closure of the cranial sutures results in a small neurocranium with relatively large orbits.

# Calvaria

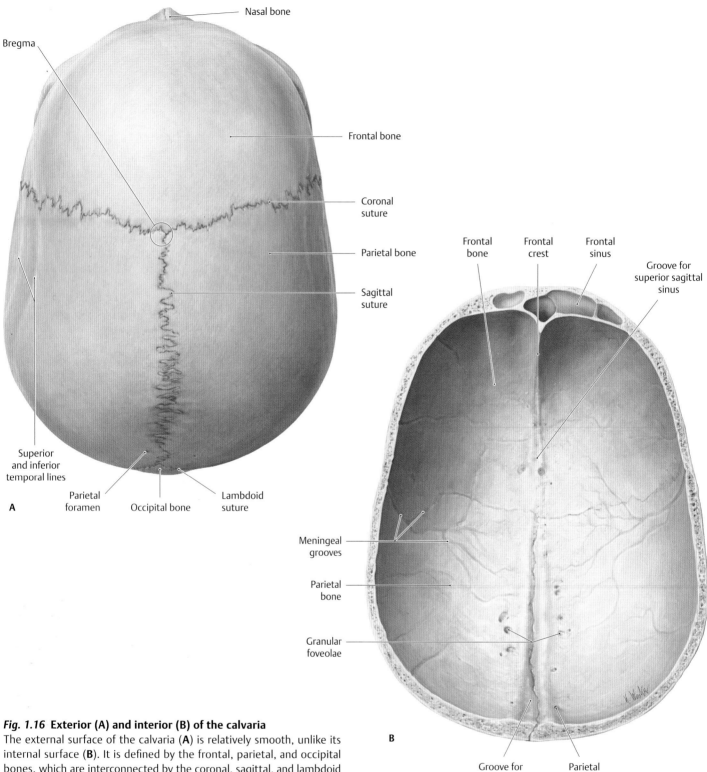

**Fig. 1.16 Exterior (A) and interior (B) of the calvaria**

The external surface of the calvaria (**A**) is relatively smooth, unlike its internal surface (**B**). It is defined by the frontal, parietal, and occipital bones, which are interconnected by the coronal, sagittal, and lambdoid sutures. The smooth external surface is interrupted by the parietal foramina, which gives passage to the parietal emissary veins (see **Fig. 1.21**). The internal surface of the calvaria bears a number of pits and grooves:

- Granular foveolae (small pits in the inner surface of the skull caused by saccular protrusions of the arachnoid membrane [arachnoid granulations] covering the brain)
- Groove for the superior sagittal sinus (a dural venous sinus of the brain, see **Fig. 1.21** and **Fig. 3.21**, p. 53)

- Arterial grooves (which mark the positions of the arterial vessels of the dura mater, such as the middle meningeal artery, which supplies most of the dura mater and overlying bone)
- Frontal crest (which gives attachment to the falx cerebri, a sickle-shaped fold of dura mater between the cerebral hemispheres).

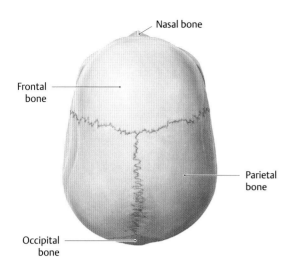

**Fig. 1.17 Exterior of the calvaria viewed from above**

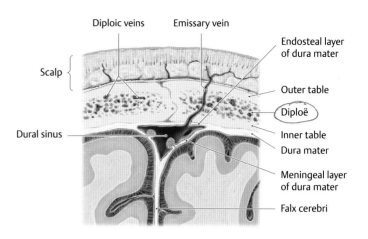

**Fig. 1.18 The scalp and calvaria**
The three-layered calvaria consists of the outer table, the diploë, and the inner table. The diploë has a spongy structure and contains red (blood-forming) bone marrow. With a plasmacytoma (malignant transformation of certain white blood cells), many small nests of tumor cells may destroy the surrounding bony trabeculae, and radiographs will demonstrate multiple lucent areas ("punched-out lesions") in the skull.

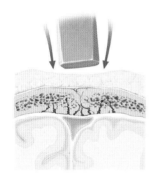

**Fig. 1.19 Sensitivity of the inner table to trauma**
The inner table of the calvaria is very sensitive to external trauma and may fracture even when the outer table remains intact (look for corresponding evidence on CT images).

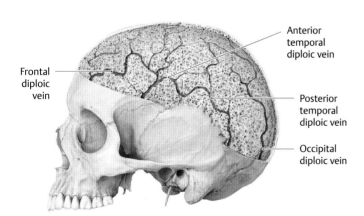

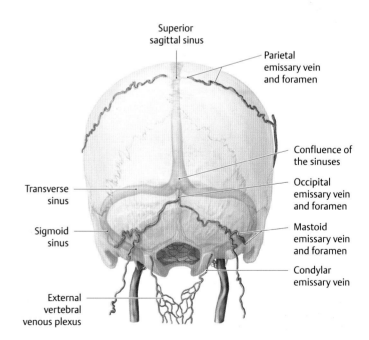

**Fig. 1.20 Diploic veins in the calvaria**
The diploic veins are located in the cancellous or spongy tissue of the cranial bones (the diploë) and are visible when the outer table is removed. The diploic veins communicate with the dural venous sinuses and scalp veins by way of the *emissary veins*, which create a potential route for the spread of infection.

**Fig. 1.21 Emissary veins of the occiput**
Emissary veins establish a direct connection between the dural venous sinuses and the extracranial veins. They pass through cranial openings such as the parietal foramen and mastoid foramen. The emissary veins are of clinical interest because they may allow bacteria from the scalp to enter the skull along these veins and infect the dura mater, causing meningitis.

**11**

# Skull Base: External View

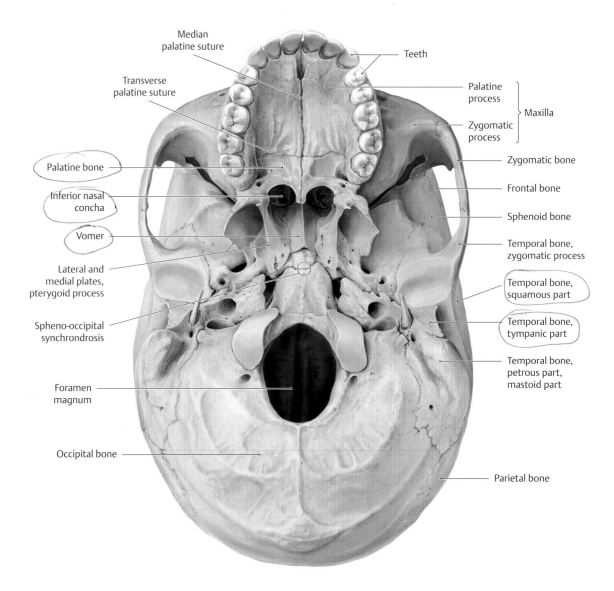

**Fig. 1.22 Bones of the base of the skull**
Inferior view. The base of the skull is composed of a mosaic-like assembly of various bones.

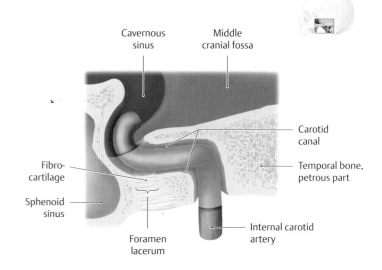

**Fig. 1.23 Relationship of the foramen lacerum to the carotid canal and internal carotid artery**
Left lateral view. The foramen lacerum is not a true aperture, being mostly occluded in life by a layer of fibrocartilage; it appears as an opening only in the dried skull. The foramen lacerum is closely related to the carotid canal and to the internal carotid artery that traverses the canal. The greater petrosal nerve and deep petrosal nerve pass across the superior surface of the foramen lacerum (see pp. 85, 94).

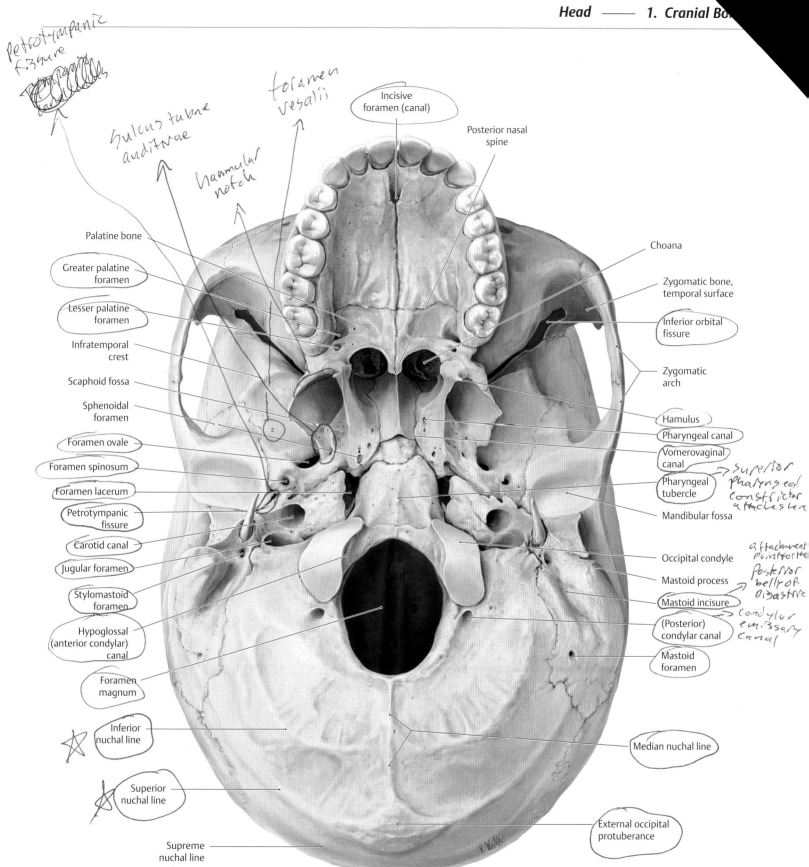

Petrotympanic fissure

Sulcus tubae auditivae

foramen vesalii

hamular notch

**Fig. 1.24 The basal aspect of the skull**
Inferior view. Note the openings that transmit nerves and vessels. With abnormalities of bone growth, these openings may remain too small or may become narrowed, compressing the neurovascular structures that pass through them. The symptoms associated with these lesions depend on the affected opening. All of the structures depicted here will be considered in more detail in subsequent pages.

The SCM inserts on the mastoid process and superior nuchal line

# Skull Base: Internal View

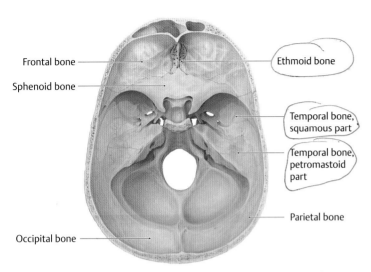

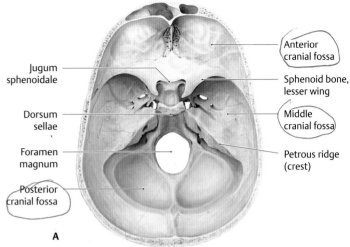

**A**

**Fig. 1.25 Bones of the base of the skull, internal view**

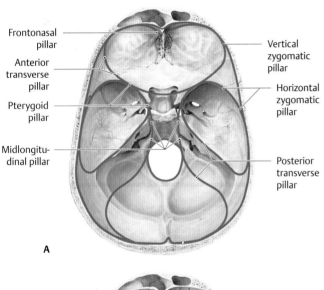

**A**

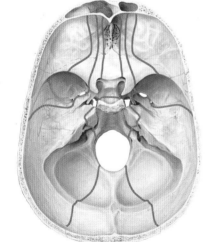

**B**

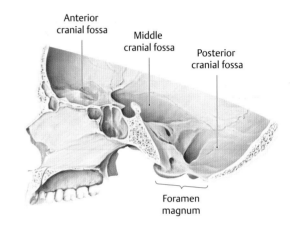

**B**

**Fig. 1.26 The cranial fossae**

**A** Interior view. **B** Midsagittal section. The interior of the skull base is deepened to form three successive fossae: the anterior, middle, and posterior cranial fossae. These depressions become progressively deeper in the frontal-to-occipital direction, forming a terraced arrangement that is displayed most clearly in **B**.

The cranial fossae are bounded by the following structures:

- Anterior to middle: lesser wings of the sphenoid bone and the jugum sphenoidale
- Middle to posterior: superior border (ridge) of the petrous part of the temporal bone and the dorsum sellae

**Fig. 1.27 Base of the skull: principal lines of force and common fracture lines**

**A** Principal lines of force. **B** Common fracture lines (interior views). In response to masticatory pressures and other mechanical stresses, the bones of the skull base are thickened to form "pillars" along the principal lines of force (compare with the force distribution in the anterior view on p. 7). The intervening areas that are not thickened are sites of predilection for bone fractures, resulting in the typical patterns of basal skull fracture lines shown here. An analogous phenomenon of typical fracture lines is found in the midfacial region (see the anterior views of Le Fort fractures on p. 7).

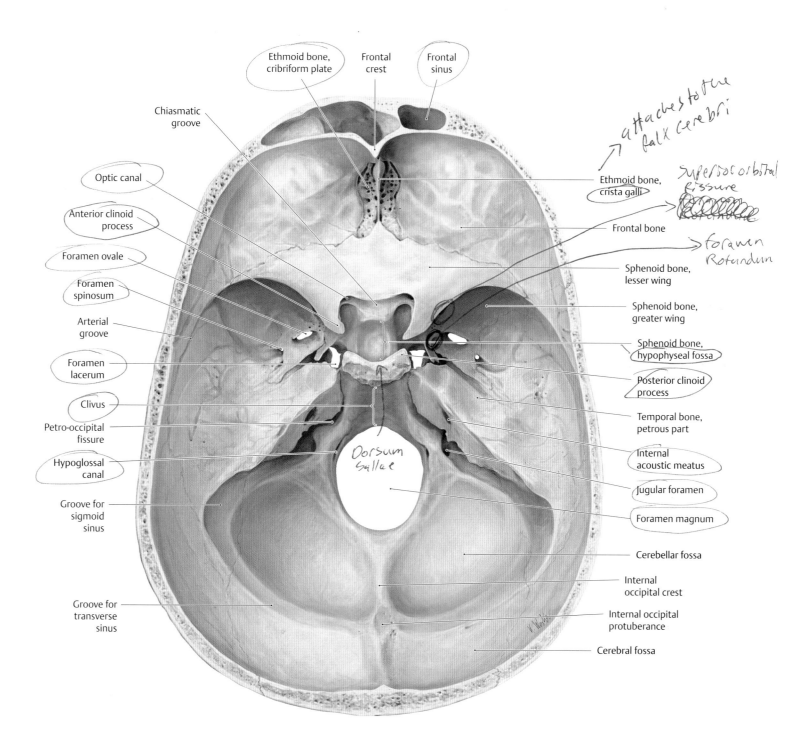

Handwritten annotations:
- attaches to the falx cerebri
- superior orbital fissure
- foramen Rotundum

**Fig. 1.28 Interior of the base of the skull**

The openings in the interior of the base of the skull do not always coincide with the openings visible in the external view because some neurovascular structures change direction when passing through the bone or pursue a relatively long intraosseous course. An example of this is the internal acoustic meatus, through which the facial nerve, among other structures, passes from the interior of the skull into the petrous part of the temporal bone. Most of its fibers then leave the petrous bone through the stylomastoid foramen, which is visible from the external aspect (see **Fig. 4.35**, p. 83, and **Fig. 4.53**, p. 94 for further details).

In learning the sites where neurovascular structures pass through the base of the skull, it is helpful initially to note whether these sites are located in the anterior, middle, or posterior cranial fossa. The arrangement of the cranial fossae is shown in **Fig. 1.26**.

The cribriform plate of the ethmoid bone connects the nasal cavity with the anterior cranial fossa and is perforated by numerous foramina for the passage of the olfactory fibers (see **Fig. 7.15**, p. 148). *Note:* Because the bone is so thin in this area, a frontal head injury may easily fracture the cribriform plate and lacerate the dura mater, allowing CSF to enter the nose. This poses a risk of meningitis, as bacteria from the nonsterile nasal cavity may enter the sterile CSF.

# Sphenoid Bone

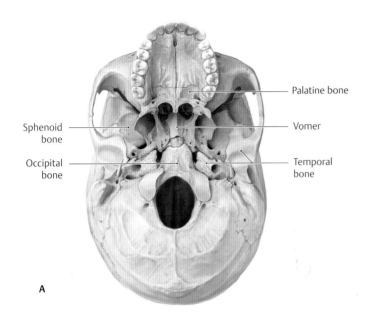

A

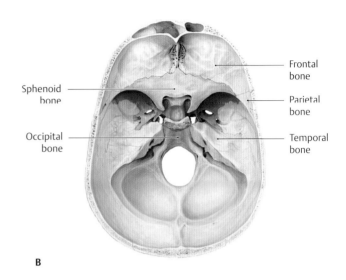

B

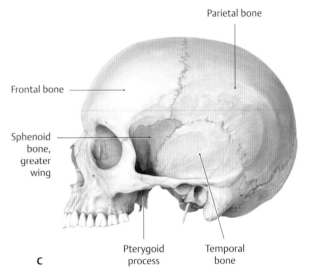

C

**Fig. 1.29 Position of the sphenoid bone in the skull**
The sphenoid bone is the most structurally complex bone in the human body. It must be viewed from various aspects in order to appreciate all its features (see also **Fig. 1.30**):

**A Base of the skull, external aspect.** The sphenoid bone combines with the occipital bone to form the load-bearing midline structure of the skull base.

**B Base of the skull, internal aspect.** The lesser wing of the sphenoid bone forms the boundary between the anterior and middle cranial fossae. The openings for the passage of nerves and vessels are clearly displayed (see details in **Fig. 1.30**).

**C Lateral view.** Portions of the greater wing of the sphenoid bone can be seen above the zygomatic arch, and portions of the pterygoid process can be seen below the zygomatic arch.

**Fig. 1.30 Isolated sphenoid bone**

**A Inferior view** (its position in situ is shown in **Fig. 1.29**). This view demonstrates the medial and lateral plates of the pterygoid process. Between them is the pterygoid fossa, which is occupied by the medial pterygoid muscle. The foramen spinosum and foramen ovale provide pathways through the base of the skull (see also in **C**).

**B Anterior view.** This view illustrates why the sphenoid bone was originally called the sphecoid bone ("wasp bone") before a transcription error turned it into the sphenoid ("wedge-shaped") bone. The apertures of the sphenoid sinus on each side resemble the eyes of the wasp, and the pterygoid processes of the sphenoid bone form its dangling legs, between which are the pterygoid fossae. This view also displays the superior orbital fissure, which connects the middle cranial fossa with the orbit on each side. The two sphenoid sinuses are separated by an internal septum (see **Fig. 7.11**, p. 145).

**C Superior view.** The superior view displays the sella turcica, whose central depression, the hypophyseal fossa, contains the pituitary gland. The foramen spinosum, foramen ovale, and foramen rotundum can be identified.

**D Posterior view.** The superior orbital fissure is seen particularly clearly in this view, whereas the optic canal is almost completely obscured by the anterior clinoid process. The foramen rotundum is open from the middle cranial fossa to the pterygopalatine fossa of the skull (the foramen spinosum is not visible in this view; compare with **A**). Because the sphenoid and occipital bones fuse together during puberty ("tribasilar bone"), a suture is no longer present between the two bones. The cancellous trabeculae are exposed and have a porous appearance.

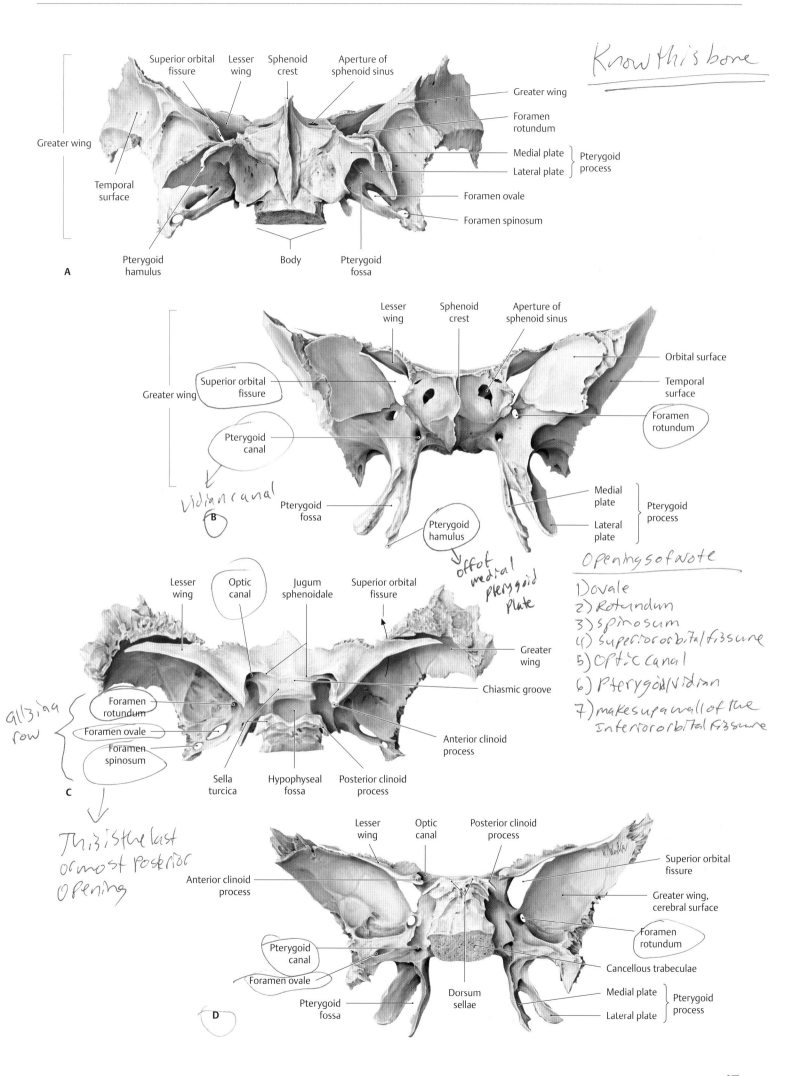

Know this bone

**A**

Greater wing — Superior orbital fissure — Lesser wing — Sphenoid crest — Aperture of sphenoid sinus — Greater wing — Foramen rotundum — Medial plate / Lateral plate } Pterygoid process — Foramen ovale — Foramen spinosum — Greater wing — Temporal surface — Pterygoid hamulus — Body — Pterygoid fossa

**B**

Greater wing — Superior orbital fissure — Lesser wing — Sphenoid crest — Aperture of sphenoid sinus — Orbital surface — Temporal surface — Foramen rotundum — Pterygoid canal — Pterygoid fossa — Pterygoid hamulus — Medial plate / Lateral plate } Pterygoid process

Vidian canal

off of medial pterygoid plate

Openings of Note
1) Ovale
2) Rotundum
3) Spinosum
4) Superior orbital fissure
5) Optic Canal
6) Pterygoid/Vidian
7) makes up a wall of the inferior orbital fissure

**C**

Lesser wing — Optic canal — Jugum sphenoidale — Superior orbital fissure — Greater wing — Chiasmic groove — Foramen rotundum — Foramen ovale — Foramen spinosum — Anterior clinoid process — Sella turcica — Hypophyseal fossa — Posterior clinoid process

9/13/99 row

This 3 is the last or most posterior opening

**D**

Lesser wing — Optic canal — Posterior clinoid process — Superior orbital fissure — Anterior clinoid process — Greater wing, cerebral surface — Foramen rotundum — Cancellous trabeculae — Pterygoid canal — Foramen ovale — Pterygoid fossa — Dorsum sellae — Medial plate / Lateral plate } Pterygoid process

# Temporal Bone

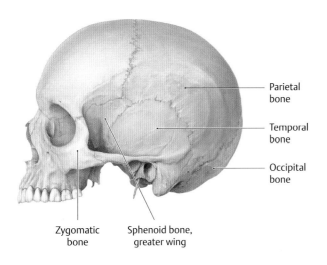

**Fig. 1.31 Position of the temporal bone in the skull**
Left lateral view. The temporal bone is a major component of the base of the skull. It forms the capsule for the auditory and vestibular apparatus and bears the articular fossa of the temporomandibular joint (TMJ).

Parietal bone

Temporal bone

Occipital bone

Zygomatic bone

Sphenoid bone, greater wing

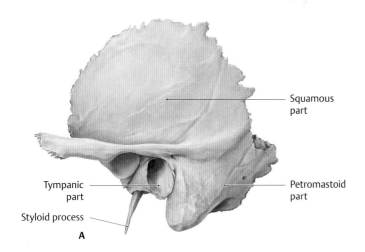

Squamous part

Tympanic part

Styloid process

Petromastoid part

**A**

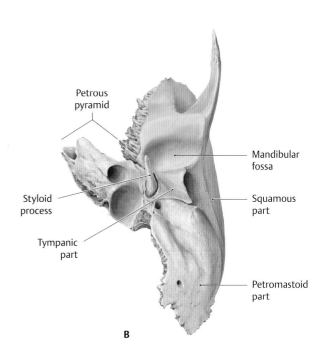

Petrous pyramid

Styloid process

Tympanic part

Mandibular fossa

Squamous part

Petromastoid part

**B**

**Fig. 1.32 Ossification centers of the left temporal bone**
**A** Left lateral view. **B** Inferior view.
The temporal bone develops from four centers that fuse to form a single bone:

- The squamous part, or temporal squama (light green), bears the articular fossa of the TMJ (mandibular fossa).

- The petromastoid part (pale green) contains the auditory and vestibular apparatus.
- The tympanic part (darker green) forms large portions of the external auditory canal.
- The styloid part (styloid process) develops from cartilage derived from the second branchial arch. It is a site of muscle attachment.

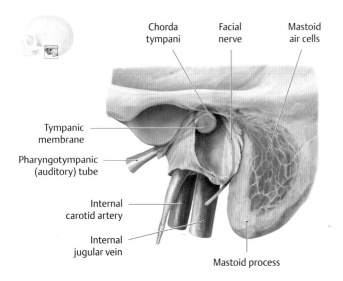

Chorda tympani

Facial nerve

Mastoid air cells

Tympanic membrane

Pharyngotympanic (auditory) tube

Internal carotid artery

Internal jugular vein

Mastoid process

**Fig. 1.33 Projection of clinically important structures onto the left temporal bone**
The tympanic membrane is shown translucent in this lateral view. Because the petrous bone contains the middle and inner ear and the tympanic membrane, a knowledge of its anatomy is of key importance in otological surgery. The internal surface of the petrous bone has openings (see **Fig. 1.34**) for the passage of the facial nerve, internal carotid artery, and internal jugular vein. A fine nerve, the chorda tympani, passes through the tympanic cavity and lies medial to the tympanic membrane. The chorda tympani arises from the facial nerve, which is susceptible to injury during surgical procedures (see **Table 4.22**, p. 82, and **Fig. 4.34**, p. 83). The mastoid process of the petrous bone forms air-filled chambers, the mastoid cells, that vary greatly in size. Because these chambers communicate with the middle ear, which in turn communicates with the nasopharynx via the pharyngotympanic (auditory) tube (also called eustachian tube), bacteria in the nasopharynx may pass up the pharyngotympanic tube and gain access to the middle ear. From there they may pass to the mastoid air cells and finally enter the cranial cavity, causing meningitis.

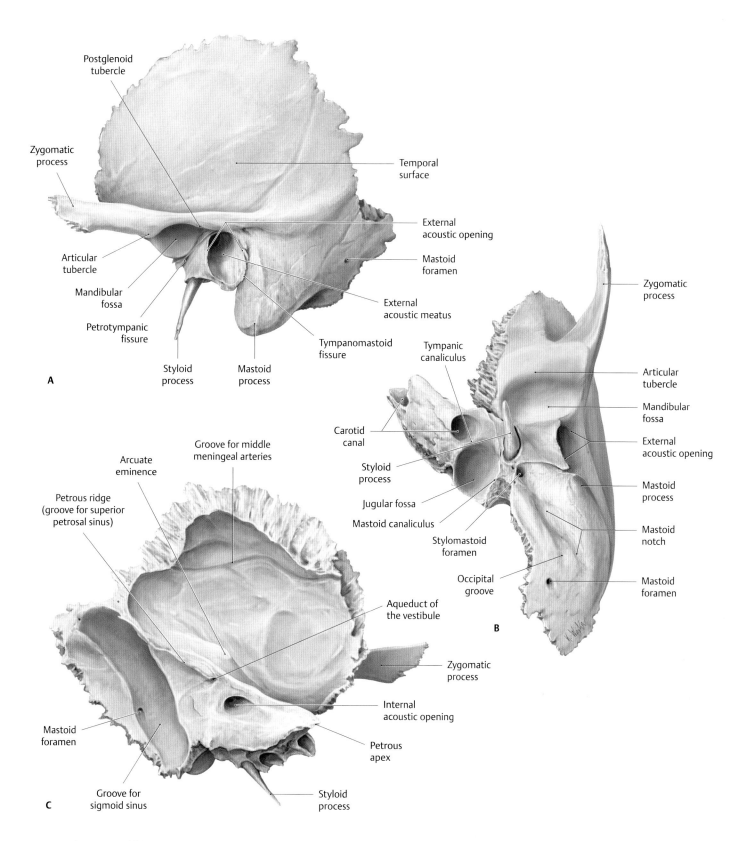

**Fig. 1.34 Left temporal bone**

**A Lateral view.** An emissary vein passes through the mastoid foramen (external orifice shown in **A**, internal orifice in **C**), and the chorda tympani passes through the medial part of the petrotympanic fissure (see **Fig. 4.35**, p. 83). The mastoid process develops gradually in life due to traction from the sternocleidomastoid muscle and is pneumatized from the inside (see **Fig. 1.33**).

**B Inferior view.** The shallow articular fossa of the temporomandibular joint (the mandibular fossa) is clearly seen from the inferior view. The facial nerve emerges from the base of the skull through the stylo-

mastoid foramen. The initial part of the superior jugular bulb is adherent to the jugular fossa, and the internal carotid artery passes through the carotid canal to enter the skull.

**C Medial view.** This view displays the internal orifice of the mastoid foramen and the internal acoustic meatus. The facial nerve and vestibulocochlear nerve are among the structures that pass through the internal meatus to enter the petrous bone. The part of the petrous bone shown here is also called the *petrous pyramid*, whose apex (often called the "petrous apex") lies on the interior of the base of the skull.

# Occipital Bone & Ethmoid Bones

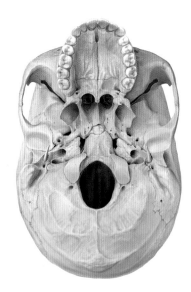

**Fig. 1.35 Integration of the occipital bone into the external base of the skull**
Inferior view.

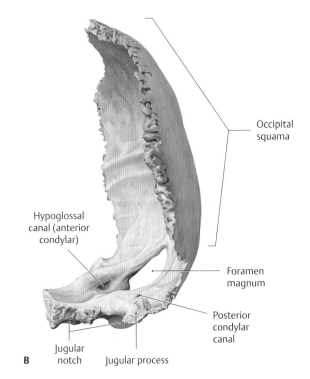

Occipital squama

Hypoglossal canal (anterior condylar)

Foramen magnum

Posterior condylar canal

Jugular notch    Jugular process

**B**

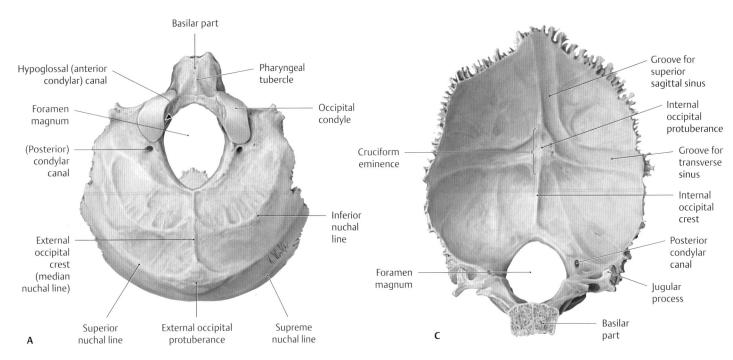

Basilar part

Hypoglossal (anterior condylar) canal

Pharyngeal tubercle

Foramen magnum

Occipital condyle

(Posterior) condylar canal

External occipital crest (median nuchal line)

Inferior nuchal line

Superior nuchal line

External occipital protuberance

Supreme nuchal line

**A**

Groove for superior sagittal sinus

Internal occipital protuberance

Cruciform eminence

Groove for transverse sinus

Internal occipital crest

Posterior condylar canal

Foramen magnum

Jugular process

Basilar part

**C**

**Fig. 1.36 Isolated occipital bone**

**A Inferior view.** This view shows the basilar part of the occipital bone, whose anterior portion is fused to the sphenoid bone. The condylar canal terminates posterior to the occipital condyles, and the hypoglossal canal passes superior and opens anterior to the occipital condyles. The condylar canal is a venous channel that begins in the sigmoid sinus and ends in the occipital vein. The hypoglossal canal contains a venous plexus in addition to the hypoglossal nerve (CN XII). The pharyngeal tubercle gives attachment to the pharyngeal raphe, and the external occipital protuberance provides a palpable bony landmark on the occiput.

**B Left lateral view.** The extent of the occipital squama, which lies above the foramen magnum, is clearly appreciated in this view. The internal openings of the condylar canal and hypoglossal canal are visible along with the jugular process, which forms part of the wall of the jugular foramen (see p. 13).

**C Internal surface.** The grooves for the dural venous sinuses of the brain can be identified in this view. The cruciform eminence overlies the confluence of the superior sagittal sinus and transverse sinuses. The configuration of the eminence shows that in some cases the sagittal sinus drains predominantly into the left transverse sinus.

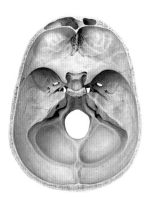

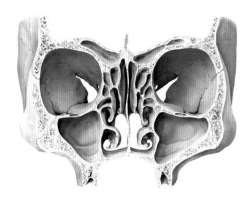

**Fig. 1.37 Integration of the ethmoid bone into the internal base of the skull**
Superior view. The superior part of the ethmoid bone forms part of the anterior cranial fossa, and its inferior portions contribute structurally to the nasal cavities and orbit. The ethmoid bone is bordered by the frontal and sphenoid bones.

**Fig. 1.38 Integration of the ethmoid bone into the facial skeleton**
Anterior view. The ethmoid bone is the central bone of the nose and paranasal sinuses. It also forms the medial wall of each orbit.

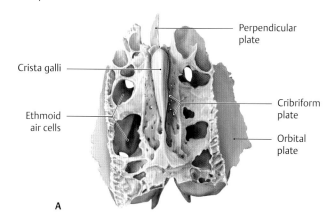

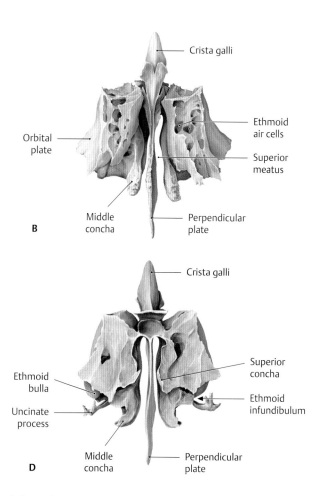

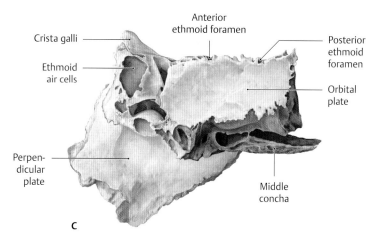

**Fig. 1.39 Isolated ethmoid bone**

**A Superior view.** This view demonstrates the crista galli, which gives attachment to the falx cerebri and the horizontally directed cribriform plate. The cribriform plate is perforated by foramina through which the olfactory fibers pass from the nasal cavity into the anterior cranial fossa (see **Fig. 7.15**, p. 148). With its numerous foramina, the cribriform plate is a mechanically weak structure that fractures easily in response to trauma. This type of fracture is manifested clinically by CSF leakage from the nose ("runny nose" in a patient with head injury).

**B Anterior view.** The anterior view displays the midline structure that separates the two nasal cavities: the perpendicular plate. Note also the middle concha, which is part of the ethmoid bone (of the conchae, only the inferior concha is a separate bone), and the ethmoid cells, which are clustered on both sides of the middle conchae.

**C Left lateral view.** Viewing the bone from the left side, we observe the perpendicular plate and the opened anterior ethmoid cells. The orbit is separated from the ethmoid cells by a thin sheet of bone called the orbital plate.

**D Posterior view.** This is the only view that displays the uncinate process, which is almost completely covered by the middle concha when in situ. It partially occludes the entrance to the maxillary sinus, the semilunar hiatus, and it is an important landmark during endoscopic surgery of the maxillary sinus. The narrow depression between the middle concha and uncinate process is called the ethmoid infundibulum. The frontal sinus, maxillary sinus, and anterior ethmoid air cells open into this "funnel." The superior concha is located at the posterior end of the ethmoid bone.

# Mandible & Hyoid Bone

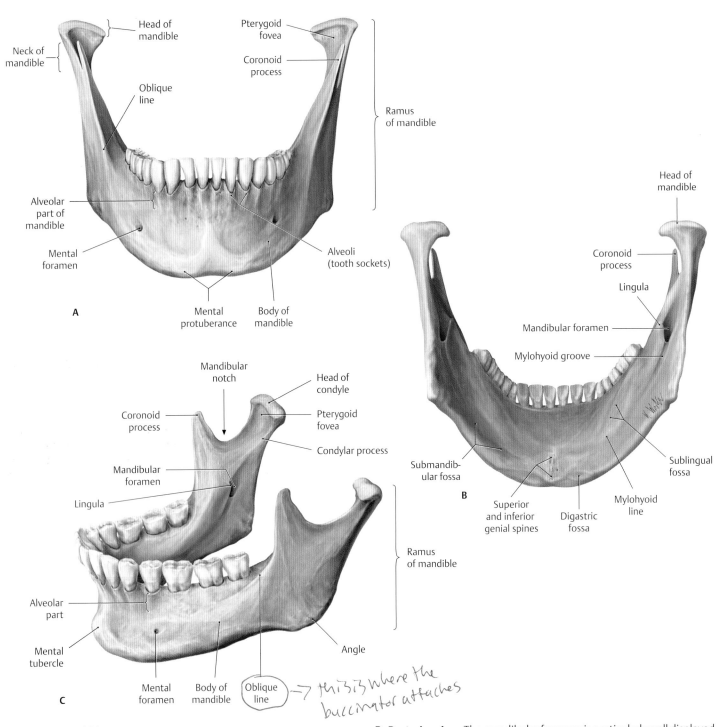

Fig. 1.40 Mandible

**A Anterior view.** The mandible is connected to the viscerocranium at the temporomandibular joint, whose convex surface is the head of the mandibular condyle. This "head of the mandible" is situated atop the vertical (ascending) ramus of the mandible, which joins with the body of the mandible at the mandibular angle. The teeth are set in the alveolar processes (alveolar part) along the upper border of the mandibular body. This part of the mandible is subject to typical age-related changes as a result of dental development (see **Fig. 1.41**). The mental branch of the trigeminal nerve exits through the mental foramen. The location of this foramen is important in clinical examinations, as the tenderness of the nerve to pressure can be tested at that location.

**B Posterior view.** The mandibular foramen is particularly well displayed in this view. It transmits the inferior alveolar nerve, which supplies sensory innervation to the mandibular teeth. Its terminal branch emerges from the mental foramen. The mandibular foramen and the mental foramen are interconnected by the mandibular canal.

**C Oblique left lateral view.** This view displays the coronoid process, the condylar process, and the mandibular notch between them. The coronoid process is a site for muscular attachments, and the condylar process bears the head of the mandible, which articulates with the articular disk in the mandibular fossa of the temporal bone. A depression on the medial side of the condylar process, the pterygoid fovea, gives attachment to portions of the lateral pterygoid muscle.

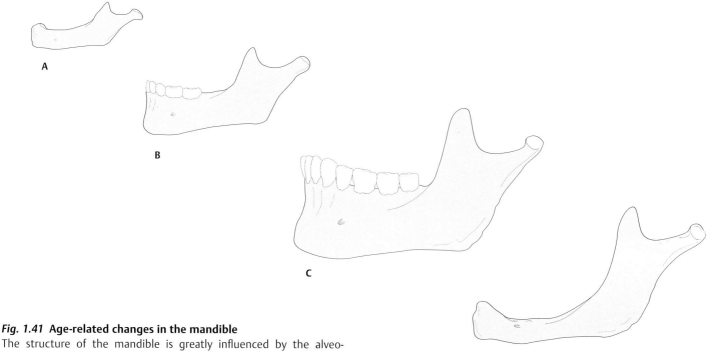

### Fig. 1.41 Age-related changes in the mandible

The structure of the mandible is greatly influenced by the alveolar processes of the teeth. Because the angle of the mandible adapts to changes in the alveolar process, the angle between the body and ramus also varies with age-related changes in the dentition. The angle measures approximately 150 degrees at birth and approximately 120 to 130 degrees in adults, decreasing to 140 degrees in the edentulous mandible of old age.

**A  At birth** the mandible is without teeth, and the alveolar part has not yet formed.
**B  In children** the mandible bears the deciduous teeth. The alveolar part is still relatively poorly developed because the deciduous teeth are considerably smaller than the permanent teeth.

**C  In adults** the mandible bears the permanent teeth, and the alveolar part of the bone is fully developed.
**D  Old age** is characterized by an edentulous mandible with resorption of the alveolar process.

*Note:* The resorption of the alveolar process with advanced age leads to a change in the position of the mental foramen (which is normally located below the second premolar tooth, as in **C**). This change must be taken into account in surgery or dissections involving the mental nerve.

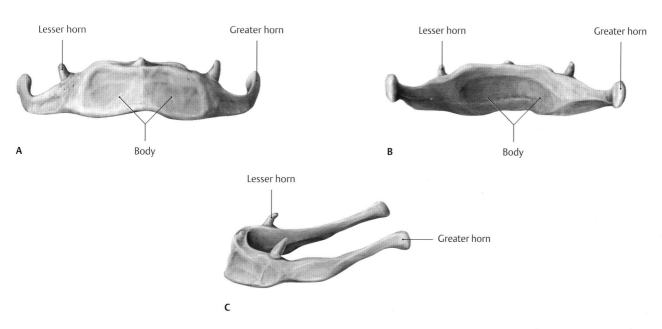

### Fig. 1.42 Hyoid bone

**A** Anterior view. **B** Posterior view. **C** Oblique left lateral view. The hyoid bone is suspended by muscles between the oral floor and larynx in the neck. The greater horn and body of the hyoid bone are palpable in the neck. The physiological movement of the hyoid bone during swallowing is also palpable.

# Muscles of Facial Expression

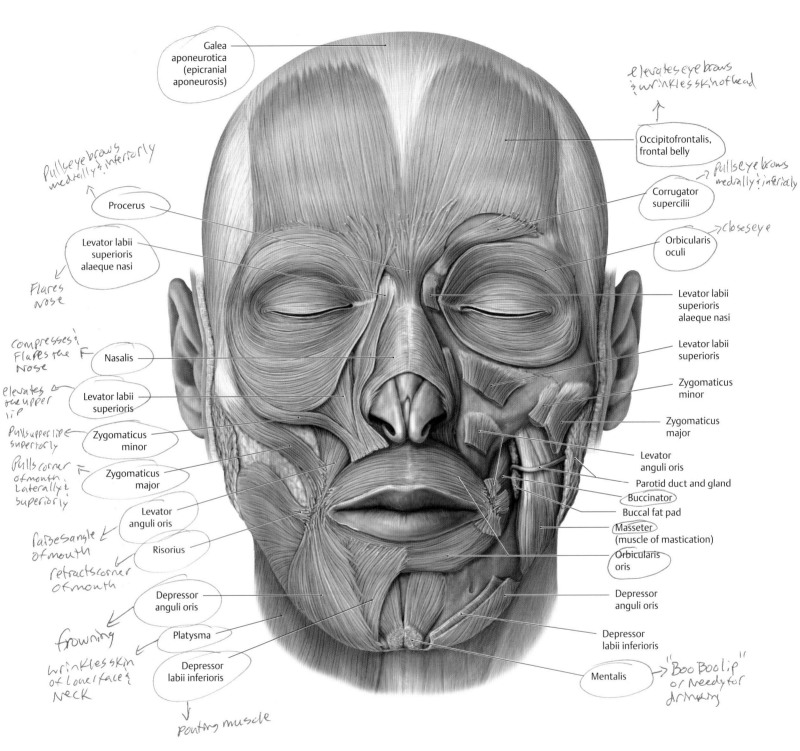

Galea aponeurotica (epicranial aponeurosis)

*elevates eyebrows & wrinkles skin of head*

Occipitofrontalis, frontal belly

*Pulls eyebrows medially & inferiorly*

Procerus

*Pulls eyebrows medially & inferiorly*

Corrugator supercilii

Levator labii superioris alaeque nasi

*close eye*

Orbicularis oculi

*Flares nose*

Levator labii superioris alaeque nasi

*compresses & flares the nose*

Nasalis

Levator labii superioris

*elevates the upper lip*

Levator labii superioris

Zygomaticus minor

*Pulls upper lip superiorly*

Zygomaticus minor

Zygomaticus major

*Pulls corner of mouth laterally & superiorly*

Zygomaticus major

Levator anguli oris

Parotid duct and gland

Buccinator

Buccal fat pad

Levator anguli oris

Masseter (muscle of mastication)

*raises angle of mouth*

Risorius

*retracts corner of mouth*

Orbicularis oris

Depressor anguli oris

Depressor anguli oris

*frowning*

Platysma

Depressor labii inferioris

*wrinkles skin of lower face & neck*

Depressor labii inferioris

Mentalis

*"Boo Boo lip" or Needy for Attention*

*pouting muscle*

**Fig. 2.1 Superficial facial muscles: anterior view**
Anterior view. The superficial layer of muscles is shown on the right side of the face. Certain muscles have been cut on the left to expose deeper muscles. The muscles of facial expression are the superficial layer of muscles that arise either directly from the periosteum or from adjacent muscles and insert onto other facial muscles or directly into the connective tissue of the skin. Because of their cutaneous attachments, the muscles of facial expression are able to move the facial skin (an action that may be temporarily abolished by botulinum toxin in-jection). They also serve a protective function (especially for the eyes) and are active during food ingestion (closing the mouth). The muscles of facial expression are innervated by branches of the facial nerve (CN VII). As these muscles terminate directly in the subcutaneous fat, and because the superficial body fascia is absent in the face, surgeons must be particularly careful when dissecting this region. The muscles of mastication lie deep to the muscles of facial expression. They control the movement of the mandible and are innervated by branches of the trigeminal nerve (CN V).

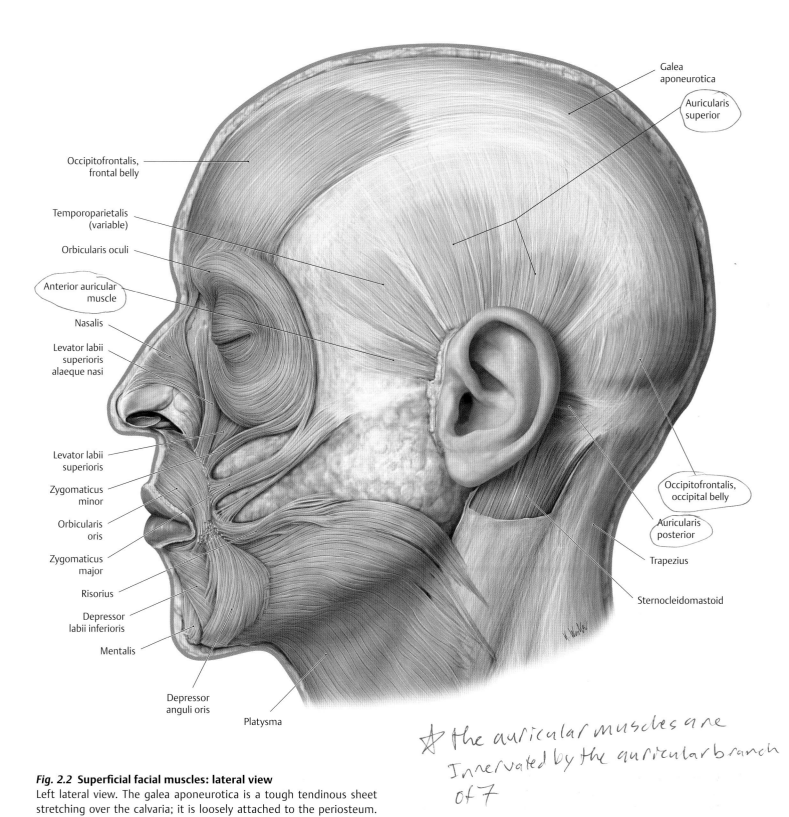

Galea
aponeurotica

Auricularis
superior

Occipitofrontalis,
frontal belly

Temporoparietalis
(variable)

Orbicularis oculi

Anterior auricular
muscle

Nasalis

Levator labii
superioris
alaeque nasi

Levator labii
superioris

Zygomaticus
minor

Orbicularis
oris

Zygomaticus
major

Risorius

Depressor
labii inferioris

Mentalis

Depressor
anguli oris

Platysma

Occipitofrontalis,
occipital belly

Auricularis
posterior

Trapezius

Sternocleidomastoid

★ the auricular muscles are
Innervated by the auricular branch
of 7

**Fig. 2.2 Superficial facial muscles: lateral view**
Left lateral view. The galea aponeurotica is a tough tendinous sheet stretching over the calvaria; it is loosely attached to the periosteum. The muscles of the calvaria that arise from the galea aponeurotica (temporoparietalis and occipitofrontalis) are collectively known as the "epicranial muscles." The occipitofrontalis has two bellies: frontal and occipital. The trapezius and sternocleidomastoid muscles are superficial neck muscles.

# Muscles of Facial Expression: Calvaria, Ear & Eye

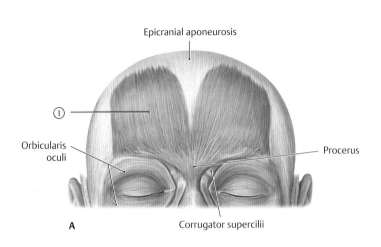

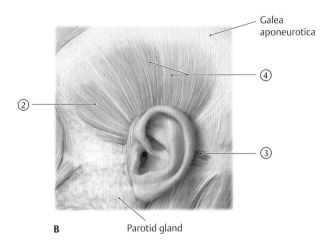

**Fig. 2.3 Muscles of facial expression: calvaria and ear**
**A** Anterior view of calvaria. **B** Left lateral view of auricular muscles.

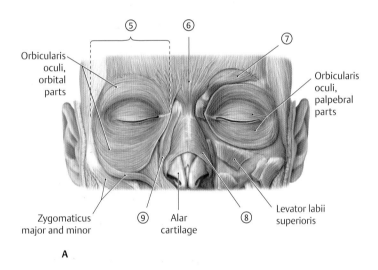

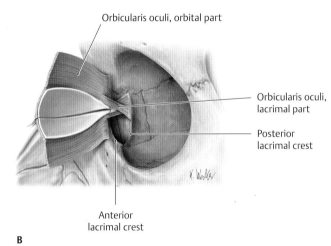

**Fig. 2.4 Muscles of facial expression: palpebral fissure and nose**
**A** Anterior view. The most functionally important muscle of this region is the orbicularis oculi, which closes the palpebral fissure (a protective reflex against foreign matter). As the orbicularis oculi closes the palpebral fissure, it does so by closing from lateral to medial, thus spreading lacrimal secretions across the cornea. If the action of the orbicularis oculi is lost because of facial nerve paralysis, the loss of this protective reflex will be accompanied by drying of the eye from prolonged exposure to the air. The function of the orbic-

ularis oculi is tested by asking the patient to squeeze the eyelids tightly shut.
**B** The orbicularis oculi has been dissected from the left orbit to the medial canthus of the eye and reflected anteriorly to demonstrate its lacrimal part (called the Horner muscle). This part of the orbicularis oculi arises mainly from the posterior lacrimal crest, and its action is a subject of debate (it may have a functional role in drainage of the lacrimal sac).

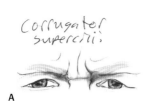

A  *Corrugator supercilii*

 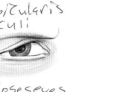

B  *Orbicularis oculi*

*closeseyes*

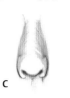

C  *Nasalis*

· *Compresses Nasal aperature*
· *Widens Nasal aperature*

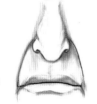

D  *Levator Labii superioris alaqui Nasi –*

· *Elares Nostrils*
· *elevates upper lip*

**Fig. 2.5 Changes of facial expression: palpebral fissure and nose**
Anterior view.
**A** Corrugator supercilii. **B** Orbicularis oculi. **C** Nasalis. **D** Levator labii superioris alaeque nasi.

**Table 2.1 Muscles of facial expression: calvaria & ear, palbebral fissure & nose**

| Muscle and parts | Origin | Insertion | I* | Main action(s) |
|---|---|---|---|---|
| **Calvaria and ear** | | | | |
| ① Occipitofrontalis, frontal belly | Epicranial aponeurosis near coronal suture | Skin and subcutaneous tissue of eyebrows and forehead | T | Elevates eyebrows; wrinkles skin of forehead |
| Auricularis muscles | | | T | Elevate ear |
| ② Anterior | Temporal fascia (anterior portion) | Helix of the ear | | • Pull ear superiorly and anteriorly |
| ③ Posterior | Epicranial aponeurosis on side of head | Upper portion of auricle | | • Elevate ear |
| ④ Superior | Temporal fascia | Helix of the ear | PA | • Pull ear superiorly and posteriorly |
| Occipitofrontalis, occipital belly | Occipital bone (highest nuchal line) and temporal bone (mastoid part) | Epicranial aponeurosis near coronal suture | | Pulls scalp backwards |
| **Palpebral fissure and nose** | | | | |
| ⑤ Orbicularis oculi | | | | Whole muscle acts as orbital sphincter (closes eyelids) |
| • Orbital part | Medial orbital margin (frontal bone and maxilla) and medial palpebral ligament | Adjacent muscles (occipitofrontalis, corrugator supercilii, levator labii, etc.) | T/Z | • Voluntary closure of eyelids, furrowing of nose and eyebrows during squinting |
| • Palpebral part | Medial palpebral ligament | Eyelids (as lateral palpebral raphe) | | • Voluntary (sleeping) and involuntary closure (blinking) of eyelids |
| • Lacrimal part | Lacrimal crest | Tarsi of eyelids, lateral palpebral raphe | | • Pulls eyelids medially |
| ⑥ Procerus | Fascial aponeurosis of lower nasal bone | Skin between eyebrows | T/Z | Pulls eyebrows medially and inferiorly (frowning) |
| ⑦ Corrugator supercilii | Bone of superciliary arch (medial end) | Skin above supraorbital margin | T | Acts with orbicularis oculi to pull eyebrows medially and inferiorly (during squinting) |
| ⑧ Nasalis | | | | |
| • Transverse part | Maxilla | Aponeurosis at bridge of nose | B/Z | • Compresses nasal aperture (compressor naris) |
| • Alar part | | Ala nasi | | • Widens nasal aperture (flares nostril) by drawing ala toward nasal septum |
| ⑨ Levator labii superioris alaeque nasi | Frontal process of maxilla | Greater alar cartilage and orbital muscles (levator labii superioris and orbicularis oris) | B/Z | Elevates upper lip, increases the curvature of the nasolabial furrow, dilates nostril |

* Innervation: The muscles of facial expression are innervated by six branches of the facial nerve (CN VII). The posterior muscles are innervated by the posterior auricular (PA) nerve, which arises before the facial nerve enters the parotid gland (see p. 84). The anterior muscles are innervated by five branches off the parotid plexus of the facial nerve: temporal (T), zygomatic (Z), buccal (B), mandibular (M), and cervical (C).

# Muscles of Facial Expression: Mouth

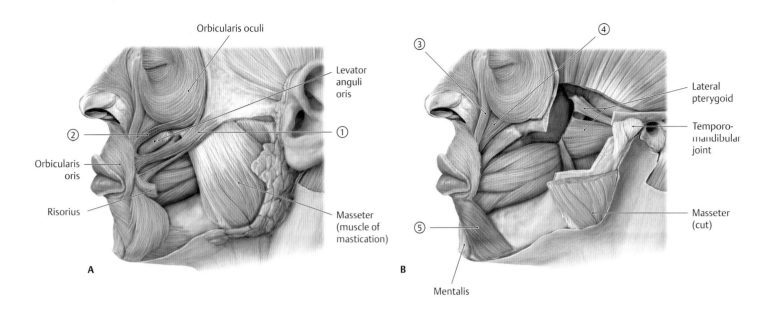

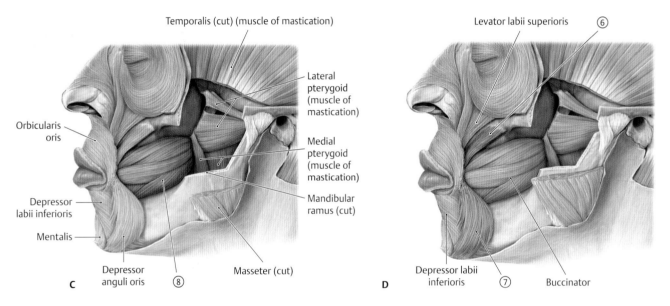

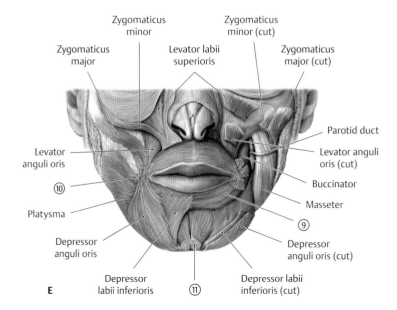

**Fig. 2.6 Muscles of facial expression: mouth**
Left lateral view.
**A** Zygomaticus major and minor. **B** Levator labii superioris and depressor labii inferioris (exposed by removal of the depressor anguli oris). **C** Buccinator. **D** Levator anguli oris and depressor anguli oris. **E** Anterior view.

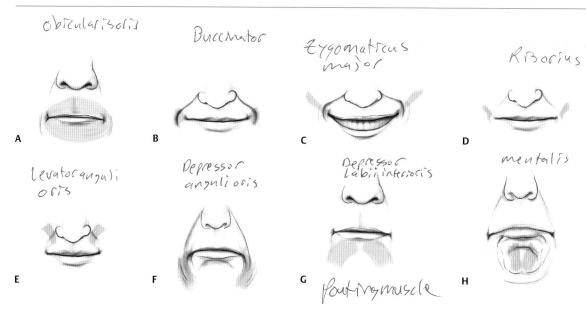

*Fig. 2.7* **Changes of facial expression: mouth**
Anterior view.
**A** Orbicularis oris. **B** Buccinator. **C** Zygomaticus major. **D** Risorius.
**E** Levator anguli oris. **F** Depressor anguli oris. **G** Depressor labii infe-
rioris. **H** Mentalis.

*Table 2.2* **Muscles of facial expression: mouth**

| Muscle | Origin | Insertion | I* | Main action(s) |
|---|---|---|---|---|
| ① Zygomaticus major | Zygomatic bone (lateral surface, posterior part) | Muscles at the angle of the mouth | Z | Pulls corner of mouth superiorly and laterally |
| ② Zygomaticus minor | | Upper lip just medial to corner of the mouth | | Pulls upper lip superiorly |
| ③ Levator labii superioris alaeque nasi (see **Fig. 2.1**) | Maxilla (frontal process) | Upper lip and alar cartilage of nose | B/Z | Elevates upper lip; flares nostril |
| ④ Levator labii superioris | Maxilla (frontal process) and infraorbital margin | Skin of upper lip | | Elevates upper lip |
| ⑤ Depressor labii inferioris | Mandible (anterior portion of oblique line) | Lower lip at midline; blends with muscle from opposite side | M | Pulls lower lip inferiorly and laterally, also contributes to eversion (pouting) |
| ⑥ Levator anguli oris | Maxilla (canine fossa, below infraorbital foramen) | Muscles at the angle of mouth | B/Z | Raises angle of mouth; helps form nasolabial furrow |
| ⑦ Depressor anguli oris | Mandible (oblique line below canine, premolar, and 1st molar teeth) | Skin at corner of mouth; blends with orbicularis oris | B/M | Pulls angle of mouth inferiorly and laterally |
| ⑧ Buccinator | Alveolar processes of maxilla and mandible (by molars); pterygomandibular raphe | Lips, orbicularis oris, submucosa of lips and cheek | B | • Suckling in nursing infant<br>• Presses cheek against molar teeth, working with tongue to keep food between occlusal surfaces and out of oral vestibule; expels air from oral cavity/resists distention when blowing<br>*Unilateral:* draws mouth to one side |
| ⑨ Orbicularis oris | Deep surface of skin Superiorly: Maxilla (median plane) Inferiorly: Mandible | Mucous membrane of lips | B/M | Acts as oral sphincter<br>• Compresses and protrudes lip (e.g., whistling, sucking, kissing)<br>• Resists distention (when blowing) |
| ⑩ Risorius | Fascia and superficial muscles over masseter | Skin of corner of mouth | B | Retracts corner of mouth as in smiling, laughing, grimacing |
| ⑪ Mentalis | Frenulum of lower lip | Skin of chin | M | Elevates and protrudes lower lip (drinking) |
| Platysma | Skin over lower neck and upper lateral thorax | Mandible (inferior border); skin over lower face; angle of mouth | C | Depresses and wrinkles skin of lower face and mouth; tenses skin of neck; aids in forced depression of the mandible |

* Innervation: The muscles of facial expression are innervated by six branches of the facial nerve (CN VII). The posterior muscles are innervated by the posterior auricular (PA) nerve, which arises before the facial nerve enters the parotid gland (see p. 84). The anterior muscles are innervated by five branches off the parotid plexus of the facial nerve: temporal (T), zygomatic (Z), buccal (B), mandibular (M), and cervical (C).

29

# Muscles of Mastication: Overview

The muscles of mastication are located at various depths in the parotid and infratemporal regions of the face. They attach to the mandible and receive their motor innervation from the mandibular division of the trigeminal nerve (CN V₃).

| Table 2.3 **Masseter and temporalis muscles** | | | | |
|---|---|---|---|---|
| **Muscle** | | **Origin** | **Insertion** | **Innervation*** | **Action** |
| Masseter | ① Superficial head | Zygomatic bone (maxillary process) and zygomatic arch (lateral aspect of anterior ⅔) | Mandibular angle and ramus (inferior lateral surface) | Masseteric n. (anterior division of CN V₃) | Elevates mandible; also assists in protraction, retraction, and side-to-side motion |
| | Middle head | Zygomatic arch (medial aspect of anterior ⅔) | Mandibular ramus (central part of occlusal surface) | | |
| | ② Deep head | Zygomatic arch (deep surface of posterior ⅓) | Mandibular ramus (superior lateral surface) and inferior coronoid process | | |
| Temporalis | ③ Superficial head | Temporal fascia | Coronoid process of mandible (apex, medial surface, and anterior surface of mandibular ramus) | Deep temporal nn. (anterior division of CN V₃) | *Vertical (anterior) fibers:* Elevate mandible<br>*Horizontal (posterior) fibers:* Retract (retrude) mandible<br>*Unilateral:* Lateral movement of mandible (chewing) |
| | ④ Deep head | Temporal fossa (inferior temporal line) | | | |

\* The muscles of mastication are innervated by motor branches of the mandibular nerve (CN V₃), the 3rd division of the trigeminal nerve (CN V).

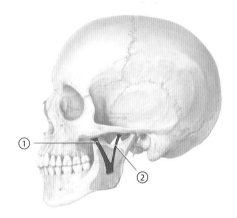

**Fig. 2.8 Masseter**

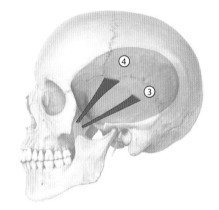

**Fig. 2.9 Temporalis**

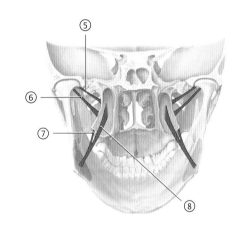

**Fig. 2.10 Pterygoids**

| Table 2.4 **Lateral and medial pterygoid muscles** | | | | |
|---|---|---|---|---|
| **Muscle** | | **Origin** | **Insertion** | **Innervation** | **Action** |
| Lateral pterygoid | ⑤ Superior (upper) head | Greater wing of sphenoid bone (infratemporal crest) | Mandible (pterygoid fovea) and temporomandibular joint (articular disk) | Mandibular n. (anterior division of CN V₃) via lateral pterygoid n. | *Bilateral:* Protrudes mandible (pulls articular disk forward)<br>*Unilateral:* Lateral movements of mandible (chewing) |
| | ⑥ Inferior (lower) head | Lateral pterygoid plate (lateral surface) | Mandible (pterygoid fovea and condylar process) | | |
| Medial pterygoid | ⑦ Superficial (external) head | Maxilla (maxillary tuberosity) and palatine bone (pyramidal process) | Pterygoid rugosity on medial surface of the mandibular angle | Mandibular n. (anterior division of CN V₃) via medial pterygoid n. | Elevates (adducts) mandible |
| | ⑧ Deep (internal) head | Medial surface of lateral pterygoid plate and pterygoid fossa | | | |

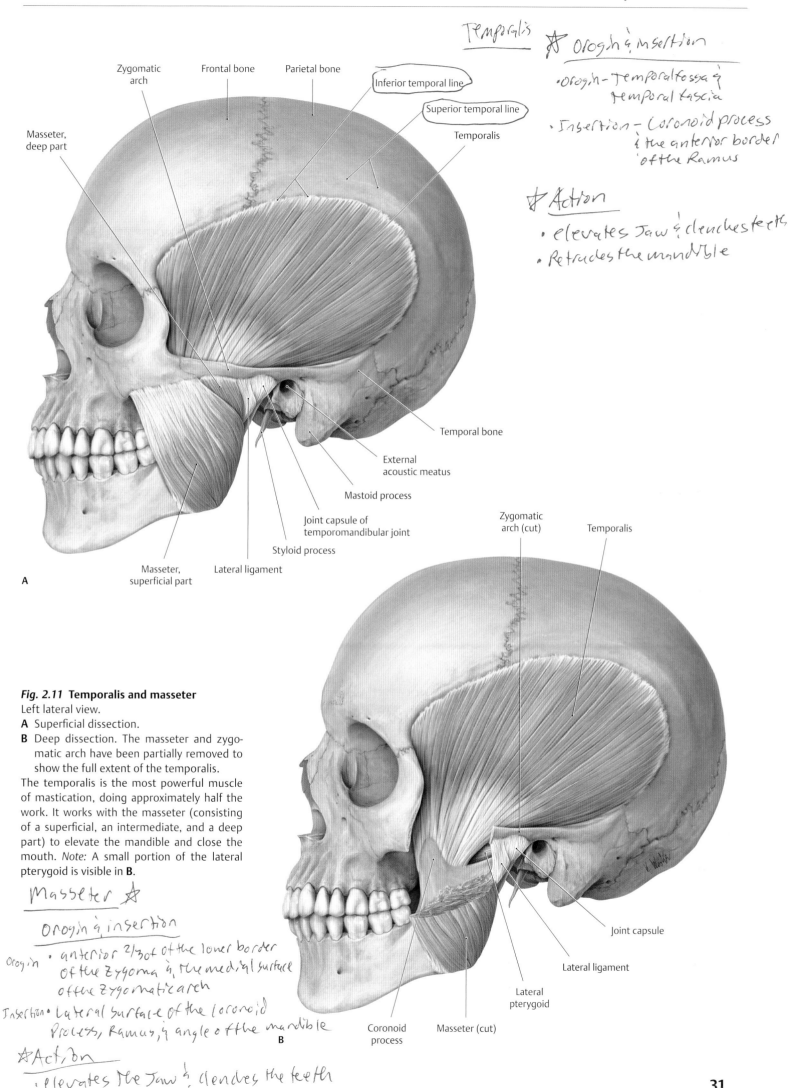

Temporalis

☆ Origin & insertion

• Origin - Temporal fossa &
  temporal fascia

• Insertion - Coronoid process
  & the anterior border
  of the Ramus

☆ Action

• elevates Jaw & clenches teeth
• Retracts the mandible

**Fig. 2.11 Temporalis and masseter**
Left lateral view.
**A** Superficial dissection.
**B** Deep dissection. The masseter and zygomatic arch have been partially removed to show the full extent of the temporalis.
The temporalis is the most powerful muscle of mastication, doing approximately half the work. It works with the masseter (consisting of a superficial, an intermediate, and a deep part) to elevate the mandible and close the mouth. *Note:* A small portion of the lateral pterygoid is visible in **B**.

Masseter ☆

Origin & insertion

Origin • anterior 2/3 of the lower border
  of the Zygoma & the medial surface
  of the Zygomatic arch

Insertion • Lateral surface of the coronoid
  Process, Ramus, & angle of the mandible

☆ Action
• elevates the Jaw & clenches the teeth

**31**

*Lateral Pterygoid*
- *origin*
  - *Superior head - Infratemporal site of sphenoid greater wing*
  - *Inferior head - Lateral surface of Lateral Pterygoid plate*
- *Insertion*
  - *superior belly - articular disk*
  - *Inferior belly - Pterygoid fovea*
- *Action - protrusion, assists in rotation*

# Muscles of Mastication: Deep Muscles

★ *Medial Pterygoid*
- *origin - medial surface of lateral pterygoid plate, max. tuberosity, Pyramidal Process of the palatine bones*
- *Insertion - posterior and lower part of the medial surface of the ramus & angle of mandible.*
- *Action - Protrusion, elevation, assists in rotation*

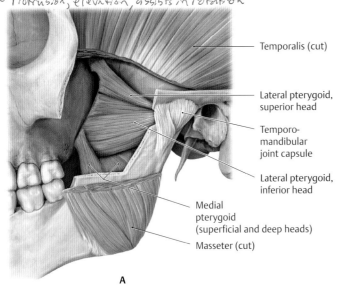
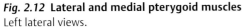

A — Temporalis (cut)
Lateral pterygoid, superior head
Temporo-mandibular joint capsule
Lateral pterygoid, inferior head
Medial pterygoid (superficial and deep heads)
Masseter (cut)

**A**

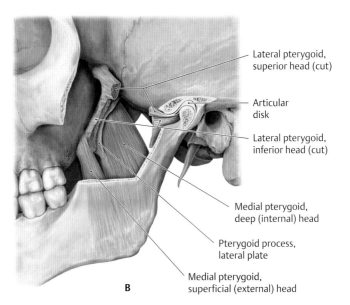

Lateral pterygoid, superior head (cut)
Articular disk
Lateral pterygoid, inferior head (cut)
Medial pterygoid, deep (internal) head
Pterygoid process, lateral plate
Medial pterygoid, superficial (external) head

**B**

**Fig. 2.12 Lateral and medial pterygoid muscles**
Left lateral views.

A The coronoid process of the mandible has been removed here along with the lower part of the temporalis so that both pterygoid muscles are observed (see **Fig. 2.11B**).

B Here the temporalis has been completely removed, and the inferior head of the lateral pterygoid has been windowed. The *lateral* pterygoid initiates depression of the mandible, which is then continued by the suprahyoid and infrahyoid muscles and gravity. With

the temporomandibular joint opened, we can see that fibers from the superior head of the lateral pterygoid blend with the articular disk. The lateral pterygoid functions as the guide muscle of the temporomandibular joint. The *medial* pterygoid runs almost perpendicular to the lateral pterygoid and contributes to the formation of a muscular sling that partially encompasses the mandible (see **Fig. 2.13**). Note how the inferior head of the lateral pterygoid originates between the two heads of the medial pterygoid.

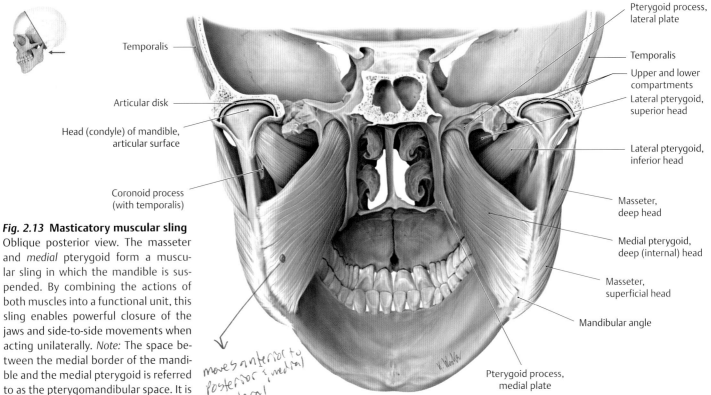

Temporalis
Articular disk
Head (condyle) of mandible, articular surface
Coronoid process (with temporalis)

Pterygoid process, lateral plate
Temporalis
Upper and lower compartments
Lateral pterygoid, superior head
Lateral pterygoid, inferior head
Masseter, deep head
Medial pterygoid, deep (internal) head
Masseter, superficial head
Mandibular angle
Pterygoid process, medial plate

**Fig. 2.13 Masticatory muscular sling**
Oblique posterior view. The masseter and *medial* pterygoid form a muscular sling in which the mandible is suspended. By combining the actions of both muscles into a functional unit, this sling enables powerful closure of the jaws and side-to-side movements when acting unilaterally. *Note:* The space between the medial border of the mandible and the medial pterygoid is referred to as the pterygomandibular space. It is important as it is the target area for administering local anesthesia to the inferior alveolar nerve.

*moves anterior to Posterior & medial to Lateral*

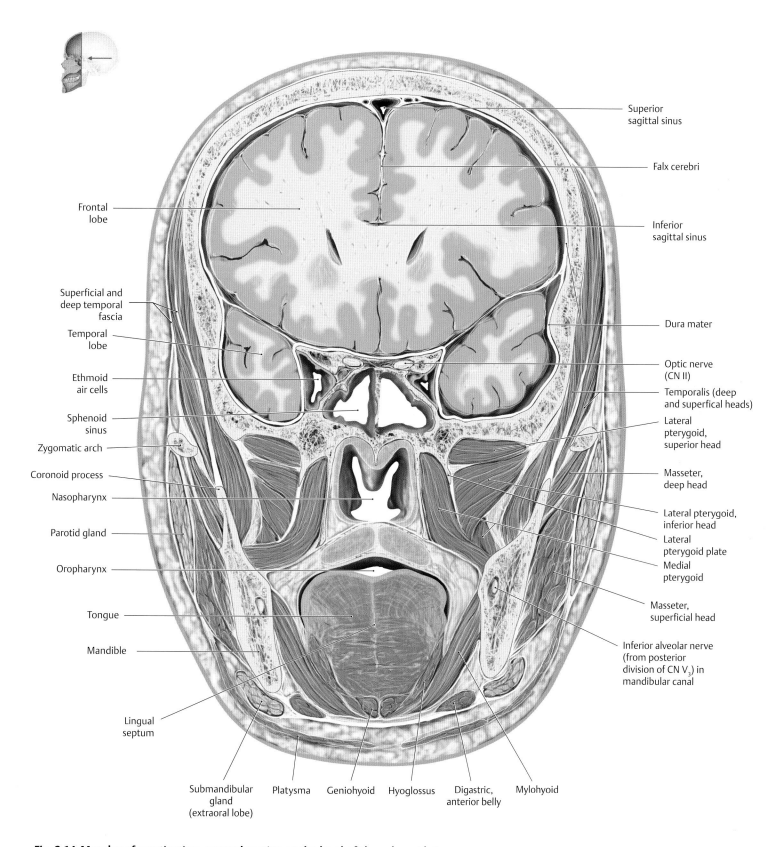

**Fig. 2.14 Muscles of mastication, coronal section at the level of the sphenoid sinus**
Posterior view. The topography of the muscles of mastication and neighboring structures is particularly well displayed in this section.

# Temporomandibular Joint (TMJ): Biomechanics

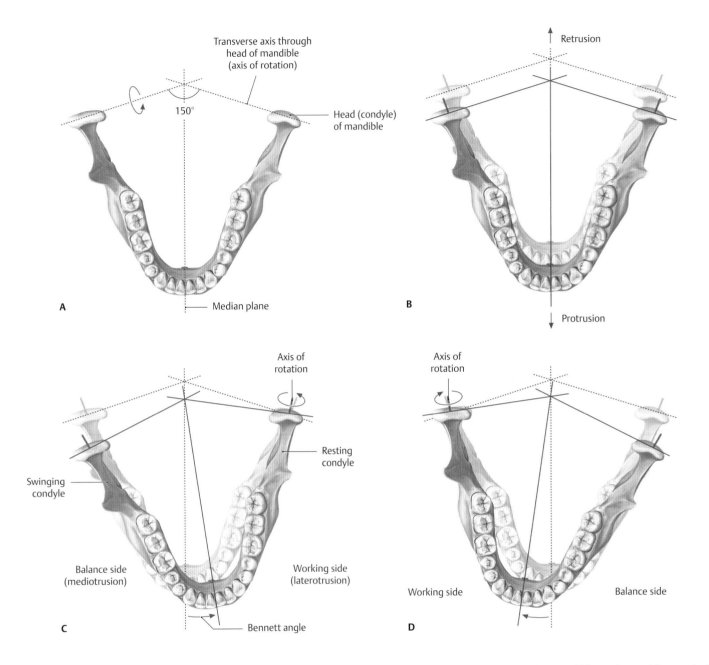

**Fig. 2.15 Movements of the mandible in the TMJ**
Superior view. Most of the movements in the TMJ are complex motions that have three main components:

- Rotation (opening and closing the mouth)
- Translation (protrusion and retrusion of the mandible)
- Grinding movements during mastication

**A Rotation.** The axis for joint rotation runs transversely through both heads of the mandible. The two axes intersect at an angle of approximately 150 degrees (range of 110–180 degrees between individuals). During this movement the TMJ acts as a hinge joint (abduction/depression and adduction/elevation of the mandible). In humans, pure rotation in the TMJ usually occurs only during sleep with the mouth slightly open (aperture angle up to approximately 15 degrees, see **Fig. 2.16B**). When the mouth is opened past 15 degrees, rotation is combined with translation (gliding) of the mandibular head.

**B Translation.** In this movement the mandible is advanced (protruded) and retracted (retruded). The axes for this movement are parallel to the median axes through the center of the mandibular heads.

**C Grinding movements in the left TMJ.** In describing these lateral movements, a distinction is made between the "resting condyle" and the "swinging condyle." The resting condyle on the left working side rotates about an almost vertical axis through the head of the mandible (also a rotational axis), whereas the swinging condyle on the right balance side swings forward and inward in a translational movement. The lateral excursion of the mandible is measured in degrees and is called the Bennett angle. During this movement the mandible moves in laterotrusion on the working side and in mediotrusion on the balance side.

**D Grinding movements in the right TMJ.** Here, the right TMJ is the working side. The right resting condyle rotates about an almost vertical axis, and the left condyle on the balance side swings forward and inward.

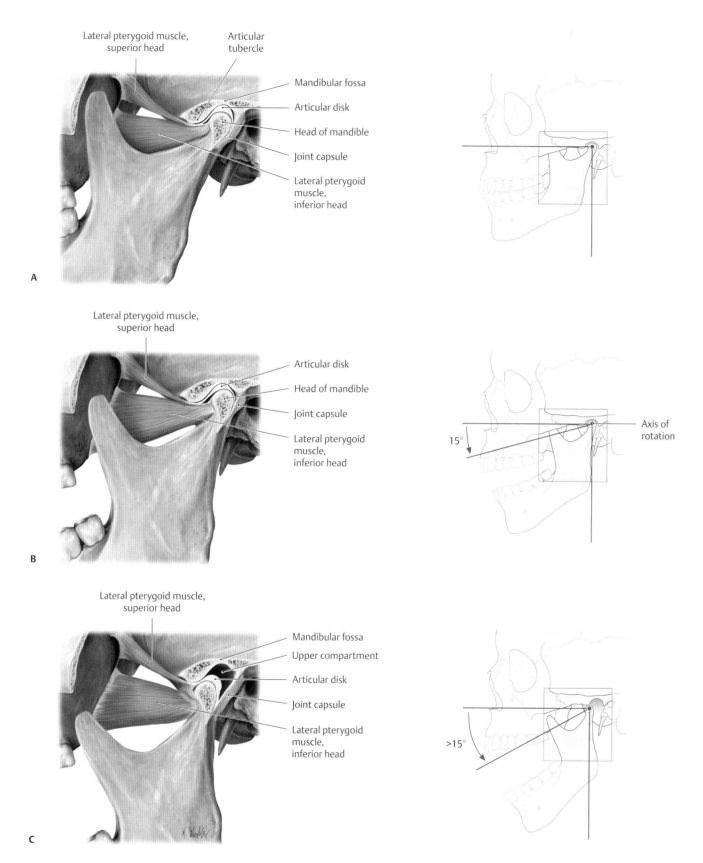

**A** Lateral pterygoid muscle, superior head
Articular tubercle
Mandibular fossa
Articular disk
Head of mandible
Joint capsule
Lateral pterygoid muscle, inferior head

**B** Lateral pterygoid muscle, superior head
Articular disk
Head of mandible
Joint capsule
Lateral pterygoid muscle, inferior head
15°
Axis of rotation

**C** Lateral pterygoid muscle, superior head
Mandibular fossa
Upper compartment
Articular disk
Joint capsule
Lateral pterygoid muscle, inferior head
>15°

*Fig. 2.16* **Movements of the TMJ**
Left lateral view. Each drawing shows the left TMJ (including the artic-ular disk and capsule) and the lateral pterygoid muscle. *Note:* The gap between the heads of the lateral pterygoid is exaggerated. Each sche-matic diagram at right shows the corresponding axis of joint move-ment. The muscle, capsule, and disk form a functionally coordinated musculo-disco-capsular system and work closely together when the mouth is opened and closed.

**A Mouth closed.** When the mouth is in a closed position, the head of the mandible rests against the mandibular (glenoid) fossa of the tempo-ral bone.

**B Mouth opened to 15 degrees.** Up to 15 degrees of abduction, the head of the mandible remains in the mandibular fossa.

**C Mouth opened past 15 degrees.** At this point the head of the man-dible glides forward onto the articular tubercle. The joint axis that runs transversely through the mandibular head is shifted forward. The articular disk is pulled forward by the superior part of the lateral pterygoid muscle, and the head (condyle) of the mandible is drawn forward by the inferior part of that muscle.

# Temporomandibular Joint (TMJ)

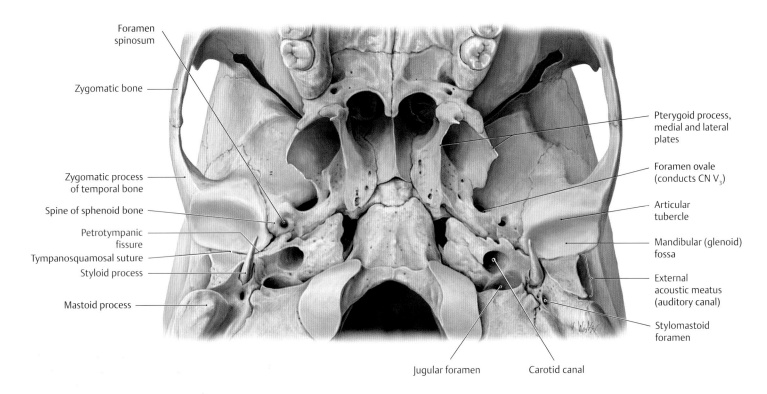

Foramen spinosum

Zygomatic bone

Zygomatic process of temporal bone

Spine of sphenoid bone

Petrotympanic fissure

Tympanosquamosal suture

Styloid process

Mastoid process

Pterygoid process, medial and lateral plates

Foramen ovale (conducts CN V₃)

Articular tubercle

Mandibular (glenoid) fossa

External acoustic meatus (auditory canal)

Stylomastoid foramen

Jugular foramen          Carotid canal

**Fig. 2.17 Mandibular (glenoid) fossa of the TMJ**
Inferior view. The head of the mandible articulates with the articular disk in the mandibular (glenoid) fossa of the temporal bone. The mandibular fossa is a depression in the squamous part of the temporal bone. The articular tubercle is located on the anterior side of the mandibular fossa. The head of the mandible is markedly smaller than the mandibular fossa, allowing it to have an adequate range of movement (see p. 35). Unlike other articular surfaces, the mandibular fossa is covered by fibrocartilage rather than hyaline cartilage. As a result, it is not

as clearly delineated on the skull as other articular surfaces. The external auditory canal lies just posterior to the mandibular fossa. Trauma to the mandible may damage the auditory canal. *Note:* The mandibular fossa is divided into two compartments (anterior and posterior), separated by the tympanosquamosal and petrotympanic fissures. The posterior compartment is nonarticulatory, and the chorda tympani nerve and inferior tympanic artery are able to pass through this space without being compressed. The glenoid lobe of the parotid gland may also project into the posterior compartment.

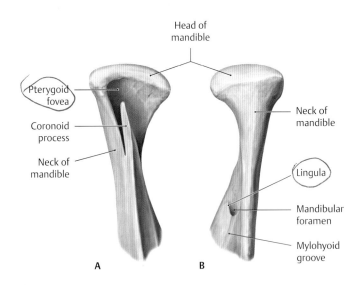

Head of mandible

Pterygoid fovea

Coronoid process

Neck of mandible

Neck of mandible

Lingula

Mandibular foramen

Mylohyoid groove

A          B

**Fig. 2.18 Processes of the mandible**
**A** Anterior view. **B** Posterior view. The head of the mandible not only is markedly smaller than the articular fossa but also has a cylindrical shape. This shape increases the mobility of the mandibular head, as it allows rotational movements about a vertical axis.

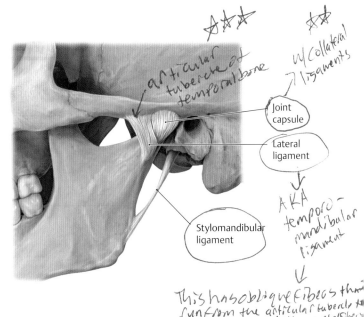

*[handwritten annotations: ⋆⋆⋆ articular tubercle of temporal bone; ⋆⋆ w/ collateral ligaments]*

Joint capsule

Lateral ligament

*[handwritten: AKA temporo-mandibular ligament]*

Stylomandibular ligament

*[handwritten: This has oblique fibers that run from the articular tubercle to the condylar neck. And horizontal fibers that run the same course]*

**Fig. 2.19 Ligaments of the left TMJ**
Lateral view. The TMJ is surrounded by a relatively lax capsule, which permits physiological dislocation during jaw opening. The joint is stabilized by three ligaments: lateral (temporomandibular), stylomandibular, and sphenomandibular. This lateral view demonstrates the strongest of these ligaments, the lateral ligament, which stretches over the capsule and is blended with it.

*movement restrictions* ☆☆☆☆
- *Lateral (temporomandibular) ligament — limits posterior & interior movement.*
- *Stylomandibular ligament — limits downward and forward movement.*
- *Sphenomandibular ligament — limits downward and lateral movement.*

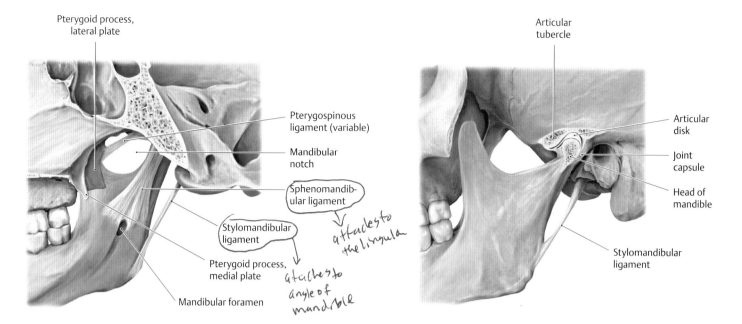

**Fig. 2.20 Ligaments of the right TMJ**
Medial view. The sphenomandibular ligament can be identified in this view.

*attaches to the lingula*

*attaches to angle of mandible*

**Fig. 2.21 Opened left TMJ**
Lateral view. The capsule extends posteriorly to the petrotympanic fissure (not shown here). Interposed between the mandibular head and fossa is the articular disk, which is attached to the joint capsule on all sides. *Note:* The articular disk (meniscus) divides the TMJ into upper and lower compartments. Gliding (translational) movement occcurs in the upper compartment, hinge (rotational) movement in the lower compartment.

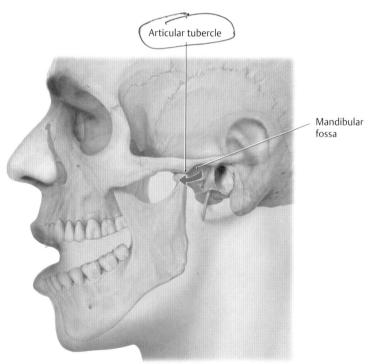

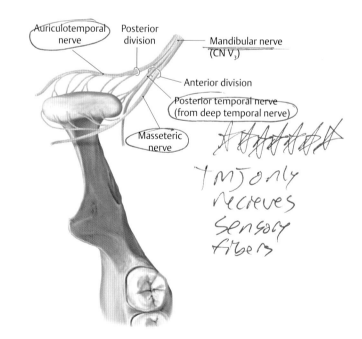

*TMJ only recieves sensory fibers*

**Fig. 2.22 Dislocation of the TMJ**
The head of the mandible may slide past the articular tubercle when the mouth is opened, dislocating the TMJ. This may result from heavy yawning or a blow to the opened mandible. When the joint dislocates, the mandible becomes locked in a protruded position and can no longer be closed. This condition is easily diagnosed clinically and is reduced by pressing on the mandibular row of teeth.

**Fig. 2.23 Sensory innervation of the TMJ capsule** (after Schmidt)
Superior view. The TMJ capsule is supplied by articular branches arising from three branches of the mandibular division of the trigeminal nerve (CN $V_3$):

- Auriculotemporal nerve (posterior division of CN $V_3$)
- Posterior deep temporal nerve (anterior division of CN $V_3$)
- Masseteric nerve (anterior division of CN $V_3$)

*Note:* While the masseteric and posterior deep temporal nerves are generally considered to be motor nerves, they also innervate the TMJ.

# Muscles of the Head: Origins & Insertions

The bony origins and insertions of the muscles are indicated by color shading: origins (red) and insertions (blue).

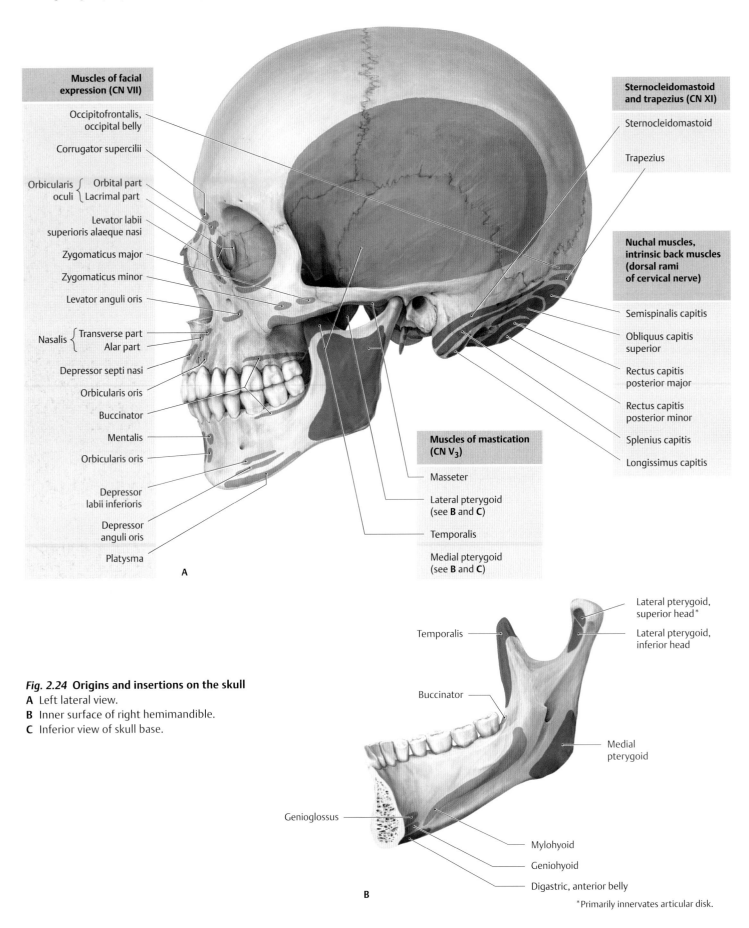

**Muscles of facial expression (CN VII)**

- Occipitofrontalis, occipital belly
- Corrugator supercilii
- Orbicularis oculi { Orbital part / Lacrimal part
- Levator labii superioris alaeque nasi
- Zygomaticus major
- Zygomaticus minor
- Levator anguli oris
- Nasalis { Transverse part / Alar part
- Depressor septi nasi
- Orbicularis oris
- Buccinator
- Mentalis
- Orbicularis oris
- Depressor labii inferioris
- Depressor anguli oris
- Platysma

**A**

**Sternocleidomastoid and trapezius (CN XI)**

- Sternocleidomastoid
- Trapezius

**Nuchal muscles, intrinsic back muscles (dorsal rami of cervical nerve)**

- Semispinalis capitis
- Obliquus capitis superior
- Rectus capitis posterior major
- Rectus capitis posterior minor
- Splenius capitis
- Longissimus capitis

**Muscles of mastication (CN V₃)**

- Masseter
- Lateral pterygoid (see **B** and **C**)
- Temporalis
- Medial pterygoid (see **B** and **C**)

- Lateral pterygoid, superior head*
- Temporalis
- Lateral pterygoid, inferior head
- Buccinator
- Medial pterygoid
- Genioglossus
- Mylohyoid
- Geniohyoid
- Digastric, anterior belly

**B**

***Fig. 2.24 Origins and insertions on the skull***
**A** Left lateral view.
**B** Inner surface of right hemimandible.
**C** Inferior view of skull base.

*Primarily innervates articular disk.

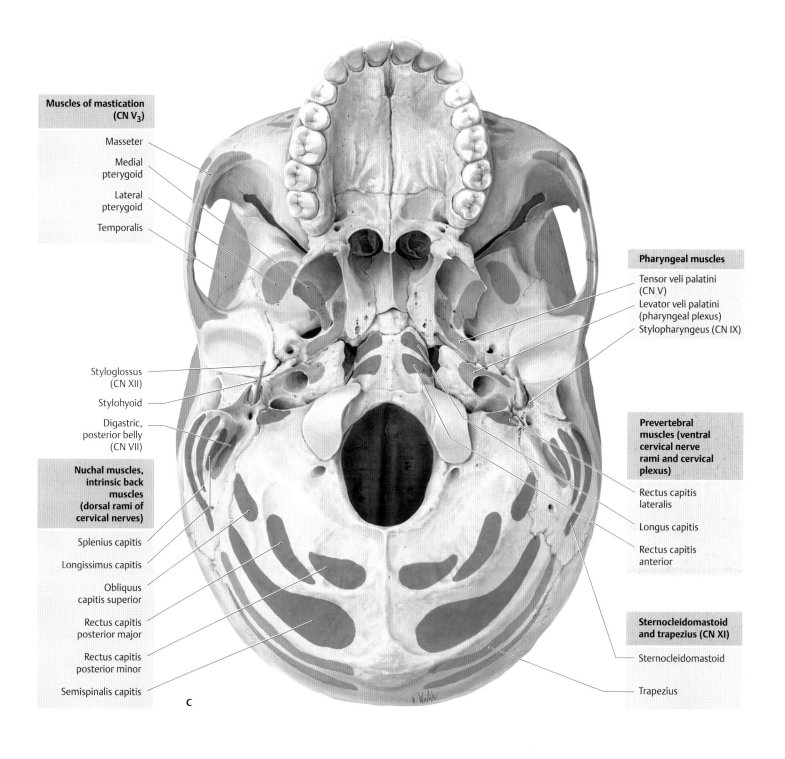

**Muscles of mastication (CN V₃)**

Masseter

Medial pterygoid

Lateral pterygoid

Temporalis

Styloglossus (CN XII)

Stylohyoid

Digastric, posterior belly (CN VII)

**Nuchal muscles, intrinsic back muscles (dorsal rami of cervical nerves)**

Splenius capitis

Longissimus capitis

Obliquus capitis superior

Rectus capitis posterior major

Rectus capitis posterior minor

Semispinalis capitis

**Pharyngeal muscles**

Tensor veli palatini (CN V)

Levator veli palatini (pharyngeal plexus)

Stylopharyngeus (CN IX)

**Prevertebral muscles (ventral cervical nerve rami and cervical plexus)**

Rectus capitis lateralis

Longus capitis

Rectus capitis anterior

**Sternocleidomastoid and trapezius (CN XI)**

Sternocleidomastoid

Trapezius

C

# Arteries of the Head: Overview

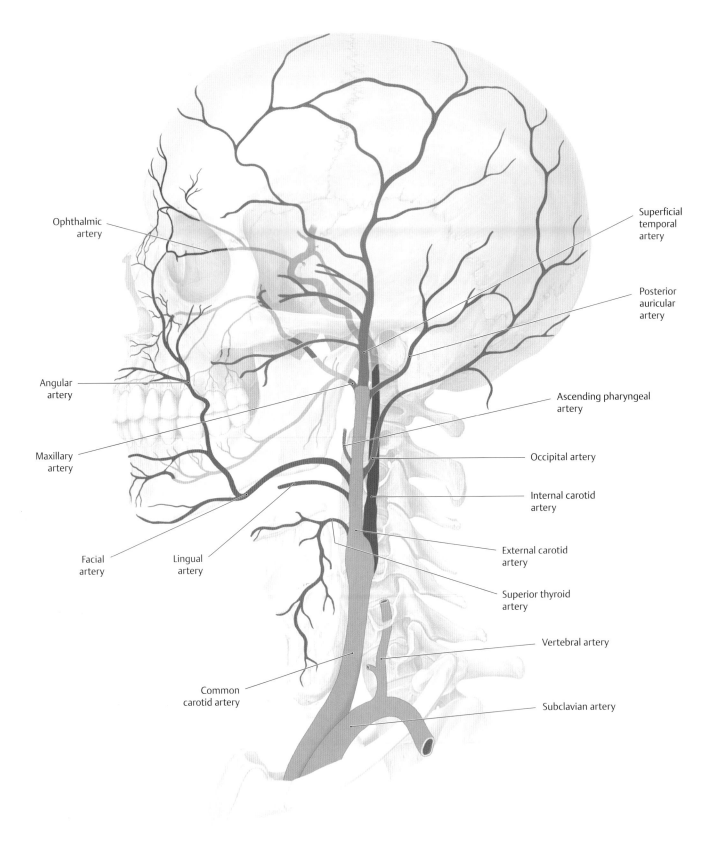

Ophthalmic
artery

Superficial
temporal
artery

Posterior
auricular
artery

Angular
artery

Ascending pharyngeal
artery

Occipital artery

Maxillary
artery

Internal carotid
artery

External carotid
artery

Facial
artery

Lingual
artery

Superior thyroid
artery

Vertebral artery

Common
carotid artery

Subclavian artery

**Fig. 3.1 Arteries of the head**

Left lateral view. The common carotid artery divides into the internal carotid artery (purple) and the external carotid artery (gray) at the carotid bifurcation (at the level of the C4 vertebra, between the thyroid cartilage and hyoid bone). The external carotid artery divides into eight major branches that supply the scalp, face, and structures of the head and neck. These eight branches can be arranged into four groups: anterior (red), medial (blue), posterior (green), and terminal (yellow). The internal carotid artery does not branch before entering the skull. It gives off branches within the cranial cavity. The ophthalmic branch of the internal carotid artery provides branches that will anastomose with branches of the facial artery on the face (see **Fig. 3.2**).

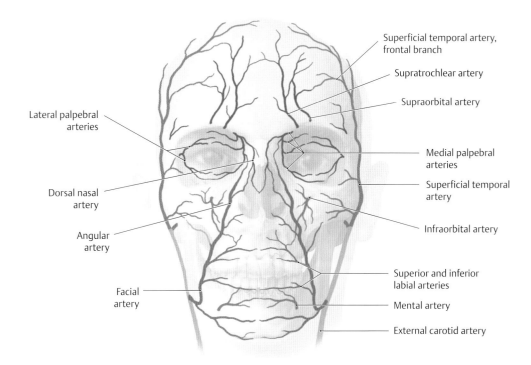

**Fig. 3.2 Branches of the carotid arteries**
The external carotid artery may be arranged into four groups of branches. The facial artery (red) communicates with certain branches of the ophthalmic artery, which arises from the internal carotid artery (purple).

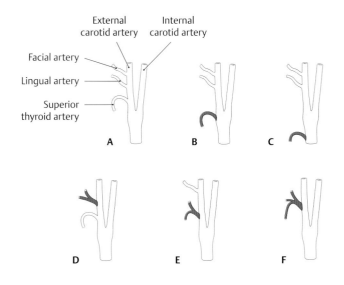

**Fig. 3.3 Variants in external carotid artery branching**
**A** Typically (50%), the anterior branches (facial, lingual, and superior thyroid arteries) arise from the external carotid artery above the carotid bifurcation.

   *Variants:*

**B, C** The superior thyroid artery arises at the level of the carotid bifurcation (20%) or from the common carotid artery (10%).

**D–F** Two or three branches combine to form a common trunk: linguofacial (18%), thyrolingual (2%), or thyrolinguofacial (1%).

| **Table 3.1 Branches of the external carotid artery** | |
|---|---|
| **Anterior branches (red)** | **Region supplied** |
| Superior thyroid a. | Larynx, thyroid gland, pharynx |
| Lingual a. | Oral cavity, tongue |
| Facial a. | Superficial facial region, submandibular gland, neck |
| **Medial branch (blue)** | **Region supplied** |
| Ascending pharyngeal a. | Pharynx |
| **Posterior branches (green)** | **Region supplied** |
| Occipital a. | Occipital region |
| Posterior auricular a. | Ear, posterior scalp |
| **Terminal branches (yellow)** | **Region supplied** |
| Maxillary a. | Mandibular (via inferior alveolar branch) and maxillary dentition, masticatory muscles, posteromedial facial skeleton, meninges, nasal cavity and face (via infraorbital and mental arteries) |
| Superficial temporal a. | Temporal region, ear, parotid gland |

# External Carotid Artery: Anterior, Medial & Posterior Branches

*✳ Some losers fail anatomy, others post magnificent scores*

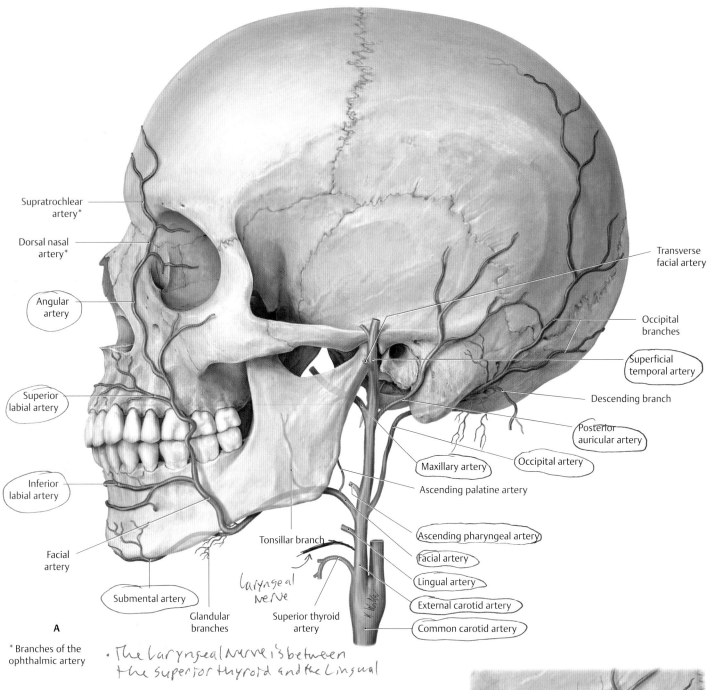

Supratrochlear artery*

Dorsal nasal artery*

Angular artery

Superior labial artery

Inferior labial artery

Facial artery

Submental artery

Glandular branches

**A**

Transverse facial artery

Occipital branches

Superficial temporal artery

Descending branch

Posterior auricular artery

Occipital artery

Maxillary artery

Ascending palatine artery

Ascending pharyngeal artery

Facial artery

Lingual artery

External carotid artery

Common carotid artery

Tonsillar branch

*Laryngeal Nerve*

Superior thyroid artery

* Branches of the ophthalmic artery

• The Laryngeal Nerve is between the superior thyroid and the Lingual

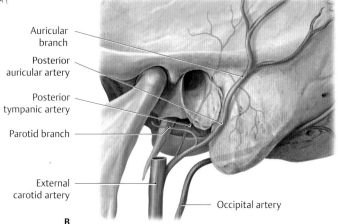

Auricular branch

Posterior auricular artery

Posterior tympanic artery

Parotid branch

External carotid artery

Occipital artery

**B**

**Fig. 3.4 Anterior and posterior branches**
Left lateral view.
**Anterior branches (A):** The facial artery has four cervical and four facial branches. The four cervical branches (ascending palatine, tonsillar,
glandular, and submental arteries) arise in the neck before the facial
artery crosses the mandible to reach the face. The four facial branches
(inferior and superior labial, lateral nasal, and angular arteries) supply
the superficial face. The facial branches anastomose with branches of
the internal carotid artery. Due to the extensive arterial anastomoses,
facial injuries tend to bleed profusely but also heal quickly.
**Posterior branches (B):** The two posterior branches of the external carotid artery are the occipital artery and the posterior auricular artery.

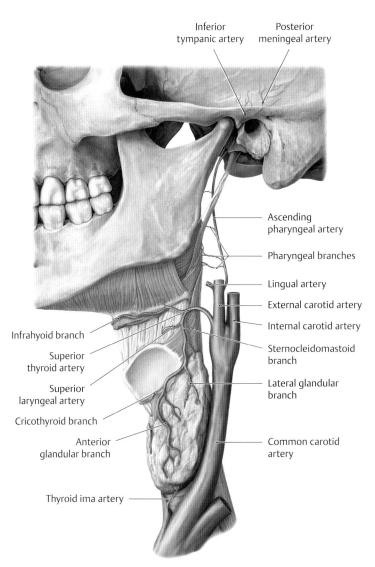

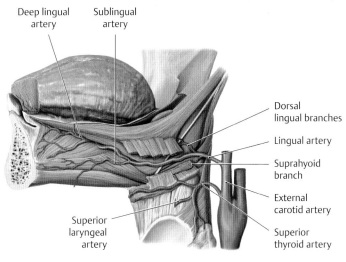

## Fig. 3.7 Lingual artery and its branches

Left lateral view. The lingual artery is the second anterior branch of the external carotid artery. It has a relatively large caliber, providing the tongue and oral cavity with its rich blood supply. It also gives off branches to the tonsils.

### Fig. 3.5 Anterior and medial branches

Left lateral view. The superior thyroid artery is typically the first branch to arise from the external carotid artery. One of the anterior branches, it supplies the larynx (via the superior laryngeal branch) and thyroid gland. The ascending pharyngeal artery springs from the medial side of the external carotid artery, usually arising above the level of the superior thyroid artery.

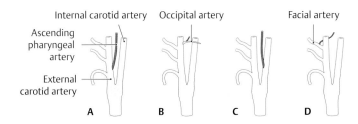

### Fig. 3.6 Origin of the ascending pharyngeal artery: typical case and variants (after Lippert and Pabst)

**A** In **typical cases** (70%) the ascending pharyngeal artery arises from the external carotid artery.

**B–D Variants:**
The ascending pharyngeal artery arises from **B** the occipital artery (20%), **C** the internal carotid artery (8%), or **D** the facial artery (2%).

| Table 3.2 Anterior, medial, and posterior branches | |
|---|---|
| **Branch** | **Branches and distribution** |
| **Anterior** | |
| Superior thyroid a. | Glandular branches: thyroid gland |
| | Superior laryngeal a.: larynx |
| | Sternocleidomastoid branch: sternocleidomastoid m. |
| | Pharyngeal branches: pharynx |
| Lingual a. | Dorsal lingual branches: base of tongue, epiglottis |
| | Suprahyoid branch: suprahyoid mm. |
| | Sublingual a.: sublingual gland, tongue, floor of oral cavity |
| | Deep lingual a.: tongue |
| Facial a. | Ascending palatine a.: pharyngeal wall, soft palate, pharyngotympanic tube, palatine tonsil |
| | Tonsillar a.: tonsils |
| | Glandular branch: submandibular gland |
| | Submental a.: anterior digastric and mylohyoid, submandibular gland |
| | Superior and inferior labial aa.: lips |
| | Lateral nasal branch: dorsum of nose |
| | Angular a.: nasal root |
| **Medial** | |
| Ascending pharyngeal a. | Pharyngeal branches: pharyngeal wall |
| | Inferior tympanic a.: mucosa of middle ear |
| | Posterior meningeal a.: dura, posterior cranial fossa |
| **Posterior** | |
| Occipital a. | Occipital branches: scalp of occipital region |
| | Descending branch: posterior neck muscles |
| Posterior auricular branch | Stylomastoid a.: facial n. in facial canal, tympanic cavity |
| | Posterior tympanic a.: tympanic cavity |
| | Auricular branch: posterior side of auricle |
| | Occipital branch: occiput |
| | Parotid branch: parotid gland |

*Note:* The two terminal branches are covered in Table 3.4.

**43**

# External Carotid Artery: Maxillary Artery

The maxillary artery is the largest of the two terminal branches of the external carotid artery (see p. 42). It supplies the maxilla and mandible (including the teeth), the muscles of mastication, the palate, the nose, and the dural covering of the brain.

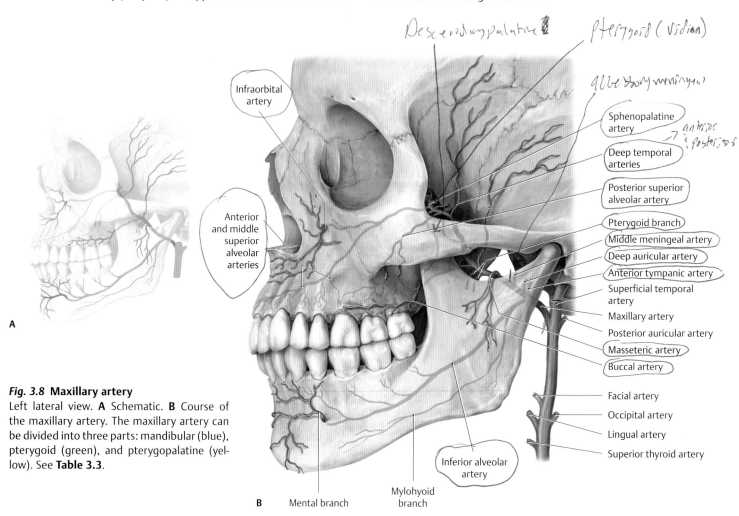

*Descending palatine*

*Pterygoid (Vidian)*

*accessory meningeal*

Infraorbital artery

Sphenopalatine artery

*anterior & posterior*

Deep temporal arteries

Posterior superior alveolar artery

Anterior and middle superior alveolar arteries

Pterygoid branch

Middle meningeal artery

Deep auricular artery

Anterior tympanic artery

Superficial temporal artery

Maxillary artery

Posterior auricular artery

Masseteric artery

Buccal artery

Facial artery

Occipital artery

Lingual artery

Superior thyroid artery

Inferior alveolar artery

Mylohyoid branch

Mental branch

**A**

**B**

**Fig. 3.8 Maxillary artery**
Left lateral view. **A** Schematic. **B** Course of the maxillary artery. The maxillary artery can be divided into three parts: mandibular (blue), pterygoid (green), and pterygopalatine (yellow). See **Table 3.3**.

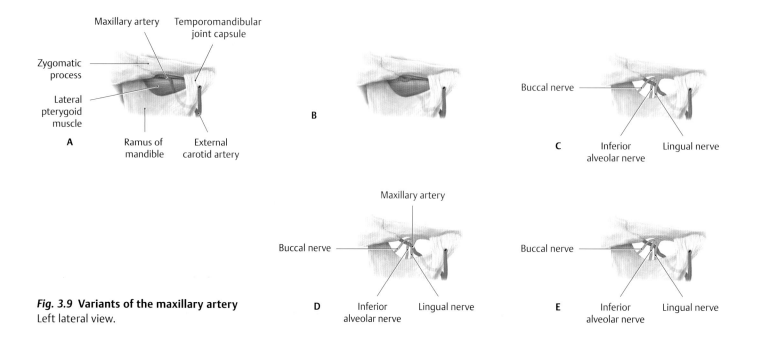

Maxillary artery

Temporomandibular joint capsule

Zygomatic process

Lateral pterygoid muscle

**A**

Ramus of mandible

External carotid artery

**B**

Buccal nerve

**C**

Inferior alveolar nerve

Lingual nerve

Maxillary artery

Buccal nerve

**D**

Inferior alveolar nerve

Lingual nerve

Buccal nerve

**E**

Inferior alveolar nerve

Lingual nerve

**Fig. 3.9 Variants of the maxillary artery**
Left lateral view.

**44**

## Table 3.3 Branches of the maxillary artery

| Branch | Course | Distribution |
|---|---|---|
| Mandibular part (blue): Also known as the bony part or 1st part, this portion runs medial to the neck of the mandible and gives off 5 major branches, all of which enter bone. | | |
| Inferior alveolar a. | Gives off a lingual and a mylohyoid branch before entering the mandibular foramen to travel along the mandibular canal; it splits into 2 terminal branches (incisive and mental) | Mandibular molars and premolars with associated gingiva, mandible |
| | • Lingual branch | Lingual mucous membrane |
| | • Mylohyoid branch | Mylohyoid |
| | • Incisive branch | Mandibular incisors |
| | • Mental branch | Chin |
| Anterior tympanic a. | Runs through the petrotympanic fissure along with the chorda tympani | Middle ear |
| Deep auricular a. | Travels through the wall of the external acoustic meatus | Lateral tympanic membrane, skin of external acoustic meatus |
| | • Branch to temporomandibular joint | Temporomandibular joint |
| Middle meningeal a. | Runs through the foramen spinosum to the middle cranial cavity | Bones of the cranial vault, dura of anterior and middle cranial fossae |
| Accessory meningeal a. | Runs through the foramen ovale to the middle cranial fossa | Medial and lateral pterygoid, tensor veli palatini, sphenoid bone, dura, trigeminal ganglion |
| Pterygoid part (green): Also known as the muscular part or 2nd part, this portion runs between the temporalis and lateral pterygoid. It gives off 5 major branches, all of which supply muscle. | | |
| Masseteric a. | Runs through the mandibular incisure (notch) | Masseter, temporomandibular joint |
| Deep temporal aa. | Consist of anterior, middle, and posterior branches, which course deep to the temporalis | Temporalis |
| Lateral pterygoid a. | Runs directly to the lateral pterygoid muscle | Lateral pterygoid |
| Medial pterygoid a. | Runs directly to the medial pterygoid muscle | Medial pterygoid |
| Buccal a. | Accompanies the buccal n. | Buccal mucosa and skin, buccinator |
| Pterygopalatine part or 3rd part (yellow): This portion runs through the pterygomaxillary fissure to enter the pterygopalatine fossa. It gives off 6 major branches, which accompany the branches of the maxillary nerve (CN V$_2$).* | | |
| Posterior superior alveolar a. | Runs through the pterygomaxillary fissure; may arise from the infraorbital a. | Maxillary molars and premolars, with associated gingiva; maxillary sinus |
| Infraorbital a. | Runs through the inferior orbital fissure into the orbit, where it runs along the infraorbital groove and canal, exiting onto the face via the infraorbital foramen | Cheek, upper lip, nose, lower eyelid |
| | • Anterior and middle superior alveolar aa. | Maxillary teeth and maxillary sinus |
| Descending palatine a. | Greater palatine a.: runs via the greater (anterior) palatine canal; in the canal it gives off several lesser palatine aa.; continues through greater palatine foramen onto hard palate | Roof of hard palate, nasal cavity (inferior meatus), maxillary gingiva |
| | • Lesser palatine aa.: run via the lesser palatine foramen | Soft palate |
| | • Anastomosing branch: runs via the incisive canal; joins with the sphenopalatine a. | Nasal septum |
| Sphenopalatine a. | Runs via the sphenopalatine foramen to the nasal cavity; gives off posterior lateral nasal branches, then travels to the nasal septum, where it terminates as posterior septal branches | |
| | • Posterior lateral nasal aa.: anastomose with the ethmoidal aa. and nasal branches of the greater palatine a. | Nasal air sinuses (frontal, maxillary, ethmoidal, and sphenoidal) |
| | • Posterior septal branches: anastomose with the ethmoidal arteries on the nasal septum | Nasal conchae and nasal septum |
| A. of the pterygoid canal | Runs through the pterygoid canal | Pharyngotympanic tube, tympanic cavity, upper pharynx |
| Pharyngeal a. | Runs through the palatovaginal canal | Nasopharynx, sphenoidal sinus, and pharyngotympanic tube; mucosa of nasal cavity |

*All branches are named for the nerve they travel with except for the sphenopalatine artery, which travels with the nasopalatine nerve.

# External Carotid Artery: Terminal Branches

There are two terminal branches of the external carotid artery: the maxillary artery and the superficial temporal artery. The external carotid artery divides into the maxillary and superficial temporal arteries

within the substance of the parotid gland. The extent of the maxillary artery makes it difficult to visualize. Three clinically relevant branches have been included here in greater detail.

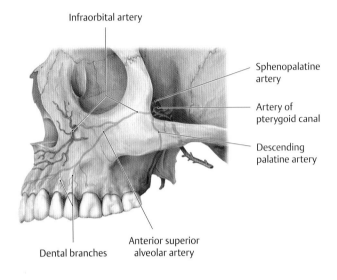

**Fig. 3.10 Infraorbital artery**
Left lateral view. The infraorbital artery arises from the pterygopalatine part of the maxillary artery (a terminal branch of the external carotid artery), and the supraorbital artery (not shown) arises from the internal carotid artery (via the ophthalmic branch). These vessels therefore provide a path for potential anastomosis between the internal and external carotid arteries on the face.

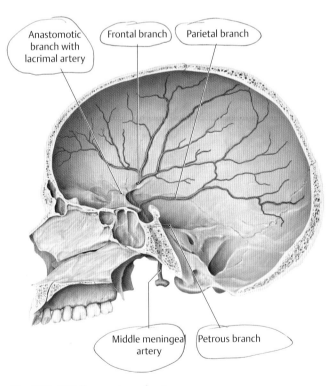

**Fig. 3.12 Middle meningeal artery**
Medial view of right middle meningeal artery. The middle meningeal artery arises from the mandibular portion of the maxillary artery. It passes through the foramen spinosum into the middle cranial fossa. Despite its name, it supplies blood not just to the meninges, but also to the overlying calvaria. Rupture of the middle meningeal artery by head trauma results in an epidural hematoma.

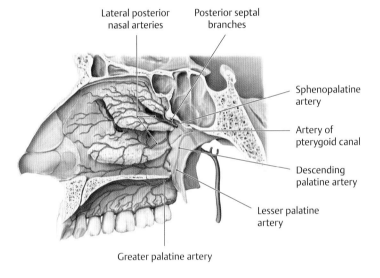

**Fig. 3.11 Sphenopalatine artery**
Medial view of right nasal wall and right sphenopalatine artery. The sphenopalatine artery enters the nasal cavity through the sphenopalatine foramen. The anterior portion of the nasal septum contains a highly vascularized region (Kiesselbach's area), which is supplied by both the posterior septal branches of the sphenopalatine artery (external carotid artery) and the anterior septal branches of the anterior ethmoidal artery (internal carotid artery via ophthalmic artery). When severe nasopharyngeal bleeding occurs, it may be necessary to ligate the maxillary artery in the pterygopalatine fossa.

### Fig. 3.13 Superficial temporal artery

Left lateral view. The superficial temporal artery is the second of the two terminal branches of the external carotid artery. Particularly in elderly or cachectic patients, the often tortuous course of the frontal branch of this vessel can be easily traced across the temple. The superficial temporal artery may be involved in an inflammatory immune disease (temporal arteritis), which can be confirmed by biopsy of this vessel. The patients, usually elderly men, complain of severe headaches.

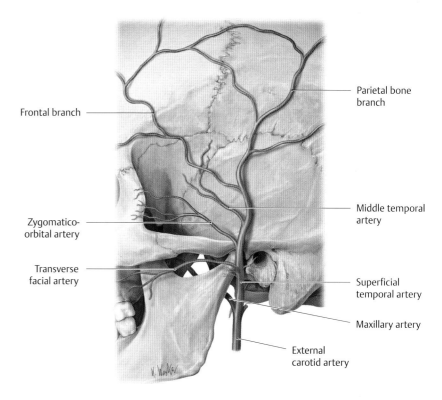

| Table 3.4 Terminal branches of the external carotid artery | | | |
|---|---|---|---|
| **Branch** | **Parts/Branches** | | **Distribution** |
| Maxillary a. (see p. 45) | Mandibular (1st; bony) part | Inferior alveolar a. | Mandibular teeth and gingiva, mandible |
| | | Anterior tympanic a. | Middle ear |
| | | Deep auricular a. | Temporomandibular joint and external auditory canal |
| | | Middle meningeal a. | Cranial vault, dura, anterior and middle cranial fossae |
| | | Accessory meningeal a. | Dura, trigeminal ganglion |
| | Pterygoid (2nd; muscular) part | Masseteric a. | Masseter, temporomandibular joint |
| | | Deep temporal branches | Temporalis |
| | | Medial pterygoid branches | Medial pterygoid |
| | | Lateral pterygoid branches | Lateral pterygoid |
| | | Buccal a. | Buccal mucosa and skin, buccinator |
| | Pterygopalatine (3rd) part | Posterior superior alveolar a. | Maxillary molars and gingiva, maxillary sinus |
| | | Infraorbital a. | Maxillary alveoli, maxillary dentition (via anterior and middle superior alveolar arteries) |
| | | Descending palatine a. | Nasal cavity (inferior meatus), roof of hard palate, maxillary gingiva, soft palate, nasal septum |
| | | Sphenopalatine a. | Lateral wall of nasal cavity, conchae, nasal septum |
| | | A. of the pterygoid canal | Pharyngotympanic tube, tympanic cavity, upper pharynx |
| | | Pharyngeal a. | Nasopharynx, sphenoidal sinus, and pharyngotympanic tube; mucosa of nasal cavity |
| Superficial temporal a. | Transverse facial a. | | Soft tissues below zygomatic arch |
| | Frontal branches | | Scalp of forehead |
| | Parietal branches | | Scalp of vertex |
| | Zygomatico-orbital a. | | Lateral external orbital wall |

# Internal Carotid Artery

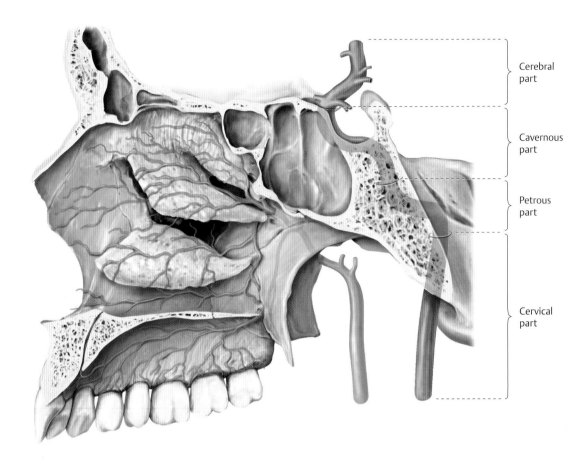

**A**

**Fig. 3.14 Subdivisions of the internal carotid artery**

**A** Medial view of the right internal artery in its passage through the bones of the skull. **B** Anatomical segments of the internal carotid artery and their branches. The internal carotid artery is distributed chiefly to the brain but also supplies extracerebral regions of the head. It consists of four parts (listed from bottom to top):

- Cervical part
- Petrous part
- Cavernous part
- Cerebral part

The petrous part of the internal carotid artery (traversing the carotid canal) and the cavernous part (traversing the cavernous sinus) have a role in supplying extracerebral structures of the head. They give off additional small branches that supply local structures and are usually named for the areas they supply. Of the branches not supplying the brain, of special importance is the ophthalmic artery, which arises from the cerebral part of the internal carotid artery. *Note:* The ophthalmic artery forms an anastomosis with the artery of the pterygoid canal derived from the maxillary artery.

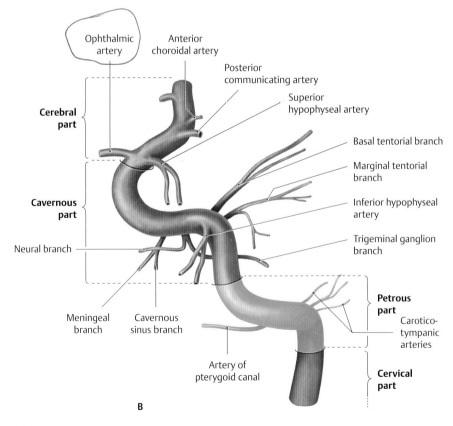

**B**

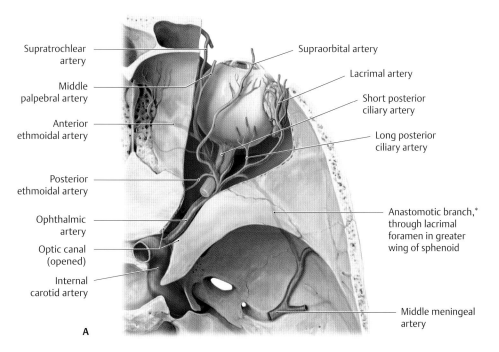

Supratrochlear artery
Middle palpebral artery
Anterior ethmoidal artery
Posterior ethmoidal artery
Ophthalmic artery
Optic canal (opened)
Internal carotid artery

Supraorbital artery
Lacrimal artery
Short posterior ciliary artery
Long posterior ciliary artery
Anastomotic branch,* through lacrimal foramen in greater wing of sphenoid
Middle meningeal artery

**A**

* See **Fig. 3.12**

### Fig. 3.15 Ophthalmic artery

**A** Superior view of the right orbit. **B** Anterior view of the facial branches of the right ophthalmic artery.

The ophthalmic artery supplies blood to the eyeball itself and to the orbital structures. Some of its terminal branches are distributed to portions of the face (e.g., forehead, eyelids, and nose). Other terminal branches (anterior and posterior ethmoidal arteries) contribute to the supply of the nasal septum (see **Fig. 3.16**).

*Note:* Branches of the lateral palpebral artery and supraorbital artery may form an anastomosis with the frontal branch of the superficial temporal artery (territory of the external carotid artery). With atherosclerosis of the internal carotid artery, this anastomosis may become an important alternative route for blood to the brain. In addition, there are anastomoses between the dorsal nasal artery and the angular artery.

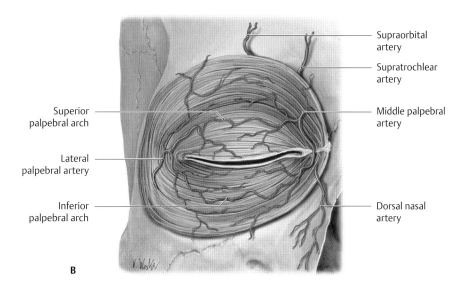

Superior palpebral arch
Lateral palpebral artery
Inferior palpebral arch

Supraorbital artery
Supratrochlear artery
Middle palpebral artery
Dorsal nasal artery

**B**

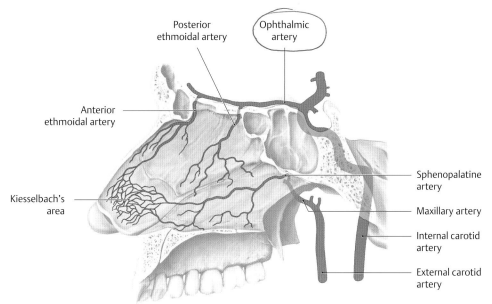

Posterior ethmoidal artery
Ophthalmic artery
Anterior ethmoidal artery
Kiesselbach's area

Sphenopalatine artery
Maxillary artery
Internal carotid artery
External carotid artery

### Fig. 3.16 Vascular supply of the nasal septum

Left lateral view. The nasal septum is another region in which the internal carotid artery (anterior and posterior ethmoidal arteries, green) meets the external carotid artery (sphenopalatine artery, yellow). A richly vascularized area on the anterior part of the nasal septum, called Kiesselbach's area (blue), is the most common site of nosebleed. Because Kiesselbach's area is an area of anastomosis, it may be necessary to ligate the sphenopalatine/maxillary artery and/or the ethmoidal arteries through an orbital approach, depending on the source of the bleeding. (See also **Fig. 7.17.**)

**49**

# Veins of the Head: Overview

*Lazy*
✳ Super fat rappers pimp out manly skanks

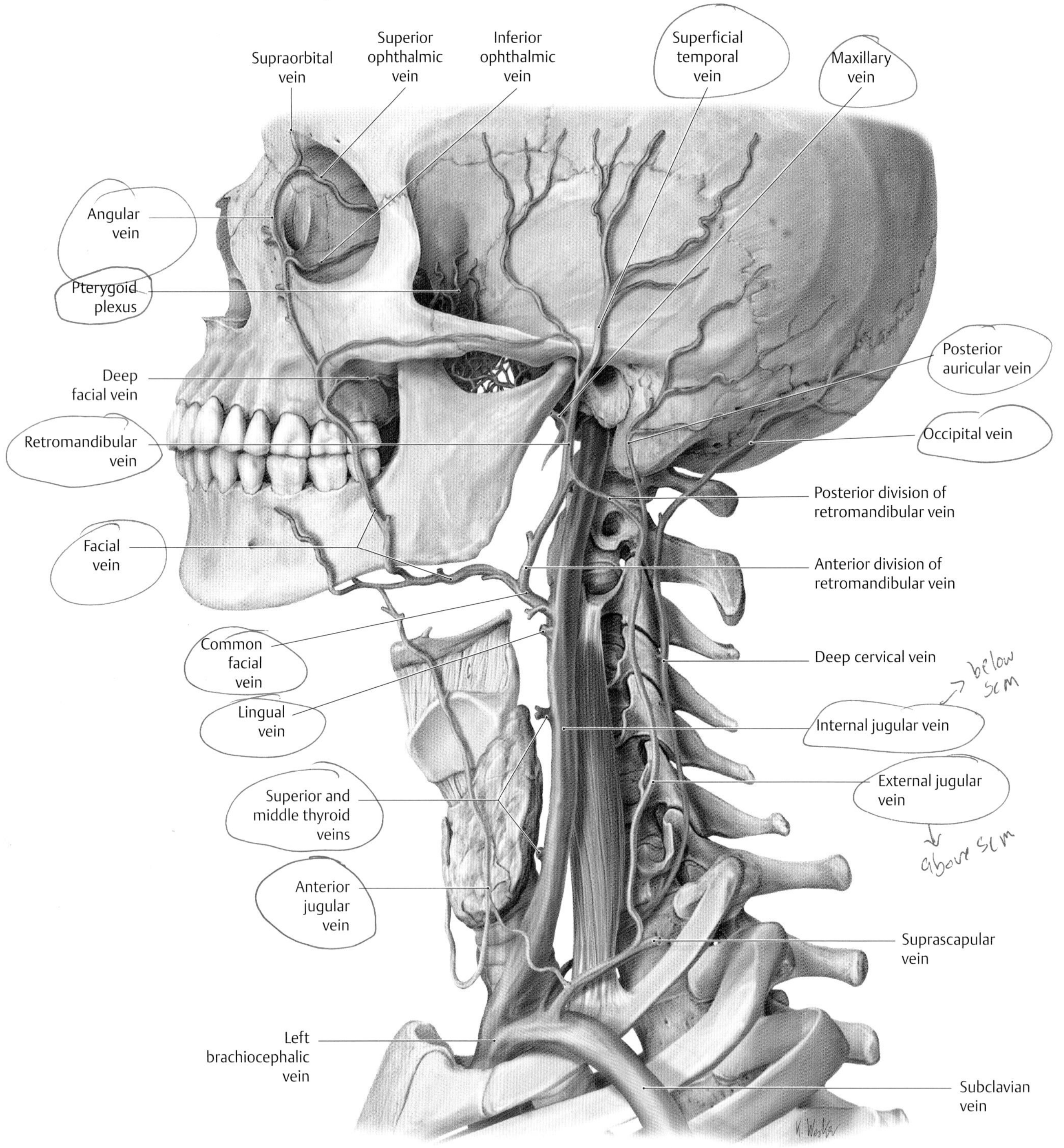

**Fig. 3.17 Veins of the head and neck**

Left lateral view. The principal vein of the head and neck is the internal jugular vein. This drains blood from both the exterior and the interior of the skull (including the brain) in addition to receiving venous blood from the neck. It receives blood from the common facial vein (formed by the union of the facial vein and the anterior division of the retromandibular vein), the lingual, superior thyroid, and middle thyroid veins, and the inferior petrosal sinus. Enclosed in the carotid sheath, the internal jugular vein descends from the jugular foramen to its union with the subclavian vein to form the brachiocephalic vein. The external jugular vein receives blood from the posterior division of the retromandibular vein and the posterior auricular vein. The occipital vein normally drains to the deep cervical veins.

✳ For Just the internal Jugular
Super Lazy fat Rappers meet Skanks

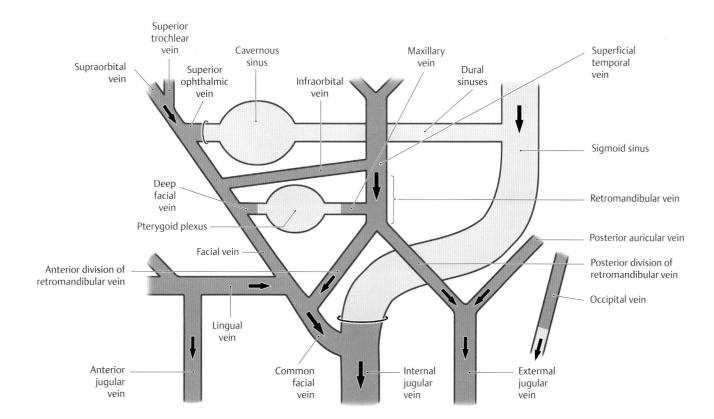

**Fig. 3.18 Veins of the head: overview**

The superficial veins of the head communicate with each other and with the dural sinuses via the deep veins of the head (pterygoid plexus and cavernous sinus). The pterygoid plexus connects the facial vein and the retromandibular vein (via the deep facial vein and maxillary vein, respectively). The cavernous sinus connects the facial vein to the sigmoid sinus (via the ophthalmic veins and the petrosal sinuses, respectively).

**Table 3.5 Venous drainage of the head and neck**

| Vein | Location | Tributaries | Region drained |
|---|---|---|---|
| Internal jugular v. | Within carotid sheath | Common facial v.<br>— Facial v.<br>— Retromandibular v., anterior division<br>— Lingual v.<br>— Superior and middle thyroid vv. | Skull, anterior and lateral face, oral cavity, neck |
| | | Sigmoid sinus and inferior petrosal sinuses | Interior of skull (including brain) |
| External jugular v. | Within superficial cervical fascia | Retromandibular v., posterior division | Lateral skull |
| | | Posterior auricular v. | Occiput |
| Anterior jugular v. | | | Anterior neck |

# Veins of the Head: Deep Veins

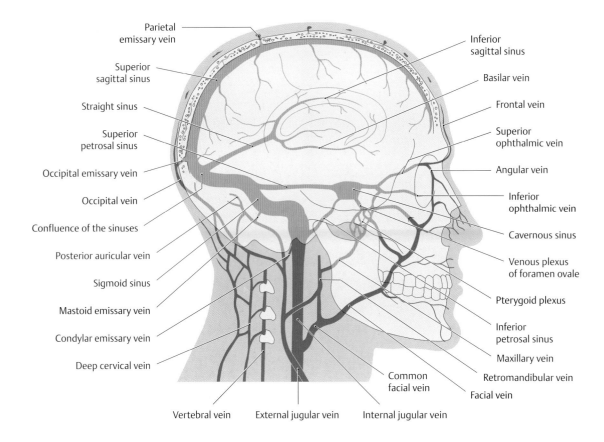

**Fig. 3.19 Venous drainage of the head**
The superficial veins of the head have extensive connections with the deep veins of the head and the dural sinuses. The meninges and brain are drained by the dural sinuses, which lie within the skull. Emissary veins connect the superficial veins of the skull directly to the dural sinuses. In addition, the deep veins of the head (e.g., pterygoid plexus) are intermediaries between the superficial veins of the face and the dural venous sinuses.

**Table 3.6 Venous anastomoses as portals of infection**

The extracranial veins of the head are connected to the deep veins and dural sinuses. Patients who sustain midfacial fractures may bleed profusely due to the extensive venous anastomoses. Because the veins are generally valveless, extracranial bacteria may migrate to the deep veins, causing infections (e.g., bacteria from boils on the upper lip or nose may enter the angular vein and travel to the cavernous sinus). Bacteria in the cavernous sinus may cause thrombosis.

| Extracranial vein | Connecting vein | Venous sinus |
|---|---|---|
| Angular v. | Superior ophthalmic v. | Cavernous sinus |
| Vv. of palatine tonsil | Pterygoid plexus, inferior ophthalmic v. | |
| Superficial temporal v. | Parietal emissary v. | Superior sagittal sinus |
| Occipital v. | Occipital emissary v. | Transverse sinus, confluence of the sinuses |
| | Mastoid emissary v. | Sigmoid sinus |
| Posterior auricular v. | | |
| External vertebral venous plexus | Condylar emissary v. | |

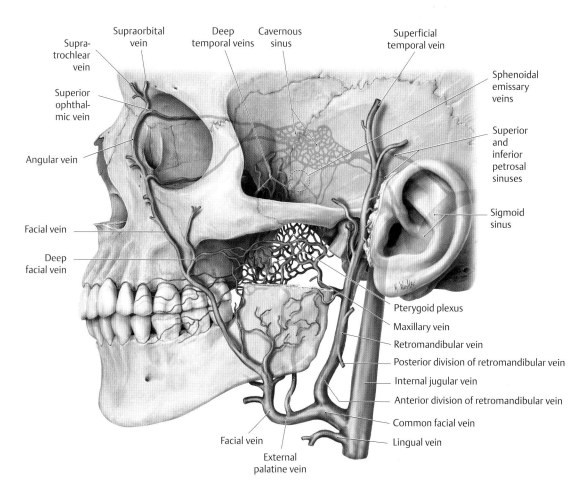

**Fig. 3.20 Deep veins of the head**

Left lateral view. The pterygoid plexus is a venous network situated behind the mandibular ramus and embedded in the pterygoid muscles. Because the veins of the face have no valves (small valves may be present but are generally nonfunctional), the movement of the pterygoid muscles forces blood from the pterygoid plexus into the jugular veins.

The pterygoid plexus is linked to the facial vein via the deep facial vein and to the retromandibular vein via the maxillary vein. The plexus is also linked to the cavernous sinus via the sphenoidal emissary vein. The cavernous sinus receives blood from the superior and inferior ophthalmic veins.

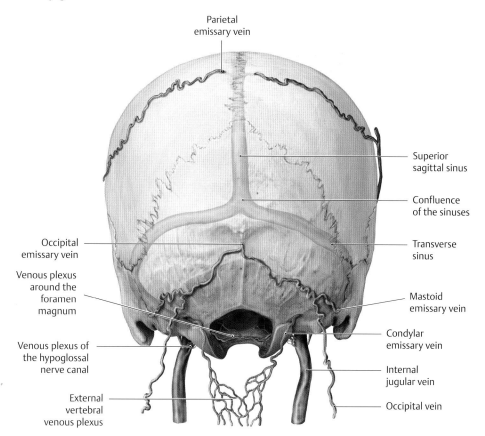

**Fig. 3.21 Veins of the occiput**

Posterior view. The dural sinuses are the series of venous channels that drain the brain (see p. 302). The superficial veins of the occiput communicate with the dural sinuses by way of the emissary veins. The emissary veins enter a similarly named foramen to communicate with the dural sinuses.

**53**

# Organization of the Nervous System

### Fig. 4.1 Nervous system

**A** Anterior view. **B** Posterior view. The nervous system is a collection of neurons that can be divided anatomically into two groups:

- **Central nervous system** (CNS, pink): Brain and spinal cord.
- **Peripheral nervous system** (PNS, yellow): Nerves emerging from the CNS. These are divided into two types depending on their site of emergence:
  - **Cranial nerves:** 12 pairs of nerves emerge from the brain (telencephalon, diencephalon, and brainstem only). These nerves may contain sensory and/or motor fibers.
  - **Spinal nerves:** 31 pairs of nerves emerge from the spinal cord. Spinal nerves contain both sensory and motor fibers that emerge from the spinal cord as separate roots and unite to form the mixed nerve. In certain regions, the spinal nerves may combine to form plexuses (e.g., cervical, brachial, or lumbosacral).

The cranial nerves are discussed in this chapter. The spinal nerves and CNS are discussed in Chapter 13: Neuroanatomy. The innervation of the neck is discussed in Chapter 12: Neurovascular Topography of the Neck.

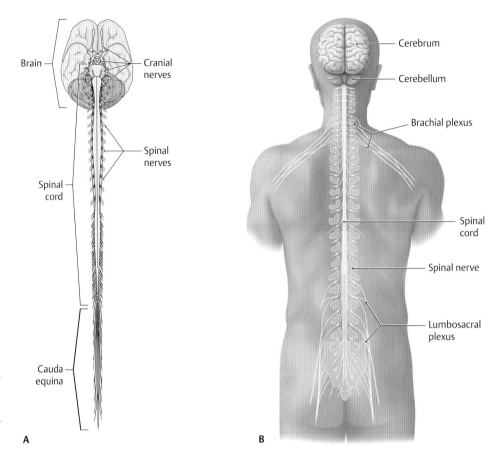

A

B

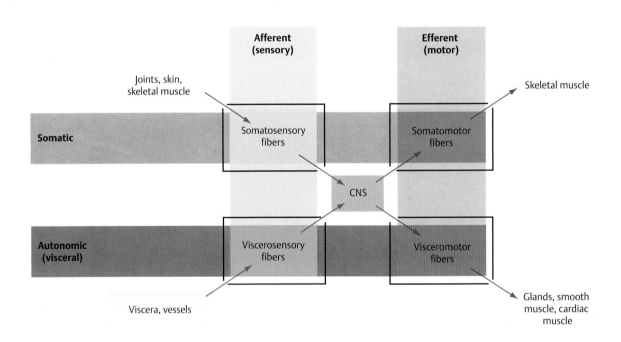

### Fig. 4.2 Organization of the nervous system

The nervous system is a vast network that can be divided according to two criteria:

1. Type of information: Afferent (sensory) cells and pathways receive information and transmit it to the CNS. Efferent (motor) cells and pathways convey information from the CNS.

2. Destination/origin: The somatic division of the nervous system primarily mediates interaction with the external environment. These processes are often voluntary. The autonomic (visceral) nervous system primarily mediates regulation of the internal environment. These processes are frequently involuntary.

The two criteria yield four types of nerve fibers that connect the CNS to the PNS.

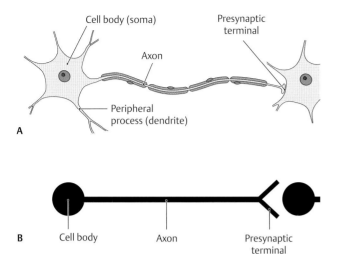

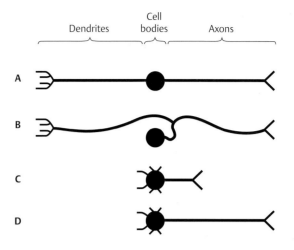

## Fig. 4.3 Neurons and nerves

**A** Neuron structure. **B** Convention of drawing neurons.

Neurons are the specialized cells of the nervous system that convey information in the CNS and PNS. Neurons consist of a cell body (soma) with two types of projections:

- Dendrites: Receptor segments that receive impulses from other neurons or cells.
- Axons: Projecting segments that transmit impulses to other neurons or cells.

The number and organization of the projections reflect the function of the neuron (see **Fig. 4.4**). Neurons convey impulses to each other at synapses: neurotransmitters released from the presynaptic terminal (bouton) of the axon are bound by receptors on the postsynaptic membrane of the next neuron's dendrite. The impulse can then be relayed along the axon.

## Fig. 4.4 Types of neurons

Neurons are divided functionally into three main groups: sensory neurons, interneurons, and motor neurons. The structure of the neurons reflects their function.

**Sensory neurons:** Collect sensory information and transport it to the CNS. These neurons tend to have long peripheral processes (dendrites) and long central processes (axons).

- Bipolar neuron (**A**): Named for the two long processes (peripheral and central) on opposite sides of the cell body. (E.g., retinal cells.)
- Pseudounipolar neuron (**B**): The dendrite and axon appear to arise from the same projection from the cell body. (E.g., primary afferent neurons.)

**Interneurons** (**C**): Convey information between sensory and motor neurons within the CNS. This multipolar interneuron has numerous dendrites and a short axon.

**Motor neurons** (**D**): Originate motor impulses and transmit them from the CNS. This multipolar motor neuron has numerous dendrites and a long axon.

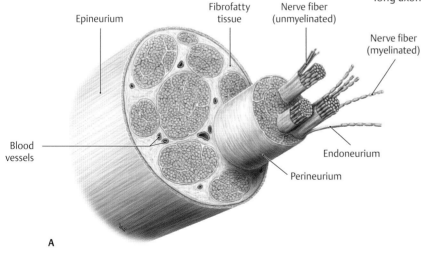

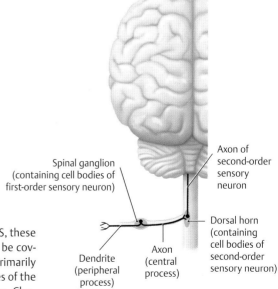

## Fig. 4.5 Neurons in the CNS and PNS

**A** Nerve fibers. **B** Nerves/tracts and ganglia/nuclei.

Bundles of axons travel together to synapse on the cell bodies of other neurons. In the PNS, these axon bundles are called nerves; in the CNS, they are called tracts. The axon bundles can be covered with myelin to increase the speed of impulse transmission. As myelin is composed primarily of fatty acids, myelinated areas appear white (white matter). The unmyelinated cell bodies of the neurons appear darker (gray matter). Cell bodies are considerably larger than cell processes. Clusters of cell bodies therefore produce characteristic bulges: in the PNS these are called ganglia; in the CNS they are called nuclei.

# Sensory Pathways

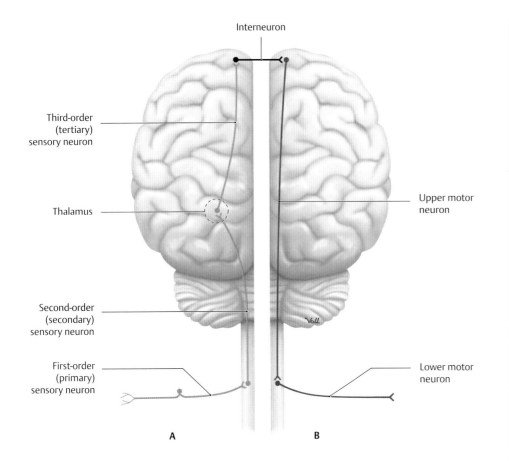

**Fig. 4.6 Sensory and motor pathways: overview**

**A** Sensory (afferent) pathways. **B** Motor (efferent) pathways.

The sensory (afferent) pathways detect and relay information from sensory organs to the cerebral cortex, generally via a three-neuron pathway (see **Table 4.1**). The motor (efferent) pathways produce and transmit impulses from the cortex via a two-neuron (motor) pathway or a three-neuron (autonomic) pathway (see **Fig. 4.8**). The sensory and motor pathways are connected by interneurons.

| Table 4.1 Sensory (afferent) pathways | |
|---|---|
| Sensory information is traditionally relayed from sensory organs to the cortex by a three-neuron pathway: | |
| 1st order | **Primary (first-order) neurons:** Collect sensory data from the sensory organ and convey it to the CNS. These neurons are often pseudounipolar (with cell bodies located in sensory ganglia). *Note:* Although most neurons are activated by the release of neurotransmitters, first-order neurons may be activated by other inputs (e.g., photons [sight], vibrations [sound], olfactory stimuli [smell]). The axons of first-order neurons enter the CNS to synapse on second-order neurons. |
| 2nd order | **Secondary (second-order) neurons:** Located in the CNS, these neurons receive impulses from first-order neurons in the PNS. The axons of second-order neurons ascend as tracts to synapse on third-order neurons in the thalamus. |
| 3rd order | **Tertiary (third-order) neurons:** Located in the thalamus, these neurons project to the appropriate area of the sensory cortex. |

| Table 4.2 Sensory pathways in the spinal and cranial nerves | | |
|---|---|---|
| Both the spinal and cranial nerves use the three-neuron sensory pathway. | | |
| **Neuron** | **Location of cell body (soma)** | |
| | **Spinal nerve** | **Cranial nerve** |
| 1st order | **Spinal ganglia of dorsal root:** All 31 spinal nerve pairs have a dorsal sensory root and a ventral motor root. Only the dorsal root has the characteristic bulge of a sensory ganglion (motor cells are not pseudounipolar). | **Sensory ganglia near brainstem:** Of the 12 cranial nerves, only 7 are sensory (CN I, II, V, VII, VIII, IX, and X). These seven nerves are associated with eight sensory ganglia; two cranial nerves (CN V and VII) have a single sensory ganglion, while three (CN VIII, IX, and X) have two sensory ganglia each. |
| 2nd order | **Sensory nuclei in dorsal horn of the spinal cord:** The dorsal horn is the posterior portion of the gray matter of the spinal cord. It contains exclusively sensory neurons. Axons ascend via white matter tracts to the thalamus. | **Sensory nuclei in dorsolateral brainstem:** The sensory nuclei are arranged as a longitudinal nuclear column in the dorsolateral portion of the brainstem. Axons ascend via white matter tracts to the thalamus. |
| 3rd order | Thalamus | |
| Cortical | Sensory cortex | |

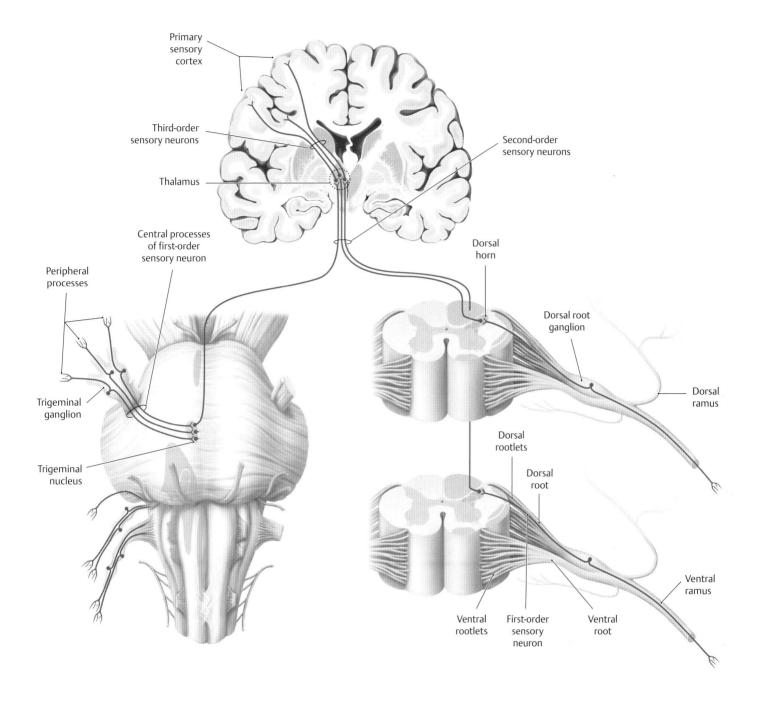

**Fig. 4.7 Sensory pathways: cranial and spinal nerves**
Left: Cranial nerves. Right: Spinal nerves.
Sensory information is relayed to the sensory cortex via a three-step pathway.

1. First-order pseudounipolar neurons receive impulses from the periphery. They convey these impulses along their peripheral processes to their central process (axons) that synapse in the CNS. The cell bodies of first-order neurons are located in sensory ganglia.

2. Second-order neurons with cell bodies in the gray matter of the CNS receive impulses from first-order neurons. The axons of second-order neurons ascend as white matter tracts to the thalamus.

3. Third-order neurons with cell bodies in the thalamus receive impulses from ascending tracts. The axons of third-order neurons ascend to the sensory cortex.

# Motor Pathways

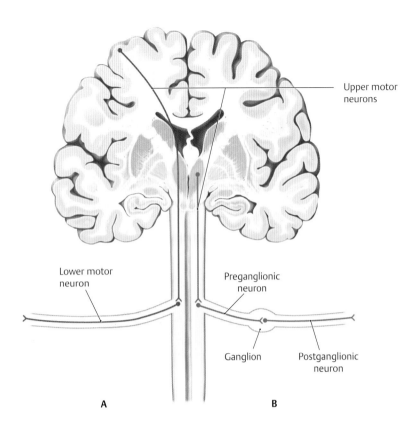

**Table 4.3 Motor (efferent) pathways**

Skeletal muscle is innervated by a traditional two-neuron motor pathway.

| | |
|---|---|
| **Upper motor neuron** | Upper motor neurons are located in the motor cortex. Their axons descend via white matter tracts to lower motor neurons in the brainstem and spinal cord. |
| **Lower motor neuron** | Lower motor neurons are located in the brainstem (cranial nerves) and spinal cord (spinal nerves). Their axons leave the CNS to synapse on target cells. Autonomic lower motor neurons synapse *before* they reach their target cells (see p. 62). |

*Fig. 4.8* **Motor pathways**
**A** Two-neuron motor pathway. **B** Three-neuron (autonomic) motor pathway.

The two major types of skeletal muscle (somatic and branchial, see pp. 60–61) are innervated by the classic two-neuron motor pathway (somatomotor and branchiomotor, respectively), with impulses originating in the cortex. Smooth muscle, cardiac muscle, and glands are innervated by autonomic motor pathways that involve a third neuron, with impulses originating in the hypothalamus (see p. 62).

*Note:* Outside of the CNS (spinal cord and brain), the ANS involves two neurons (one preganglionic and one postganglionic), whereas the branchial and somatic motor pathways have a single neuron (the lower motor neuron).

**Table 4.4 Motor (efferent) pathways**

| Neuron | Location of cell body (soma) | |
|---|---|---|
| | **Spinal nerve** | **Cranial nerve** |
| Upper motor neuron | **Motor cortex:** The cell bodies of skeletal muscle upper motor neurons are located in the gray matter of the cortex. Their axons descend via white matter tracts. | |
| | **Hypothalamus:** The cell bodies of autonomic upper motor neurons are located in the hypothalamus. Their axons descend via white matter tracts. | |
| Lower motor neuron | **Motor nuclei in ventral horn of spinal cord:** The ventral horn is the anterior portion of the gray matter of the spinal cord. It contains exclusively motor neurons. The axons of these neurons leave the CNS as the motor root of the spinal nerves. The motor root combines with the dorsal root outside the spinal cord to form the mixed spinal nerve. *Note:* Unlike the dorsal root, the motor root has no ganglion. | **Motor nuclei in dorsomedial margin of brainstem:** Of the 12 cranial nerves, all but 3 have motor nuclei. The motor nuclei are arranged in longitudinal nuclear columns. The axons of these neurons leave the CNS as the motor roots of the cranial nerves. Unlike the spinal nerves, the motor and sensory roots of the cranial nerves combine before exiting the CNS. *Note:* CN V is the only exception to this: its motor root combines with the sensory root of CN V$_3$ as it passes through the foramen ovale. |

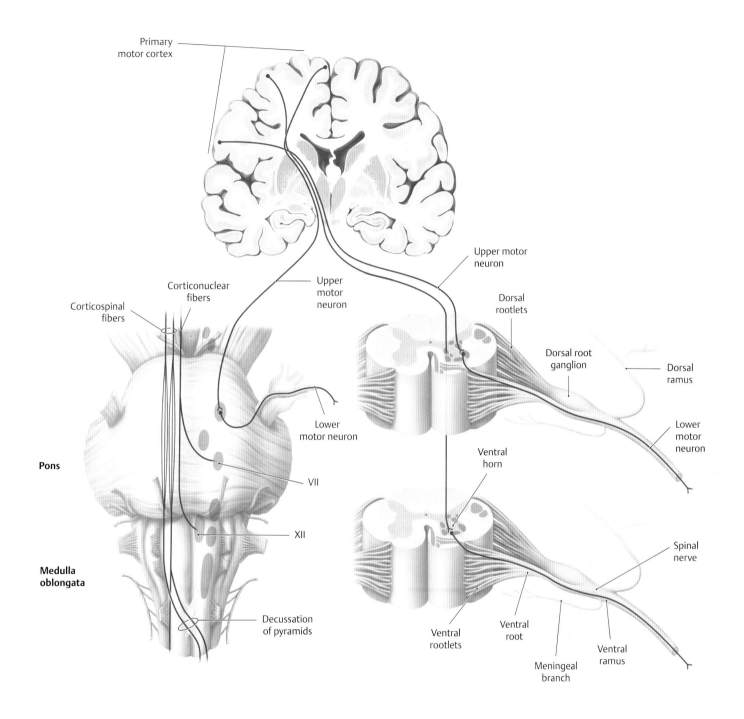

Primary
motor cortex

Corticonuclear
fibers

Corticospinal
fibers

Upper
motor
neuron

Upper motor
neuron

Dorsal
rootlets

Dorsal root
ganglion

Dorsal
ramus

Lower
motor neuron

Lower
motor
neuron

**Pons**

VII

Ventral
horn

**Medulla
oblongata**

XII

Spinal
nerve

Decussation
of pyramids

Ventral
rootlets

Ventral
root

Meningeal
branch

Ventral
ramus

**Fig. 4.9 Motor pathways: cranial and spinal nerves**
Left: Cranial nerves. Right: Spinal nerves.
Motor information is relayed from the motor cortex via a two-step pathway.

1. Upper motor neurons: Neurons in the gray matter of the motor cortex project axons that descend via white matter tracts to the brain and spinal cord.

2. Lower motor neurons: Neurons in the motor nuclei of the brainstem (cranial nerves) or ventral horn of the spinal cord (spinal nerves) project axons that emerge from the CNS as the motor roots of the nerves. These axons synapse on target skeletal muscle cells. *Note:* Lower motor neurons in the autonomic nervous system synapse *before* reaching their targets (smooth muscle, cardiac muscle, and glands).

# Skeletal Muscle: Innervation & Embryonic Development

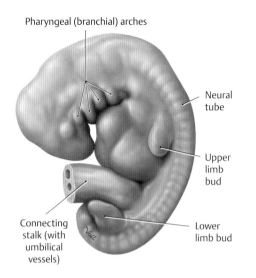

Pharyngeal (branchial) arches

Neural tube

Upper limb bud

Connecting stalk (with umbilical vessels)

Lower limb bud

**Fig. 4.10 Five-week-old embryo**

*Table 4.5* **Skeletal muscle: development and innervation**

Skeletal muscle has one of two embryonic origins: somites or branchial (pharyngeal) arches. Nerves migrate with muscle cells during embryonic development, explaining the pattern of adult innervation.

| Muscle | Somatic muscle | Branchial muscle |
|---|---|---|
| Derivation | Somites | Branchial (pharyngeal) arches |
| Germ layer | Mesoderm (paraxial mesenchyme) | |
| Location | Throughout body (including head and neck) | Head and neck |
| Nerve fibers | Somatomotor fibers | Branchiomotor fibers |
| Nerves | Spinal and cranial nerves | Cranial nerves |

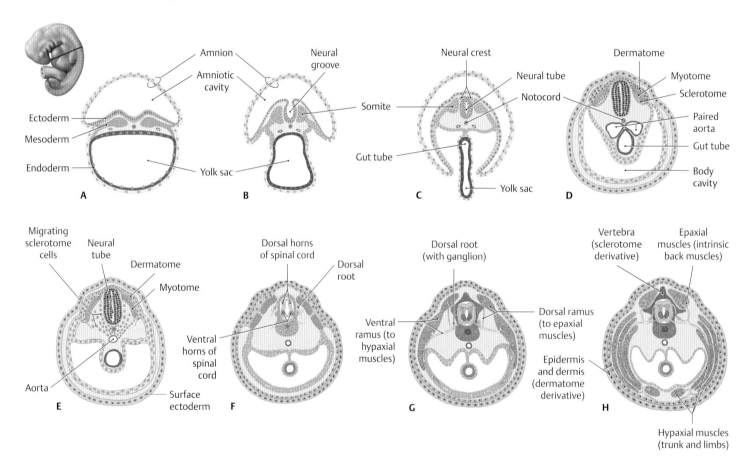

**Fig. 4.11 Somatic muscle: embryonic development**

Gastrulation occurs in week 3 of human embryonic development. It produces three germ layers in the embryonic disk: ectoderm (light gray), mesoderm (red), and endoderm (dark gray). Somatic muscle develops from the mesoderm. **A** Day 19: The three layers are visible in the embryonic disk. The amnion forms the amniotic cavity dorsally, and the endoderm encloses the yolk sac. **B** Day 20: Somites form, and the neural groove begins to close. **C** Day 22: Eight pairs of somites flank the closed neural tube (CNS precursor). The yolk sac elongates ventrally to form the gut tube and yolk sac. **D** Day 24: Each somite divides into a dermatome (cutaneous), myotome (muscular), and sclerotome (vertebral). This section does not cut the connecting stalk (derived from the yolk sac). **E** Day 28: Sclerotomes migrate to form the vertebral column around the notocord (primitive spinal cord). **F** Day 30: All 34 or 35 somite pairs have formed. The neural tube differentiates into a primitive spinal cord. Motor and sensory neurons differentiate in the ventral and dorsal horns of the spinal cord, respectively. **G** By day 40: The dorsal and ventral roots form the mixed spinal nerve. The dorsal branch supplies the epaxial muscles (future intrinsic back muscles); the ventral branch supplies the hypaxial muscles (ventral muscles, including all muscles except the intrinsic back musculature). **H** Week 8: The epaxial and hypaxial muscles have differentiated into the skeletal muscles of the trunk. Cells from the sclerotomes also migrate into the limbs. During this migration, the spinal nerves form plexuses (cervical, brachial, and lumbosacral), which innervate the muscles of the neck, upper limb, and lower limb, respectively.

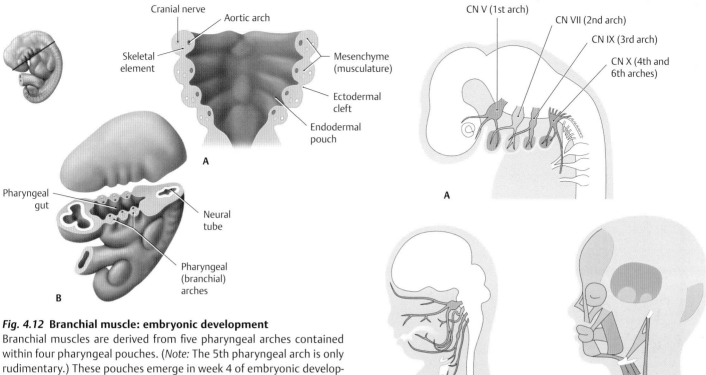

**Fig. 4.12 Branchial muscle: embryonic development**
Branchial muscles are derived from five pharyngeal arches contained within four pharyngeal pouches. (*Note:* The 5th pharyngeal arch is only rudimentary.) These pouches emerge in week 4 of embryonic development and give rise to structures of the head and face. **A** Each pharyngeal arch consists of mesodermal cells (future branchial muscles) with an embedded nerve, artery, and skeletal element. The mesodermal mesenchyme is surrounded by an outer ectodermal layer and an inner endodermal layer. **B** The paired pharyngeal pouches surround the pharyngeal gut.

**Fig. 4.13 Branchial derivatives**
Each of the four pharyngeal pouches contains a cranial nerve (**A**), which, during the course of development, migrates to its final position (**B**) with the branchial muscles derived from that arch (**C**).

| Table 4.6 Skeletal muscle of the head |
|---|

The vast majority of the muscles of the head are derived from the pharyngeal arches (the extraocular muscles and extrinsic and intrinsic lingual muscles are somite derivatives). However, of the eight cranial nerves that innervate the skeletal muscle of the head, four convey somatomotor fibers to these somatic derivatives, and four convey branchiomotor fibers to the branchial arch derivatives.

| Muscle origin | | Muscles | | Cranial nerve |
|---|---|---|---|---|
| Somatic | Prochordal mesenchyme | • Levator palpebrae superioris<br>• Inferior oblique* | • Superior rectus*<br>• Medial rectus*<br>• Inferior rectus* | Oculomotor n. (CN III) |
| | Maxillomandibular mesenchyme | • Superior oblique* | | Trochlear n. (CN IV) |
| | | • Lateral rectus* | | Abducent n. (CN VI) |
| | Occipital somites | • Extrinsic muscles of the tongue (except palatoglossus)<br>• Intrinsic muscles of the tongue | | Hypoglossal n. (CN XII) |
| Branchial | 1st branchial arch | • Temporalis**<br>• Masseter**<br>• Lateral pterygoid**<br>• Medial pterygoid** | • Mylohyoid<br>• Digastric (anterior belly)<br>• Tensor tympani<br>• Tensor veli palatini | Trigeminal n., mandibular division (CN V₃) |
| | 2nd branchial arch | • Muscles of facial expression<br>• Stylohyoid<br>• Digastric (posterior belly) and stapedius | | Facial n. (CN VII) |
| | 3rd branchial arch | • Stylopharyngeus | | Glossopharyngeal n. (CN IX) |
| | 4th and 6th branchial arches | • Pharyngeal muscles<br>• Levator veli palatini<br>• Muscule uvulae | • Palatoglossus<br>• Laryngeal muscles | Vagus n. (CN X) |

*Extraocular muscle (six total).

**Muscle of mastication (four total).

# Autonomic Motor Pathways

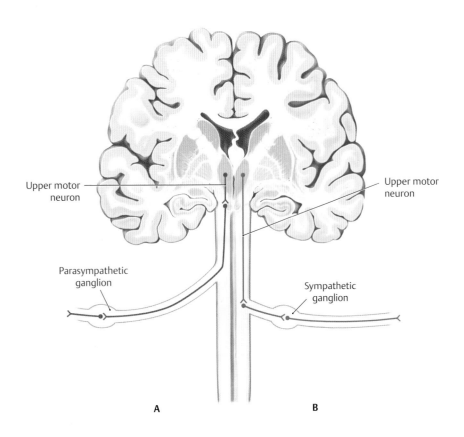

Upper motor
neuron

Upper motor
neuron

Parasympathetic
ganglion

Sympathetic
ganglion

A  B

**Fig. 4.14 Autonomic pathways**
Unlike skeletal muscle, which is innervated by a two-neuron motor pathway, viscera (smooth muscle, cardiac muscle, and glands) are innervated by the three-neuron motor pathways of the autonomic nervous system. The autonomic nervous system is divided into two parts: parasympathetic (**A**) and sympathetic (**B**). The parasympathetic ganglia are usually located close to their target structures (longer preganglionic and shorter postganglionic axons); the sympathetic ganglia are usually located close to the CNS (shorter preganglionic and longer postganglionic axons).

| Table 4.7 Autonomic (efferent) pathways | |
|---|---|
| Viscera (smooth muscle, cardiac muscle, and glands) are innervated by a three-neuron motor pathway. | |
| **Upper motor neuron** | In the two-neuron pathway, the axon of an upper motor neuron descends from the hypothalamus to synapse on a lower motor neuron located in the brainstem or spinal cord. |
| **Preganglionic neuron** | Lower motor neurons are located in the brainstem nuclei (cranial nerves) or lateral horn of the spinal cord (spinal nerves). The axons of these secondary neurons emerge from the CNS and synapse *before* reaching the target cells. |
| **Postganglionic neuron** | The cell bodies of the tertiary (postganglionic) neurons form the autonomic ganglia. In general, sympathetic ganglia are located close to the CNS, and parasympathetic ganglia are located close to their target organs. |

| Table 4.8 Sympathetic pathways | | |
|---|---|---|
| **Neuron** | **Location of cell body (soma)** | |
| Upper motor neuron | **Hypothalamus:** The cell bodies of autonomic upper motor neurons are located in the hypothalamus. Their axons descend via white matter tracts. | |
| Preganglionic neuron | **Lateral horn of spinal cord (T1–L2):** The lateral horn is the middle portion of the gray matter of the spinal cord, situated between the ventral and dorsal horns. It contains exclusively autonomic (sympathetic) neurons. The axons of these neurons leave the CNS as the motor root of the spinal nerves and enter the paravertebral ganglia via the white rami communicantes (myelinated). | |
| Preganglionic neurons in paravertebral ganglia | All preganglionic sympathetic neurons enter the sympathetic chain. There they may synapse in a chain ganglion or ascend or descend to synapse. Preganglionic sympathetic neurons synapse in one of two places, yielding two types of sympathetic ganglia. | |
| | Synapse *in* the paravertebral ganglia | Pass without synapsing *through* the parasympathetic ganglia. These fibers travel in the thoracic, lumbar, and sacral splanchnic nerves to synapse in the prevertebral ganglia. |
| Postganglionic neuron | **Paravertebral ganglia:** These ganglia form the sympathetic nerve trunks that flank the spinal cord. Postganglionic axons leave the sympathetic trunk via the gray rami communicantes (unmyelinated). | **Prevertebral ganglia:** Associated with peripheral plexuses, which spread along the abdominal aorta. There are three primary prevertebral ganglia:<br>• Celiac ganglion<br>• Superior mesenteric ganglion<br>• Inferior mesenteric ganglion |
| Distribution of postganglionic fibers | Postganglionic fibers are distributed in two ways:<br>1. Spinal nerves: Postganglionic neurons may re-enter the spinal nerves via the gray rami communicantes. These sympathetic neurons induce constriction of blood vessels, sweat glands, and arrector pili (muscle fibers attached to hair follicles, "goose bumps").<br>2. Arteries and ducts: Nerve plexuses may form along existing structures. Postganglionic sympathetic fibers may travel with arteries to target structures. Viscera are innervated by this method (e.g., sympathetic innervation concerning vasoconstriction, bronchial dilatation, glandular secretions, pupillary dilatation, smooth muscle contraction). | |

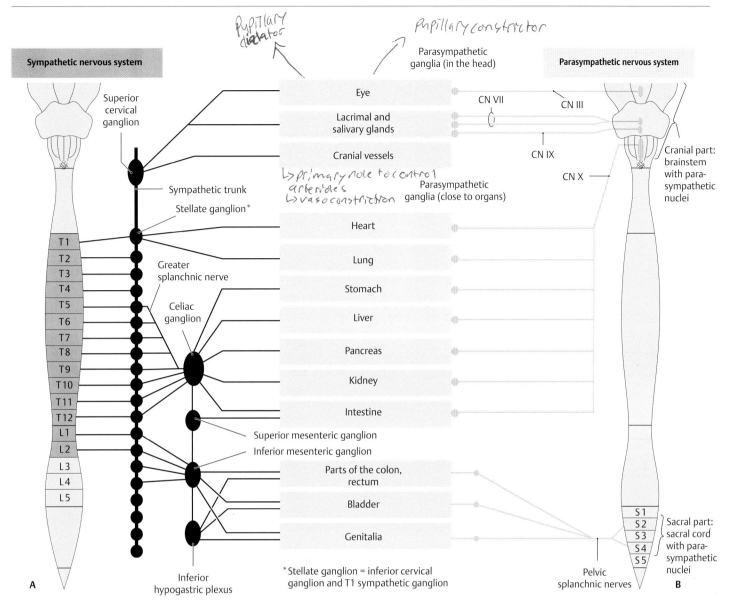

**Fig. 4.15 Autonomic nervous system**
A Sympathetic nervous system. B Parasympathetic nervous system.

*Table 4.9 Parasympathetic pathways*

| Neuron | Location of cell body (soma) | |
|---|---|---|
| Upper motor neuron | **Hypothalamus:** The cell bodies of autonomic upper motor neurons are located in the hypothalamus. Their axons descend via white matter tracts. | |
| Preganglionic neuron | The parasympathetic nervous system is divided into two parts (cranial and sacral), based on the location of the preganglionic parasympathetic neurons. | |
| | **Brainstem cranial nerve nuclei:** The axons of these secondary neurons leave the CNS as the motor root of cranial nerves III, VII, IX, and X. | **Spinal cord (S2–S4):** The axons of these secondary neurons leave the CNS (S2–S4) as the pelvic splanchnic nerves. These nerves travel in the dorsal rami of the S2–S4 spinal nerves and are distributed via the sympathetic plexuses to the pelvic viscera. |
| Postganglionic neuron | **Cranial nerve parasympathetic ganglia:** The parasympathetic cranial nerves of the head each have at least one ganglion:<br>• CN III: Ciliary ganglion<br>• CN VII: Pterygopalatine ganglion and submandibular ganglion<br>• CN IX: Otic ganglion<br>• CN X: Small unnamed ganglia close to target structures | |
| Distribution of postganglionic fibers | Parasympathetic fibers course with other fiber types to their targets. In the head, the postganglionic fibers from the pterygopalatine ganglion (CN VII) and otic ganglion (CN IX) are distributed via branches of the trigeminal nerve (CN V). Postganglionic fibers from the ciliary ganglion (CN III) course with sympathetic and sensory fibers in the short ciliary nerves (preganglionic fibers travel with the somatomotor fibers of CN III). In the thorax, abdomen, and pelvis, preganglionic parasympathetic fibers from CN X and the pelvic splanchnic nerves combine with postganglionic sympathetic fibers to form plexuses (e.g., cardiac, pulmonary, esophageal). | |

# Peripheral Nerves & Nerve Lesions

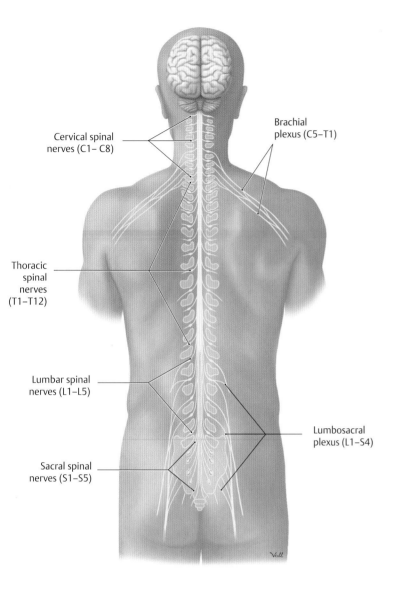

Cervical spinal nerves (C1– C8)

Brachial plexus (C5–T1)

Thoracic spinal nerves (T1–T12)

Lumbar spinal nerves (L1–L5)

Lumbosacral plexus (L1–S4)

Sacral spinal nerves (S1–S5)

### Fig. 4.16 Peripheral nerves

Peripheral nerves emerge from the CNS (brain and spinal cord) at various levels. These nerves may convey afferent (sensory) and/or efferent (motor) neurons to regions of the body. The patterns of innervation can be understood through the embryonic migration of cell populations (see p. 60). The least invasive way of exploring nerve territories is by examining the sensory innervation of the skin. The patterns of cutaneous sensory innervation may be used to determine the level of nerve lesions (see **Fig. 4.18**).

**Cutaneous sensory innervation:** With the exception of the face (see **Fig. 4.17**), the body receives cutaneous sensory innervation (touch, pain, and temperature) from branches of the spinal nerves. Sensory fibers emerge from the spinal cord as the dorsal root, which combines with the ventral (motor) root in the intervertebral foramen to form the mixed spinal nerve.

**Embryonic development** (see p. 60): During development, each spinal nerve is associated with a somite pair on either side of the spinal cord. Each somite divides into a dermatome (cutaneous), myotome (muscular), and sclerotome (vertebral). As these cells migrate, the spinal nerves migrate with them. Due to migration patterns, the regions of the body can be divided into two groups:

- **Trunk:** In the trunk, the spinal nerves course reasonably horizontally to innervate a narrow strip of bone, muscle, and skin corresponding to their spinal cord level (e.g., intercostal nerves). This is due to the segmental migration of the trunk muscles during development. In this region, the peripheral nerves are therefore the ventral and dorsal rami of the spinal nerves. They will give off direct cutaneous branches.
- **Limbs:** In the limbs, the migration of the muscle cells causes the spinal nerves to form plexuses (cervical, brachial, and lumbosacral). These plexuses subsequently give off peripheral nerves, which innervate specific regions of the body (see **Fig. 4.18**). Peripheral nerves in the limbs may be derived from multiple spinal cord levels.

*Note:* Motor lesions cause paralysis of the innervated muscle. Depending on the level of the lesion, this may or may not coincide with sensory loss.

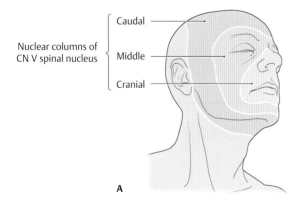

Nuclear columns of CN V spinal nucleus

Caudal

Middle

Cranial

**A**

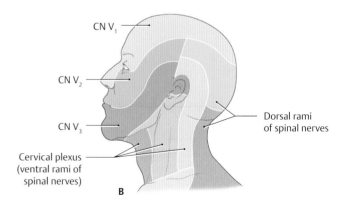

CN V₁

CN V₂

CN V₃

Cervical plexus (ventral rami of spinal nerves)

Dorsal rami of spinal nerves

**B**

### Fig. 4.17 Cutaneous sensory innervation of the face

Unlike the rest of the skin, the face is derived from the pharyngeal arches. Like all structures derived from the pharyngeal arches, it receives innervation from cranial nerves. The trigeminal nerve (CN V) provides general sensory innervation (touch, pain, and temperature) to most of the face. If a nerve lesion occurs in the peripheral nerve (CN V₁, CN V₂, or CN V₃), the pattern of general sensory loss will resemble

**B**. If a nerve lesion occurs *within* the CNS (in the spinal nucleus of the trigeminal nerve), the pattern of sensory loss will resemble **A**. The concentric pattern corresponds to the organization of the spinal nucleus: the higher (more cranial) portion of the nucleus innervates the periphery, and the lower (more caudal) portion innervates the center of the face.

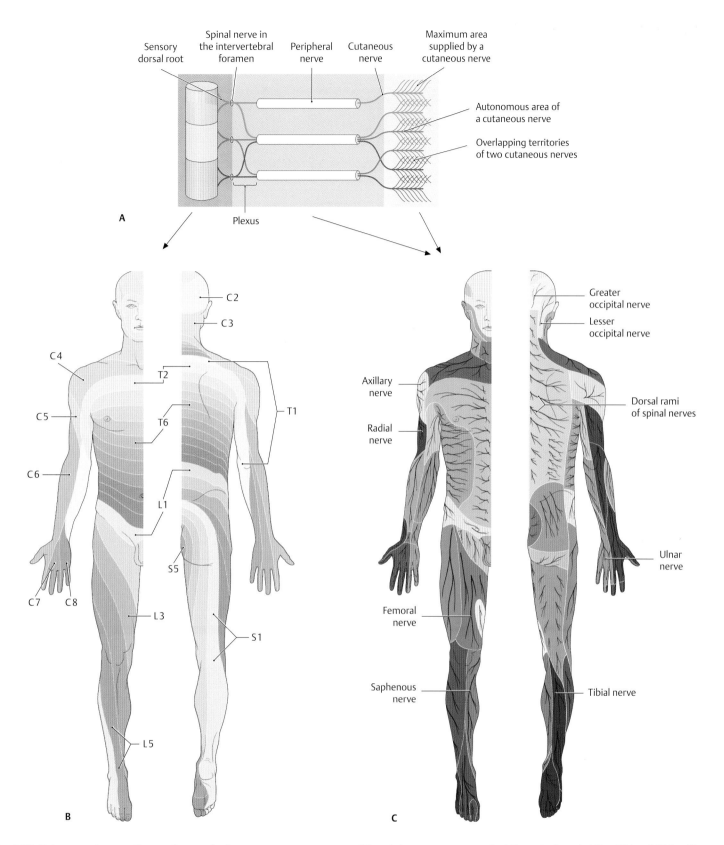

**Fig. 4.18 Cutaneous innervation and nerve lesions**

Cutaneous sensory innervation occurs via cutaneous branches of peripheral nerves (**A**). In the trunk, the peripheral nerves are the rami of the spinal nerves. In the limbs (neck, upper limb, and lower limb), the peripheral nerves are formed by nerve plexuses, in which the ventral rami fibers from multiple spinal cord levels combine (e.g., the femoral nerve contains fibers from L2–L4). Lesions can occur at the segmental (dark gray), peripheral (light gray), or cutaneous (white) level.

**Segmental (radicular) sensory innervation** (**B**): The superficial skin area corresponding to a specific spinal cord root is called a *dermatome*. Lesions of the dorsal root of a spinal nerve or of the corresponding sensory nuclei in the spinal cord (dark gray area in **A**) will cause this pattern of sensory loss. For example, a herniated disk between the C4 and

C5 vertebrae may press against the spinal cord at the C6 level. This will cause sensory loss in the C6 dermatome (lateral forearm and hand).

**Peripheral sensory innervation** (**C**): Lesions of a peripheral nerve (light gray area in **A**) will produce sensory loss in its cutaneous territories. (*Note:* These are not necessarily contiguous.) For example, chronic use of crutches may compress the radial nerve (which contains fibers from C5–T1). This will result in sensory loss in the territory of the radial nerve (i.e., posterior arm and forearm [dark red]). Contrast this to sensory loss of the C5–T1 dermatomes (i.e., no cutaneous sensation in entire arm).

**Cutaneous sensory innervation:** Lesions of a cutaneous nerve (white area in **A**) will affect only the territory of that branch (see individual lines in **C**).

# Cranial Nerves: Overview

**Table 4.10  Cranial nerves**

| Cranial nerve | Attachment to brain | Afferent | | | | Efferent | | |
|---|---|---|---|---|---|---|---|---|
| | | GSA | GVA | SSA | SVA | GSE | GVE | SVE |
| CN I: Olfactory n. | Telencephalon | | | | ○ | | | |
| CN II: Optic n. | Diencephalon | ● | | | | | | |
| CN III: Oculomotor n. | Mesencephalon | | | | | ● | ○ | |
| CN IV: Trochlear n. | | | | | | ● | | |
| CN V: Trigeminal n. | Pons | ○ | | | | | | ● |
| CN VI: Abducent n. | Pontomedullary junction | | | | | ● | | |
| CN VII: Facial n. | | ○ | | ○ | | ○ | | ● |
| CN VIII: Vestibulocochlear n. | | | ● | | | | | |
| CN IX: Glossopharyngeal n. | Medulla oblongata | ○ | ○ | ● | | ○ | | ● |
| CN X: Vagus n. | | ○ | ○ | ● | | ○ | | ● |
| CN XI: Accessory n. | | | | | | ● | | ● |
| CN XII: Hypoglossal n. | | | | | | ● | | |

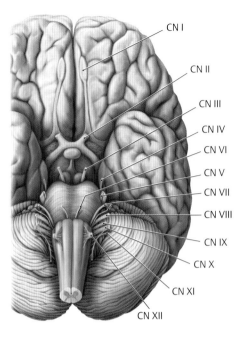

**Fig. 4.19  Cranial nerves**
Whereas the 31 spinal nerve pairs emerge from the spinal cord, the 12 pairs of cranial nerves emerge from the brain at various levels (**Table 4.10**). They are numbered according to the order of their emergence. (*Note:* Cranial nerves I and II are not true peripheral nerves but are instead extensions of the telencephalon [CN I] and diencephalon [CN II].) Unlike the spinal nerves, which each have a dorsal sensory and a ventral motor root, the cranial nerves may contain afferent (sensory) and/or efferent (motor) fibers. The types of fibers (**Table 4.11**) correspond to the function of the nerve (**Table 4.12**).

**Table 4.11  Cranial nerve fiber types**

The seven types of cranial nerve fibers are classified according to three criteria (reflected in the three-letter codes): 1. General (G) vs. Special (S), 2. Somatic (S) vs. Visceral (V), 3. Afferent (A) vs. Efferent (E). Each fiber type has an associated color used throughout this chapter.

| | Afferent (sensory) fibers | | | | Efferent (motor) fibers | | |
|---|---|---|---|---|---|---|---|
| General fibers | GSA | General somatosensory | General sensation (touch, pain, and temperature) from somite derivatives (skin, skeletal muscle, and mucosa) | | GSE | Somatomotor | Motor innervation to striated (skeletal) muscle derived from somites |
| | GVA | General viscerosensory | General sensation from viscera (smooth muscle, cardiac muscle, and glands) | | GVE | Parasympathetic | Motor innervation to viscera (smooth muscle, cardiac muscle, glands, etc.) |
| Special fibers | SSA | Special somatosensory | Sight, hearing, and balance | | | | |
| | SVA | Special viscerosensory | Taste and smell | | SVE | Branchiomotor | Fibers to striated (skeletal) muscle derived from the branchial arches |

**Table 4.12 Cranial nerve function**

| Cranial nerve | | Passage through skull | Fiber | | Sensory territory (afferent) / Target organ (efferent) |
|---|---|---|---|---|---|
| | | | A | E | |
| CN I: Olfactory n. (p. 70) | | Ethmoid bone (cribriform plate) | ○ | | Smell: special viscerosensory fibers from olfactory mucosa of nasal cavity |
| CN II: Optic n. (p. 71) | | Optic canal | ● | | Sight: special somatosensory fibers from retina |
| CN III: Oculomotor n. (pp. 72–73) | | Superior orbital fissure | | ● | Somatomotor innervation: to levator palpebrae superioris and four extraocular mm. (superior, medial, and inferior rectus, and inferior oblique) |
| | | | | ◐ | Parasympathetic innervation: preganglionic fibers to ciliary ganglion; postganglionic fibers to intraocular mm. (ciliary mm. and pupillary sphincter) |
| CN IV: Trochlear n. (pp. 72–73) | | Superior orbital fissure | | ● | Somatomotor innervation: to one extraocular m. (superior oblique) |
| CN V: Trigeminal n. (pp. 74–75) | CN V₁ (pp. 76–77) | Superior orbital fissure | ○ | | General somatic sensation: from orbit, nasal cavity, paranasal sinuses, and face |
| | CN V₂ (pp. 78–79) | Foramen rotundum | ○ | | General somatic sensation: from nasal cavity, paranasal sinuses, superior nasopharynx, upper oral cavity, internal skull, and face |
| | CN V₃ (pp. 80–81) | Foramen ovale | ○ | | General somatic sensation: from lower oral cavity, ear, internal skull, and face |
| | | | | ● | Branchiomotor innervation: to the eight mm. derived from the 1st branchial arch (including mm. of mastication) |
| CN VI: Abducent n. (pp. 72–73) | | Superior orbital fissure | | ● | Somatomotor innervation: to one extraocular m. (lateral rectus) |
| CN VII: Facial n. (pp. 82–85) | | Internal acoustic meatus | ○ | | General somatic sensation: from external ear |
| | | | ○ | | Taste: special viscerosensory fibers from tongue (anterior ⅔) and soft palate |
| | | | | ◐ | Parasympathetic innervation: preganglionic fibers to submandibular and pterygopalatine ganglia; postganglionic fibers to glands (e.g., lacrimal, submandibular, sublingual, palatine) and mucosa of nasal cavity, palate, and paranasal sinuses |
| | | | | ● | Branchiomotor innervation: to mm. derived from the 2nd branchial arch (including mm. of facial expression, stylohyoid, and stapedius) |
| CN VIII: Vestibulocochlear n. (pp. 86–87) | | Internal acoustic meatus | ● | | Hearing and balance: special somatosensory fibers from cochlea (hearing) and vestibular apparatus (balance) |
| CN IX: Glossopharyngeal n. (pp. 88–89) | | Jugular foramen | ○ | | General somatic sensation: from oral cavity, pharynx, tongue (posterior ⅓), and middle ear |
| | | | ○ | | Taste: special visceral sensation from tongue (posterior ⅓) |
| | | | ● | | General visceral sensation: from carotid body and sinus |
| | | | | ◐ | Parasympathetic innervation: preganglionic fibers to otic ganglion; postganglionic fibers to parotid gland and inferior labial glands |
| | | | | ● | Branchiomotor innervation: to the one m. derived from the 3rd branchial arch (stylopharyngeus) |
| CN X: Vagus n. (pp. 90–91) | | Jugular foramen | ○ | | General somatic sensation: from ear and internal skull |
| | | | ○ | | Taste: special visceral sensation from epiglottis |
| | | | ● | | General visceral sensation: from aortic body, laryngopharynx and larynx, respiratory tract, and thoracoabdominal viscera |
| | | | | ◐ | Parasympathetic innervation: preganglionic fibers to small, unnamed ganglia near target organs or embedded in smooth muscle walls; postganglionic fibers to glands, mucosa, and smooth muscle of pharynx, larynx, and thoracic and abdominal viscera |
| | | | | ● | Branchiomotor innervation: to mm. derived from the 4th and 6th branchial arches; also distributes branchiomotor fibers from CN XI |
| CN XI: Accessory n. (p. 92) | | Jugular foramen | | ● | Somatomotor innervation: to trapezius and sternocleidomastoid |
| | | | | ● | Branchiomotor innervation: to laryngeal mm. (except cricothyroid) via pharyngeal plexus and CN X (*Note:* The branchiomotor fibers from the cranial root of CN XI are distributed by CN X [vagus n.].) |
| CN XII: Hypoglossal n. (p. 93) | | Hypoglossal canal | | ● | Somatomotor innervation: to all intrinsic and extrinsic lingual mm. (except palatoglossus) |

# Cranial Nerve Nuclei

**Fig. 4.20 Cranial nerve nuclei: topographic arrangement**
Cross sections through the spinal cord and brainstem, superior view. Yellow = Somatic sensation. Green = Visceral sensation. Blue = Viscero-motor function. Red = Somatomotor function.
The nuclei of the spinal and cranial nerves have a topographic arrangement based on embryonic migration of neuron populations.

**A** Embryonic spinal cord: Initially, the developing spinal cord demonstrates a dorsoventral arrangement in which the sensory (afferent) neurons are dorsal and the motor (efferent) neurons are ventral. This pattern is continued into the adult spinal cord: the cell bodies of afferent neurons (generally secondary neurons) are located in the dorsal horn, and the cell bodies of efferent neurons (lower motor neurons and preganglionic autonomic neurons) are located in the ventral and lateral horns, respectively.

**B** Early embryonic brainstem: Sensory neurons (in the alar plate) migrate laterally, whereas motor nuclei (in the basal plate) migrate medially. This produces a mediolateral arrangement of nuclear columns (functionally similar nuclei stacked longitudinally).

**C** Adult brainstem: The four longitudinal nuclear columns have a mediolateral arrangement (from medial to lateral): somatic efferent, visceral efferent, visceral afferent, and somatic afferent.

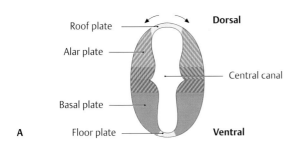

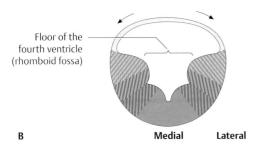

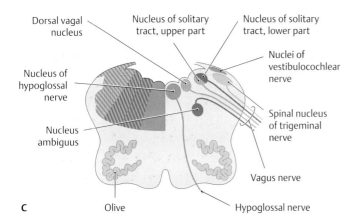

**Table 4.13 Cranial nerve nuclei**

There is not a 1-to-1 relationship between cranial nerve fiber types and cranial nerve nuclei. Some nerves derive similar fibers from multiple nuclei (e.g., CN V and CN VIII). Other nuclei are associated with multiple nerves. *Note:* The five sensory cranial nerves have eight associated sensory ganglia (cell bodies of first-order sensory neurons). The three parasympathetic cranial nerves have four associated autonomic ganglia (cell bodies of postganglionic neurons).

| Nuclei | Cranial nerve |
|---|---|
| **Somatic afferent nuclear column** (yellow) | |
| **General somatosensory:** Three nuclei that are primarily associated with CN V but receive fibers from other nerves. | |
| • Mesencephalic nucleus | CN V (via trigeminal ganglion) |
| • Principal (pontine) sensory nucleus | CN IX (via superior ganglion) |
| | CN X (via superior ganglion) |
| • Spinal nucleus | Possibly CN VII (via geniculate ganglion) |
| **Special somatosensory:** Six nuclei that are associated with CN VIII.* The nerve and nuclei are divided into a vestibular part (balance) and a cochlear part (hearing). | |
| • Medial, lateral, superior, and inferior vestibular nuclei | CN VIII, vestibular root (via vestibular ganglion) |
| • Anterior and posterior cochlear nuclei | CN VIII, cochlear root (via spiral ganglia) |
| **Visceral afferent nuclear column** (green) | |
| **General and special viscerosensory:** One nuclear complex in the brainstem that consists of a superior (taste) and inferior (general visceral sensation) part and is associated with three cranial nerves.** | |
| • Nucleus of the solitary tract, inferior part | CN IX (via inferior ganglion) |
| | CN X (via inferior ganglion) |
| • Nucleus of the solitary tract, superior part | CN VII (via geniculate ganglion) |
| | CN IX (via inferior ganglion) |
| | CN X (via inferior ganglion) |
| **Visceral motor nuclear column** (blue) | |
| **Parasympathetic** (general visceromotor): Four nuclei that each have an associated cranial nerve and one or more ganglia. | |
| • Edinger-Westphal nucleus | CN III (via ciliary ganglion) |
| • Superior salivatory nucleus | CN VII (via submandibular and pterygopalatine ganglia) |
| • Inferior salivatory nucleus | CN IX (via otic ganglion) |
| • Dorsal motor nucleus | CN X (via myriad unnamed ganglia near target organs) |
| **Branchiomotor** (special visceromotor): Three nuclei that innervate the muscles of the pharyngeal arches via four cranial nerves. | |
| • Trigeminal motor nucleus | CN V |
| • Facial nucleus | CN VII |
| • Nucleus ambiguus | CN IX |
| | CN X (with fibers from CN XI) |
| **Somatomotor nuclear column** (red) | |
| Five nuclei, each associated with a separate nerve. | |
| • Nucleus of the oculomotor n. | CN III |
| • Nucleus of the trochlear n. | CN IV |
| • Nucleus of the abducent n. | CN VI |
| • Nucleus of the accessory n. | CN XI |
| • Nucleus of the hypoglossal n. | CN XII |

*There are no brainstem nuclei associated with CN II because it emerges from the diencephalon.

**The special visceral afferent fibers in the olfactory nerve (CN I) project to the telencephalon.

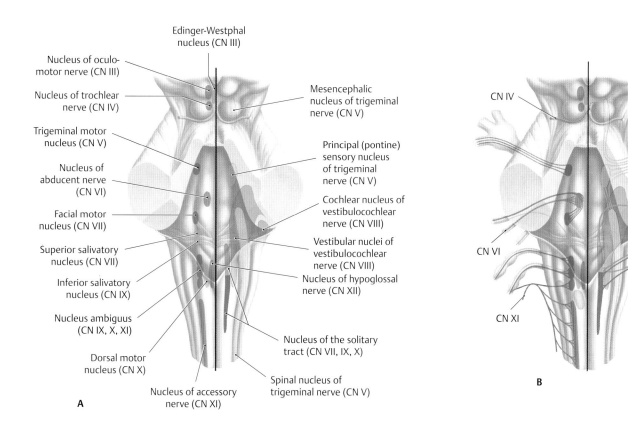

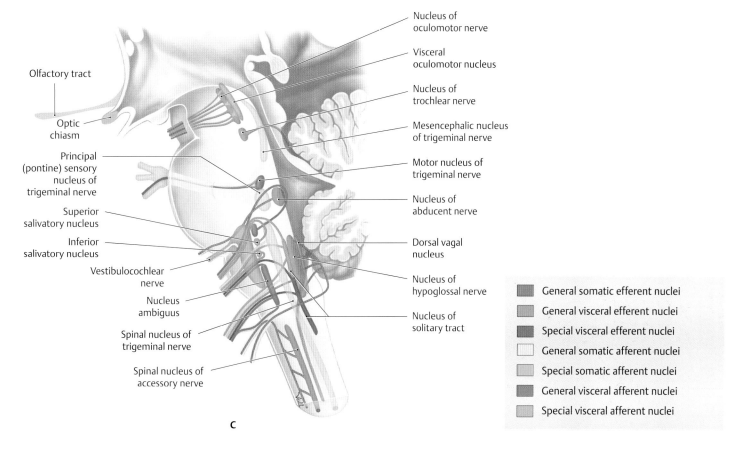

| | |
|---|---|
| ▓ | General somatic efferent nuclei |
| ▓ | General visceral efferent nuclei |
| ▓ | Special visceral efferent nuclei |
| ░ | General somatic afferent nuclei |
| ░ | Special somatic afferent nuclei |
| ▓ | General visceral afferent nuclei |
| ▓ | Special visceral afferent nuclei |

**Fig. 4.21 Cranial nerve nuclei: location**

**A,B** Posterior view of brainstem (cerebellum removed). **C** Left lateral view of midsagittal section. *Note:* The cranial nerves are numbered and described according to the level of their *emergence* from the brainstem. This does not necessarily correspond to the level of the cranial nerve nuclei associated with the nerve.

# CN I & II: Olfactory & Optic Nerves

Neither the olfactory nerve nor the optic nerve is a true peripheral nerve. They are extensions of the brain (telencephalon and diencephalon, respectively). They are therefore both sheathed in meninges (removed here) and contain CNS-specific cells (oligodendrocytes and microglia).

*Fig. 4.22* **Olfactory nerve (CN I)**
**A** Left lateral view of left nasal septum and right lateral nasal wall (the posterior part of the nasal septum is cut). **B** Inferior view of brain. (*Shaded structures are deep to the basal surface.)
The olfactory nerve relays smell information (special visceral afferent) to the cortex via a classical three-neuron pathway.

1. First-order sensory neurons are located in the mucosa of the upper nasal septum and superior nasal concha (**A**). These bipolar neurons form 20 or so fiber bundles collectively called the olfactory nerves (CN I). As the "olfactory region" is limited by the extent of these fibers (2–4 cm²), the nasal conchae create turbulence, which ensures that air (and olfactory stimuli) passes over this area. The thin, unmyelinated olfactory fibers enter the anterior cranial fossa via the cribriform plate of the ethmoid bone.
2. Second-order sensory neurons are located in the olfactory bulb (**B**). Their axons course in the olfactory tract to the medial or lateral olfactory striae. These axons synapse in the amygdala, the prepiriform area, or neighboring areas (see p. 152).
3. Third-order neurons relay the information to the cerebral cortex.

The first-order neurons have a limited lifespan (several months) and are continuously replenished from a pool of precursor cells in the olfactory mucosa. The regenerative capacity of the olfactory mucosa diminishes with age. Injuries to the cribriform plate may damage the meningeal covering of the olfactory fibers, causing olfactory disturbances and cerebrospinal fluid leakage ("runny nose" after head trauma). See p. 153 for the mechanisms of smell.

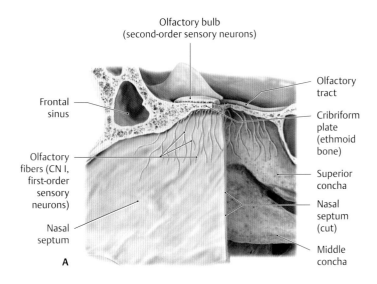

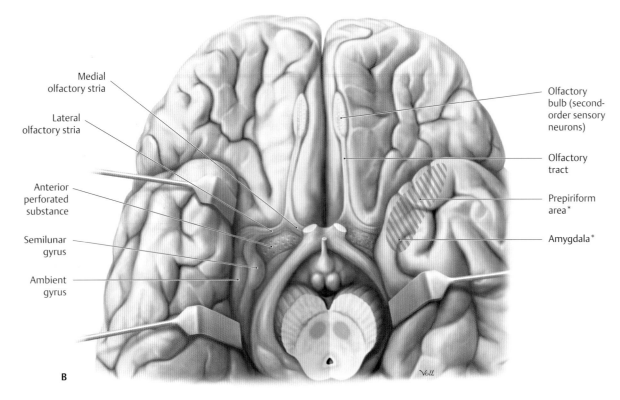

### Fig. 4.23 Optic nerve (CN II)

**A** Inferior view of brain. **B** Left lateral view of opened orbit. **C** Left posterolateral view of brainstem. The optic nerve (special somatic afferent) relays sight information from the retina to the visual cortex (striate area) via a four-neuron pathway (see p. 134). First-order neurons (rods and cones) in the retina translate incoming photons into impulses, which are relayed to second-order bipolar neurons and third-order ganglion cells. These retinal ganglion cells combine to form the optic nerve (CN II). The optic nerve passes from the orbit into the middle cranial fossa via the optic canal (the optic canal is medial to the superior orbital fissure by which the other cranial nerves enter the orbit, **B**). Ninety percent of the third-order neurons in the optic nerve synapse in the lateral geniculate body (**C**), which then projects to the striate area. Ten percent of the third-order neurons synapse in the mesencephalon. This nongeniculate part of the visual pathway functions in unconscious and reflex action. See p. 133 for the mechanisms of sight.

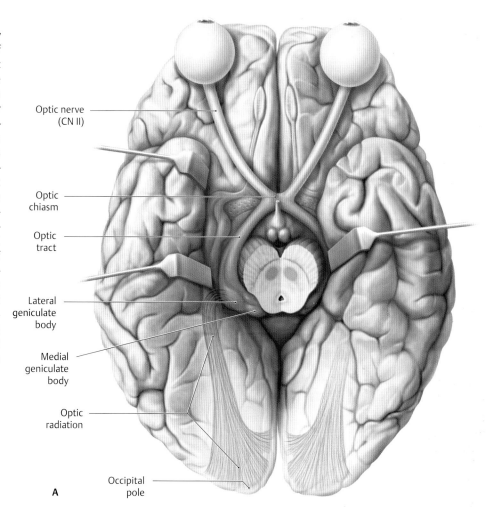

A

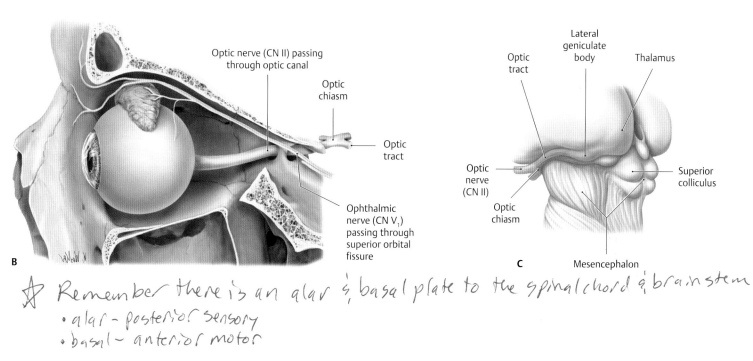

B

C

☆ Remember there is an alar & basal plate to the spinal chord & brainstem
• alar - posterior sensory
• basal - anterior motor

# CN III, IV & VI: Oculomotor, Trochlear & Abducent Nerves

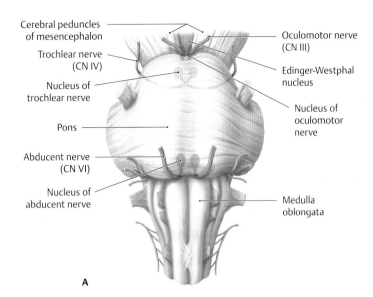

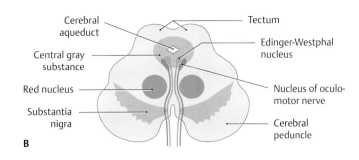

**Fig. 4.24 Cranial nerves of the extraocular muscles**

**A** Anterior view of brainstem. **B** Superior view of cross section through the mesencephalon.

CN III, IV, and VI are the three cranial nerves that collectively innervate the six extraocular muscles. (*Note:* CN III is also involved with the parasympathetic supply to the intraocular muscles.) CN III and IV arise from nuclei in the mesencephalon (midbrain, the highest level of the brainstem) and emerge at roughly the same level. CN VI arises from nuclei in the pons and emerges from the brainstem at the pontomedullary junction.

### Table 4.14 Oculomotor nerve (CN III)

**Nuclei, ganglion, and fiber distribution**

**Somatomotor** (red)

| | |
|---|---|
| Nucleus of the oculomotor nerve (mesencephalon) | Lower motor neurons innervate:<br>• Levator palpebrae superioris<br>• Superior, medial, and inferior rectus muscles<br>• Inferior oblique |

**Parasympathetic** (blue)

| | |
|---|---|
| Edinger-Westphal nucleus (mesencephalon) | Preganglionic neurons travel in the inferior division of CN III |
| | Postganglionic neurons in the **ciliary ganglion** innervate:<br>Intraocular muscles (pupillary sphincter and ciliary muscle) |

**Course**

CN III emerges from the mesencephalon, the highest level of the brainstem. It runs anteriorly through the lateral wall of the cavernous sinus to enter the orbit through the **superior orbital fissure**. After passing *through* the common tendinous ring, CN III divides into a superior and an inferior division.

**Lesions**

Lesions cause oculomotor palsy of various extents. Complete oculomotor palsy is marked by paralysis of all the innervated muscles, causing:
• Ptosis (drooping of eyelid) = disabled levator palpebrae superioris
• Inferolateral deviation of affected eye, causing diplopia (double vision) = disabled extraocular muscles
• Mydriasis (pupil dilation) = disabled pupillary sphincter
• Accommodation difficulties (difficulty focusing) = disabled ciliary muscle

### Table 4.15 Trochlear nerve (CN IV)

**Nucleus and fiber distribution**

**Somatomotor** (red)

| | |
|---|---|
| Nucleus of the trochlear nerve (mesencephalon) | Lower motor neurons innervate:<br>• Superior oblique |

**Course**

CN IV is the only cranial nerve to emerge from the dorsal side (posterior surface) of the brainstem. After emerging from the mesencephalon, it courses anteriorly around the cerebral peduncle. CN IV then enters the orbit through the **superior orbital fissure**, passing *lateral* to the common tendinous ring. It has the longest *intra*dural course of the three extraocular motor nerves.

**Lesions**

Lesions cause trochlear nerve palsy:
• Superomedial deviation of the affected eye, causing diplopia = disabled superior oblique
*Note:* Because CN IV crosses to the opposite side, lesions close to the nucleus result in trochlear nerve palsy on the opposite side (contralateral palsy). Lesions past the site where the nerve crosses the midline cause palsy on the same side (ipsilateral palsy).

### Table 4.16 Abducent nerve (CN VI)

**Nucleus and fiber distribution**

**Somatomotor** (red)

| | |
|---|---|
| Nucleus of the abducent nerve (pons) | Lower motor neurons innervate:<br>• Lateral rectus |

**Course**

CN VI follows a long *extra*dural path. It emerges from the pontomedullary junction (inferior border of pons) and runs through the cavernous sinus in close proximity to the internal carotid artery. CN VI enters the orbit through the **superior orbital fissure** and courses *through* the common tendinous ring.

**Lesions**

Lesions cause abducent nerve palsy:
• Medial deviation of the affected eye, causing diplopia = disabled lateral rectus
*Note:* The path of CN VI through the cavernous sinus exposes it to injury. Cavernous sinus thrombosis, aneurysms of the internal carotid artery, meningitis, and subdural hemorrhage may all compress the nerve, resulting in nerve palsy. Excessive fall in CSF pressure (e.g., due to lumbar puncture) may cause the brainstem to descend, exerting traction on the nerve.

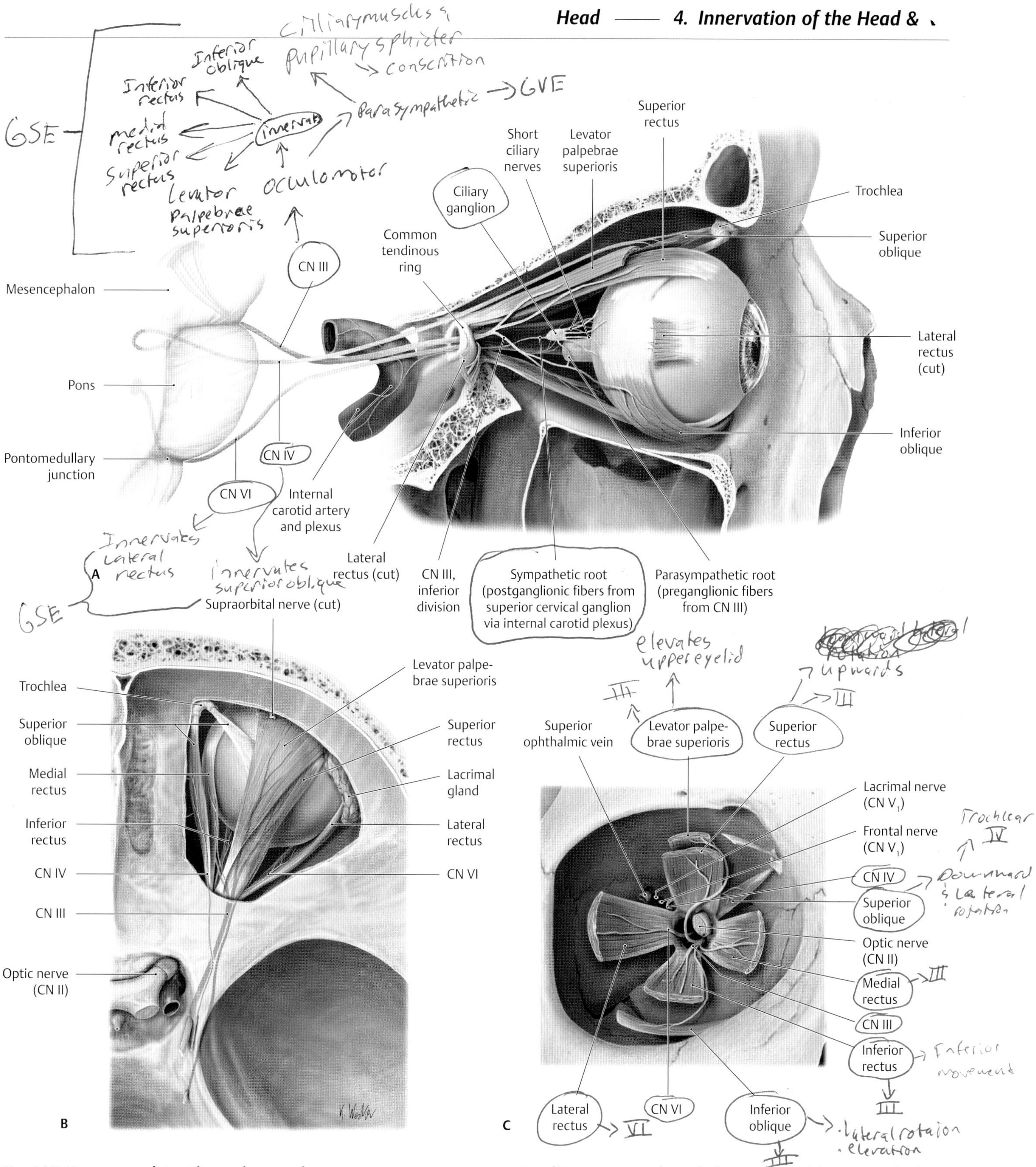

*Handwritten annotations (top area):*

Ciliary muscles &
Pupillary sphincter
→ consctrtion

Inferior oblique

Inferior rectus

medial rectus

Superior rectus

Innervate

Parasympathetic → GVE

Oculomotor

Levator palpebrae superioris

GSE

Labels on Figure A:

Mesencephalon

Pons

Pontomedullary junction

CN III

CN IV

CN VI

Internal carotid artery and plexus

Innervates Lateral rectus

GSE

Innervates superior oblique

A

Supraorbital nerve (cut)

Lateral rectus (cut)

CN III, inferior division

Short ciliary nerves

Levator palpebrae superioris

Ciliary ganglion

Superior rectus

Common tendinous ring

Trochlea

Superior oblique

Lateral rectus (cut)

Inferior oblique

Sympathetic root (postganglionic fibers from superior cervical ganglion via internal carotid plexus)

Parasympathetic root (preganglionic fibers from CN III)

*Handwritten:* elevates upper eyelid ; III ↑ ; ⟩ upwards ; ⟩ III ; Levator palpebrae superioris ; Superior rectus

**Figure B labels:**

Trochlea

Superior oblique

Medial rectus

Inferior rectus

CN IV

CN III

Optic nerve (CN II)

B

Levator palpebrae superioris

Superior rectus

Lacrimal gland

Lateral rectus

CN VI

K. Wesker

**Figure C labels:**

Superior ophthalmic vein

Levator palpebrae superioris

Superior rectus

Lacrimal nerve (CN V₁)

Frontal nerve (CN V₁)

CN IV

Superior oblique

Optic nerve (CN II)

Medial rectus

CN III

Inferior rectus

Lateral rectus

CN VI

Inferior oblique

C

*Handwritten (right side):* Trochlear IV ↑ ⟩ Downward & lateral rotation ; ⟩ III ; ⟩ Inferior movement ; III ; ⟩ lateral rotation, elevation ; ⟩ VI

---

## Fig. 4.25 Nerves supplying the ocular muscles

Right orbit. **A** Lateral view with temporal wall removed. **B** Superior view of opened orbit. **C** Anterior view. Cranial nerves III, IV, and VI enter the orbit through the superior orbital fissure, lateral to the optic canal (CN IV then passes lateral to the common tendinous ring, and CN III and VI pass through it). All three nerves supply somatomotor innervation to the extraocular muscles. The ciliary ganglion communicates three types of fibers (parasympathetic, sympathetic, and sensory) to and from the intraocular muscles via the short ciliary nerves. (Only parasympathetics synapse in the ciliary ganglion. All other fibers pass through without synapsing.) The ciliary ganglion therefore has three roots:

- Parasympathetic (motor) root: Preganglionic parasympathetic fibers travel with the inferior division of CN III to the ciliary ganglion. Only the parasympathetic fibers synapse in the ciliary ganglion (the other

two fiber types pass through the ganglion without synapsing).
- Sympathetic root: Postganglionic sympathetic fibers from the superior cervical ganglion travel on the internal carotid artery to enter the superior orbital fissure, where they may course along the ophthalmic artery to enter the short ciliary nerves via the ciliary ganglion.
- Sensory root: Sensory fibers (from the eyeball) travel to the nasociliary nerve (CN V₁) via the ciliary ganglion.

The short ciliary nerves therefore contain sensory fibers from the eyeball and postganglionic sympathetic and parasympathetic fibers from the superior cervical and ciliary ganglion, respectively. *Note:* Sympathetic fibers from the superior cervical ganglion may also travel with the nasociliary nerve (CN V₁) and reach the intraocular muscles via the long ciliary nerves.

*Handwritten (bottom left):* ganglion has 3
1) Parasympathetic preganglionic & postganglionic from III
2) sympathetic from the carotid plexus
3) sensory from the eye to V₁

# CN V: Trigeminal Nerve, Nuclei & Divisions

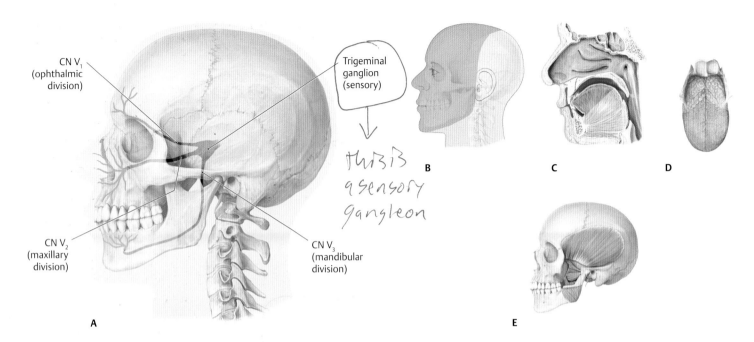

**Fig. 4.26 Trigeminal nerve divisions and distribution**
**A** Left lateral view of trigeminal divisions. **B–D** Somatosensory nerve territories. **E** Branchiomotor nerve territories.
The trigeminal nerve is the major sensory nerve of the face. It has three major divisions (**A**) that convey general somatic sensation (touch, pain, and proprioception) from the face (**B**) and select mucosa (**C** and **D**). The trigeminal nerve also contains branchiomotor fibers that innervate the eight muscles derived from the first branchial arch (**E**).

| Table 4.17 Trigeminal nerve (CN V) divisions and distribution | | | |
|---|---|---|---|
| CN V consists of a large sensory root and a small motor root, which emerge from the brainstem separately in the middle cranial fossa at the level of the pons. | | | |
| **Sensory root** | | | |
| **Fibers** | **General somatosensory** (yellow): Convey general sensation (touch, pain, and temperature) from the sensory territories of CN V (see **Fig. 4.26**). The cell bodies of these first-order pseudounipolar neurons are primarily located in the trigeminal ganglion. | | |
| **Course** | The sensory root is formed by three divisions that unite as the **trigeminal ganglion** in the middle cranial fossa. | **Division** | **Distribution** |
| | | CN V₁ (ophthalmic division) | From orbit via superior orbital fissure (see p. 76) |
| | | CN V₂ (maxillary division) | From pterygopalatine fossa via foramen rotundum (see p. 94) |
| | | CN V₃ (mandibular division) | From inferior skull base via foramen ovale (see pp. 80, 94) |
| **Nuclei** | Afferent axons from all three divisions synapse on three brainstem nuclei located in the mesencephalon, pons, and medulla oblongata of the spinal cord. | **Nuclei** | **Sensation** |
| | | Mesencephalic nucleus | Proprioception (see **Table 4.18**) |
| | | Principal (pontine) sensory nucleus | Touch |
| | | Spinal nucleus | Pain and temperature |
| **Motor root** | | | |
| **Fibers** | **Branchiomotor** (purple): Conveys motor fibers to the eight muscles derived from the 1st branchial (pharyngeal) arch: | • Masseter<br>• Temporalis<br>• Lateral pterygoid<br>• Medial pterygoid | • Tensor veli palatini<br>• Tensor tympani<br>• Mylohyoid<br>• Digastric, anterior belly |
| **Course** | The motor root emerges separately from the pons and unites with CN V₃ in the foramen ovale. | | |
| **Nucleus** | Motor nucleus (located in pons) | | |
| **"Scaffolding":** CN V is used as scaffolding for the distribution of autonomic (sympathetic and parasympathetic) and taste fibers from other cranial nerves. | | | |
| **Para-sympathetic** | All three branches of CN V are used to convey postganglionic parasympathetic fibers from parasympathetic ganglia.<br>• CN VII: Preganglionic fibers from CN VII synapse in the pterygopalatine or the submandibular ganglion, associated with CN V₂ and CN V₃, respectively. Postganglionic parasympathetic fibers then travel with the sensory branches of CN V to reach their targets.<br>• CN IX: Preganglionic fibers synapse in the otic ganglion; postganglionic fibers are distributed along branches of CN V₃. | | |
| **Sympathetic** | Postganglionic sympathetic fibers from the superior cervical ganglion may also be distributed by the sensory branches of CN V. | | |
| **Taste** | Taste fibers from the presulcal tongue travel via the lingual nerve (CN V₃) to the chorda tympani (CN VII) and nuclei of CN VII. | | |

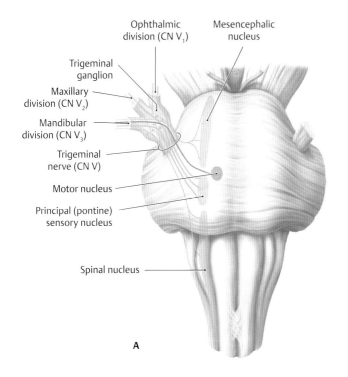

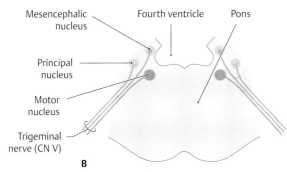

**Fig. 4.27 Trigeminal nerve nuclei**
**A** Anterior view of brainstem. **B** Superior view of cross section through the pons.
Afferent neurons in the trigeminal nerve divisions convey general somatic sensation (touch, pain, and temperature) to the CNS. The neurons from all three divisions synapse in three brainstem nuclei named for their locations (see **Table 4.18**):

- **Mesencephalic nucleus**
- **Principal (pontine) sensory nucleus**
- **Spinal nucleus**

Efferent fibers arise from lower motor neurons in the **motor nucleus**. These fibers exit at the motor root of the trigeminal nerve and unite with the mandibular division (CN V$_3$) in the foramen ovale. The branchiomotor fibers innervate the muscles of the first branchial arch.

**Fig. 4.28 Trigeminal nerve lesions**
Lesions of the trigeminal nerve divisions (peripheral nerves) will produce sensory loss following the pattern in **Fig. 4.26B** and potentially motor paralysis. Lesions of the spinal nucleus of the trigeminal cord will produce sensory loss (pain and temperature) in the pattern shown here (Sölder lines). These concentric circles correspond to the somatotopic organization of the spinal cord nucleus: more cranial portions receive axons from the center of the face, and more caudal portions receive axons from the periphery.

**Table 4.18 Trigeminal nerve nuclei and lesions**

**Nuclei**

**Somatosensory** (yellow)

Afferent neurons from the sensory territories of all three trigeminal divisions synapse in three brainstem nuclei named for their location.

| Nucleus | Location | Sensation |
|---|---|---|
| Mesencephalic nucleus | Mesencephalon | Proprioception (*Note:* The first-order sensory cell bodies of proprioceptive fibers associated with CN V have their cell bodies located in the mesencephalic nucleus.) |
| Principal (pontine) sensory nucleus | Pons | Touch |
| Spinal nucleus | Medulla oblongata | Pain and temperature |

*Note:* These sensory nuclei contain the cell bodies of second-order neurons. The mesencephalic nucleus is an exception — it contains the cell bodies of first-order pseudounipolar neurons, which have migrated into the brain.

**Branchiomotor** (purple)

Lower motor neurons are located in the motor nucleus of the trigeminal nerve. They innervate the eight muscles derived from the 1st branchial arch:

- Masseter
- Temporalis
- Lateral pterygoid
- Medial pterygoid
- Tensor veli palatini
- Tensor tympani
- Mylohyoid
- Digastric, anterior belly

**Lesions**

Traumatic lesions of the trigeminal nerve may cause sensory loss in corresponding territories or paralysis to the target muscles. *Note:* The afferent fibers of the trigeminal nerve compose the afferent limb of the corneal reflex (reflex eyelid closure).
- Trigeminal neuralgia is a disorder of CN V causing intense, crippling pain in the sensory territories.

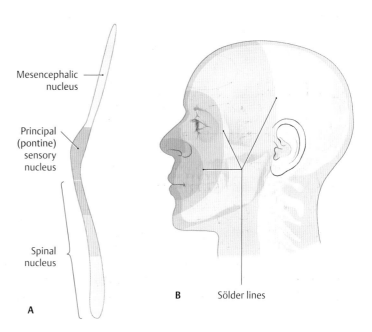

# CN V₁: Trigeminal Nerve, Ophthalmic Division

**Fig. 4.29 Ophthalmic division (CN V₁) of the trigeminal nerve**

Lateral view of the partially opened right orbit. The ophthalmic nerve divides into three major branches *before* reaching the superior orbital fissure: the lacrimal (L), frontal (F), and nasociliary (N) nerves. These nerves run roughly in the lateral, middle, and medial portions of the upper orbit, respectively. The lacrimal and frontal nerves enter the orbit superior to the common tendinous ring, and the nasociliary nerve enters through it. See **Table 4.19** for labels.

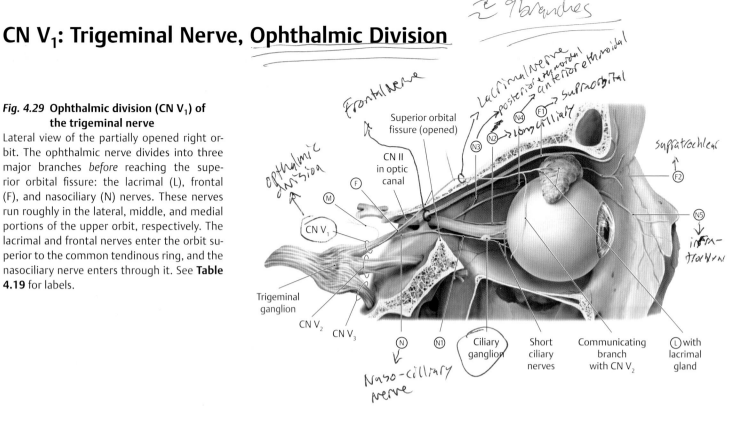

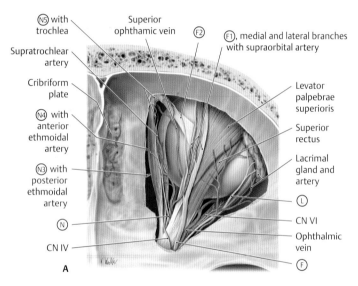

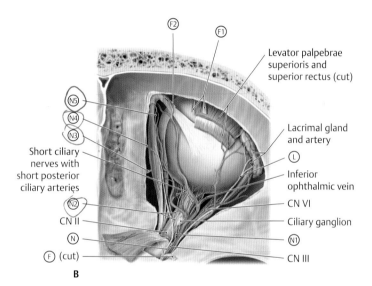

**Fig. 4.30 Ophthalmic nerve divisions in the orbit**

Superior view of orbit. (*Removed:* Bony roof, periorbita, and periorbital fat.) See **Table 4.19** for labels. **A** Lacrimal, frontal, and nasociliary divisions. **B** Nasociliary nerve and ciliary ganglion. (*Removed:* Superior rectus and levator palpebrae superioris.)

The *extraocular* muscles receive somatomotor innervation from the oculomotor (CN III), trochlear (CN IV), and abducent (CN VI) nerves. The *intraocular* muscles receive autonomic (sympathetic and parasympathetic) innervation via the short and long ciliary nerves. Sympathetic fibers from the superior cervical ganglion ascend on the internal carotid artery and travel in two manners: they may join the nasociliary nerve (CN V₁), which distributes them as the long ciliary nerves, or they may course along the ophthalmic artery to enter the ciliary ganglion as the *sympathetic root*. The ciliary ganglion also receives parasympathetic fibers from CN III (via the *parasympathetic root*). The ganglion distributes these sympathetic and parasympathetic fibers via the short ciliary nerves. The short ciliary nerves contain sensory fibers, which enter the nasociliary nerve via the *sensory root* of the ciliary ganglion.

## Table 4.19 Ophthalmic nerve (CN V₁)

The ophthalmic nerve (CN V₁) is a sensory nerve* that conveys fibers from structures of the superior facial skeleton to the trigeminal ganglion. CN V₁ gives off one branch in the middle cranial fossa before dividing into three major branches, which pass through the superior orbital fissure into the orbit. The lacrimal, frontal, and nasociliary nerves travel in the lateral, middle, and medial portions of the upper orbit, respectively.

| | |
|---|---|
| Ⓜ **Meningeal n.** | Sensory: Dura mater of the middle cranial fossa. |
| Ⓛ **Lacrimal n.** | The smallest of the three major branches, the lacrimal nerve runs in the superolateral orbit. |
| Opening | Superior orbital fissure (above the common tendinous ring). |
| Course | Runs (with the lacrimal artery) along the superior surface of the lateral rectus, through the lacrimal gland and orbital septum to the skin of the upper eyelid. |
| Innervation | Sensory: Upper eyelid (skin and conjunctiva) and lacrimal gland. |
| | Sensory and parasympathetic:  Lacrimal gland. Postganglionic parasympathetic secretomotor fibers from the pterygopalatine ganglion of the facial nerve (CN VII) travel with the zygomatic and zygomaticotemporal nerves (CN V₂). They enter the sensory lacrimal nerve (CN V₁) via a communicating branch and are distributed to the gland. Postganglionic sympathetic fibers follow a similar path. |
| Ⓕ **Frontal n.** | The largest of the three major branches, the lacrimal nerve runs in the middle of the upper orbit. |
| Opening | Superior orbital fissure (above the common tendinous ring). |
| Course and branches | Runs along the superior surface of the levator palpebrae superioris, below the periosteum. At roughly the level of the posterior eyeball, the frontal nerve divides into two terminal branches: |

| | | |
|---|---|---|
| | Ⓕ₁ **Supraorbital n.** | Continues on the superior surface of the levator palpebrae superioris and passes through the supraorbital foramen (notch). |
| | Ⓕ₂ **Supratrochlear n.** | Courses anteromedially with the supratrochlear artery toward the trochlea (tendon of superior oblique) and passes through the frontal notch. |

| | |
|---|---|
| Innervation | Sensory: Upper eyelid (skin and conjunctiva) and the skin of the forehead (both branches). The supraorbital n. also receives fibers from frontal sinus mucosa; the supratrochlear n. communicates with the infratrochlear nerve. |
| Ⓝ **Nasociliary n.** | The nasociliary nerve runs in the middle and medial parts of the upper orbit. |
| Opening | Superior orbital fissure (via the common tendinous ring). |
| Course and branches | Runs medially (across the optic nerve [CN II]) and then anteriorly between the superior oblique and medial rectus. Gives off three branches (two sensory and one sympathetic) before dividing into two terminal branches (anterior ethmoid and infratrochlear nerves). |

| | | |
|---|---|---|
| | Ⓝ₁ **Sensory root of the ciliary ganglion** | Sensory: Fibers from the **short ciliary nerves** pass without synapsing through the ciliary ganglion and enter the nasociliary nerve via the sensory root. |
| | Ⓝ₂ **Long ciliary nn.** | Sensory: Eye (e.g., cornea and sclera). |
| | Ⓝ₃ **Posterior ethmoid n.** | Sensory: Ethmoid air cells and sphenoid sinus. Fibers run in the ethmoid bone (posterior ethmoid canal) to the nasociliary nerve. |
| | Ⓝ₄ **Anterior ethmoid n.** | Sensory: Superficial nose and anterior nasal cavity.<br>• **Internal nasal n.:** Mucosa of the anterior portions of the nasal septum (medial internal nasal n.) and lateral nasal wall (lateral internal nasal n.).<br>• **External nasal n.:** Skin of the nose (courses under the nasalis muscle).<br>Fibers from these two terminal branches ascend via the nasal bone, course posteriorly in the cranial cavity over the cribriform plate, and enter the orbit via the anterior ethmoid canal. |
| | Ⓝ₅ **Infratrochlear n.** | Sensory: Medial aspect of the upper eyelid (skin and conjunctiva) and the lacrimal sac. Fibers enter the orbit near the trochlea (tendon of superior oblique) and course posteriorly to the nasociliary nerve. |

| | |
|---|---|
| Innervation | Sensory: Ethmoid air cells, sphenoid sinus, anterior nasal cavity, superficial nose, upper eyelid, lacrimal sac, and eye. |

*Note: Nerve courses are traditionally described proximal to distal (CNS to periphery). However, for sensory nerves, the sensory relay is in the opposite direction. It is more appropriate to talk of sensory nerves collecting fibers than to talk of them branching to supply a region.

# CN V₂: Trigeminal Nerve, Maxillary Division

*~ 15 branches*

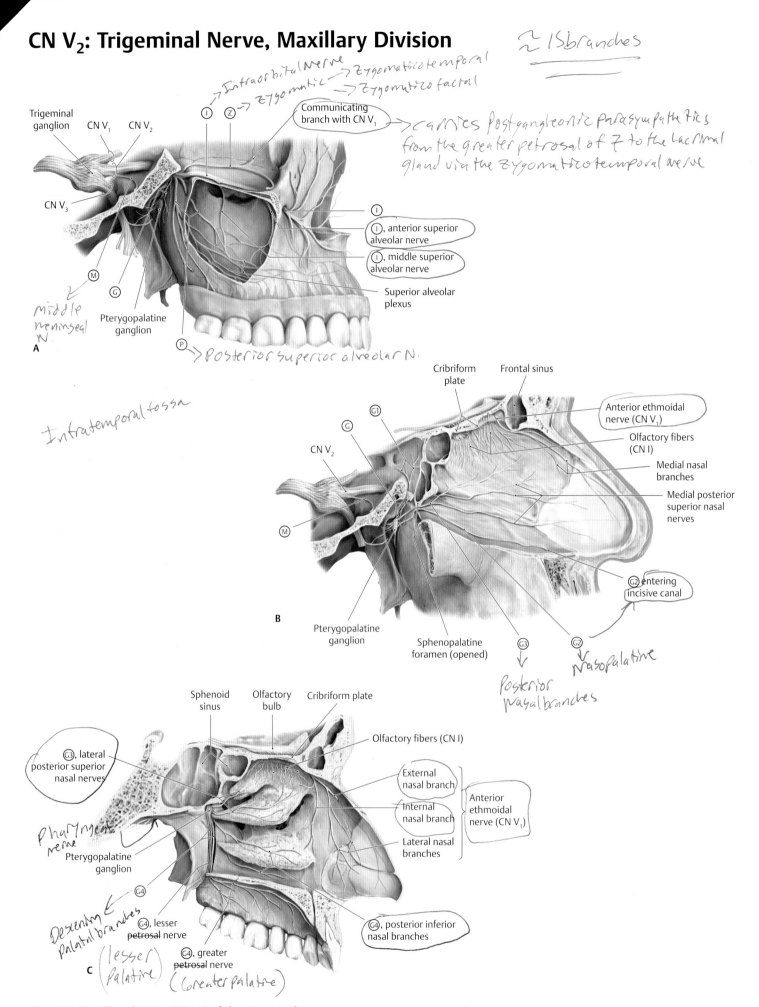

Handwritten annotations:
- Intraorbital Nerve → Zygomaticotemporal
- Zygomatic → Zygomaticofacial
- carries postganglionic parasympathetics from the greater petrosal of 7 to the Lacrimal gland via the Zygomaticotemporal nerve
- middle meningeal N.
- Posterior superior alveolar N.
- Intratemporal fossa
- Posterior nasal branches
- Nasopalatine
- Pharyngeal nerve
- Descending Palatal branches
- (lesser Palatine)
- (Greater Palatine)

Labels (printed):
- Trigeminal ganglion
- CN V₁, CN V₂
- CN V₃
- Communicating branch with CN V₁
- ①, anterior superior alveolar nerve
- ①, middle superior alveolar nerve
- Superior alveolar plexus
- Pterygopalatine ganglion
- A
- Cribriform plate
- Frontal sinus
- Anterior ethmoidal nerve (CN V₁)
- Olfactory fibers (CN I)
- Medial nasal branches
- Medial posterior superior nasal nerves
- CN V₂
- G1, G
- M
- G2 entering incisive canal
- G3
- Pterygopalatine ganglion
- Sphenopalatine foramen (opened)
- B
- Sphenoid sinus
- Olfactory bulb
- Cribriform plate
- Olfactory fibers (CN I)
- G3, lateral posterior superior nasal nerves
- External nasal branch
- Internal nasal branch
- Anterior ethmoidal nerve (CN V₁)
- Lateral nasal branches
- Pterygopalatine ganglion
- G4
- G4, lesser petrosal nerve
- G4, greater petrosal nerve
- G4, posterior inferior nasal branches
- C

***Fig. 4.31* Maxillary division (CN V₂) of the trigeminal nerve**
Right lateral view. See **Table 4.20** for labels. **A** Opened right maxillary sinus. **B** Nasal septum in right nasal cavity. **C** Left lateral nasal wall.

**Table 4.20 Maxillary nerve (CN V₂)**

Like the ophthalmic nerve (CN V₁), the maxillary nerve (CN V₂) is a sensory nerve* that conveys fibers from structures of the facial skeleton to the trigeminal ganglion. CN V₂ gives off one branch in the middle cranial fossa before entering the foramen rotundum to the pterygopalatine fossa. In the pterygopalatine fossa, the maxillary nerve divides into branches (e.g., zygomatic, posterior superior alveolar, and infraorbital nerves) and receives ganglionic branches from the pterygopalatine ganglion. This ganglion has five major branches, which distribute CN V₂ fibers. These sensory CN V₂ fibers convey autonomic fibers from the pterygopalatine ganglion.

**Direct branches of the maxillary n. (CN V₂)**

| | |
|---|---|
| Ⓜ **Middle meningeal n.** | Sensory: Meninges of the middle cranial fossa. |
| Ⓖ **Ganglionic branches** | Generally, two ganglionic branches suspend (pass through) the **pterygopalatine ganglion** from CN V₂ (see below). |
| Ⓩ **Zygomatic n.** | Sensory: Skin of the temple (**zygomaticotemporal nerve**) and cheek (**zygomaticofacial nerve**). Fibers enter the orbit via canals in the zygomatic bone and course in the lateral orbit wall to CN V₂ via the inferior orbital fissure. |
| Ⓟ **Posterior superior alveolar n.** | Sensory: Maxillary molars (with associated gingivae and buccal mucosa) and maxillary sinus. Fibers course on the infratemporal surface of the maxilla. The posterior superior alveolar nerve contributes to the **superior alveolar plexus** (anterior, middle, and superior alveolar nn.). |
| Ⓘ **Infraorbital n.** | Sensory: Lower eyelid (skin and conjunctiva), maxillary sinus, and maxillary teeth (via anterior and middle superior alveolar branches). <br> • **Middle superior alveolar nerve:** Sensory fibers from the maxillary premolars (with associated gingivae, buccal mucosa, and maxillary sinus). <br> • **Anterior superior alveolar nerve:** Sensory fibers from the maxillary incisors and canines (with associated gingivae, lingual mucosa, and maxillary sinus). Nasal branch: Sensory fibers from anterior portions of the nasal wall, floor, and septum. <br> These fibers enter the infraorbital canal and emerge from the infraorbital groove. |

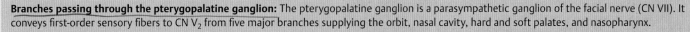

**Branches passing through the pterygopalatine ganglion:** The pterygopalatine ganglion is a parasympathetic ganglion of the facial nerve (CN VII). It conveys first-order sensory fibers to CN V₂ from five major branches supplying the orbit, nasal cavity, hard and soft palates, and nasopharynx.

| | |
|---|---|
| Ⓖ₁ **Orbital branches** | Sensory: Orbital periosteum (via inferior orbital fissure) and paranasal sinuses (ethmoid air cells and sphenoid sinus, via the posterior ethmoid canal). |
| Ⓖ₂ **Nasopalatine n.** | Sensory: Anterior hard palate and the inferior nasal septum. The left and right nasopalatine nerves ascend (in the anterior and posterior incisive foramina, respectively) and converge in the incisive fossa. They travel posterosuperiorly on the nasal septum (vomer) through the sphenopalatine foramen. |
| Ⓖ₃ **Posterior superior nasal nn.** | Sensory: Posterosuperior nasal cavity. (*Note:* The anterior ethmoid nerve [CN V₁] conveys fibers from the anterosuperior portion.) <br> • **Lateral posterior superior nasal nn.:** Posterior ethmoid air cells and mucosa in the posterior of the superior and middle nasal conchae. <br> • **Medial posterior superior nasal nn.:** Mucosa of the posterior nasal roof and septum. |
| Ⓖ₄ **Palatine (descending, greater) nn.** | Sensory: Hard and soft palates. <br> • **Greater palatine n.:** Hard palate (gingivae, mucosa, and glands) and soft palate via greater palatine canal. Receives fibers from the inferior nasal concha and walls of the middle and inferior nasal meatuses through the perpendicular plate of the ethmoid bone (posterior inferior nasal branches). <br> • **Lesser palatine n.:** Soft palate, palatine tonsils, and uvula via lesser palatine canal. <br> The greater and lesser palatine nerves converge in the greater palatine canal. |
| Ⓖ₅ **Pharyngeal n.** | Sensory: Mucosa of the superior nasopharynx via palatovaginal (pharyngeal) canal. |

**Autonomic scaffolding:** The pterygopalatine ganglion is affiliated with the sensory CN V₂. Postganglionic autonomic fibers are distributed by sensory fibers of CN V₂.

| | |
|---|---|
| **Pterygopalatine ganglion (CN VII)** | **Motor root:** Preganglionic parasympathetic fibers from the facial nerve (CN VII) travel in the **greater petrosal nerve** (joins with deep petrosal nerve to form nerve of pterygoid canal). |
| | **Sympathetic root:** Postganglionic sympathetic fibers from the superior cervical ganglion ascend (via the internal carotid plexus) and travel in the **deep petrosal nerve** (joins with greater petrosal nerve to form nerve of pterygoid canal). |
| | **Sensory root:** Sensory fibers pass through the ganglion from five sensory branches (see above). |

• **Lacrimal gland:** Postganglionic parasympathetic secretomotor fibers to the lacrimal gland leave the pterygopalatine ganglion on the zygomatic nerve (CN V₂). They travel with the zygomaticotemporal nerve to the lacrimal nerve (CN V₁) via a communicating branch.
• **Glands of the oral cavity:** Postganglionic parasympathetic fibers to the glands of the palatine, pharyngeal, and nasal mucosa reach their targets via corresponding sensory branches of CN V₂.
• **Blood vessels:** Postganglionic sympathetic fibers are distributed by CN V₂.
• **Taste (CN VII):** Taste fibers (special visceral afferent) associated with CN VII ascend from the palate to the greater petrosal nerve and geniculate ganglion of CN VII via the palatine nerves.

*Note: Nerve courses are traditionally described proximal to distal (CNS to periphery). However, for sensory nerves, the sensory relay is in the opposite direction. It is more appropriate to talk of sensory nerves collecting fibers than to talk of them branching to supply a region.

# CN V₃: Trigeminal Nerve, Mandibular Division

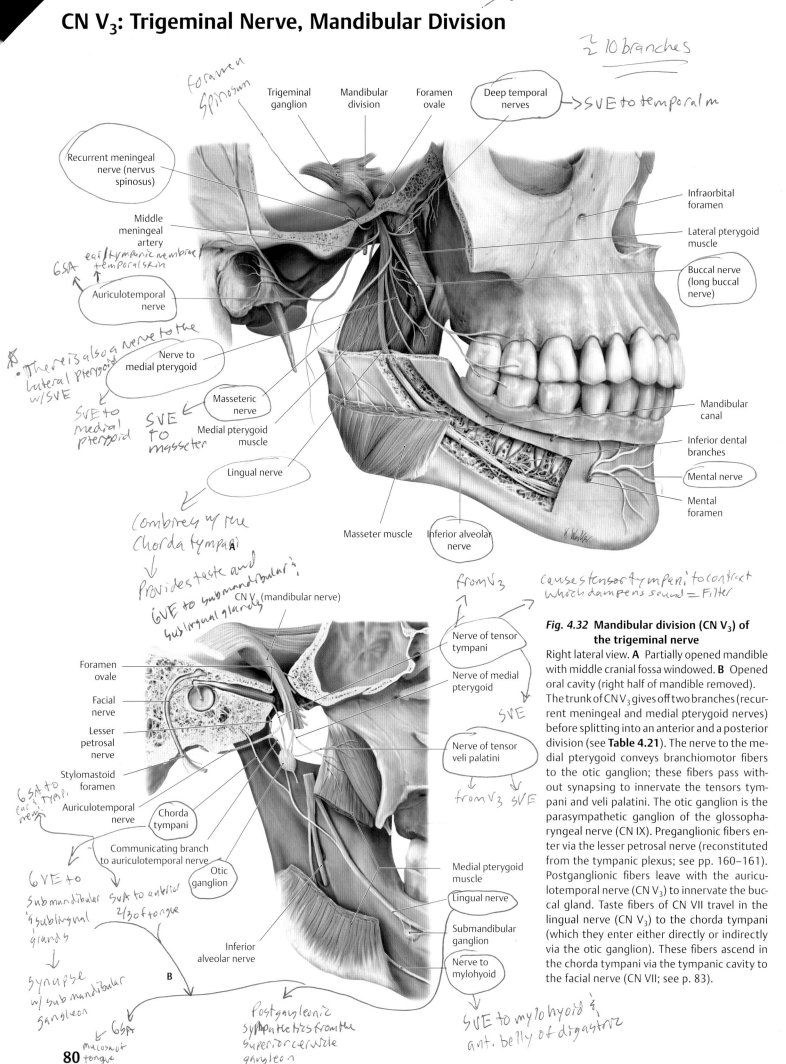

Handwritten annotations:
- → only DIVISION w/ SVE
- ⫽ 10 branches
- → SVE to temporal m
- GSA to ear/tympanic membrane/temporal skin
- ✱ There is also a nerve to the lateral pterygoid w/ SVE
- SVE to medial pterygoid
- SVE to medial pterygoid
- SVE to masseter
- Combines w/ the Chorda tympani ↓ Provides taste and GVE to submandibular & sublingual glands
- from V₃
- causes tensor tympani to contract which dampens sound = Filter
- GSA to ear, tymp. mem.
- GVE to submandibular & sublingual glands ↓ synapse w/ submandibular ganglion ← GSA mucosa of tongue
- SVA to anterior ⅔ of tongue
- Postganglionic sympathetics from the superior cervical ganglion
- from V₃ SVE
- SVE to mylohyoid & ant. belly of digastric

Labels (Figure A):
- Foramen spinosum
- Recurrent meningeal nerve (nervus spinosus)
- Trigeminal ganglion
- Mandibular division
- Foramen ovale
- Deep temporal nerves
- Infraorbital foramen
- Middle meningeal artery
- Lateral pterygoid muscle
- Auriculotemporal nerve
- Buccal nerve (long buccal nerve)
- Nerve to medial pterygoid
- Masseteric nerve
- Medial pterygoid muscle
- Lingual nerve
- Mandibular canal
- Inferior dental branches
- Mental nerve
- Mental foramen
- Masseter muscle
- Inferior alveolar nerve
- K. Wesker
- **A**

Labels (Figure B):
- CN V₃ (mandibular nerve)
- Nerve of tensor tympani
- Nerve of medial pterygoid
- Foramen ovale
- Facial nerve
- Lesser petrosal nerve
- Nerve of tensor veli palatini
- Stylomastoid foramen
- Auriculotemporal nerve
- Chorda tympani
- Communicating branch to auriculotemporal nerve
- Otic ganglion
- Medial pterygoid muscle
- Lingual nerve
- Submandibular ganglion
- Inferior alveolar nerve
- Nerve to mylohyoid
- **B**

## Fig. 4.32 Mandibular division (CN V₃) of the trigeminal nerve

Right lateral view. **A** Partially opened mandible with middle cranial fossa windowed. **B** Opened oral cavity (right half of mandible removed). The trunk of CN V₃ gives off two branches (recurrent meningeal and medial pterygoid nerves) before splitting into an anterior and a posterior division (see **Table 4.21**). The nerve to the medial pterygoid conveys branchiomotor fibers to the otic ganglion; these fibers pass without synapsing to innervate the tensors tympani and veli palatini. The otic ganglion is the parasympathetic ganglion of the glossopharyngeal nerve (CN IX). Preganglionic fibers enter via the lesser petrosal nerve (reconstituted from the tympanic plexus; see pp. 160–161). Postganglionic fibers leave with the auriculotemporal nerve (CN V₃) to innervate the buccal gland. Taste fibers of CN VII travel in the lingual nerve (CN V₃) to the chorda tympani (which they enter either directly or indirectly via the otic ganglion). These fibers ascend in the chorda tympani via the tympanic cavity to the facial nerve (CN VII; see p. 83).

## Table 4.21 Mandibular nerve (CN V₃)

The mandibular nerve (CN V₃) is the mixed afferent-efferent branch of CN V, containing general sensory fibers and branchiomotor fibers to the eight muscles derived from the 1st pharyngeal arch. The large sensory and small motor roots of CN V leave the middle cranial fossa via the foramen ovale. In the infratemporal fossa, they unite to form the CN V₃ trunk. The trunk gives off two branches before splitting into an anterior and a posterior division. Of the eight branchial arch muscles, three are supplied by the trunk, three by the anterior division, and two by the posterior division.

**Trunk:** The trunk of CN V₃ gives off one sensory and one motor branch. The motor branch conveys branchiomotor fibers to three of the eight muscles of the 1st pharyngeal arch.

| | |
|---|---|
| ® **Recurrent meningeal branch** (nervus spinosus) | Sensory: Dura of the middle cranial fossa (also anterior cranial fossa and calvarium). The nervus spinosum arises in the infratemporal fossa and re-enters the middle cranial fossa via the foramen spinosum. |
| ⓂⓅ **Medial pterygoid n.** | *SVE*<br>Branchiomotor: Directly to the **medial pterygoid**. Certain fibers enter the otic ganglion via the motor root and pass without synapsing to:<br>• N. to tensor veli palatini: **Tensor veli palatini**.<br>• N. to tensor tympani: **Tensor tympani**. |

**Anterior division:** The anterior division of CN V₃ contains predominantly efferent fibers (with one sensory branch, the buccal nerve.) The branchio-motor fibers innervate three of the eight muscles of the 1st pharyngeal arch.

| | |
|---|---|
| Ⓜ **Masseter n.** | Branchiomotor: **Masseter**. |
| | Sensory: Temporomandibular joint (articular branches). |
| Ⓣ **Deep temporal nn.** | Branchiomotor: **Temporalis** via two branches:<br>• Anterior deep temporal n.<br>• Posterior deep temporal n. |
| ⓁⓅ **Lateral pterygoid n.** | Branchiomotor: **Lateral pterygoid**. |
| Ⓑ **Buccal (long buccal) n.** | Sensory: Cheek (skin and mucosa) and buccal gingivae of the molars. |

**Posterior division:** The larger posterior division of CN V₃ contains predominantly afferent fibers (with one motor branch, the mylohyoid nerve). The mylohyoid nerve arises from the inferior alveolar nerve and supplies the remaining two muscles of the 1st pharyngeal arch.

| | |
|---|---|
| Ⓐ **Auriculotemporal n.** | Sensory: Skin of the ear and temple. Fibers pass through the parotid gland, behind the temporomandibular joint, and into the infratemporal fossa. The nerve typically splits around the middle meningeal artery (a branch of the maxillary artery) before joining the posterior division.<br>Distributes postganglionic parasympathetic fibers from the otic ganglion. |
| Ⓛ **Lingual n.** | Sensory: Mucosa of the oral cavity (presulcal tongue, oral floor, and gingival covering of lingual surface of mandibular teeth). In the infratemporal fossa, the lingual nerve combines with the chorda tympani (CN VII). |
| Ⓘ **Inferior alveolar n.** | Sensory: Mandibular teeth and chin:<br>• **Incisive branch:** Incisors, canines, and 1st premolars (with associated labial gingivae).<br>• **Mental n.:** Labial gingivae of the incisors and the skin of the lower lip and chin.<br>The mental nerve enters the mental foramen and combines with the incisive branch in the mandibular canal. The inferior alveolar nerve exits the mandible via the mandibular foramen and combines to form the posterior division of CN V₃.<br>*Note:* 2nd premolars and mandibular molars are supplied by the inferior alveolar nerve before it splits into its terminal branches.<br><br>Branchiomotor: Fibers branch just proximal to the mandibular foramen:<br>• **Mylohyoid n.: Mylohyoid** and anterior belly of the **digastric**. |

**Autonomic scaffolding:** The parasympathetic ganglia of CN VII (submandibular ganglion) and CN IX (otic ganglion) are functionally associated with CN V₃.

| | | |
|---|---|---|
| **Submandibular ganglion** (CN VII) | Parasympathetic root | Preganglionic parasympathetic fibers from the facial nerve (CN VII) travel to the ganglion in the **chorda tympani**, facial nerve, and lingual nerve (CN V₃). |
| | Sympathetic root | Sympathetic fibers from the **superior cervical ganglion** ascend (via the internal carotid plexus) and travel in a plexus on the facial artery. |
| **Otic ganglion** (CN IX) | Parasympathetic root | Preganglionic parasympathetic fibers enter from CN IX via the **lesser petrosal nerve**. |
| | Sympathetic root | Postganglionic sympathetic fibers from the **superior cervical ganglion** enter via a plexus on the middle meningeal artery. |

*[handwritten annotations: "Parasymp → to parotid", "from CN9"]*

• **Parotid gland:** Postganglionic parasympathetic fibers from the otic ganglion travel to the parotid gland via the auriculotemporal n. (CN V₃).
• **Submandibular and sublingual glands:** Postganglionic autonomic fibers to the submandibular and sublingual glands travel from the submandibular ganglion via glandular branches.

• **Taste** (CN VII): Taste fibers (special viscerosensory fibers) to CN VII may travel via the lingual nerve (CN V₃) to the chorda tympani (CN VII).

*Note:* Nerve courses are traditionally described proximal to distal (CNS to periphery). However, for sensory nerves, the sensory relay is in the opposite direction. It is more appropriate to talk of sensory nerves collecting fibers than to talk of them branching to supply a region.

# CN VII: Facial Nerve, Nuclei & Internal Branches

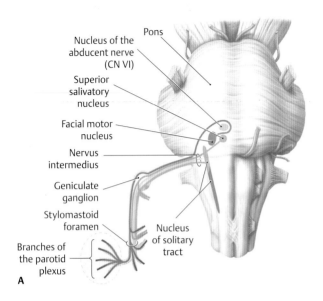

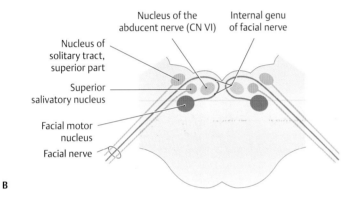

**Fig. 4.33 Facial nerve (CN VII)**
**A** Anterior view of brainstem. **B** Superior view of cross section through pons.
**Fibers:** The facial nerve provides branchiomotor innervation to the muscles of the second branchial arch and parasympathetic motor innervation to most salivary glands (via the pterygopalatine and submandibular ganglia). Taste fibers are conveyed via pseudounipolar sensory neurons with cell bodies in the geniculate ganglion. The facial nerve also receives general sensation from the external ear.
**Branches:** The superficial branches of CN VII are primarily branchiomotor (only the posterior auricular nerve may contain sensory fibers as well as motor). Taste and preganglionic parasympathetic fibers travel in both the chorda tympani and greater petrosal nerves. These fibers converge in the external genu and enter the brainstem together as the nervus intermedius.

| *Table 4.22* **Facial nerve (CN VII)** | |
| --- | --- |
| **Nuclei, ganglia, and fiber distribution** | |
| **Branchiomotor** (purple) | |
| Facial motor nucleus | Lower motor neurons innervate all muscles of the 2nd branchial (pharyngeal) arch: <br> • Muscles of facial expression <br> • Stylohyoid <br> • Digastric, posterior belly <br> • Stapedius |
| **Parasympathetic** (blue) | |
| Superior salivatory nucleus | Preganglionic neurons synapse in the **pterygopalatine** or **submandibular ganglion**. |
| | Postganglionic neurons innervate: <br> • Lacrimal gland <br> • Submandibular and sublingual glands <br> • Small glands of the oral and nasal cavities |
| **Special visceral afferent** (light green) | |
| Nucleus of the solitary tract, superior part | First-order pseudounipolar cells in the **geniculate ganglion** relay taste sensation from the presulcal tongue and soft palate (via the chorda tympani and greater petrosal nerve). |
| **General somatic afferent** (not shown) | |
| First-order pseudounipolar cells in the **geniculate ganglion** relay general sensation from the external ear (auricle and skin of the auditory canal) and lateral tympanic membrane. | |
| **Course** | |
| **Emergence:** Axons from the superior salivatory nucleus and the nucleus of the solitary tract form the **nervus intermedius**. These combine with the branchiomotor and somatosensory fibers to emerge from the brainstem as CN VII. <br> **Internal branches:** CN VII enters the petrous bone via the internal acoustic meatus. Within the facial canal, it gives off one branchiomotor branch (nerve to the stapedius) and two nerves (greater petrosal nerve and chorda tympani) containing both parasympathetic and taste fibers. <br> **External branches:** The remaining fibers emerge via the stylomastoid foramen. Three direct branches arise before the fibers enter the parotid gland (nerve to posterior digastric, nerve to stylohyoid, and posterior auricular nerve). In the gland, the branchiomotor fibers branch to form the parotid plexus, which innervates the muscles of the 2nd branchial arch. | |
| **Lesions** | |
| CN VII is most easily injured in its distal portions (after emerging from the parotid gland). Nerve lesions of the parotid plexus cause muscle paralysis. Temporal bone fractures may injure the nerve within the facial canal, causing disturbances of taste, lacrimation, salivation, etc. (see **Fig. 4.34**). | |

### Fig. 4.34 Branches of the facial nerve

The facial nerve enters the facial canal of the petrous bone via the internal acoustic meatus. Most branchiomotor fibers and all somatosensory fibers emerge via the stylomastoid foramen. Within the facial canal, CN VII gives off one branchiomotor branch and two nerves containing both parasympathetic and taste fibers (greater petrosal nerve and chorda tympani). Temporal bone fractures may injure the facial nerve at various levels:

1 Internal acoustic meatus: Lesions affect CN VII and the vestibulocochlear nerve (CN VIII). Peripheral motor facial paralysis is accompanied by hearing loss and dizziness.
2 External genu of facial nerve: Peripheral motor facial paralysis is accompanied by disturbances of taste sensation, lacrimation, and salivation (greater petrosal nerve).
3 Motor paralysis is accompanied by disturbances of salivation and taste (chorda tympani). Paralysis of the stapedius causes hyperacusis (hypersensitivity to normal sounds).
4 Facial paralysis is accompanied by disturbances of taste and salivation (chorda tympani).
5 Facial paralysis is the only manifestation of a lesion at this level.

Internal acoustic meatus
CN VIII
Greater petrosal nerve
Nerve to the stapedius
Chorda tympani
Stylo-mastoid foramen
Posterior auricular nerve
Nerves to the stylohyoid and posterior digastric
Parotid plexus

1
2
3
4
5

### Fig. 4.35 Course of the facial nerve

Right lateral view of right temporal bone (petrous part). Both the facial nerve and vestibulocochlear nerve (CN VIII, not shown) pass through the internal acoustic meatus on the posterior surface of the petrous bone. The facial nerve courses laterally in the bone to the external genu, which contains the **geniculate ganglion** (cell bodies of first-order pseudounipolar sensory neurons). At the genu (L. *genu* = knee), CN VII bends and descends in the facial canal. It gives off three branches between the geniculate ganglion and the stylomastoid foramen:

- **Greater petrosal nerve:** Parasympathetic and taste (special visceral afferent) fibers branch from the geniculate ganglion in the greater petrosal canal. They emerge on the anterior surface of the petrous pyramid and continue across the surface of the foramen lacerum. The greater petrosal nerve combines with the deep petrosal nerve in the pterygoid canal (nerve of the pterygoid canal, vidian). The greater petrosal nerve contains the fibers that form the motor root of the pterygopalatine ganglion (the parasympathetic ganglion of CN VII). The pterygopalatine ganglion distributes autonomic fibers via the trigeminal nerve (primarily the maxillary division, CN V₂).
- **Stapedial nerve:** Branchiomotor fibers innervate the stapedius muscle.
- **Chorda tympani:** The remaining parasympathetic and taste fibers leave the facial nerve as the chorda tympani. This nerve runs through the tympanic cavity and petrotympanic fissure to the infratemporal fossa, where it unites with the lingual nerve (CN V₃).

The remaining fibers (branchiomotor with some general sensory) exit via the stylomastoid foramen.

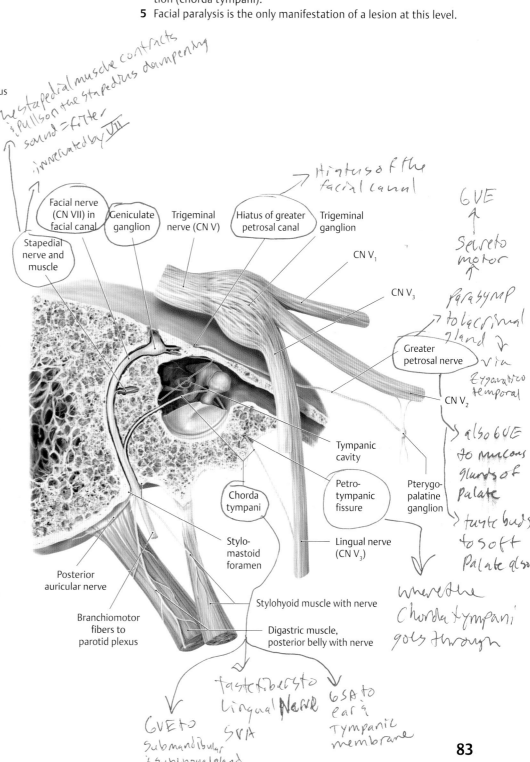

Facial nerve (CN VII) in facial canal
Geniculate ganglion
Trigeminal nerve (CN V)
Hiatus of greater petrosal canal
Trigeminal ganglion
Stapedial nerve and muscle
CN V₁
CN V₃
Greater petrosal nerve
CN V₂
Tympanic cavity
Petro-tympanic fissure
Pterygo-palatine ganglion
Chorda tympani
Stylo-mastoid foramen
Lingual nerve (CN V₃)
Posterior auricular nerve
Stylohyoid muscle with nerve
Branchiomotor fibers to parotid plexus
Digastric muscle, posterior belly with nerve

*[handwritten annotations:]* The stapedial muscle contracts; Pull's on the stapedius dampening; sound = filter; innervated by VII

Hiatus of the facial canal

GVE ↑ Secreto motor ↑ parasymp → to lacrimal gland via zygomatico temporal

→ also GVE to mucous glands of palate → taste buds to soft palate also

Where the chorda tympani goes through

taste fibers to lingual Nerve SVA

GSA to ear & tympanic membrane

GVE to submandibular & sublingual gland

# CN VII: Facial Nerve, External Branches & Ganglia

*6 superficial branches*

### Fig. 4.36 Innervation of the second branchial arch muscles

Left lateral view. The branchiomotor fibers of CN VII innervate all the muscles derived from the second branchial arch. With the exception of the stapedial nerve (to the stapedius), all branchiomotor fibers in the facial nerve emerge from the facial canal via the stylomastoid foramen. Three branches arise *before* the parotid plexus:

- Posterior auricular nerve (*Note:* This may also contain general somatosensory fibers.)
- Nerve to the digastric (posterior belly)
- Nerve to the stylohyoid

The remaining branchiomotor fibers then enter the parotid gland where they divide into two trunks (temporofacial and cervicofacial) and five major branches, which innervate the muscles of facial expression:

- Temporal
- Zygomatic
- Buccal
- Mandibular (marginal mandibular)
- Cervical

The branching of the plexus is variable.

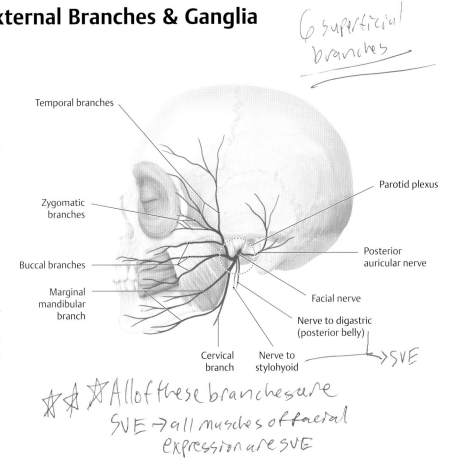

Temporal branches

Zygomatic branches

Buccal branches

Marginal mandibular branch

Parotid plexus

Posterior auricular nerve

Facial nerve

Nerve to digastric (posterior belly)

Cervical branch

Nerve to stylohyoid

→ SVE

*✱✱ ✱ All of these branches are SVE → all muscles of facial expression are SVE*

### Fig. 4.37 Facial paralysis

**A** Upper motor neurons in the primary somatomotor cortex (precentral gyrus) descend to the cell bodies of lower motor neurons in the facial motor nucleus. The axons of these lower motor neurons innervate the muscles derived from the second branchial arch. The facial motor nucleus has a "bipartite" structure: its cranial (upper) part supplies the muscles of the calvaria and palpebral fissure, and its caudal (lower) part supplies the muscles of the lower face. The cranial part of the nucleus receives bilateral innervation (from upper motor neurons in both hemispheres). The caudal part receives contralateral innervation (from cortical neurons on the other side).

**B** Central (supranuclear) paralysis: Loss of upper motor neurons (shown here for the left hemisphere) causes contralateral paralysis in the lower half of the face but no paralysis in the upper half. For example, the patient's mouth will sag on the right (contralateral paralysis of lower muscles), but the ability to wrinkle the forehead and close the eyes is intact.

**C** Peripheral (infranuclear) paralysis: Loss of lower motor neurons (shown here for right brainstem) causes complete ipsilateral paralysis. For example, the whole right side of the face is paralyzed. Depending on the site of the lesion, additional deficits may be present (decreased lacrimation or salivation, loss of taste sensation in the presulcal tongue).

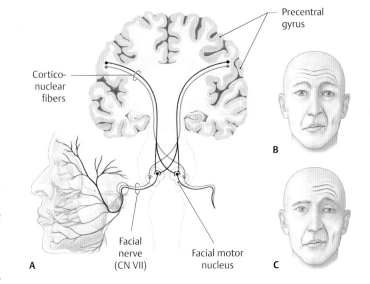

Precentral gyrus

Cortico-nuclear fibers

Facial nerve (CN VII)

Facial motor nucleus

A

B

C

*8 total branches for VII (main branches)*
- *the superficial 6 – SVE*
- *greater petrosal – GVE*
- *chordae tympany – GSA, GVE, SVA*

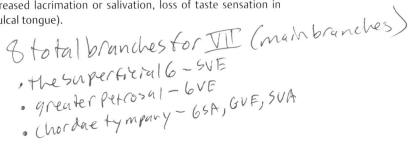

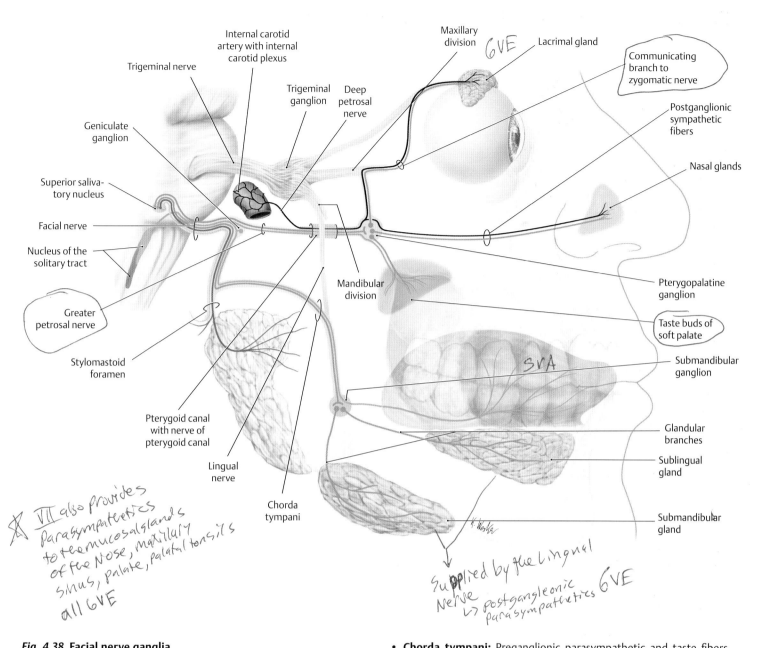

*Handwritten annotations on figure:* 6VE (near Maxillary division); Communicating branch to zygomatic nerve (circled); SVA (on tongue); 6VE (near top); "VII also provides Parasympathetics to the mucosal glands of the Nose, maxillary sinus, palate, palatal tonsils — all 6VE"; "Supplied by the Lingual Nerve ↳ postganglionic parasympathetics 6VE"

**Fig. 4.38 Facial nerve ganglia**
Autonomic and taste fibers often travel with sensory fibers from other nerves to reach their targets. Parasympathetic and taste fibers leave the facial nerve via two branches: the greater petrosal nerve and the chorda tympani.

- **Greater petrosal nerve:** Preganglionic parasympathetic and taste fibers from the geniculate ganglion course in the greater petrosal canal. They are joined by the deep petrosal nerve, which conveys postganglionic sympathetic fibers from the superior cervical ganglion (via the internal carotid plexus). The greater and deep petrosal nerves combine to form the nerve of the pterygoid canal (vidian), which conveys sympathetic, parasympathetic, and taste fibers to the pterygopalatine ganglion (only parasympathetics will synapse at the ganglion; all other fiber types pass through without synapsing). Branches of CN V$_2$ then distribute the fibers to their targets:
  - **Lacrimal gland:** Autonomic fibers (sympathetic and parasympathetic) run with branches of CN V$_2$ (zygomatic and zygomaticotemporal nerves) to a communicating branch, which conveys them to the lacrimal nerve (CN V$_1$) and thus to the lacrimal gland.
  - **Small glands of the nasal and oral cavities:** Autonomic fibers run with branches of CN V$_2$ to the small glands in the mucosa of the nasal cavity, maxillary sinuses, and palatine tonsils.
  - **Taste:** Taste fibers run with branches of CN V$_2$ to the soft palate.

- **Chorda tympani:** Preganglionic parasympathetic and taste fibers course through the chorda tympani. They emerge from the petrotympanic fissure and combine with the lingual nerve (CN V$_3$) in the infratemporal fossa. They are conveyed to the submandibular ganglion by the lingual nerve, and from there, postganglionic branches travel to their targets via branches of CN V$_3$.
  - **Submandibular and sublingual glands:** Postganglionic parasympathetic fibers run with branches of CN V$_3$ to the glands.
  - **Taste buds of tongue:** The taste buds on the presulcal portion of the tongue receive taste fibers from the chorda tympani via the lingual nerve (CN V$_3$). *Note:* The postsulcal portion of the tongue and the oropharynx receive taste fibers from CN IX. The root of the tongue and epiglottis receive taste fibers from CN X.

*Note:* The **lesser petrosal nerve** runs in the lesser petrosal canal roughly parallel to the greater petrosal nerve. The lesser petrosal nerve conveys preganglionic parasympathetic fibers from the tympanic plexus (CN IX) to the otic ganglion. These fibers innervate the parotid, buccal, and inferior labial glands, with postganglionic fibers distributed via branches of CN V$_3$.

*Handwritten note:* "The lesser petrosal runs preganglionic Parasympathetics to the otic ganglion which then runs to the parotid gland"

# CN VIII: Vestibulocochlear Nerve → NO Sensory

*[handwritten: CN 5, 7, 9, 10 Provide Sensory to ear & tympanic membrane vestibule]*

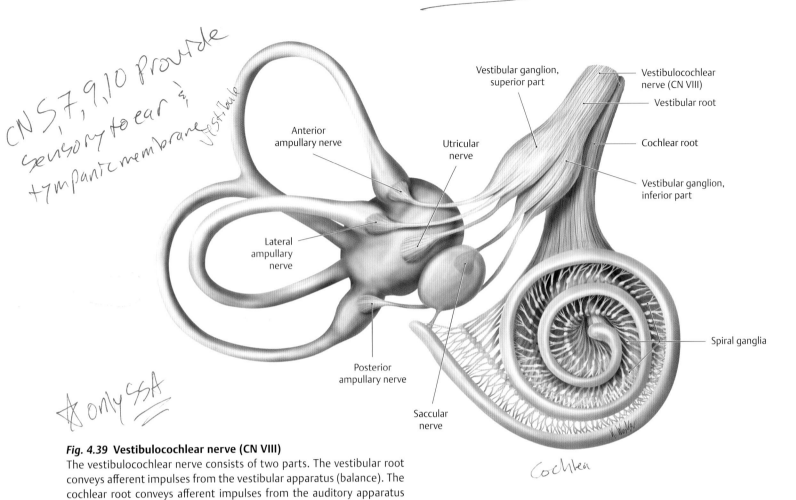

*[handwritten: # only SSA]*

**Fig. 4.39 Vestibulocochlear nerve (CN VIII)**
The vestibulocochlear nerve consists of two parts. The vestibular root conveys afferent impulses from the vestibular apparatus (balance). The cochlear root conveys afferent impulses from the auditory apparatus (hearing).

*[handwritten: Cochlea]*

| Table 4.23 Vestibulocochlear nerve (CN VIII) | | |
|---|---|---|
| **Nuclei, ganglia, and fiber distribution** | | |
| **Special somatic afferent** (orange): Special somatic sensory neurons convey sensory fibers from the vestibular apparatus (balance) and auditory apparatus (hearing). Both parts of the nerve contain first-order bipolar sensory neurons. | | |
| **Neurons** | **Vestibular root** | **Cochlear root** |
| Peripheral processes | In the sensory cells of the semicircular canals, the saccule, and the utricle. | In the hair cells of the organ of Corti. |
| Cell bodies | **Vestibular ganglion**<br>• Inferior part: Peripheral processes from saccule and posterior semicircular canal.<br>• Superior part: Peripheral processes from anterior and lateral semicircular canals and utricle. | **Spiral ganglia.** The peripheral processes from the neurons in these myriad ganglia radiate outward to receive sensory input from the spiral modiolus. |
| Central processes (axons) | To four **vestibular nuclei** in the medulla oblongata (floor of the rhomboid fossa). A few pass directly to the cerebellum via the inferior cerebellar peduncle. | To two **cochlear nuclei** lateral to the vestibular nuclei. |
| Nuclei | Superior, lateral, medial, and inferior vestibular nuclei. | Anterior and posterior cochlear nuclei. |
| Lesions | Dizziness. | Hearing loss (ranging to deafness). |
| **Course** | | |
| The vestibular and cochlear roots unite in the internal acoustic meatus to form the vestibulocochlear nerve, which is covered by a common connective tissue sheath. The nerve emerges from the internal acoustic meatus on the medial surface of the petrous bone and enters the brainstem at the level of the pontomedullary junction, in particular at the cerebellopontine angle. | | |

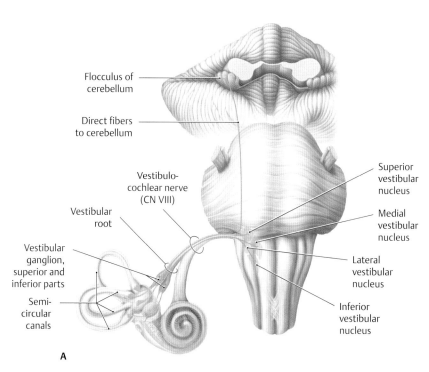

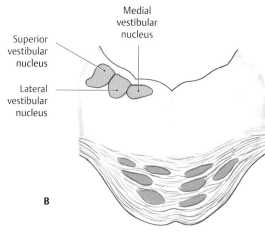

**Fig. 4.40 Vestibular root and nuclei**
**A** Anterior view of the medulla oblongata and pons. **B** Cross section through the upper medulla oblongata.

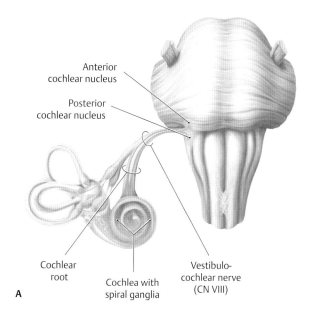

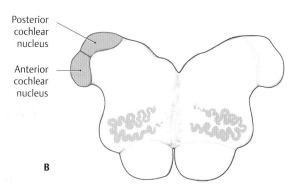

**Fig. 4.41 Cochlear root and nuclei**
**A** Anterior view of the medulla oblongata and pons. **B** Cross section through the upper medulla oblongata.

**Fig. 4.42 Acoustic neuroma in the cerebellopontine angle**
Acoustic neuromas (more accurately, vestibular schwannomas) are benign tumors of the cerebellopontine angle arising from the Schwann cells of the vestibular root of CN VIII. As they grow, they compress and displace the adjacent structures and cause slowly progressive hearing loss and gait ataxia. Large tumors can impair the egress of CSF from the 4th ventricle, causing hydrocephalus and symptomatic intracranial hypertension (vomiting, impairment of consciousness).

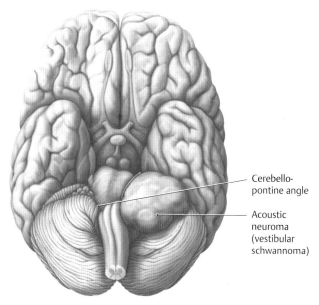

**87**

# CN IX: Glossopharyngeal Nerve

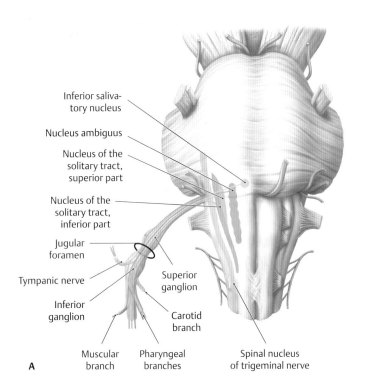

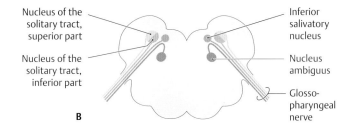

**Fig. 4.43 Glossopharyngeal nerve nuclei**
**A** Anterior view of brainstem. **B** Cross section through the medulla oblongata.

| Table 4.24 Glossopharyngeal nerve (CN IX) | |
|---|---|
| **Nuclei, ganglia, and fiber distribution** | |
| **Branchiomotor** (purple) | |
| Nucleus ambiguus | Lower motor neurons innervate the muscles derived from the 3rd, 4th, and 6th branchial arches via CN IX, X, and XI.<br>• CN IX innervates the derivative of the 3rd branchial arch (stylopharyngeus) |
| **Parasympathetic** (blue) | |
| Inferior salivatory nucleus | Preganglionic neurons synapse in the **otic ganglion**. |
| | Postganglionic neurons innervate:<br>• Parotid gland (**Fig. 4.44A**)<br>• Buccal glands<br>• Inferior labial glands |
| **General somatic afferent** (yellow) | |
| Spinal nucleus of CN V | First-order pseudounipolar cells in the **superior ganglion** of CN IX innervate:<br>• Nasopharynx, oropharynx, postsulcal tongue, palatine tonsils, and uvula (**Fig. 4.44B,C**). These fibers include the afferent limb of the gag reflex.<br>• Tympanic cavity and pharyngotympanic tube (**Fig. 4.44D**). |
| **Viscerosensory** (green) | |
| First-order pseudounipolar cells in the **inferior ganglion** relay taste and visceral sensation to the **nucleus of the solitary tract**. This nuclear complex consists of a superior part (taste) and inferior part (general visceral sensation). | |
| Nucleus of the solitary tract | Taste (**Fig. 4.44E**): Special viscerosensory fibers from the postsulcal tongue synapse in the **superior part**. |
| | Visceral sensation (**Fig. 4.44F**): General viscerosensory fibers from the carotid body (chemoreceptors) and carotid sinus (pressure receptors) synapse in the **inferior part**. |
| **Course** | |
| The glossopharyngeal nerve arises from the medulla oblongata and exits the skull by passing through the jugular foramen. It has two sensory ganglia with first-order pseudounipolar sensory cells: the superior ganglion (somatosensory) is within the cranial cavity, and the inferior ganglion (viscerosensory) is distal to the jugular foramen. | |
| **Lesions** | |
| Isolated CN IX lesions are rare. Lesions tend to occur during basal skull fractures, which disrupt the jugular foramen. Such injuries would affect CN IX, X, and XI. | |

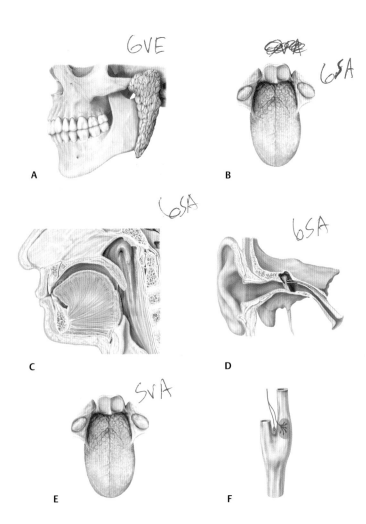

**Fig. 4.44 Distribution of CN IX fibers**

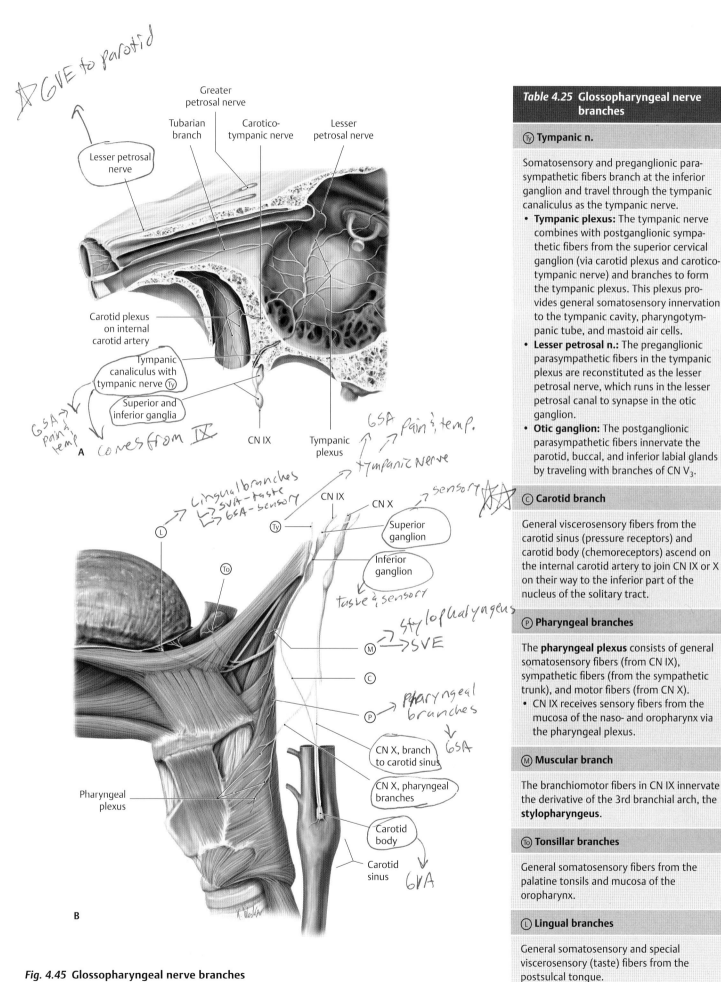

*Fig. 4.45* **Glossopharyngeal nerve branches**
**A** Left anterolateral view of opened tympanic cavity. **B** Left lateral view.

*Table 4.25* **Glossopharyngeal nerve branches**

**ⓉⓎ Tympanic n.**

Somatosensory and preganglionic para-sympathetic fibers branch at the inferior ganglion and travel through the tympanic canaliculus as the tympanic nerve.
- **Tympanic plexus:** The tympanic nerve combines with postganglionic sympathetic fibers from the superior cervical ganglion (via carotid plexus and carotico-tympanic nerve) and branches to form the tympanic plexus. This plexus provides general somatosensory innervation to the tympanic cavity, pharyngotympanic tube, and mastoid air cells.
- **Lesser petrosal n.:** The preganglionic parasympathetic fibers in the tympanic plexus are reconstituted as the lesser petrosal nerve, which runs in the lesser petrosal canal to synapse in the otic ganglion.
- **Otic ganglion:** The postganglionic parasympathetic fibers innervate the parotid, buccal, and inferior labial glands by traveling with branches of CN V₃.

**Ⓒ Carotid branch**

General viscerosensory fibers from the carotid sinus (pressure receptors) and carotid body (chemoreceptors) ascend on the internal carotid artery to join CN IX or X on their way to the inferior part of the nucleus of the solitary tract.

**Ⓟ Pharyngeal branches**

The **pharyngeal plexus** consists of general somatosensory fibers (from CN IX), sympathetic fibers (from the sympathetic trunk), and motor fibers (from CN X).
- CN IX receives sensory fibers from the mucosa of the naso- and oropharynx via the pharyngeal plexus.

**Ⓜ Muscular branch**

The branchiomotor fibers in CN IX innervate the derivative of the 3rd branchial arch, the **stylopharyngeus**.

**Ⓣⓞ Tonsillar branches**

General somatosensory fibers from the palatine tonsils and mucosa of the oropharynx.

**Ⓛ Lingual branches**

General somatosensory and special viscerosensory (taste) fibers from the postsulcal tongue.

89

# CN X: Vagus Nerve

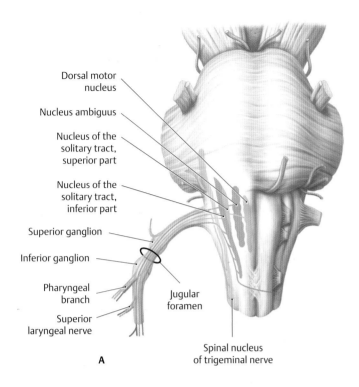

**A**

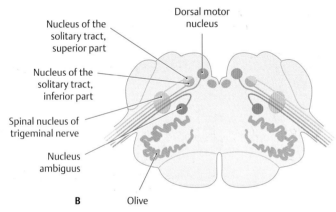

**B**      Olive

**Fig. 4.46 Vagus nerve nuclei**
**A** Anterior view of medulla oblongata. **B** Cross section through the medulla oblongata.
The vagus nerve has the most extensive distribution of all the cranial nerves (L. *vagus* = vagabond). Parasympathetic fibers descend into the thorax and abdomen. These fibers form autonomic plexuses with post-ganglionic sympathetic fibers (from the sympathetic trunk and abdominal ganglia). The plexuses extend along organs and blood vessels and provide motor innervation to the thoracic and abdominal viscera. General viscerosensory fibers ascend via CN X to the inferior part of the nucleus of the solitary tract.

**Table 4.26** Vagus nerve (CN X)

**Nuclei, ganglia, and fiber distribution**

**Branchiomotor** (purple)

| | |
|---|---|
| Nucleus ambiguus | Lower motor neurons innervate the muscles derived from the 3rd, 4th, and 6th branchial arches via CN IX, X, and XI. CN X innervates the derivatives of the 4th and 6th branchial arches:<br>• Pharyngeal muscles (pharyngeal constrictors)<br>• Muscles of the soft palate (levator veli palatini, musculus uvulae, palatoglossus, palatopharyngeus)<br>• Intrinsic laryngeal muscles |

**Parasympathetic** (blue)

| | |
|---|---|
| Dorsal motor nucleus | Preganglionic neurons synapse in small, unnamed ganglia close to target structures. |
| | Postganglionic neurons innervate:<br>• Smooth muscles and glands of thoracic and abdominal viscera (**Fig. 4.48G**) |

**General somatic afferent** (yellow)

| | |
|---|---|
| Spinal nucleus of CN V | First-order pseudounipolar cells in the **superior (jugular) ganglion** innervate:<br>• Dura of the posterior cranial fossa (**Fig. 4.48F**)<br>• Auricle, external auditory canal, and lateral tympanic membrane (**Fig. 4.48B,C**)<br>• Mucosa of the oropharynx and laryngopharynx |

**Viscerosensory** (green)

First-order pseudounipolar cells in the **inferior (nodose) ganglion** relay taste and visceral sensation to the **nucleus of the solitary tract**. This nuclear complex consists of a superior part (taste) and inferior part (general visceral sensation).

| | |
|---|---|
| Nucleus of the solitary tract | Taste (**Fig. 4.48D**): Fibers from the epiglottis and the root of the tongue are conveyed to the **superior part** of the nucleus of the solitary tract. |
| | Visceral sensation (**Fig. 4.48G**): Fibers are relayed to the **inferior part** of the nucleus of the solitary tract from:<br>• Mucosa of the laryngopharynx and larynx (**Fig. 4.48A**)<br>• Aortic arch (pressure receptors) and para-aortic body (chemoreceptors) (**Fig. 4.48E**)<br>• Thoracic and abdominal viscera (**Fig. 4.48G**) |

**Course**

The vagus nerve arises from the medulla oblongata and emerges from the skull via the jugular foramen. It has two sensory ganglia with first-order pseudounipolar cells: the superior (jugular) ganglion (soma-tosensory) is within the cranial cavity, and the inferior (nodose) ganglion (viscerosensory) is distal to the jugular foramen.

**Lesions**

The recurrent laryngeal nerve supplies parasympathetic innervation to the intrinsic laryngeal muscles (except the cricothyroid). This includes the posterior cricoarytenoid, the only muscle that abducts the vocal cords. Unilateral lesions of this nerve cause hoarseness; bilateral destruction leads to respiratory distress (dyspnea).

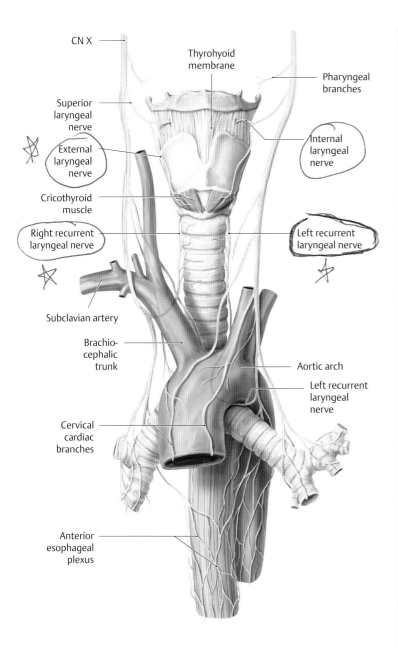

**Fig. 4.47 Vagus nerve branches in the neck**
Anterior view.

CN X
Thyrohyoid membrane
Pharyngeal branches
Superior laryngeal nerve
Internal laryngeal nerve
External laryngeal nerve
Cricothyroid muscle
Right recurrent laryngeal nerve
Left recurrent laryngeal nerve
Subclavian artery
Brachio-cephalic trunk
Aortic arch
Left recurrent laryngeal nerve
Cervical cardiac branches
Anterior esophageal plexus

### Table 4.27 Vagus nerve branches

**Meningeal branches**

General somatosensory fibers from the dura of the posterior cranial fossa.

**Auricular branch**

General somatosensory fibers from external ear (auricle, external acoustic canal, and part of lateral side of tympanic membrane).

**Pharyngeal branches**

The **pharyngeal plexus** consists of general somatosensory fibers (from CN IX), sympathetic fibers (from the sympathetic trunk), and motor fibers (from CN X).
• CN X conveys branchiomotor fibers to the pharyngeal muscles.

**Carotid branch**

General viscerosensory fibers from the carotid body (chemoreceptors) ascend on the internal carotid artery to join CN IX or X on their way to the inferior part of the nucleus of the solitary tract.

**Superior laryngeal n.**

Combines with a sympathetic branch from the superior cervical ganglion and divides into:
• **Internal laryngeal n.:** Sensory fibers from the mucosa of the laryngopharynx and larynx.
• **External laryngeal n.:** Parasympathetic motor innervation to the cricothyroid.

**Recurrent laryngeal n.**

The recurrent laryngeal nerve is asymmetrical:
• Right recurrent laryngeal n.: Recurs behind the right subclavian artery.
• Left recurrent laryngeal n.: Recurs behind the aortic arch.
Ascends between the trachea and esophagus. The recurrent laryngeal nerves supply:
• Motor innervation to the laryngeal muscles (except the cricothyroid).
• Viscerosensory innervation to the laryngeal mucosa.

**Branches to the thorax and abdomen**

The vagus nerve also conveys parasympathetic and general viscerosensory fibers from the cardiac, pulmonary, esophageal, celiac, renal, hepatic, and gastric plexuses (**Fig. 4.48G**)

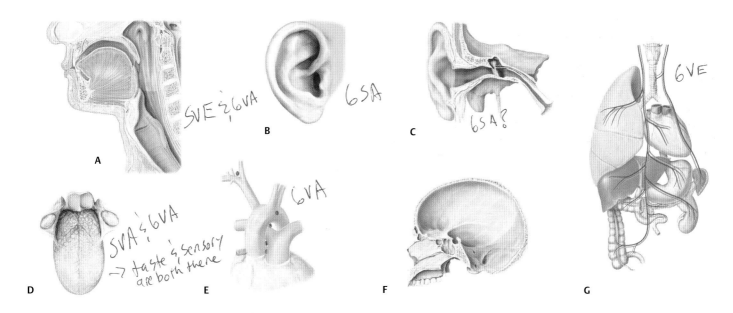

**Fig. 4.48 Distribution of the vagus nerve (CN X)**

# CN XI & XII: Accessory Spinal & Hypoglossal Nerves

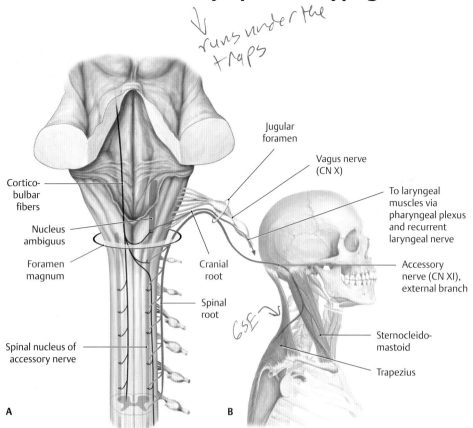

*Fig. 4.49 Accessory nerve*
**A** Posterior view of brainstem. **B** Right lateral view of sternocleidomastoid and trapezius.

(*Note:* For didactic reasons, the right muscles are displayed though they are innervated by the right cranial nerve nuclei.)

| Table 4.28 Accessory nerve (CN XI) |
|---|
| **Nuclei, ganglia, and fiber distribution** |

**Branchiomotor** (purple)

| Nucleus ambiguus | Lower motor neurons innervate the muscles derived from the 3rd, 4th, and 6th branchial arches via CN IX, X, and XI.<br>• CN XI innervates the laryngeal muscles (except cricoarytenoid). |
|---|---|

**General somatomotor** (red)

| Spinal nucleus of CN XI | Lower motor neurons in the lateral part of the ventral horn of C2–C6 spinal cord segments innervate:<br>• Trapezius (upper part).<br>• Sternocleidomastoid. |
|---|---|

**Course**

CN XI arises and courses in two parts that unite briefly distal to the jugular foramen:

**Cranial root:** Branchiomotor fibers emerge from the medulla oblongata and pass through the jugular foramen. They briefly unite with the spinal root before joining CN X at the inferior ganglion. CN X distributes the branchiomotor fibers via the pharyngeal plexus and the external and recurrent laryngeal nerves.

**Spinal root:** General somatomotor fibers emerge as rootlets from the spinal medulla. They unite and ascend through the foramen magnum. The spinal root then passes through the jugular foramen, courses briefly with the cranial root, and then descends to innervate the sternocleidomastoid and trapezius.

**Lesions**

The sternocleidomastoid is exclusively innervated by CN XI, and the lower portions of the trapezius are innervated by C3–C5. Accessory nerve lesions therefore cause complete (flaccid) sternocleidomastoid paralysis but only partial trapezius paralysis.

**Trapezius paralysis:** Unilateral lesions may occur during operations in the neck (e.g., lymph node biopsies), causing:
• Drooping of the shoulder on the affected side.
• Difficulty raising the arm above the horizontal.

**Sternocleidomastoid paralysis:**
• Unilateral lesions: Flaccid paralysis causes torticollis (wry neck, i.e., difficulty turning the head to the opposite side).
• Bilateral lesions: Difficulty holding the head upright.

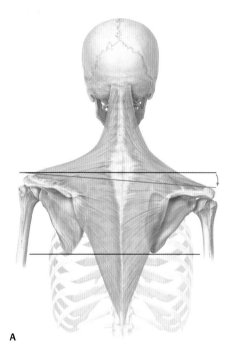

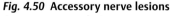

*Fig. 4.50 Accessory nerve lesions*
Accessory nerve lesions cause partial paralysis of the trapezius and complete (flaccid) paralysis of the sternocleidomastoid (see **Table 4.28**). Both lesions shown here are unilateral (right side). **A** Posterior view. Partial paralysis of the trapezius causes drooping of the shoulder on the affected side. **B** Right anterolateral view. Flaccid paralysis of the sternocleidomastoid causes torticollis (wry neck).

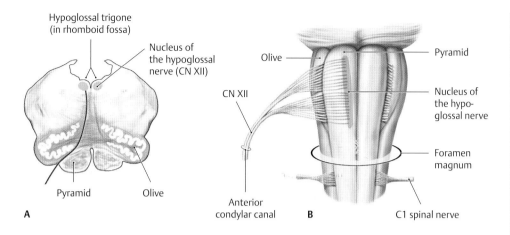

Hypoglossal trigone
(in rhomboid fossa)

Nucleus of
the hypoglossal
nerve (CN XII)

Olive

Pyramid

CN XII

Nucleus of
the hypo-
glossal nerve

Pyramid

Olive

Foramen
magnum

**A**

Anterior
condylar canal

**B**

C1 spinal nerve

### Fig. 4.51 Hypoglossal nerve nuclei

The nucleus of the hypoglossal nerve is located in the floor of the rhomboid fossa. Rootlets emerge between the pyramid and the olive.

**A** Cross section through the medulla oblongata. The proximity of the nuclei to the midline causes extensive lesions to involve both nuclei. **B** Anterior view of medulla oblongata.

### Table 4.29 Hypoglossal nerve (CN XII)

**Nuclei, ganglia, and fiber distribution**

**General somatomotor** (red)

| | |
|---|---|
| Nucleus of CN XII | Lower motor neurons innervate:<br>• Extrinsic lingual muscles (except palatoglossus).<br>• Intrinsic lingual muscles. |

**Course**

The hypoglossal nerve emerges from the medulla oblongata as rootlets between the olive and pyramid. These rootlets combine into CN XII, which courses through the hypoglossal (anterior condylar) canal. CN XII enters the root of the tongue superior to the hyoid bone and lateral to the hyoglossus.
• C1 motor fibers from the cervical plexus travel with the hypoglossal nerve: some branch to form the superior root of the ansa cervicalis (not shown), whereas others continue with CN XII to supply the geniohyoid and thyrohyoid muscles.

**Lesions**

Upper motor neurons innervate the lower motor neurons in the contralateral nucleus of the hypoglossal nerve. Supranuclear lesions (central hypoglossal paralysis) will therefore cause the tongue to deviate away from the affected side. Nuclear or peripheral lesions will cause the tongue to deviate toward the affected side (**Fig. 4.52C**).

Precentral
gyrus

Left and right
genioglossus muscles

Paralyzed
genioglossus

**B**

**C**

Cortico-
bulbar
fibers

Styloglossus
muscle

Tongue

### Fig. 4.52 Hypoglossal nerve

**A** Course of the hypoglossal nerve. Upper motor neurons synapse on lower motor neurons on the contralateral nucleus of the hypoglossal nerve. Supranuclear lesions will therefore cause contralateral paralysis; peripheral lesions will cause ipsilateral paralysis (same side). **B** The functional genioglossus extends the tongue anteriorly. **C** Unilateral paralysis due to a peripheral lesion causes the tongue to deviate *toward* the affected side (dominance of the intact genioglossus).

CN X

C1

CN XII

Nucleus of
the hypoglossal
nerve

Anterior
condylar
canal

Genioglossus muscle

Hyoglossus
muscle

**A**

*only GSE* (handwritten)

*→ Innervates the intrinsic muscles of the tongue & the extrinsic muscles of the tongue* (handwritten)

# Neurovascular Pathways through the Skull Base

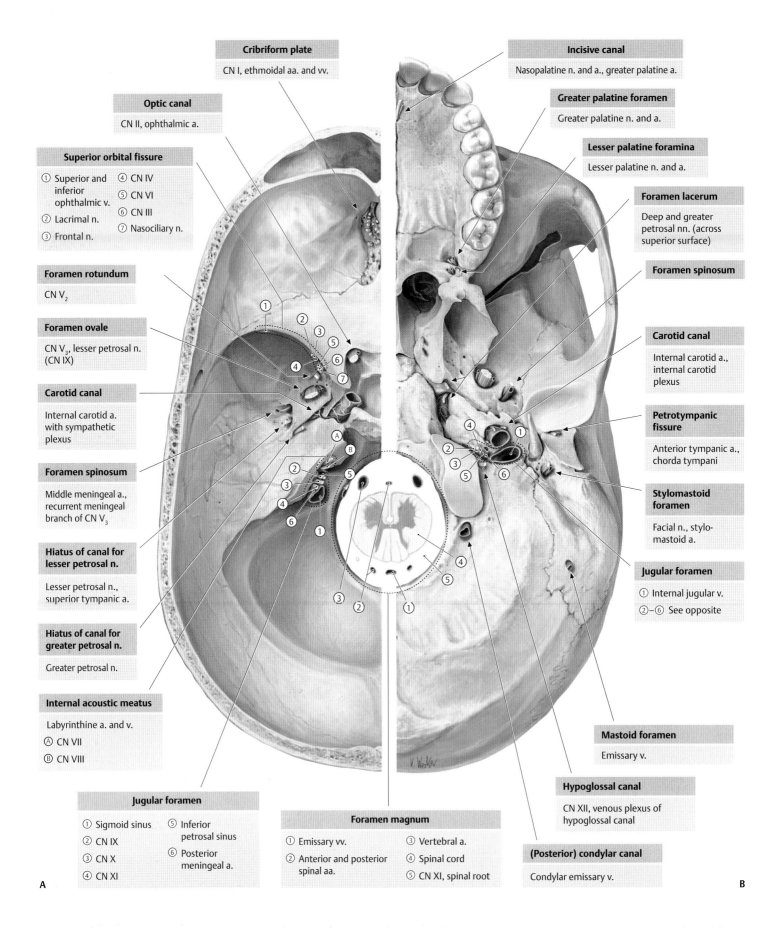

**Cribriform plate**
CN I, ethmoidal aa. and vv.

**Optic canal**
CN II, ophthalmic a.

**Superior orbital fissure**
① Superior and inferior ophthalmic v.
② Lacrimal n.
③ Frontal n.
④ CN IV
⑤ CN VI
⑥ CN III
⑦ Nasociliary n.

**Foramen rotundum**
CN V₂

**Foramen ovale**
CN V₃, lesser petrosal n. (CN IX)

**Carotid canal**
Internal carotid a. with sympathetic plexus

**Foramen spinosum**
Middle meningeal a., recurrent meningeal branch of CN V₃

**Hiatus of canal for lesser petrosal n.**
Lesser petrosal n., superior tympanic a.

**Hiatus of canal for greater petrosal n.**
Greater petrosal n.

**Internal acoustic meatus**
Labyrinthine a. and v.
Ⓐ CN VII
Ⓑ CN VIII

**Incisive canal**
Nasopalatine n. and a., greater palatine a.

**Greater palatine foramen**
Greater palatine n. and a.

**Lesser palatine foramina**
Lesser palatine n. and a.

**Foramen lacerum**
Deep and greater petrosal nn. (across superior surface)

**Foramen spinosum**

**Carotid canal**
Internal carotid a., internal carotid plexus

**Petrotympanic fissure**
Anterior tympanic a., chorda tympani

**Stylomastoid foramen**
Facial n., stylomastoid a.

**Jugular foramen**
① Internal jugular v.
②–⑥ See opposite

**Mastoid foramen**
Emissary v.

**Hypoglossal canal**
CN XII, venous plexus of hypoglossal canal

**(Posterior) condylar canal**
Condylar emissary v.

**Jugular foramen**
① Sigmoid sinus
② CN IX
③ CN X
④ CN XI
⑤ Inferior petrosal sinus
⑥ Posterior meningeal a.

**Foramen magnum**
① Emissary vv.
② Anterior and posterior spinal aa.
③ Vertebral a.
④ Spinal cord
⑤ CN XI, spinal root

A                                                                                                    B

***Fig. 4.53* Passage of neurovascular structures through the skull base**
**A** Superior view of cranial cavity. **B** Inferior view of base of skull. This image and the corresponding table only address structures entering and exiting the skull. Many neurovascular structures pass through bony canals within the skull (to pterygopalatine fossa, infratemporal fossa, etc.).

### Table 4.30 Openings in the skull base

| Cranial cavity | Opening | Transmitted structures | |
|---|---|---|---|
| | | Nerves | Arteries and veins |
| **Internal view, base of the skull** | | | |
| Anterior cranial fossa | Cribriform plate | • CN I (olfactory fibers collected to form olfactory n.) | • Anterior and posterior ethmoidal aa. (from ophthalmic a.)<br>• Ethmoidal vv. (to superior ophthalmic v.) |
| Middle cranial fossa | Optic canal | • CN II (optic n.) | • Ophthalmic a. (from internal carotid a.) |
| | Superior orbital fissure | • CN III (oculomotor n.)<br>• CN IV (trochlear n.)<br>• CN IV (abducent n.)<br>• CN V$_1$ (ophthalmic n.) divisions (lacrimal, frontal, and nasociliary nn.) | • Superior and inferior ophthalmic vv. (to cavernous sinus) (*Note:* The inferior ophthalmic v. also drains through the inferior orbital fissure to the pterygoid plexus.) |
| | Foramen rotundum* | • CN V$_2$ (maxillary n.) | |
| | Foramen ovale | • CN V$_3$ (mandibular n.)<br>• Lesser petrosal n. (CN IX) | • Accessory meningeal a. (from mandibular part of maxillary a.) |
| | Foramen spinosum | • CN V$_3$, recurrent meningeal branch | • Middle meningeal a. (from mandibular part of maxillary a.) |
| | Carotid canal | • Carotid plexus (postganglionic sympathetics from superior cervical ganglion) | • Internal carotid a. |
| | Hiatus of canal for greater petrosal n. | • Greater petrosal n. (CN VII) | |
| | Hiatus of canal for lesser petrosal n. | • Lesser petrosal n. (CN IX) | • Superior tympanic a. (from middle meningeal a.) |
| Posterior cranial fossa | Internal acoustic meatus | • CN VII (facial n.)<br>• CN VIII (vestibulocochlear n.) | • Labyrinthine a. (from vertebral a.)<br>• Labyrinthine vv. (to superior petrosal or transverse sinus) |
| | Jugular foramen | • CN IX (glossopharyngeal n.)<br>• CN X (vagus n.)<br>• CN XI (accessory n., cranial root) | • Internal jugular v. (bulb)<br>• Sigmoid sinus (to bulb of internal jugular v.)<br>• Posterior meningeal a. (from ascending pharyngeal a.) |
| | Hypoglossal canal | • CN XII (hypoglossal n.) | • Venous plexus of hypoglossal canal |
| | Foramen magnum | • Medulla oblongata with meningeal coverings<br>• CN XI (accessory n.) | • Vertebral aa.<br>• Anterior and posterior spinal aa. (from vertebral a.)<br>• Emissary vv. |
| **External aspect, base of the skull (where different from internal aspect)** | | | |
| | Incisive canal | • Nasopalatine n. (from CN V$_2$) | • Branch of greater palatine a. |
| | Greater palatine foramen | • Greater palatine n. (from CN V$_2$) | • Greater palatine a. (from pterygopalatine part of maxillary a.) |
| | Lesser palatine foramen | • Lesser palatine n. (from CN V$_2$) | • Lesser palatine aa. (from pterygopalatine part of maxillary a. or as branch of greater palatine a. or descending palatine a.) |
| | Foramen lacerum** | • Deep petrosal n. (from superior cervical ganglion via carotid plexus)<br>• Greater petrosal n. (from CN VII) | |
| | Petrotympanic fissure | • Chorda tympani (from CN VII) | • Anterior tympanic a. (from mandibular part of maxillary a.) |
| | Stylomastoid foramen | • Facial n. (CN VII) | • Stylomastoid a. (from posterior auricular a.) |
| | (Posterior) condylar canal | | • Condylar emissary v. (to sigmoid sinus) |
| | Mastoid foramen | | • Mastoid emissary v. (to sigmoid sinus) |

*The external opening of the foramen rotundum is located in the pterygopalatine fossa, which is located deep on the lateral surface of the base of the skull and is not visible here.

**Structures travel over the superior surface of the foramen lacerum, not through it (with the possible exception of lymphatic vessels and emissary veins).

# Anterior Face

The bones and muscles of the skull are shown in isolation in **Chapter 1** and **Chapter 2**, respectively. The arteries and veins are discussed in **Chapter 3**; the nerves are found in **Chapter 4**.

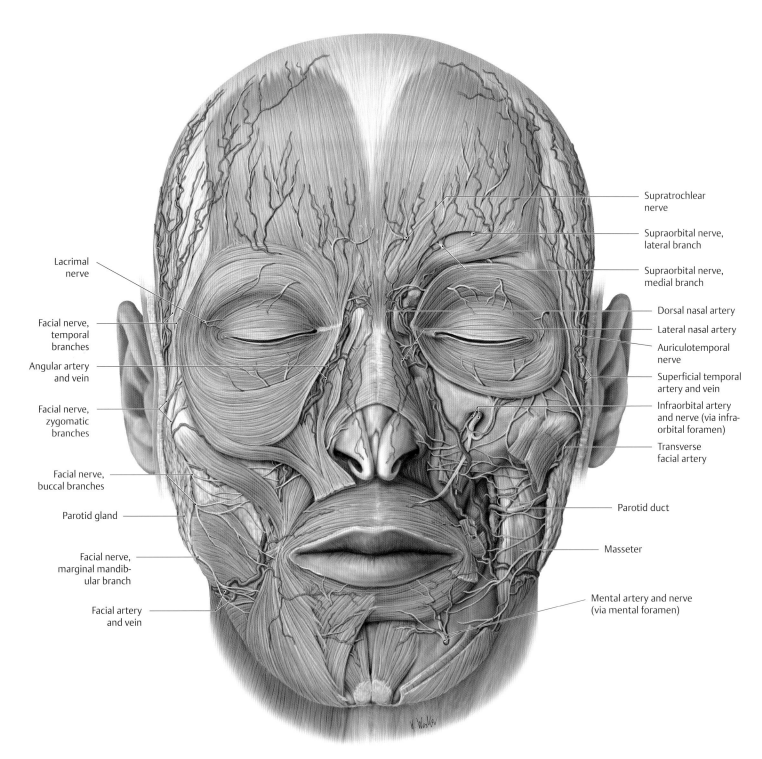

**Fig. 5.1 Superficial neurovasculature of the anterior face**
*Removed:* Skin and fatty tissue. The muscles of facial expression have been partially removed on the left side to display underlying musculature and neurovascular structures. The muscles of facial expression receive motor innervation from the facial nerve (CN VII), which emerges laterally from the parotid gland. The muscles of mastication receive motor innervation from the mandibular division of the trigemi-

nal nerve (CN V₃). The face receives sensory innervation primarily from the terminal branches of the three divisions of the trigeminal nerve (CN V), but also from the great auricular nerve, which arises from the cervical plexus (see **Fig. 5.10**). The face receives blood supply primarily from branches of the external carotid artery, though these do anastomose on the face with facial branches of the internal carotid artery (see **Fig. 5.2**).

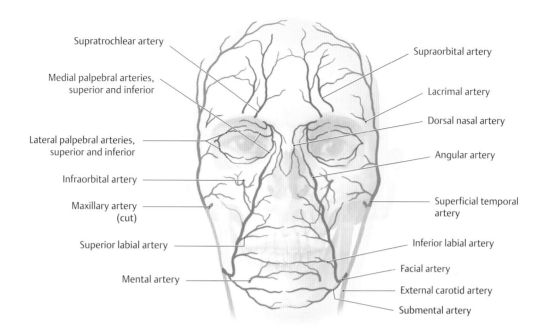

**Fig. 5.2 Arterial anastomoses in the face**
Branches of the external carotid artery (e.g., facial, superficial temporal, and maxillary arteries) and the internal carotid artery (e.g., dorsal nasal, supraorbital, and lacrimal arteries) anastomose in certain facial regions to ensure blood flow to the face and head. Anastomoses occur between the angular artery and the dorsal nasal artery, as well as between the superficial temporal artery and the supraorbital artery.

This extensive vascular supply to the face causes head injuries to bleed profusely but also heal quickly. The anastomoses are also important in cases of reduced blood flow (e.g., atherosclerosis). Cerebral ischemia, which can result from atherosclerosis of the internal carotid artery, may be avoided if there is sufficient blood flow through the superficial temporal and facial arteries.

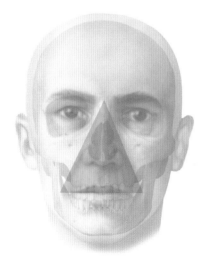

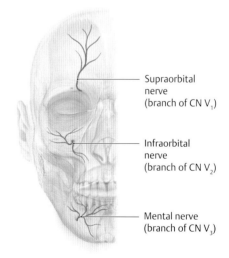

**Fig. 5.3 Venous "danger zone" in the face**
The superficial veins of the face have extensive connections with the deep veins of the head (e.g., the pterygoid plexus) and dural sinuses (e.g., the cavernous sinus) (see p. 53). Veins in the triangular danger zone are, in general, valveless. There is therefore a particularly high risk of bacterial dissemination into the cranial cavity. For example, bacteria from a boil on the lip may enter the facial vein and cause meningitis by passing through venous communications with the cavernous sinus.

**Fig. 5.4 Emergence of the trigeminal nerve**
The trigeminal nerve (CN V) is the major somatic sensory nerve of the head. Its three large sensory branches emerge from three foramina:

- CN $V_1$: Supraorbital nerve (through supraorbital foramen)
- CN $V_2$: Infraorbital nerve (through infraorbital foramen)
- CN $V_3$: Mental nerve (through mental foramen)

**97**

# Lateral Head: Superficial Layer

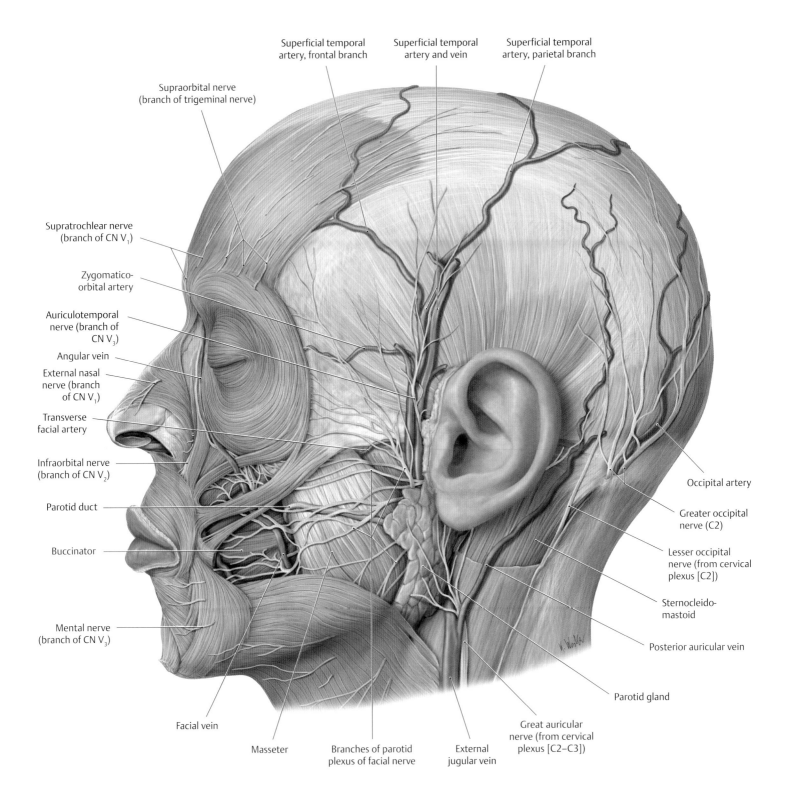

Superficial temporal artery, frontal branch

Superficial temporal artery and vein

Superficial temporal artery, parietal branch

Supraorbital nerve (branch of trigeminal nerve)

Supratrochlear nerve (branch of CN V$_1$)

Zygomatico-orbital artery

Auriculotemporal nerve (branch of CN V$_3$)

Angular vein

External nasal nerve (branch of CN V$_1$)

Transverse facial artery

Infraorbital nerve (branch of CN V$_2$)

Parotid duct

Buccinator

Mental nerve (branch of CN V$_3$)

Facial vein

Masseter

Branches of parotid plexus of facial nerve

External jugular vein

Great auricular nerve (from cervical plexus [C2–C3])

Occipital artery

Greater occipital nerve (C2)

Lesser occipital nerve (from cervical plexus [C2])

Sternocleido-mastoid

Posterior auricular vein

Parotid gland

**Fig. 5.5 Superficial neurovasculature of the lateral head**
Left lateral view. The arteries supplying the lateral head arise from branches of the external carotid artery (see **Fig. 5.6**). Blood drains primarily into the internal, external, and anterior jugular veins (see p. 52). The muscles of facial expression receive motor innervation from the facial nerve (CN VII), which emerges laterally from the parotid gland (see p. 84). The muscles of mastication receive motor innervation from the mandibular division of the trigeminal nerve (CN V$_3$, see p. 81). The sensory innervation of the face is shown in **Fig. 5.7**.

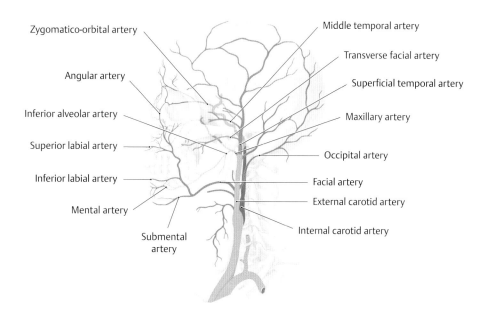

**Fig. 5.6 Superficial arteries of the head**
Left lateral view. The superficial face is supplied primarily by branches of the external carotid artery (e.g., facial, superficial temporal, and maxillary arteries). However, there is limited contribution from branches derived from the internal carotid artery in the region of the orbital rim.

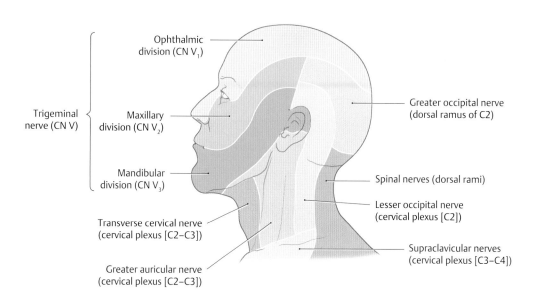

**Fig. 5.7 Sensory innervation of the lateral head and neck**
Left lateral view. The head receives sensory innervation primarily from the trigeminal nerve (orange), the cervical plexus (green and gray), and the dorsal rami of the spinal nerves (blue). Sensory supply to the face is primarily from the terminal branches of the three trigeminal nerve divisions. The occiput and nuchal region are supplied primarily by dorsal rami of the spinal nerves. The ventral rami of the first four spinal nerves combine to form the cervical plexus. The cervical plexus gives off four cutaneous branches that supply the lateral head and neck (nerves listed with their associated spinal nerve fibers): lesser occipital (C2, occasionally C3), greater auricular (C2–C3), transverse cervical (C2–C3), and supraclavicular (C3–C4) nerves.

# Lateral Head: Intermediate Layer

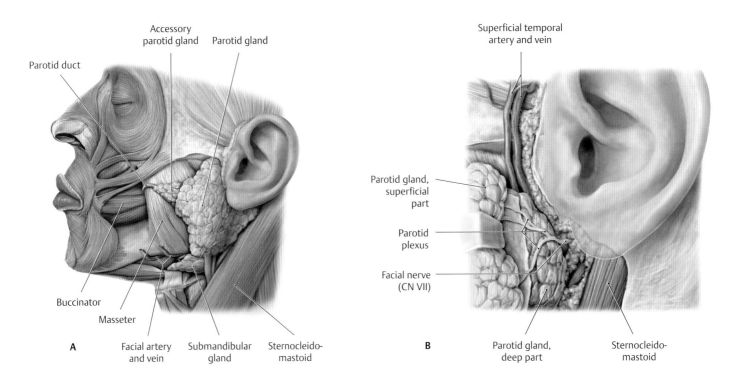

**A**  Parotid duct — Accessory parotid gland — Parotid gland — Buccinator — Masseter — Facial artery and vein — Submandibular gland — Sternocleido-mastoid

**B**  Superficial temporal artery and vein — Parotid gland, superficial part — Parotid plexus — Facial nerve (CN VII) — Parotid gland, deep part — Sternocleido-mastoid

**Fig. 5.8 Parotid bed**
Left lateral view. **A** Superficial dissection. **B** Deep dissection. The largest of the salivary glands, the parotid gland secretes saliva into the oral cavity via the parotid duct. The facial nerve divides into branches within the parotid gland and is vulnerable during the surgical removal of parotid tumors. The best landmark for locating the nerve trunk is the tip of the cartilaginous auditory canal.

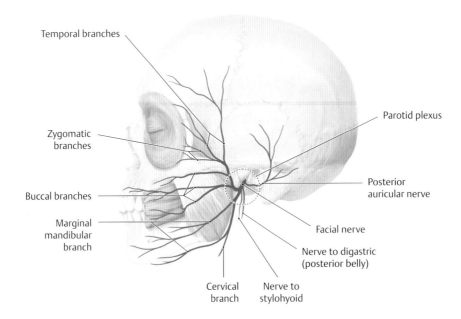

Temporal branches — Zygomatic branches — Buccal branches — Marginal mandibular branch — Cervical branch — Nerve to stylohyoid — Nerve to digastric (posterior belly) — Facial nerve — Posterior auricular nerve — Parotid plexus

**Fig. 5.9 Branching of the facial nerve (CN VII)**
Left lateral view. The large branchiomotor branch of the facial nerve (CN VII) exits the skull through the stylomastoid foramen. It gives off three branches immediately: the posterior auricular nerve and the nerves to the digastric muscle (posterior belly) and stylohyoid. It then enters the parotid gland, where it divides into two trunks: temporofacial and cervicofacial. These trunks give off five major branches that course anteriorly: temporal, zygomatic, buccal, mandibular, and cervical.

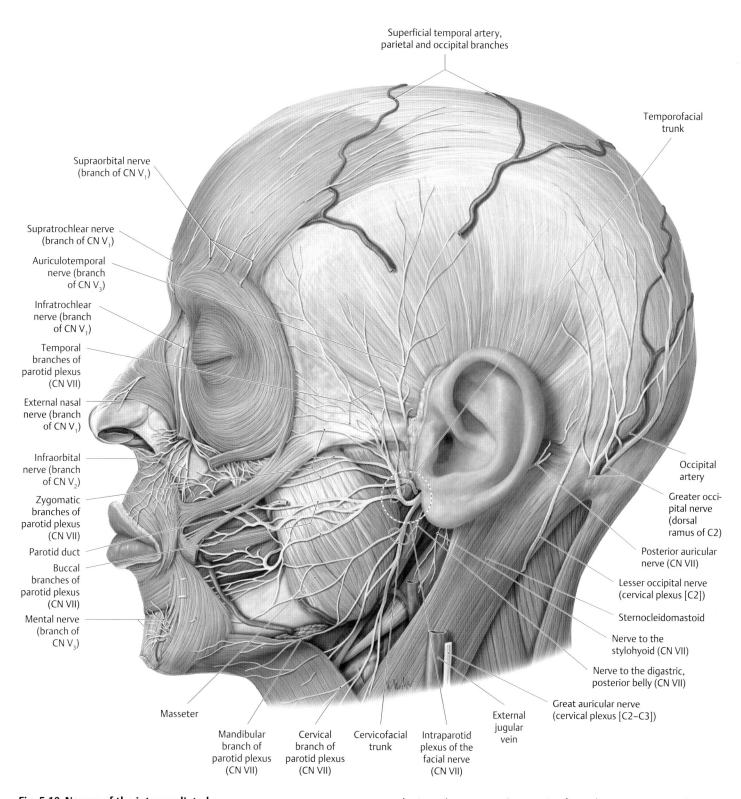

Superficial temporal artery, parietal and occipital branches

Temporofacial trunk

Supraorbital nerve (branch of CN V₁)

Supratrochlear nerve (branch of CN V₁)

Auriculotemporal nerve (branch of CN V₃)

Infratrochlear nerve (branch of CN V₁)

Temporal branches of parotid plexus (CN VII)

External nasal nerve (branch of CN V₁)

Infraorbital nerve (branch of CN V₂)

Zygomatic branches of parotid plexus (CN VII)

Parotid duct

Buccal branches of parotid plexus (CN VII)

Mental nerve (branch of CN V₃)

Masseter

Mandibular branch of parotid plexus (CN VII)

Cervical branch of parotid plexus (CN VII)

Cervicofacial trunk

Intraparotid plexus of the facial nerve (CN VII)

External jugular vein

Occipital artery

Greater occipital nerve (dorsal ramus of C2)

Posterior auricular nerve (CN VII)

Lesser occipital nerve (cervical plexus [C2])

Sternocleidomastoid

Nerve to the stylohyoid (CN VII)

Nerve to the digastric, posterior belly (CN VII)

Great auricular nerve (cervical plexus [C2–C3])

**Fig. 5.10 Nerves of the intermediate layer**
Left lateral view. The parotid gland has been removed to demonstrate the structure of the parotid plexus of the facial nerve (see **Fig. 5.9**). The occiput receives sensory innervation from the greater occipital nerve, which arises from the dorsal primary ramus of C2, and the lesser occipital nerve, which arises from the cervical plexus (ventral rami of C2).

# Infratemporal Fossa: Contents

The infratemporal fossa is located lateral to the lateral pterygoid plate of the sphenoid, medial to the ramus of the mandible, posterior to the maxilla, anterior to the styloid process (and the carotid sheath and its contents), and inferior to the greater wing of the sphenoid and a small part of the temporal bone. It is continuous with the pterygopalatine fossa (through the pterygomaxillary fissure). The maxillary artery gives rise to its mandibular (bony, first part) and pterygoid (muscular, second part) branches in the infratemporal fossa. The mandibular division of the trigeminal nerve (CN V₃) divides into its terminal branches in the infratemporal fossa.

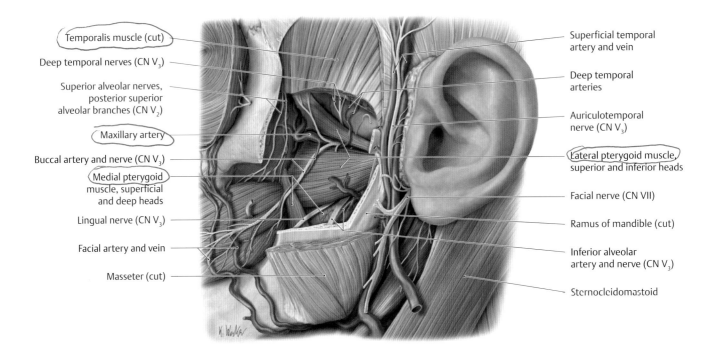

**Fig. 5.11 Infratemporal fossa, superficial dissection**
*Left lateral view. Removed:* Masseter, anterior portion of the mandibular ramus, and zygomatic arch. The pterygoid plexus normally is embedded between the medial and lateral pterygoids. It drains to the maxillary vein, a tributary of the retromandibular vein. The inferior alveolar artery and nerve can be seen entering the mandibular canal (the accompanying vein has been removed).

| Table 5.1 Muscles and vessels of the infratemporal fossa | | |
|---|---|---|
| **Muscle** | **Artery** | **Vein** |
| Lateral and medial pterygoids | Maxillary artery<br>• Mandibular branches<br>• Pterygoid branches | Pterygoid plexus |
| Temporalis tendon | | Maxillary vein |
| | | Deep facial vein (deep portion) |
| | | Emissary veins |

☆ Contents

- temporalis & Pterygoid muscles
- branches of V₃
- chorda tympani
- maxillary artery branches
- Pterygoid venous plexus

☆ *borders of the infratemporal fossa*

- Superior – Infratemporal surface of the sphenoid & temporal bones
- medial – Lateral pterygoid plate
- anterior – posterior surface of the maxilla & the buccinator
- Lateral – Ramus, coronoid, & condylar procceses
- posterior – parotid, styloid, Internal carotid artery
- Inferior – lower border of the mandible

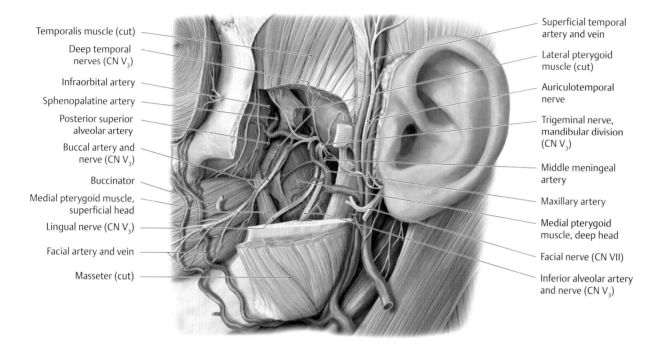

Temporalis muscle (cut)
Deep temporal nerves (CN V₃)
Infraorbital artery
Sphenopalatine artery
Posterior superior alveolar artery
Buccal artery and nerve (CN V₃)
Buccinator
Medial pterygoid muscle, superficial head
Lingual nerve (CN V₃)
Facial artery and vein
Masseter (cut)

Superficial temporal artery and vein
Lateral pterygoid muscle (cut)
Auriculotemporal nerve
Trigeminal nerve, mandibular division (CN V₃)
Middle meningeal artery
Maxillary artery
Medial pterygoid muscle, deep head
Facial nerve (CN VII)
Inferior alveolar artery and nerve (CN V₃)

***Fig. 5.12* Infratemporal fossa, deep dissection**
Left lateral view. *Removed:* Both heads of the lateral pterygoid muscle. The branches of the maxillary artery and mandibular division of the trigeminal nerve (CN V₃) can be identified. *Note:* By careful dissection, it is possible to define the site where the auriculotemporal nerve (branch of the mandibular division) splits around the middle meningeal artery before the artery enters the middle cranial fossa through the foramen spinosum (see p. 46). Branches of the third part of the maxillary artery can be observed in the pterygopalatine fossa, which is medial to the infratemporal fossa.

| *Table 5.2* Nerves in the infratemporal fossa | | | |
|---|---|---|---|
| **CN V₃** | Trunk of CN V₃ and direct branches:<br>• Recurrent meningeal branch<br>• Medial pterygoid n. | Anterior division:<br>• Masseteric n.<br>• Deep temporal nn.<br>• Buccal n.<br>• Lateral pterygoid n. | Posterior division:<br>• Auriculotemporal n.<br>• Lingual n.<br>• Inferior alveolar n.<br>• Mylohyoid n. |
| **CN V₂** | Posterior superior alveolar n. | | |
| **Other** | Otic ganglion | Lesser petrosal n. | Chorda tympani (CN VII) |

# Pterygopalatine Fossa

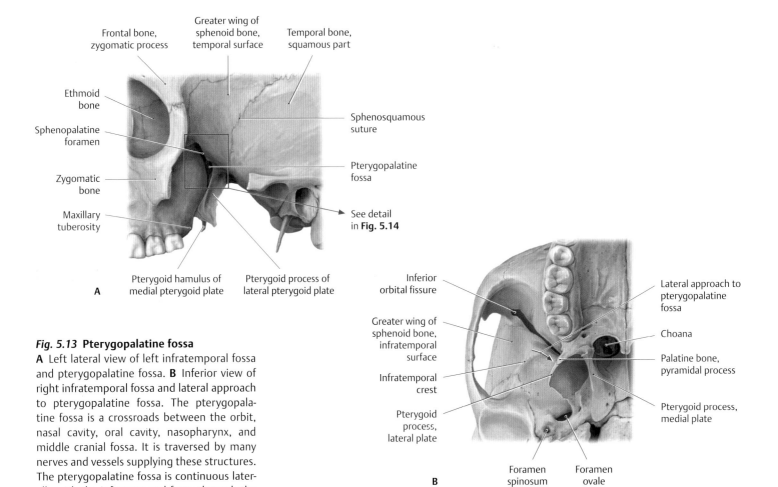

**A**

**B**

**Fig. 5.13 Pterygopalatine fossa**
**A** Left lateral view of left infratemporal fossa and pterygopalatine fossa. **B** Inferior view of right infratemporal fossa and lateral approach to pterygopalatine fossa. The pterygopalatine fossa is a crossroads between the orbit, nasal cavity, oral cavity, nasopharynx, and middle cranial fossa. It is traversed by many nerves and vessels supplying these structures. The pterygopalatine fossa is continuous laterally with the infratemporal fossa through the pterygopalatine fissure. The lateral approach through the infratemporal fossa is used in surgical operations on tumors of the pterygopalatine fossa (e.g., nasopharyngeal fibroma).

| Table 5.3 Borders of the pterygopalatine fossa | | | |
|---|---|---|---|
| **Border** | **Structure** | **Border** | **Structure** |
| Superior | Sphenoid bone (greater wing) and junction with the inferior orbital fissure | Inferior | Greater palatine canal |
| Anterior | Maxilla | Posterior | Sphenoid, root of pterygoid process |
| Medial | Palatine bone (perpendicular plate) | Lateral | Pterygomaxillary fissure |

*Fig. 5.14* **Communications of the pterygopalatine fossa**

Left lateral view of left fossa (detail from **Fig. 5.13A**). The pterygopalatine fossa contains the pterygopalatine ganglion, the parasympathetic ganglion of CN VII that is affiliated with the maxillary nerve (CN $V_2$, sensory). Sensory fibers from the face, maxillary dentition, nasal cavity, oral cavity, nasopharynx, and paranasal sinuses pass through the ganglion without synapsing and enter the middle cranial fossa as the maxillary nerve (CN $V_2$). These sensory fibers also serve as "scaffolding" for the peripheral distribution of postganglionic autonomic parasympathetic fibers from the pterygopalatine ganglion and postganglionic sympathetic fibers derived from the internal carotid plexus. See **Table 4.20** for a complete treatment of the maxillary nerve and pterygopalatine ganglion.

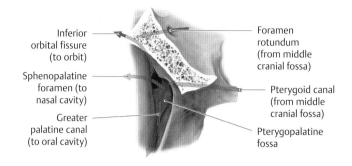

Inferior orbital fissure (to orbit)

Sphenopalatine foramen (to nasal cavity)

Greater palatine canal (to oral cavity)

Foramen rotundum (from middle cranial fossa)

Pterygoid canal (from middle cranial fossa)

Pterygopalatine fossa

| *Table 5.4* Communications of the pterygopalatine fossa | | | |
|---|---|---|---|
| **Communication** | **Direction** | **Via** | **Transmitted structures** |
| Middle cranial fossa | Posterosuperiorly | Foramen rotundum | • Maxillary n. (CN $V_2$) |
| Middle cranial fossa | Posteriorly in anterior wall of foramen lacerum | Pterygoid canal | • N. of pterygoid canal, formed from:<br>  ∘ Greater petrosal n. (preganglionic parasympathetic fibers from CN VII)<br>  ∘ Deep petrosal n. (postganglionic sympathetic fibers from internal carotid plexus)<br>• A. of pterygoid canal<br>• Vv. of pterygoid canal |
| Orbit | Anterosuperiorly | Inferior orbital fissure | • Branches of maxillary n. (CN $V_2$):<br>  ∘ Infraorbital n.<br>  ∘ Zygomatic n.<br>• Infraorbital a. and vv.<br>• Communicating vv. between inferior ophthalmic v. and pterygoid plexus of vv. |
| Nasal cavity | Medially | Sphenopalatine foramen | • Nasopalatine n. (CN $V_2$), lateral and medial superior posterior nasal branches<br>• Sphenopalatine a. and vv. |
| Oral cavity | Inferiorly | Greater palatine canal (foramen) | • Greater (descending) palatine n. (CN $V_2$) and a.<br>• Branches that emerge through lesser palatine canals:<br>  ∘ Lesser palatine nn. (CN $V_2$) and aa. |
| Nasopharynx | Inferoposteriorly | Palatovaginal (pharyngeal) canal | • CN $V_2$, pharyngeal branches, and pharyngeal a. |
| Infratemporal fossa | Laterally | Pterygomaxillary fissure | • Maxillary a., pterygoid (third) part<br>• Posterior superior alveolar n., a., and v. |

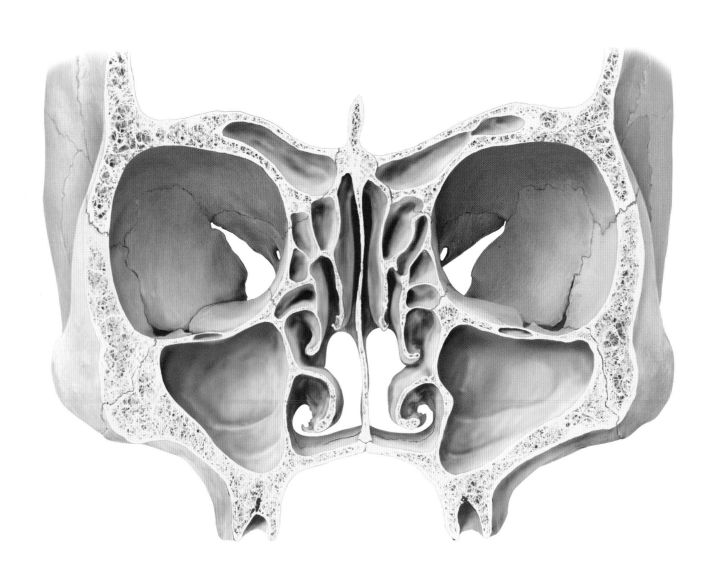

# Regions of the Head

# Bones of the Orbit

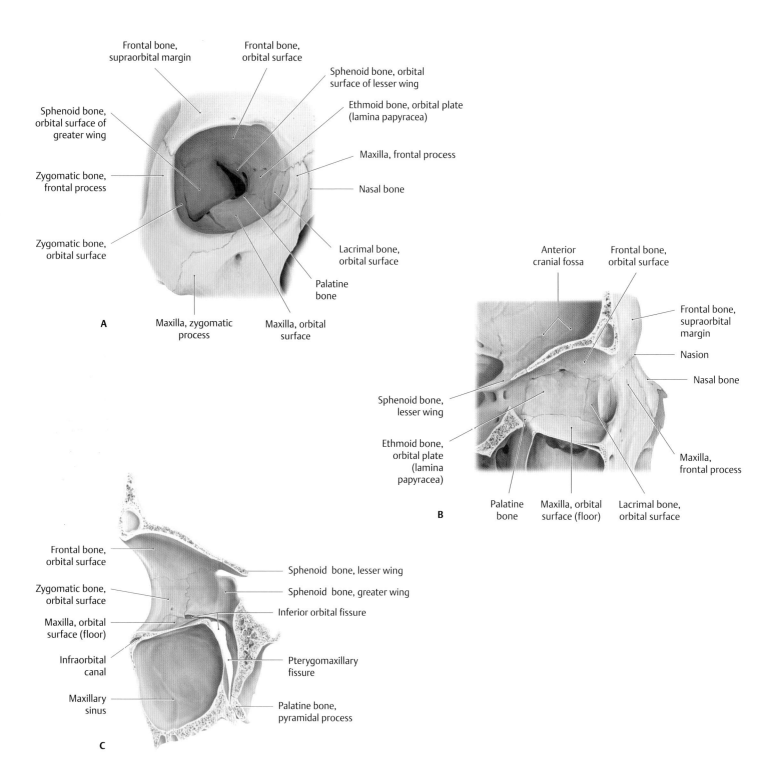

**Fig. 6.1 Bones of the orbit**

Right orbit. **A,D** Anterior view. **B,E** Lateral view with lateral orbital wall removed. **C,F** Medial view with medial orbit wall removed. The orbit is formed by seven bones: the frontal, zygomatic, ethmoid, sphenoid, lacrimal, and palatine bones, and the maxilla. The neurovascular structures of the orbit communicate with the surrounding spaces via several major passages (see **Table 6.1**): the superior and inferior orbital fissures, the optic canal, the anterior and posterior ethmoidal foramina, the infraorbital canal, and the nasolacrimal duct. The neurovascular structures of the orbit also communicate with the superficial face by passing through the orbital rim. *Note:* The exposed maxillary sinus can be seen in **E**. The maxillary hiatus contains the ostium by which the maxillary sinus opens into the nasal cavity superior to the inferior nasal concha.

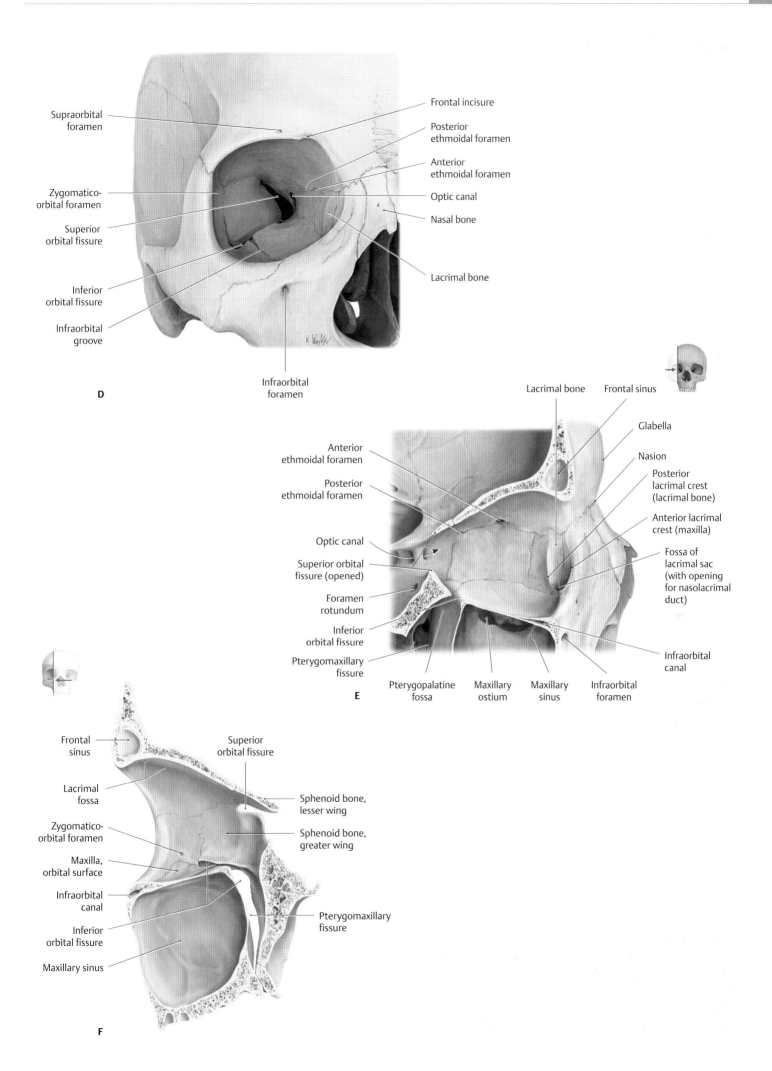

Supraorbital
foramen

Zygomatico-
orbital foramen

Superior
orbital fissure

Inferior
orbital fissure

Infraorbital
groove

Infraorbital
foramen

**D**

Frontal incisure

Posterior
ethmoidal foramen

Anterior
ethmoidal foramen

Optic canal

Nasal bone

Lacrimal bone

Lacrimal bone    Frontal sinus

Glabella

Nasion

Posterior
lacrimal crest
(lacrimal bone)

Anterior lacrimal
crest (maxilla)

Fossa of
lacrimal sac
(with opening
for nasolacrimal
duct)

Infraorbital
canal

Anterior
ethmoidal foramen

Posterior
ethmoidal foramen

Optic canal

Superior orbital
fissure (opened)

Foramen
rotundum

Inferior
orbital fissure

Pterygomaxillary
fissure

Pterygopalatine
fossa

Maxillary
ostium

Maxillary
sinus

Infraorbital
foramen

**E**

Frontal
sinus

Lacrimal
fossa

Zygomatico-
orbital foramen

Maxilla,
orbital surface

Infraorbital
canal

Inferior
orbital fissure

Maxillary sinus

Superior
orbital fissure

Sphenoid bone,
lesser wing

Sphenoid bone,
greater wing

Pterygomaxillary
fissure

**F**

# Communications of the Orbit

**Fig. 6.2 Bones of the orbits and adjacent cavities**

The bones of the orbit also form portions of the walls of neighboring cavities. The following adjacent structures are visible in the diagram:

- Anterior cranial fossa
- Frontal sinus
- Middle cranial fossa
- Ethmoid air cells
- Maxillary sinus

Disease processes may originate in the orbit and spread to these cavities, or originate in these cavities and spread to the orbit.

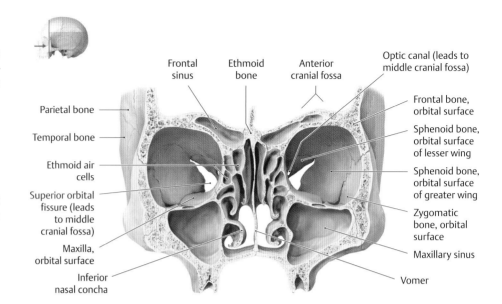

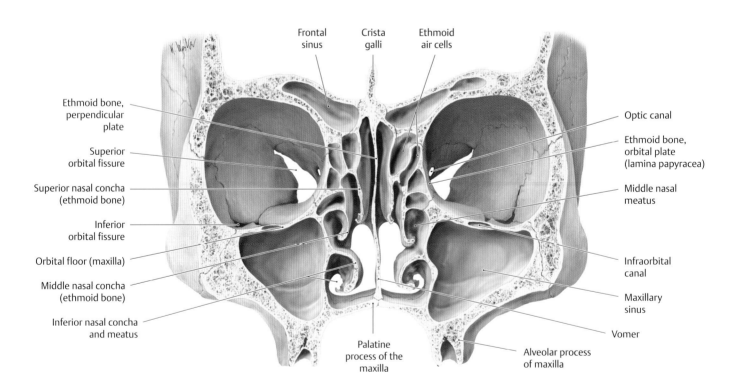

**Fig. 6.3 Orbits and neighboring structures**

Coronal section through both orbits, viewed from the front. The walls separating the orbit from the ethmoid air cells (0.3 mm, lamina papyracea) and from the maxillary sinus (0.5 mm, orbital floor) are very thin. Thus, both of these walls are susceptible to fractures and provide routes for the spread of tumors and inflammatory processes into or out of the orbit. The superior orbital fissure communicates with the middle cranial fossa, and so several structures that are not pictured here—the sphenoid sinus, pituitary gland, and optic chiasm—are also closely related to the orbit.

**Table 6.1** Communications of the orbit

| Structure | Communicates | Via | Neurovascular structures in canal/fissure |
|---|---|---|---|
| Frontal sinus and anterior ethmoid air cells | Superiorly | Unnamed canaliculi | • Sensory filaments |
| | Medially | Anterior ethmoidal canal | • Anterior ethmoidal a. (from ophthalmic a.)<br>• Anterior ethmoidal v. (to superior ophthalmic v.)<br>• Anterior ethmoidal n. (CN $V_1$) |
| Sphenoid sinus and posterior ethmoid air cells | Medially | Posterior ethmoidal canal | • Posterior ethmoidal a. (from ophthalmic a.)<br>• Posterior ethmoidal v. (to superior ophthalmic v.)<br>• Posterior ethmoidal n. (CN $V_1$) |
| Middle cranial fossa | Posteriorly | Superior orbital fissure | • Cranial nerves to the extraocular muscles (oculomotor n. [CN III], trochlear n. [CN IV], and abducent n. [CN VI])<br>• Ophthalmic n. (CN $V_1$) and branches:<br>  ◦ Lacrimal n.<br>  ◦ Frontal n. (branches into supraorbital and supratrochlear nn.)<br>  ◦ Nasociliary n.<br>• Superior (and occasionally inferior) ophthalmic v. (to cavernous sinus)<br>• Recurrent meningeal branch of lacrimal a. (anastomoses with middle meningeal a.) |
| | Posteriorly | Optic canal | • Optic n. (CN II)<br>• Ophthalmic a. (from internal carotid a.) |
| Pterygopalatine fossa | Posteroinferiorly (medially) | Inferior orbital fissure* | • Infraorbital a. (from maxillary a.)<br>• Infraorbital v. (to pterygoid plexus)*<br>• Infraorbital n. (CN $V_2$) |
| Infratemporal fossa | Posteroinferiorly (laterally) | | • Zygomatic n. (CN $V_2$)<br>• Inferior ophthalmic v. (variable, to cavernous sinus) |
| Nasal cavity | Inferomedially | Nasolacrimal canal | • Nasolacrimal duct |
| Maxillary sinus | Inferiorly | Unnamed canaliculi | • Sensory filaments |
| Face and temporal fossa | Anteriorly | Zygomaticofacial canal | • Zygomaticofacial n. (CN $V_2$)<br>• Anastomotic branch of lacrimal a. (to transverse facial and zygomatico-orbital aa.) |
| | | Zygomaticotemporal canal | • Zygomaticotemporal n. (CN $V_2$)<br>• Anastomotic branch of lacrimal a. (to deep temporal aa.) |
| Face | Anteriorly | Supraorbital foramen (notch) | • Supraorbital n., lateral branch (CN $V_1$)<br>• Supraorbital a. (from ophthalmic a.)<br>• Supraorbital v. (to angular v.) |
| | | Frontal incisure | • Supratrochlear a. (from ophthalmic a.)<br>• Supratrochlear n. (CN $V_1$)<br>• Supraorbital n., medial branch (CN $V_1$) |
| | | Orbital rim, medial aspect | • Infratrochlear n. (CN $V_1$)<br>• Dorsal nasal a. (from ophthalmic a.)<br>• Dorsal nasal v. (to angular v.) |
| | | Orbital rim, lateral aspect | • Lacrimal n. (CN $V_1$)<br>• Lacrimal a. (from ophthalmic a.)<br>• Lacrimal v. (to superior ophthalmic v.) |

* The infraorbital a., v., and n. travel in the infraorbital canal on the lateral floor of the orbit and emerge at the inferior orbital fissure. The inferior orbital fissure is continuous inferiorly with the pterygomaxillary fissure, which is the boundary between the infratemporal and the pterygopalatine fossa. The infratemporal fossa lies on the lateral side of the pterygomaxillary fissure; the pterygopalatine fossa lies on the medial side.

# Extraocular Muscles

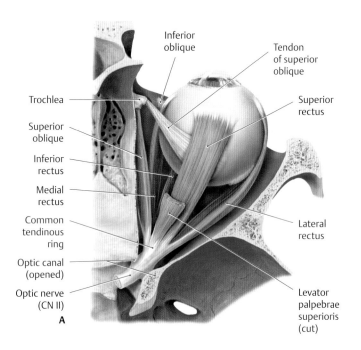

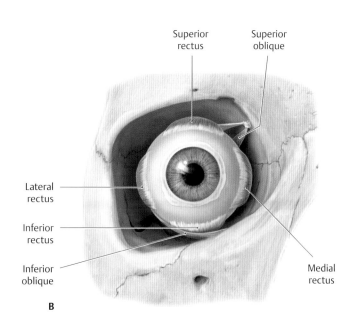

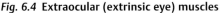

**A**

**B**

**Fig. 6.4 Extraocular (extrinsic eye) muscles**
Right eye. **A** Superior view. **B** Anterior view. The eyeball is moved in the orbit by four rectus muscles (superior, medial, inferior, lateral) and two oblique muscles (superior and inferior). The four rectus muscles arise from a tendinous ring around the optic canal (common tendinous ring, common annular tendon) and insert on the sclera of the eyeball. The superior and inferior obliques arise from the body of the sphenoid and the medial orbital margin of the maxilla, respectively. The superior oblique passes through a tendinous loop (trochlea) attached to the superomedial orbital margin (frontal bone); this redirects it at an acute angle to its insertion on the superior surface of the eyeball. The coordinated interaction of all six functionally competent extraocular muscles is necessary for directing both eyes toward the visual target. The brain then processes the two perceived retinal images in a way that provides binocular vision perception. Impaired function of one or more extraocular muscles causes deviation of the eye from its normal position, resulting in diplopia (double vision).

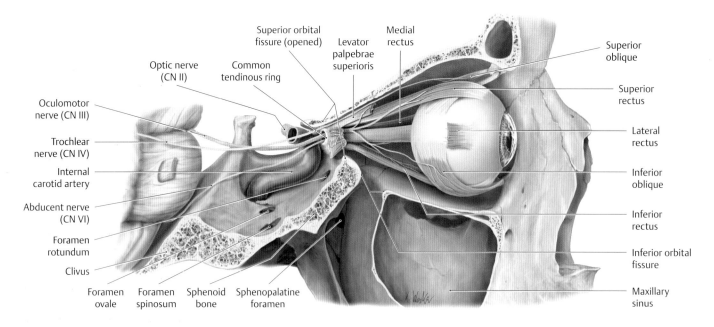

**Fig. 6.5 Innervation of the extraocular muscles**
Right eye, lateral view with the lateral wall of the orbit removed. The extraocular muscles are supplied by cranial nerves III, IV, and VI (see **Table 6.2**). *Note:* Levator palpebrae superioris is also supplied by CN III. After emerging from the brainstem, these cranial nerves first traverse the cavernous sinus, where they are in close proximity to the internal carotid artery. From there they pass through the superior orbital fissure to enter the orbit and supply their respective muscles. The optic nerve (CN II) enters the orbit via the more medially located optic canal (see **Fig. 6.1E**).

### *Fig. 6.6* Actions of the extraocular muscles

Right eye, superior view with orbital roof removed. Primary actions (red), secondary actions (blue).

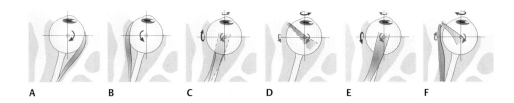

A     B     C     D     E     F

| Muscle | Primary action | Secondary action | Innervation |
|---|---|---|---|
| **A** Lateral rectus | Abduction | – | Abducent n. (CN VI) |
| **B** Medial rectus | Adduction | – | Oculomotor n. (CN III), inferior branch |
| **C** Inferior rectus | Depression | Adduction and lateral rotation | |
| **D** Inferior oblique | Elevation and abduction | Lateral rotation | |
| **E** Superior rectus | Elevation | Adduction and medial rotation | Oculomotor n. (CN III), superior branch |
| **F** Superior oblique | Depression and abduction | Medial rotation | Trochlear n. (CN IV) |

*Table 6.2* Actions and innervation of the extraocular muscles

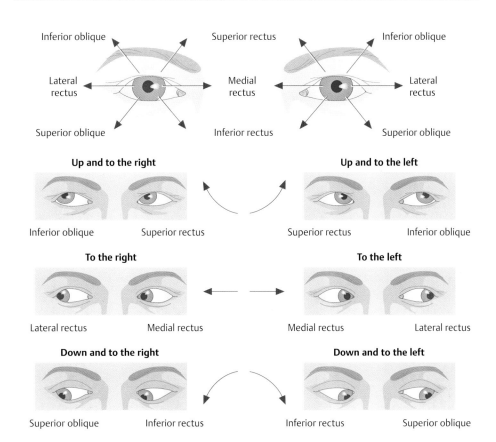

### *Fig. 6.7* The six cardinal directions of gaze

In the clinical evaluation of ocular motility to diagnose *oculomotor palsies,* six cardinal directions of gaze are tested (see arrows). Note that different muscles may be activated in each eye for any particular direction of gaze. For example, gaze to the right is effected by the com-

bined actions of the lateral rectus of the right eye and the medial rectus of the left eye. These two muscles, moreover, are supplied by different cranial nerves (VI and III, respectively).

If one muscle is weak or paralyzed, deviation of the eye will be noted during certain ocular movements (see **Fig. 6.8**).

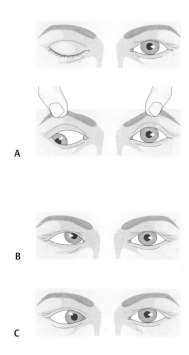

A

B

C

### *Fig. 6.8* Oculomotor palsies

Palsy of the right side shown during attempted straight-ahead gaze. **A** Complete oculomotor palsy. **B** Trochlear palsy. **C** Abducent palsy. Oculomotor palsies may result from lesions involving the cranial nerve nucleus, the course of the nerve, or the eye muscle itself. Depending on the involved muscle, symptoms may include deviated position of the affected eye and diplopia. The patient attempts to compensate for this by adjusting the position of the head.

**A** **Complete oculomotor (CN III) palsy:** Affects four extraocular muscles, two intraocular muscles (see p. 114), and the levator palpebrae superioris. Symptoms and affected muscle(s): Eyeball deviates toward lower outer quadrant = disabled superior, inferior, and medial recti and inferior oblique. Mydriasis (pupil dilation) = disabled pupillary sphincter. Loss of near accommodation = disabled ciliary muscle. Ptosis (drooping of eyelid) = disabled levator palpebrae superioris. The palpebral fissure cannot be opened during complete ptosis in which both the levator palpebrae superioris (CN III) and superior tarsus (sympathetic) muscles are paralyzed. Diplopia will therefore not be observed.

**B** **Trochlear nerve (CN IV) palsy:** Eye deviates slightly superomedially, causing diplopia = disabled superior oblique.

**C** **Abducent nerve (CN VI) palsy:** Eye deviates medially, causing diplopia = disabled lateral rectus.

# Cranial Nerves of the Extraocular Muscles: Oculomotor (CN III), Trochlear (CN IV) & Abducent (CN VI)

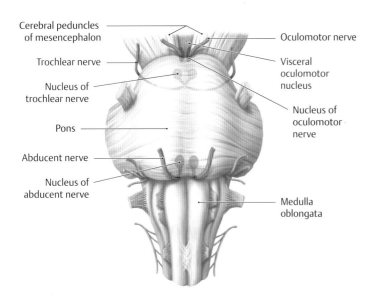

*Fig. 6.9* **Emergence of the nerves from the brainstem**
Anterior view. All three nerves that supply the extraocular muscles emerge from the brainstem. The nuclei of the oculomotor nerve and trochlear nerve are located in the midbrain (mesencephalon), and the nucleus of the abducent nerve is located in the pons.
*Note:* The oculomotor (CN III) is the only one of the three that contains somatic efferent and visceral efferent fibers and supplies multiple extraocular muscles.

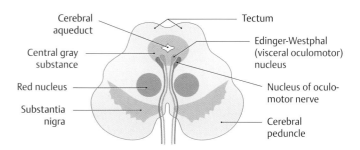

*Fig. 6.10* **Topography of the oculomotor nucleus**
Cross section through the brainstem at the level of the oculomotor nucleus, superior view. *Note:* The visceral efferent, parasympathetic nuclear complex (Edinger-Westphal [visceral oculomotor] nucleus) can be distinguished from the somatic efferent nuclear complex (nucleus of the oculomotor nerve).

---

**Table 6.4 Trochlear nerve (CN IV): overview**

**Fibers:** Somatic efferent fibers (red)

**Course:** CN IV is the only cranial nerve to emerge from the dorsal side (posterior surface) of the brainstem. It is also the only cranial nerve in which all fibers cross to the opposite side. It enters the orbit through the superior orbital fissure, passing lateral to the common tendinous ring. It has the longest *intra*dural course of the three extraocular motor nerves.

**Nuclei and distribution:**
• Somatic efferent fibers from the nucleus of the trochlear nerve emerge from the midbrain and supply motor innervation to the superior oblique.

**Lesions:** Trochlear nerve palsy:
• Superomedial deviation of the affected eye, causing diplopia = disabled superior oblique
*Note:* Because CN IV crosses to the opposite side, lesions close to the nucleus result in trochlear nerve palsy on the opposite side (contralateral palsy). Lesions past the site where the nerve crosses the midline cause palsy on the same side (ipsilateral palsy).

---

**Table 6.3 Oculomotor nerve (CN III): overview**

**Fibers:** Somatic efferent (red) and visceral efferent (blue) fibers

**Course:** CN III runs anteriorly from the mesencephalon (midbrain, highest level of the brainstem) and travels through the lateral wall of the cavernous sinus to enter the orbit through the superior orbital fissure. After passing through the common tendinous ring, CN III divides into a superior and an inferior division.

**Nuclei and distribution:**
• Somatic efferents (red): Efferents from the nucleus of the oculomotor nerve in the midbrain supply the levator palpebrae superioris and four extraocular muscles (the superior, medial, and inferior rectus muscles, and the inferior oblique).
• Visceral efferents (blue): Parasympathetic preganglionic efferents from the Edinger-Westphal (visceral oculomotor) nucleus travel with the inferior division of CN III to synapse with neurons in the ciliary ganglion. The postganglionic neurons innervate the intraocular muscles (pupillary sphincter and ciliary muscle).

**Lesions:** Oculomotor palsy of various extents. Complete oculomotor palsy is marked by paralysis of all the innervated muscles, causing:
• Ptosis (drooping of eyelid) = disabled levator palpebrae superioris
• Inferolateral deviation of affected eye causing diplopia (double vision) = disabled extraocular muscles
• Mydriasis (pupil dilation) = disabled pupillary sphincter
• Accommodation difficulties = disabled ciliary muscle

---

**Table 6.5 Abducent nerve (CN VI): overview**

**Fibers:** Somatic efferent fibers (red)

**Course:** CN VI follows a long *extra*dural path. It emerges from the pons (midlevel brainstem) and runs through the cavernous sinus in close proximity to the internal carotid artery and enters the orbit through the superior orbital fissure.

**Nuclei and distribution:**
• Somatic efferent fibers from the nucleus of the abducent nerve emerge from the inferior border of the pons (midlevel brainstem) and supply motor innervation to the lateral rectus.

**Lesions:** Abducent nerve palsy:
• Medial deviation of the affected eye, causing diplopia = disabled lateral rectus
*Note:* The long extradural path of the CN VI exposes it to injury. Cavernous sinus thrombosis, aneurysms of the internal carotid artery, meningitis, or subdural hemorrhage may all compress the nerve, resulting in nerve palsy. Excessive fall in cerebrospinal fluid (CSF) pressure (e.g., due to lumbar puncture) may cause the brainstem to descend, exerting traction on the nerve.

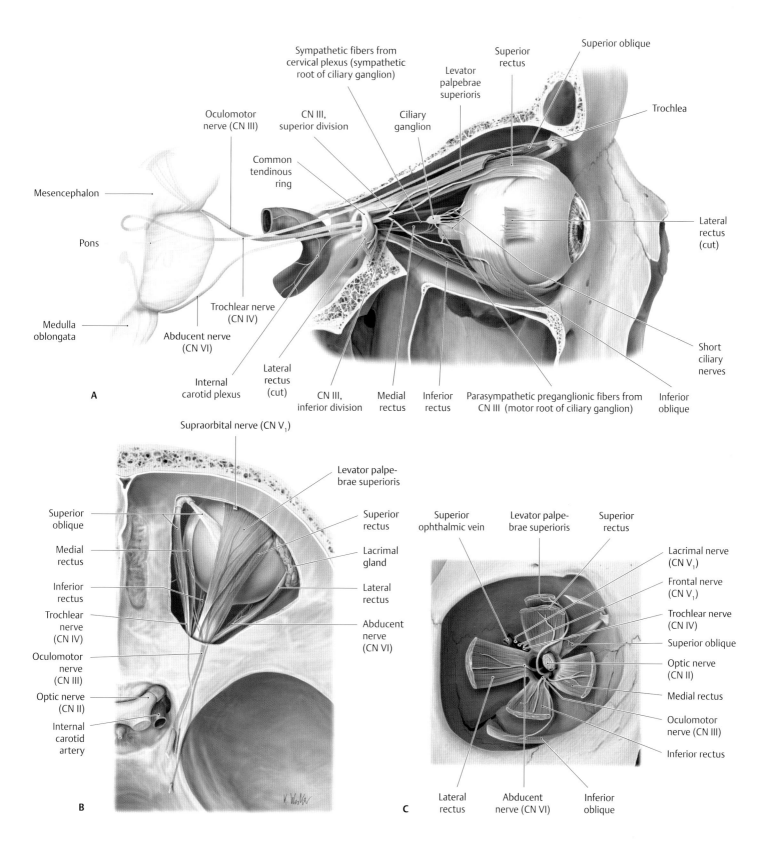

**Fig. 6.11 Nerves supplying the ocular muscles**

Right orbit. **A** Lateral view with lateral wall removed. **B** Superior view of opened orbit. **C** Anterior view. Cranial nerves III, IV, and VI enter the orbit through the superior orbital fissure, lateral to the optic canal (CN IV then passes lateral to the common tendinous ring, and CN III and VI pass through it). All three nerves supply somatic efferent fibers (somatomotor innervation) to the extraocular muscles. In addition, CN III carries parasympathetic motor innervation for the intraocular muscles. Parasympathetic preganglionic fibers travel with the inferior division of CN III, forming the parasympathetic (motor) root of the ciliary gan-

glion. Two other fiber types pass through the ciliary ganglion without synapsing: sympathetic and sensory. Sympathetic (postganglionic) fibers from the superior cervical ganglion travel on the internal carotid artery to enter the superior orbital fissure, where they run with the nasociliary nerve (CN V₁) or enter the ciliary ganglion by coursing along the ophthalmic artery. Sensory fibers from the eyeball travel to the nasociliary nerve (CN V₁) via the sensory root of the ciliary ganglion. The sensory, sympathetic, and parasympathetic fibers in the ciliary ganglion are relayed in the short ciliary nerves. *Note:* Sympathetic fibers also reach the intraocular muscles via the long ciliary nerves.

# Neurovasculature of the Orbit

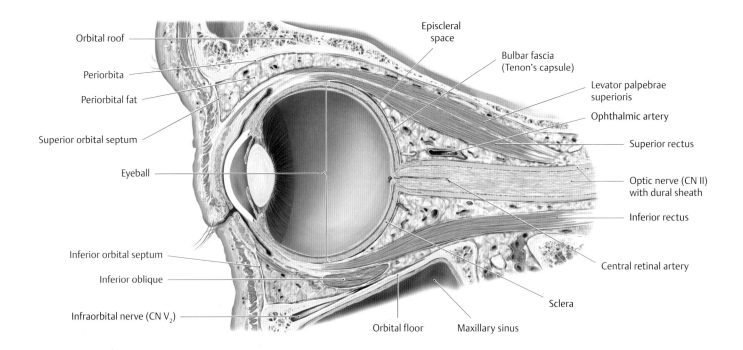

**Fig. 6.12 Upper, middle, and lower levels of the orbit**
Right orbit. Sagittal section viewed from the medial side. The orbit is lined with periosteum (periorbita) and filled with periorbital fat, which is bounded anteriorly by the orbital septa and toward the eyeball by a mobile sheath of connective tissue (bulbar fascia, Tenon's capsule). The narrow space between the bulbar fascia and sclera is called the episcleral space. Embedded in the periorbital fat are the eyeball, optic nerve, lacrimal gland, extraocular muscles, and associated neurovascular structures. Topographically, the orbit is divided into three levels:

- Upper level: orbital roof to levator palpebrae superioris
- Middle level: superior rectus to optic nerve
- Lower level: optic nerve to orbital floor

| Table 6.6 | Neurovascular contents of the orbit | |
|---|---|---|
| **Orbital level** | **Arteries and veins** | **Nerves** |
| Upper level | • Lacrimal a. (from ophthalmic a.)<br>• Lacrimal v. (to superior ophthalmic v.)<br>• Supraorbital a. (terminal branch of ophthalmic a.)<br>• Supraorbital v. (forms angular v. with supratrochlear vv.) | • Lacrimal n. (CN $V_1$)<br>• Frontal n. (CN $V_1$) and terminal branches:<br>  ○ Supraorbital n.<br>  ○ Supratrochlear n.<br>• Trochlear n. (CN IV) |
| Middle level | • Ophthalmic a. (from internal carotid a.) and branches:<br>  ○ Central retinal a.<br>  ○ Posterior ciliary aa.<br>• Superior ophthalmic v. (to cavernous sinus) | • Nasociliary n. (CN $V_1$)<br>• Abducent n. (CN VI)<br>• Oculomotor n. (CN III), superior branch and fibers from inferior branch (to ciliary ganglion)<br>• Optic n. (CN II)<br>• Ciliary ganglion and roots:<br>  ○ Parasympathetic root (presynaptic autonomic fibers from CN III)<br>  ○ Sympathetic root (postsynaptic fibers from superior cervical ganglion)<br>  ○ Sensory root (sensory fibers from eyeball to nasociliary n.)<br>• Short ciliary nn. (fibers from/to ciliary ganglion) |
| Lower level | • Infraorbital a. (terminal branch of maxillary a.)<br>• Inferior ophthalmic v. (to cavernous sinus) | • Infraorbital n. (CN $V_2$)<br>• Oculomotor n. (CN III), inferior branch |

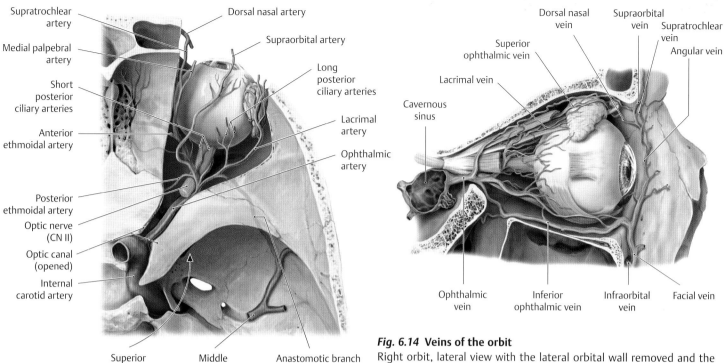

**Fig. 6.13 Branches of the ophthalmic artery**
Superior view of opened right orbit. While running below CN II in the optic canal, the ophthalmic artery gives off the central retinal artery, which pierces and travels with CN II. The ophthalmic artery then exits the canal and branches to supply the intraorbital structures (including the eyeball).

**Fig. 6.14 Veins of the orbit**
Right orbit, lateral view with the lateral orbital wall removed and the maxillary sinus opened. The veins of the orbit communicate with the veins of the superficial and deep facial region and with the cavernous sinus (potential spread of infectious pathogens, see **Fig. 3.20**).

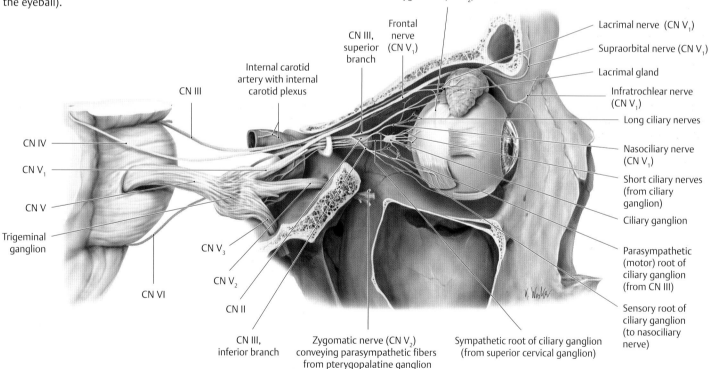

**Fig. 6.15 Innervation of the orbit**
Lateral view of opened right orbit. The extraocular muscles receive motor innervation from three cranial nerves: oculomotor (CN III), trochlear (CN IV), and abducent (CN VI). The ciliary ganglion distributes parasympathetic fibers to the intraocular muscles via the short ciliary nerves. Parasympathetic fibers reach the ganglion via the inferior branch of CN III. Sympathetic fibers from the superior cervical ganglion travel along the internal carotid artery to the superior orbital fissure. In the orbit, sympathetic fibers run with the nasociliary nerve (CN $V_1$) and/or ophthal- mic artery and pass through the ciliary ganglion (the nasociliary nerve also gives off direct sensory branches, the long ciliary nerves, which may carry postganglionic sympathetic fibers). Sensory fibers from the eyeball pass through the ciliary ganglion to the nasociliary nerve (CN $V_1$). *Note:* Parasympathetic fibers to the lacrimal gland are distributed by the lacrimal nerve (CN $V_1$), which communicates with the zygomatic nerve (CN $V_2$) via a communicating branch from the zygomaticotemporal nerve. The zygomatic nerve conveys the postganglionic fibers from the ptery- gopalatine ganglion (the preganglionic fibers arise from CN VII).

**117**

# Topography of the Orbit (I)

**Fig. 6.16 Intracavernous course of the cranial nerves that enter to the orbit**

Anterior and middle cranial fossae on the right side, superior view. The lateral and superior walls of the cavernous sinus have been opened. The trigeminal ganglion has been retracted slightly laterally, the orbital roof has been removed, and the periorbita has been fenestrated. All three of the cranial nerves that supply the ocular muscles (oculomotor nerve, trochlear nerve, and abducent nerve) enter the cavernous sinus, where they come into close relationship with the first and second divisions of the trigeminal nerve and with the internal carotid artery. While the third and fourth cranial nerves course in the lateral wall of the cavernous sinus with the ophthalmic and maxillary divisions of the trigeminal nerve, the abducent nerve runs directly through the cavernous sinus in close proximity to the internal carotid artery. Because of this relationship, the abducent nerve may be damaged as a result of sinus thrombosis or an intracavernous aneurysm of the internal carotid artery.

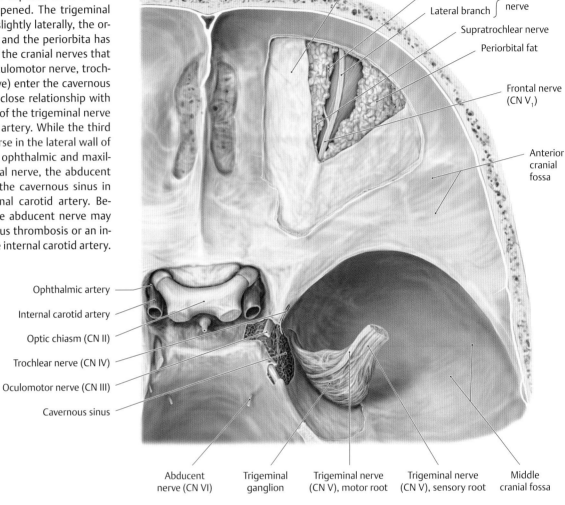

**Fig. 6.17 Neurovasculature in the optic canal and superior orbital fissure**

Right orbit, anterior view with most of the orbital contents removed.

Optic canal: optic nerve (CN II) and ophthalmic artery.

Superior orbital fissure (inside common tendinous ring): abducent (CN VI), nasociliary (CN $V_1$), and oculomotor (CN III) nerves.

Superior orbital fissure (outside common tendinous ring): superior and inferior ophthalmic veins, frontal (CN $V_1$), lacrimal (CN $V_1$), and trochlear (CN IV) nerves.

Inferior orbital fissure (contents not shown): zygomatic (CN $V_2$) nerve and branches of CN $V_2$, infraorbital artery, vein, and nerve in infraorbital canal.

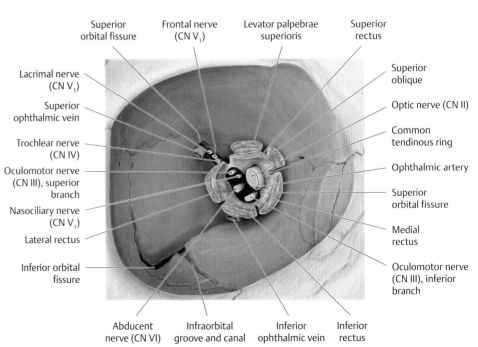

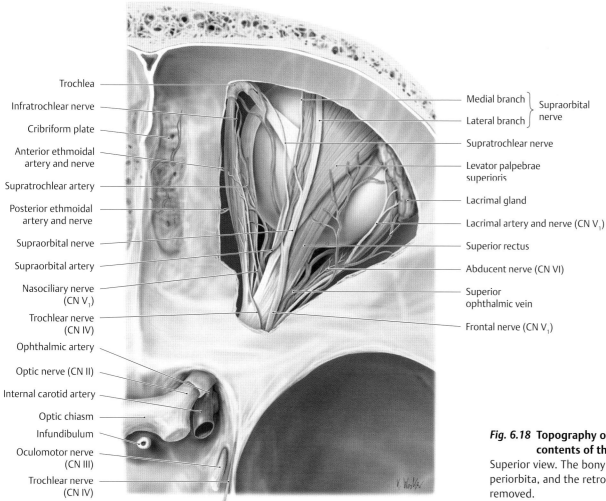

Trochlea

Infratrochlear nerve

Cribriform plate

Anterior ethmoidal
artery and nerve

Supratrochlear artery

Posterior ethmoidal
artery and nerve

Supraorbital nerve

Supraorbital artery

Nasociliary nerve
(CN V₁)

Trochlear nerve
(CN IV)

Ophthalmic artery

Optic nerve (CN II)

Internal carotid artery

Optic chiasm

Infundibulum

Oculomotor nerve
(CN III)

Trochlear nerve
(CN IV)

Medial branch ⎫ Supraorbital
Lateral branch ⎭ nerve

Supratrochlear nerve

Levator palpebrae
superioris

Lacrimal gland

Lacrimal artery and nerve (CN V₁)

Superior rectus

Abducent nerve (CN VI)

Superior
ophthalmic vein

Frontal nerve (CN V₁)

**Fig. 6.18 Topography of the right orbit:
contents of the upper level**
Superior view. The bony roof of the orbit, the
periorbita, and the retro-orbital fat have been
removed.

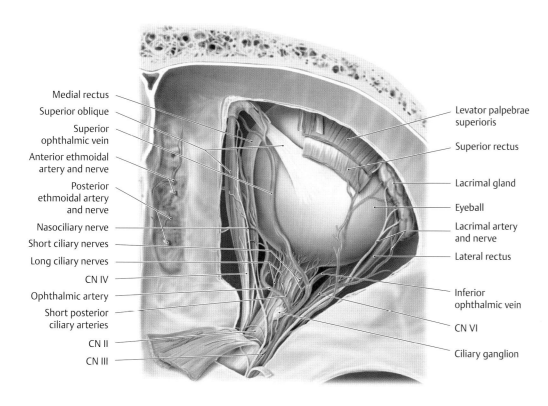

Medial rectus

Superior oblique

Superior
ophthalmic vein

Anterior ethmoidal
artery and nerve

Posterior
ethmoidal artery
and nerve

Nasociliary nerve

Short ciliary nerves

Long ciliary nerves

CN IV

Ophthalmic artery

Short posterior
ciliary arteries

CN II

CN III

Levator palpebrae
superioris

Superior rectus

Lacrimal gland

Eyeball

Lacrimal artery
and nerve

Lateral rectus

Inferior
ophthalmic vein

CN VI

Ciliary ganglion

**Fig. 6.19 Topography of the right
orbit: contents of the
middle level**
Superior view. The levator palpebrae superioris and the superior
rectus have been divided and reflected backward, and all fatty tissue has been removed to better
expose the optic nerve.
*Note:* The ciliary ganglion is approximately 2 mm in diameter and lies
lateral to the optic nerve approximately 2 cm behind the eyeball.
The ciliary ganglion relays parasympathetic fibers to the eye and intraocular muscles via the short
ciliary nerves. The short ciliary
nerves also contain sensory and
sympathetic fibers (see **Fig. 6.15**).

# Topography of the Orbit (II)

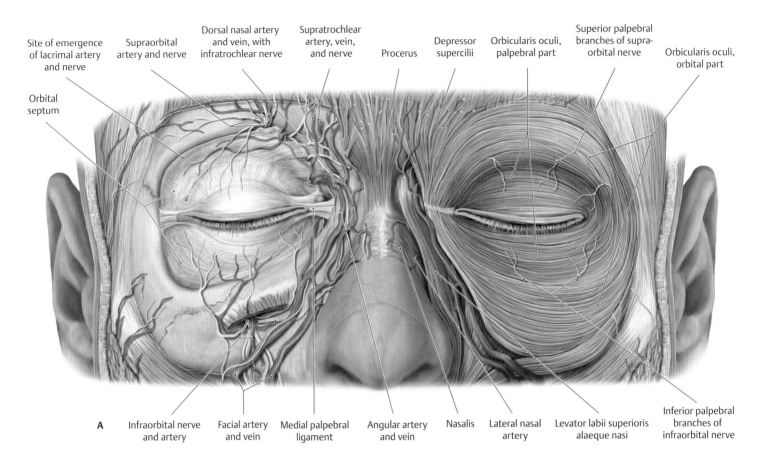

Site of emergence of lacrimal artery and nerve

Orbital septum

Supraorbital artery and nerve

Dorsal nasal artery and vein, with infratrochlear nerve

Supratrochlear artery, vein, and nerve

Procerus

Depressor supercilii

Orbicularis oculi, palpebral part

Superior palpebral branches of supra-orbital nerve

Orbicularis oculi, orbital part

**A**

Infraorbital nerve and artery

Facial artery and vein

Medial palpebral ligament

Angular artery and vein

Nasalis

Lateral nasal artery

Levator labii superioris alaeque nasi

Inferior palpebral branches of infraorbital nerve

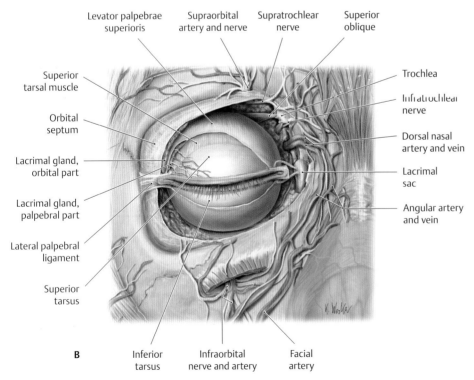

Levator palpebrae superioris

Supraorbital artery and nerve

Supratrochlear nerve

Superior oblique

Superior tarsal muscle

Orbital septum

Lacrimal gland, orbital part

Lacrimal gland, palpebral part

Lateral palpebral ligament

Superior tarsus

Trochlea

Infratrochlear nerve

Dorsal nasal artery and vein

Lacrimal sac

Angular artery and vein

**B**

Inferior tarsus

Infraorbital nerve and artery

Facial artery

**Fig. 6.20 Superficial and deep neurovascular structures of the orbital region**

Right eye, anterior view.

**A** Superficial layer. The orbital septum on the right side has been exposed by removal of the orbicularis oculi. **B** Deep layer. Anterior orbital structures have been exposed by partial removal of the orbital septum.

The regions supplied by the *internal* carotid artery (supraorbital artery) and *external* carotid artery (infraorbital artery, facial artery) meet in this region. The extensive anastomosis between the angular vein (extracranial) and superior ophthalmic veins (intracranial) creates a portal of entry by which microorganisms may reach the cavernous sinus (risk of sinus thrombosis, meningitis, see p. 53). It is sometimes necessary to ligate this anastomosis in the orbital region, as in patients with extensive infections of the external facial region.

Note the passage of the supra- and infraorbital nerves (branches of CN $V_1$ and CN $V_2$) through the accordingly named foramina. The sensory function of these two trigeminal nerve divisions can be tested at these nerve exit points.

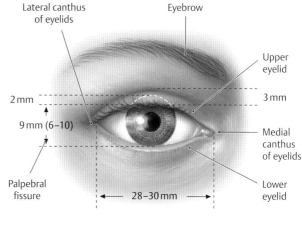

**Fig. 6.21 Surface anatomy of the eye**
Right eye, anterior view. The measurements indicate the width of the normal palpebral fissure. It is important to know these measurements because there are a number of diseases in which they are altered. For example, the palpebral fissure may be widened in peripheral facial paralysis or narrowed in ptosis (= drooping of the eyelid) due to oculomotor palsy.

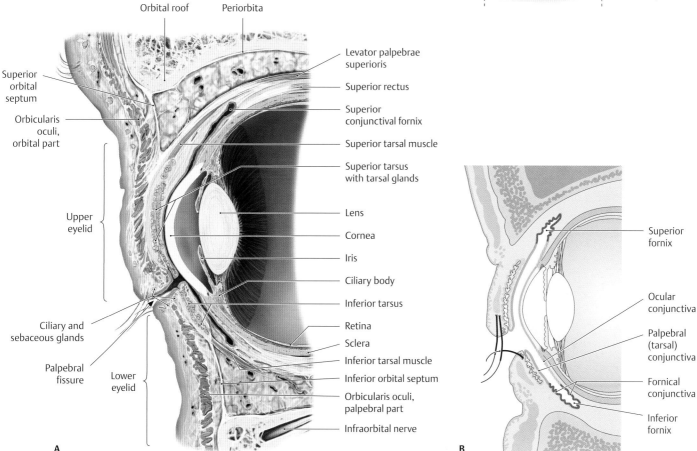

A

B

**Fig. 6.22 Structure of the eyelids and conjunctiva**
**A** Sagittal section through the anterior orbital cavity. **B** Anatomy of the conjunctiva.
The eyelid consists clinically of an outer and an inner layer with the following components:

- Outer layer: palpebral skin, sweat glands, ciliary glands (= modified sweat glands, Moll glands), sebaceous glands (Zeis glands), and two striated muscles, the orbicularis oculi and levator palpebrae (upper eyelid only), innervated by the facial nerve and the oculomotor nerve, respectively.
- Inner layer: the tarsus (fibrous tissue plate), the superior and inferior tarsal muscles (of Müller; *smooth* muscle innervated by sympathetic fibers), the tarsal or palpebral conjunctiva, and the tarsal glands (meibomian glands).

Regular blinking (20 to 30 times per minute) keeps the eyes from drying out by evenly distributing the lacrimal fluid and glandular secretions. Mechanical irritants (e.g., grains of sand) evoke the *blink reflex,* which also serves to protect the cornea and **conjunctiva**. The conjunctiva (tunica conjunctiva) is a vascularized, thin, glistening mucous membrane that is subdivided into the *palpebral conjunctiva* (green), *fornical conjunctiva* (red), and *ocular conjunctiva* (yellow). The ocular conjunctiva borders directly on the corneal surface and combines with it to form the **conjunctival sac**, whose functions include:

- facilitating ocular movements,
- enabling painless motion of the palpebral conjunctiva and ocular conjunctiva relative to each other (lubricated by lacrimal fluid), and
- protecting against infectious pathogens (collections of lymphocytes along the fornices).

The superior and inferior fornices are the sites where the conjunctiva is reflected from the upper and lower eyelid, respectively, onto the eyeball. They are convenient sites for the instillation of ophthalmic medications. *Inflammation of the conjunctiva* is common and causes a dilation of the conjunctival vessels resulting in "pink eye." Conversely, a deficiency of red blood cells (anemia) may lessen the prominence of vascular markings in the conjunctiva. This is why the conjunctiva should be routinely inspected in every clinical examination.

# Lacrimal Apparatus

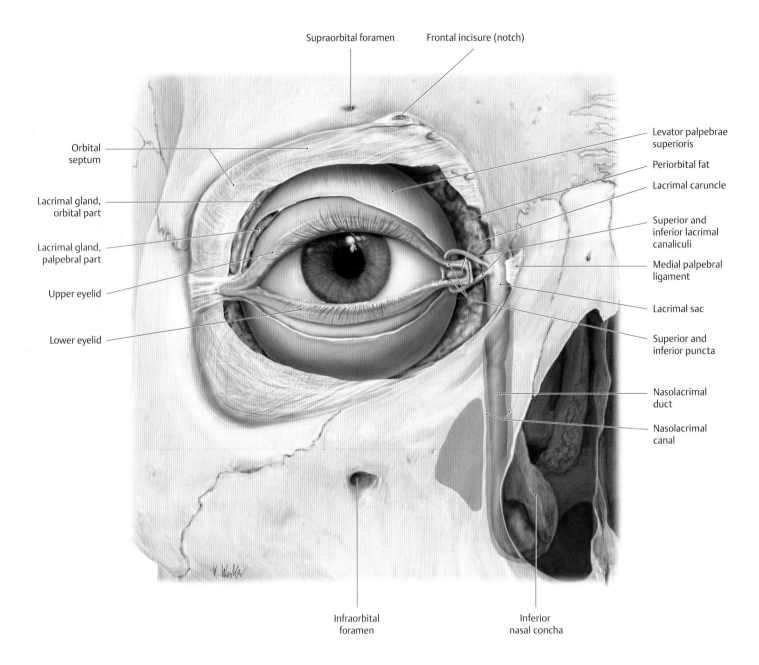

Supraorbital foramen    Frontal incisure (notch)

Levator palpebrae superioris

Periorbital fat

Lacrimal caruncle

Orbital septum

Superior and inferior lacrimal canaliculi

Lacrimal gland, orbital part

Medial palpebral ligament

Lacrimal gland, palpebral part

Lacrimal sac

Upper eyelid

Superior and inferior puncta

Lower eyelid

Nasolacrimal duct

Nasolacrimal canal

Infraorbital foramen

Inferior nasal concha

**Fig. 6.23 Lacrimal apparatus**

Right eye, anterior view. The orbital septum has been partially removed, and the tendon of insertion of the levator palpebrae superioris has been divided. The hazelnut-sized **lacrimal gland** is located in the lacrimal fossa of the frontal bone and produces most of the lacrimal fluid. Smaller *accessory lacrimal glands* (Krause or Wolfring glands) are also present. The tendon of levator palpebrae subdivides the lacrimal gland, which normally is not visible or palpable, into an *orbital lobe* (two thirds of gland) and a *palpebral lobe* (one third). The sympathetic fibers innervating the lacrimal gland originate from the superior cervical ganglion and travel along arteries to reach the lacrimal gland. Parasympathetic fibers reach the lacrimal gland via the lacrimal nerve (CN $V_1$). The lacrimal nerve communicates with the zygomatic nerve (CN $V_2$), which re-

lays postganglionic parasympathetic fibers from the pterygopalatine ganglion. The preganglionic parasympathetic fibers that synapse in the pterygopalatine ganglion travel as the greater petrosal nerve, which arises from the genu of the facial nerve (CN VII) (see **Fig. 4.38**). The **lacrimal apparatus** can be understood by tracing the flow of lacrimal fluid obliquely downward from the superolateral margin of the orbit (by the lacrimal gland) to the inferomedial margin (see **Fig. 6.25**). From the superior and inferior *puncta,* the lacrimal fluid enters the superior and inferior *lacrimal canaliculi,* which direct the fluid into the *lacrimal sac.* Finally, it drains through the *nasolacrimal duct* to an outlet below the inferior concha of the nose. "Watery eyes" are a typical cold symptom caused by obstruction of the inferior opening of the nasolacrimal duct.

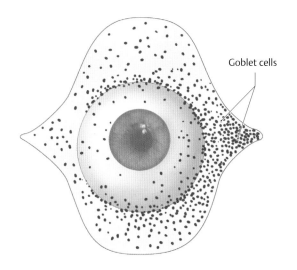

**Fig. 6.24 Distribution of goblet cells in the conjunctiva**
Goblet cells are mucus-secreting cells with an epithelial covering. Their secretions (mucins) are an important constituent of the lacrimal fluid. Mucins are also secreted by the main lacrimal gland.

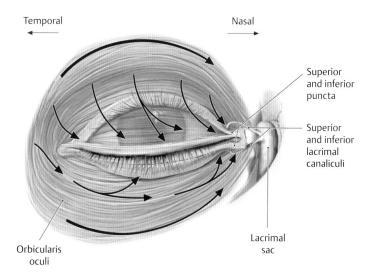

**Fig. 6.25 Mechanical propulsion of the lacrimal fluid**
During closure of the eyelids, contraction of the orbicularis oculi proceeds in a temporal-to-nasal direction. The successive contraction of these muscle fibers propels the lacrimal fluid toward the lacrimal passages. *Note:* Facial paralysis prevents closure of the eyelids, causing the eye to dry out.

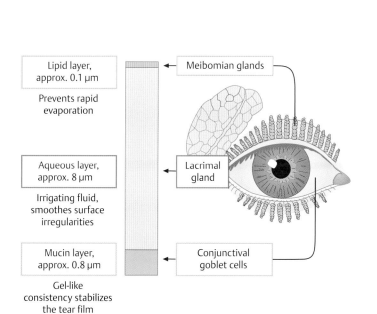

**Fig. 6.26 Structure of the tear film**
The tear film is a complex fluid with several morphologically distinct layers, whose components are produced by individual glands. The outer lipid layer, produced by the meibomian glands, protects the aqueous middle layer of the tear film from evaporating.

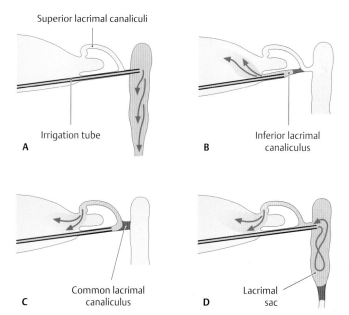

**Fig. 6.27 Obstructions to lacrimal drainage**
Sites of obstruction in the lacrimal drainage system can be located by irrigating the system with a special fluid.

**A** No obstruction to lacrimal drainage.
**B,C** Stenosis in the inferior or common lacrimal canaliculus. The stenosis causes a damming back of lacrimal fluid behind the obstructed site. In **B** the fluid refluxes through the inferior lacrimal canaliculus, and in **C** it flows through the superior lacrimal canaliculus.
**D** Stenosis below the level of the lacrimal sac (postlacrimal sac stenosis). When the entire lacrimal sac has filled with fluid, the fluid begins to reflux into the superior lacrimal canaliculus. In such cases, the lacrimal fluid often has a purulent, gelatinous appearance.

# Eyeball

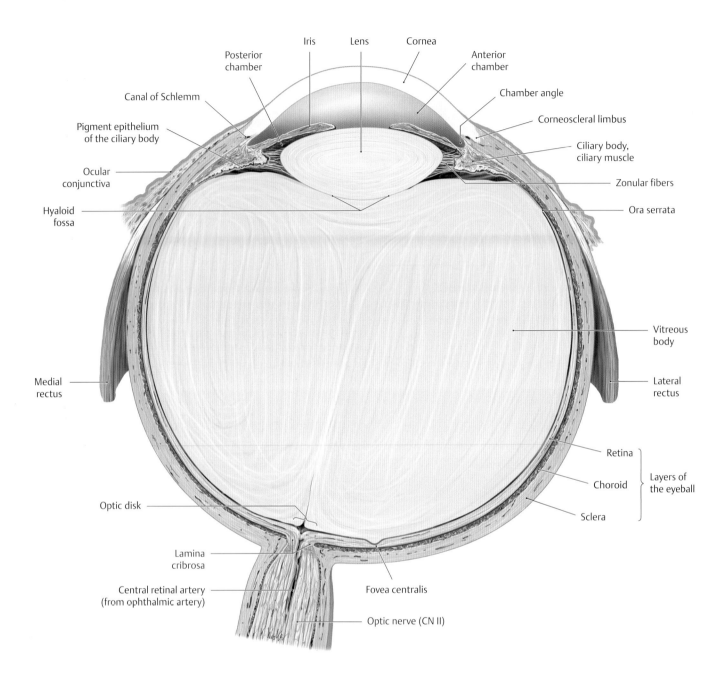

**Fig. 6.28 Eyeball**

Right eye, superior view of transverse section. Most of the eyeball is composed of three concentric layers surrounding vitreous humor: the sclera, the choroid, and the retina.

*Posterior portion of the eyeball:* The **sclera** is the posterior portion of the outer coat of the eyeball. It is a firm layer of connective tissue that gives attachment to the tendons of all the extraocular muscles. The middle layer of the eye, the **choroid**, is the most highly vascularized region in the body and serves to regulate the temperature of the eye and to supply blood to the outer layers of the retina. The inner layer of the eye, the **retina**, includes an inner layer of photosensitive cells (sensory retina) and an outer layer of retinal pigment epithelium. The axons of the optic nerve (CN II) pierce the lamina cribrosa of the sclera at the optic disk. The *fovea centralis* is a depressed area in the central retina approximately 4 mm temporal to the optic disk. Incident light is normally focused on the fovea centralis, the site of greatest visual acuity.

*Anterior portion:* The anterior portion of the eyeball has a different structure that is continuous with the posterior portion. The outer fibrous coat is the cornea, the "window of the eye," which bulges forward. At the corneoscleral limbus, the cornea is continuous with the less convex sclera. In the angle of the anterior chamber, the sclera forms the trabecular meshwork, which is connected to the canal of Schlemm. Beneath the sclera is the vascular coat of the eye, also called the uveal tract. It consists of three parts: the iris, ciliary body, and choroid. The iris shields the eye from excessive light and covers the lens. Its root is continuous with the ciliary body, which contains the ciliary muscle for visual accommodation (alters the refractive power of the lens). The epithelium of the ciliary body produces the aqueous humor. The ciliary body is continuous at the ora serrata with the choroid. The outer layer of the retina (pigment epithelium) is continued forward as the pigment epithelium of the ciliary body and the epithelium of the iris.

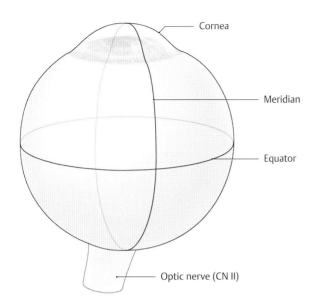

**Fig. 6.29 Reference lines and points on the eye**
The line marking the greatest circumference of the eyeball is the *equator*. Lines perpendicular to the equator are called *meridians*.

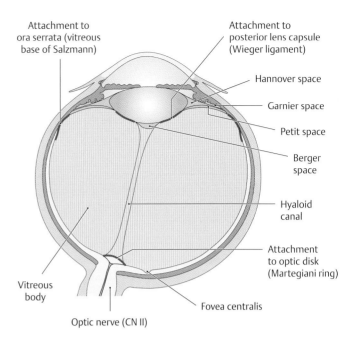

**Fig. 6.30 Vitreous body (vitreous humor)**
Right eye, transverse section viewed from above. Sites where the vitreous body is attached to other ocular structures are shown in red, and adjacent spaces are shown in green. The vitreous body stabilizes the eyeball and protects against retinal detachment. Devoid of nerves and vessels, it consists of 98% water and 2% hyaluronic acid and collagen. The "hyaloid canal" is an embryological remnant of the hyaloid artery. For the treatment of some diseases, the vitreous body may be surgically removed (vitrectomy) and the resulting cavity filled with physiological saline solution.

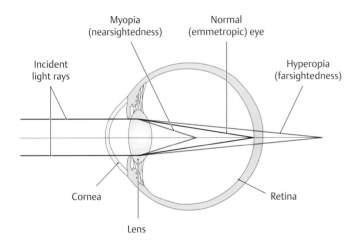

**Fig. 6.31 Light refraction**
In a normal (emmetropic) eye, parallel rays from a distant light source are refracted by the cornea and lens to a focal point on the retinal surface.

- In myopia (nearsightedness), the rays are focused to a point *in front* of the retina.
- In hyperopia (farsightedness), the rays are focused *behind* the retina.

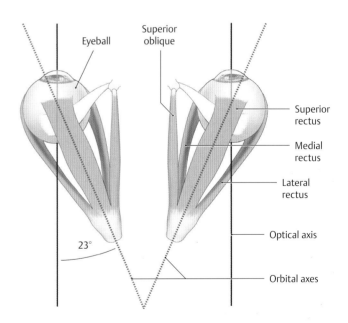

**Fig. 6.32 Optical axis and orbital axis**
Superior view of both eyes showing the medial, lateral, and superior recti and the superior oblique. The optical axis deviates from the orbital axis by 23 degrees. Because of this disparity, the point of maximum visual acuity, the fovea centralis, is lateral to the "blind spot" of the optic disk.

**125**

# Eye: Blood Supply

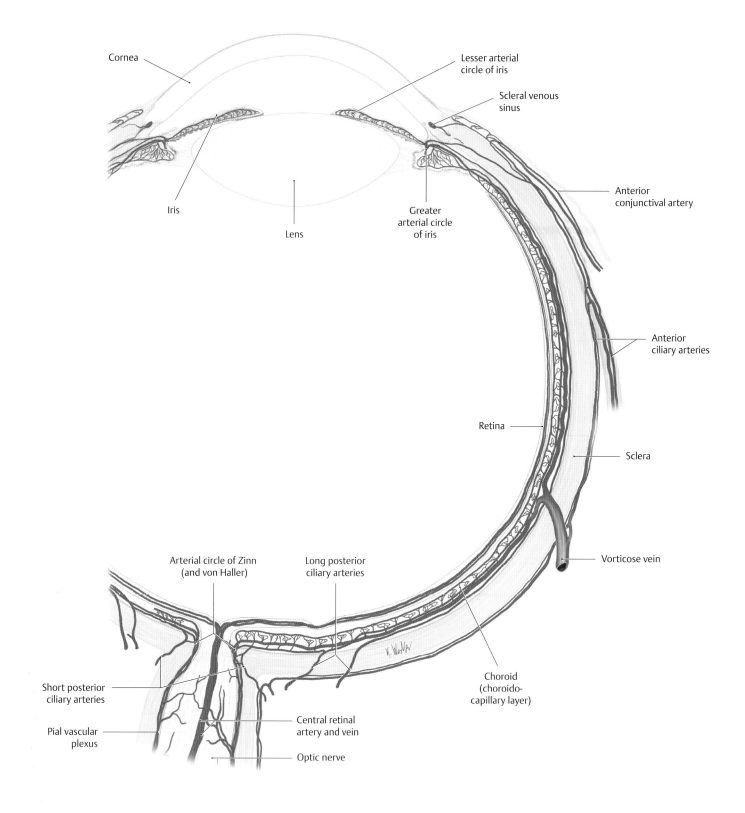

**Fig. 6.33 Blood supply of the eye**
Horizontal section through the right eye at the level of the optic nerve, viewed from above. All of the arteries that supply the eye arise from the *ophthalmic artery,* a branch of the internal carotid artery. Its ocular branches are:

- Central retinal artery to the retina
- Short posterior ciliary arteries to the choroid

- Long posterior ciliary arteries to the ciliary body and iris, where they supply the greater and lesser arterial circles of the iris (see **Fig. 6.43**)
- Anterior ciliary arteries, which arise from the vessels of the rectus muscles of the eye and anastomose with the posterior ciliary vessels

Blood is drained from the eyeball by four to eight vorticose veins, which pierce the sclera behind the equator and open into the superior or inferior ophthalmic vein.

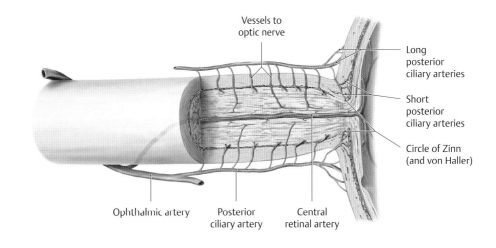

**Fig. 6.34 Arteries of the optic nerve (CN II)**
Lateral view. The central retinal artery, the first branch of the ophthalmic artery, enters the optic nerve from below approximately 1 cm behind the eyeball and courses with it to the retina while giving off multiple small branches. The posterior ciliary artery also gives off several small branches that supply the optic nerve. The distal part of the optic nerve receives its arterial blood supply from an arterial ring (circle of Zinn and von Haller) formed by anastomoses among the side branches of the short posterior ciliary arteries and central retinal artery.

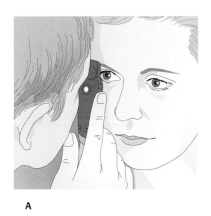

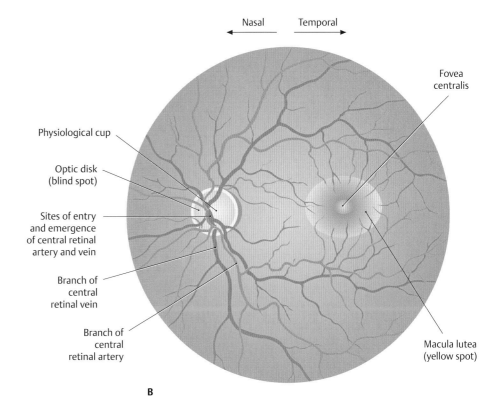

**A**

**B**

**Fig. 6.35 Ophthalmoscopic examination of the optic fundus**
**A** Examination technique (direct ophthalmoscopy). **B** Normal appearance of the optic fundus.
In direct ophthalmoscopy, the following structures of the optic fundus can be directly evaluated at approximately 16 x magnification:

- The condition of the retina
- The blood vessels (particularly the central retinal artery)
- The optic disk (where the optic nerve emerges from the eyeball)
- The macula lutea and fovea centralis

Because the retina is transparent, the color of the optic fundus is determined chiefly by the pigment epithelium and the blood vessels of the choroid. It is uniformly pale red in light-skinned persons and is considerably browner in dark-skinned persons. Abnormal detachment of the retina is usually associated with a loss of retinal transparency, and the retina assumes a yellowish white color. The central retinal artery and vein can be distinguished from each other by their color and caliber: arteries have a brighter red color and a smaller caliber than the veins. This provides a means for the early detection of vascular changes (e.g., stenosis, wall thickening, microaneurysms), such as those occurring in diabetes mellitus (diabetic retinopathy) or hypertension. The *optic disk* normally has sharp margins, a yellow-orange color, and a central depression, the physiological cup. The disk is subject to changes in pathological conditions such as elevated intracranial pressure (papilledema with ill-defined disk margins). On examination of the *macula lutea,* which is 3 to 4 mm temporal to the optic disk, it can be seen that numerous branches of the central retinal artery radiate toward the macula but do not reach its center, the fovea centralis (the fovea receives its blood supply from the choroid). A common age-related disease of the macula lutea is macular degeneration, which may gradually lead to blindness.

# Eye: Lens & Cornea

**Fig. 6.36  Position of the lens and cornea**
Histological section through the cornea, lens, and suspensory apparatus of the lens. The normal lens is clear, transparent, and only 4 mm thick. It is suspended in the hyaloid fossa of the vitreous body. The lens is attached by rows of fibrils (zonular fibers) to the ciliary muscle, whose contractions alter the shape and focal length of the lens. Thus, the lens is a dynamic structure that can change its shape in response to visual requirements. The anterior chamber of the eye is situated in front of the lens, and the posterior chamber is located between the iris and the anterior epithelium of the lens. The lens, like the vitreous body, is devoid of nerves and blood vessels and is composed of elongated epithelial cells (lens fibers).

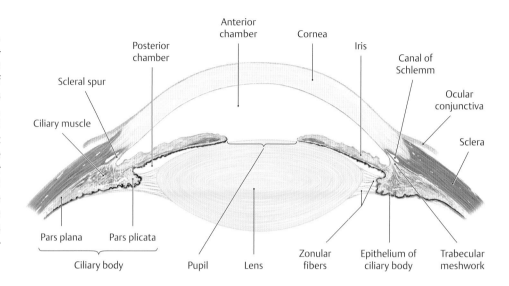

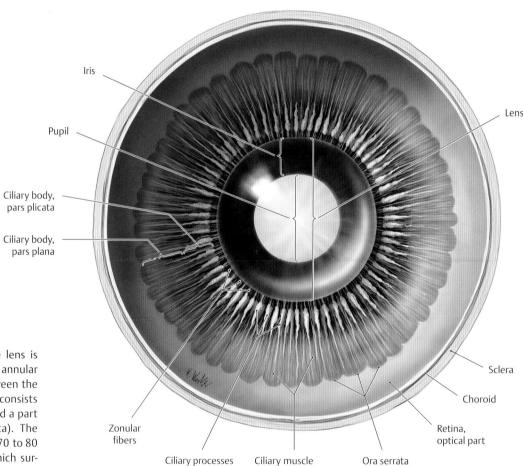

**Fig. 6.37  Lens and ciliary body**
Posterior view. The curvature of the lens is regulated by the muscle fibers of the annular ciliary body. The *ciliary body* lies between the ora serrata and the root of the iris and consists of a relatively flat part (pars plana) and a part that is raised into folds (pars plicata). The latter part is ridged by approximately 70 to 80 radially oriented ciliary processes, which surround the lens like a halo when viewed from behind. The ciliary processes contain large capillaries, and their epithelium secretes the aqueous humor. Very fine *zonular fibers* extend from the basal layer of the ciliary processes to the equator of the lens. These fibers and the spaces between them constitute the suspensory apparatus of the lens, called the *zonule*. Most of the ciliary body is occupied by the ciliary muscle, a smooth muscle composed of meridional, radial, and circular fibers. It arises mainly from the scleral spur (a reinforcing ring of sclera just below the canal of Schlemm), and it attaches to structures including the Bruch membrane of the choroid and the inner surface of the sclera. When the ciliary muscle contracts, it pulls the choroid forward and relaxes the zonular fibers. As these fibers become lax, the intrinsic resilience of the lens causes it to assume the more convex relaxed shape that is necessary for near vision. This is the basic mechanism of visual accommodation.

128

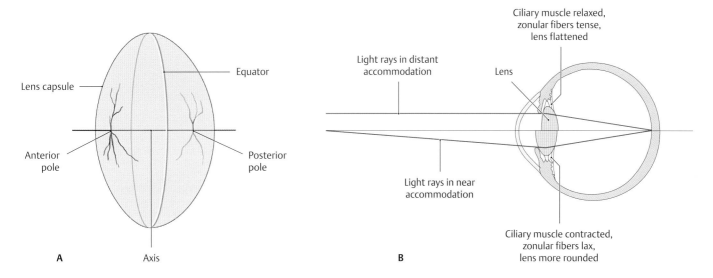

**Fig. 6.38 Reference lines and dynamics of the lens**

**A Principal reference lines of the lens:** The lens has an a*nterior* and *posterior pole,* an *axis* passing between the poles, and an *equator*. The lens has a biconvex shape with a greater radius of curvature posteriorly (16 mm) than anteriorly (10 mm). Its function is to transmit light rays and make fine adjustments in refraction. Its refractive power ranges from 10 to 20 diopters, depending on the state of accommodation. The cornea has a considerably higher refractive power of 43 diopters.

**B Light refraction and dynamics of the lens:**
- Upper half of diagram: fine adjustment of the eye for *far vision*. Parallel light rays arrive from a distant source, and the lens is flattened.
- Lower half of diagram: For *near vision* (accommodation to objects less than 5 m from the eye), the lens assumes a more rounded shape. This is effected by contraction of the ciliary muscle (parasympathetic innervation from the oculomotor nerve), causing the zonular fibers to relax and allowing the lens to assume a more rounded shape because of its intrinsic resilience.

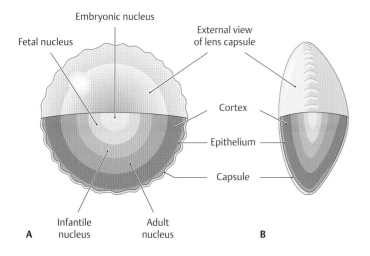

**Fig. 6.39 Growth of the lens and zones of discontinuity**

**A** Anterior view. **B** Lateral view.

The lens continues to grow throughout life, doing so in a manner opposite to that of other epithelial structures (i.e., the youngest cells are at the surface of the lens, whereas the oldest cells are deeper). Due to the constant proliferation of epithelial cells, which are all firmly incorporated in the lens capsule, the tissue of the lens becomes increasingly dense with age. A slit-lamp examination will demonstrate zones of varying cell density (zones of discontinuity). The zone of highest cell density, the *embryonic nucleus,* is at the center of the lens. With further growth, it becomes surrounded by the *fetal nucleus*. The *infantile nucleus* develops after birth, and finally the *adult nucleus* begins to form during the third decade of life. These zones are the basis for the morphological classification of cataracts, a structural alteration in the lens, causing opacity, that is more or less normal in old age (present in 10% of all 80-year-olds).

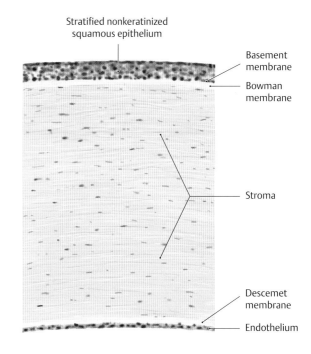

**Fig. 6.40 Structure of the cornea**

The cornea is covered externally by stratified, nonkeratinized squamous epithelium whose basal lamina borders on the anterior limiting lamina (Bowman membrane). The stroma (substantia propria) makes up approximately 90% of the corneal thickness and is bounded on its deep surface by the posterior limiting lamina (Descemet membrane). Beneath is a single layer of corneal endothelium. The cornea does have a nerve supply (for corneal reflexes), but it is not vascularized and therefore has an immunologically privileged status: normally, a corneal transplant can be performed without fear of a host rejection response.

**129**

# Eye: Iris & Ocular Chambers

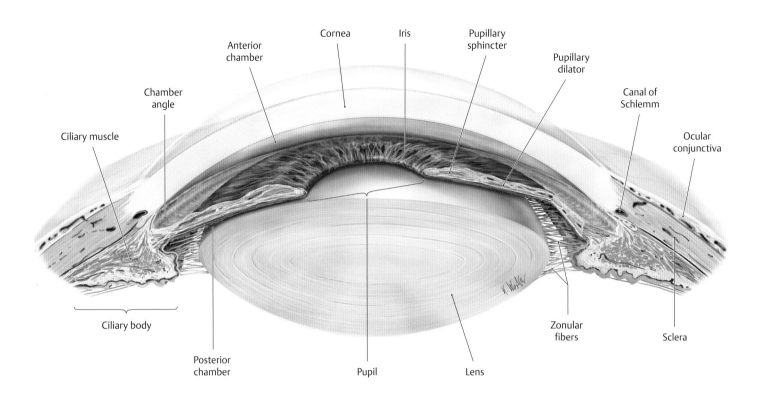

**Fig. 6.41 Iris and chambers of the eye**

Transverse section through the anterior segment of the eye, superior view. The iris, the choroid, and the ciliary body at the periphery of the iris are part of the uveal tract. In the iris, the pigments are formed that determine eye color. The iris is an optical diaphragm with a central aperture, the pupil, placed in front of the lens. The pupil is 1 to 8 mm in diameter; it constricts on contraction of the pupillary sphincter (*parasympathetic* innervation via the oculomotor nerve and ciliary ganglion) and dilates on contraction of the pupillary dilator (*sympathetic* innervation from the superior cervical ganglion via the internal carotid plexus). Together, the iris and lens separate the anterior chamber of the eye from the posterior chamber. The posterior chamber behind the iris is bounded posteriorly by the vitreous body, centrally by the lens, and laterally by the ciliary body. The anterior chamber is bounded anteriorly by the cornea and posteriorly by the iris and lens.

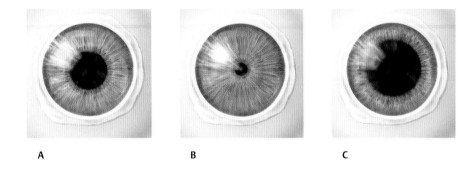

**A**          **B**          **C**

**Fig. 6.42 Pupil size**

**A** Normal pupil size. **B** Maximum constriction (miosis). **C** Maximum dilation (mydriasis).

The regulation of pupil size is aided by the two intraocular muscles, the pupillary sphincter and pupillary dilator. The pupillary sphincter (parasympathetic innervation) narrows the pupil, and the pupillary dilator (sympathetic innervation) enlarges the pupil. Pupil size is normally adjusted in response to incident light and serves mainly to optimize visual acuity.

Normally, the pupils are circular in shape and equal in size (3 to 5 mm). Various influences may cause the pupil size to vary over a range from 1.5 mm (miosis) to 8 mm (mydriasis). A greater than 1 mm discrepancy of pupil size between the right and left eyes is called *anisocoria*. Mild anisocoria is physiological in some individuals. Pupillary reflexes such as convergence and the consensual light response are described on p. 138.

| Table 6.7 Changes in pupil size: causes | |
| --- | --- |
| **Pupil constriction (parasympathetic)** | **Pupil dilation (sympathetic)** |
| Light | Darkness |
| Sleep, fatigue | Pain, excitement |
| Miotic agents:<br>• Parasympathomimetics (e.g., tear gas, VX and sarin, Alzheimer's drugs such as rivastigmine)<br>• Sympatholytics (e.g., antihypertensives) | Mydriatic agents:<br>• Parasympatholytics (e.g., atropine)<br>• Sympathomimetics (e.g., epinephrine) |
| Horner syndrome (also causes ptosis and narrowing of palpebral fissure) | Oculomotor palsy |
| General anesthesia, morphine | Migraine attack, glaucoma attack |

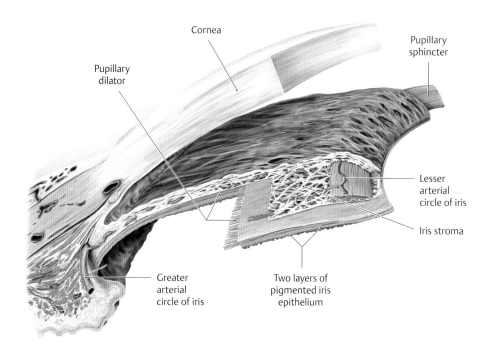

**Fig. 6.43 Structure of the iris**
The basic structural framework of the iris is the vascularized stroma, which is bounded on its deep surface by two layers of pigmented iris epithelium. The loose, collagen-containing stroma of the iris contains outer and inner vascular circles (greater and lesser arterial circles), which are interconnected by small anastomotic arteries. The pupillary sphincter is an annular muscle located in the stroma bordering the pupil. The radially disposed pupillary dilator is not located in the stroma; rather, it is composed of numerous myofibrils in the iris epithelium (myoepithelium). The stroma of the iris is permeated by pigmented connective tissue cells (melanocytes). When heavily pigmented, these melanocytes of the anterior border zone of the stroma render the iris brown or "black." Otherwise, the characteristics of the underlying stroma and epithelium determine eye color, in a manner that is not fully understood.

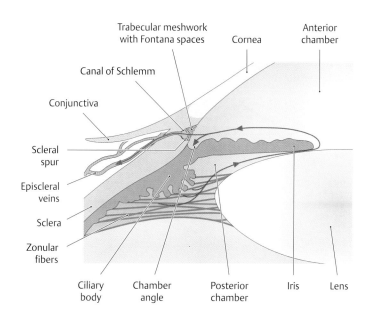

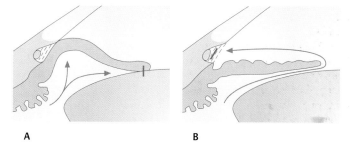

**Fig. 6.45 Obstruction of aqueous drainage and glaucoma**
Normal function of the optical system requires normal intraocular pressure (15 mm Hg in adults). This maintains a smooth curvature of the corneal surface and helps keep the photoreceptor cells in contact with the pigment epithelium. Obstruction of the normal drainage of aqueous humor causes an increase in intraocular pressure. This constricts the optic nerve at the lamina cribrosa, where it emerges from the eyeball through the sclera. Such constriction eventually leads to blindness. There are two types of glaucoma:

**A** Acute (closed-angle) glaucoma: The chamber angle is obstructed by iris tissue. Aqueous fluid cannot drain into the anterior chamber and pushes portions of the iris upward, blocking the chamber angle. This type of glaucoma often develops quickly.
**B** Chronic (open-angle) glaucoma: The chamber angle is open, but drainage through the trabecular meshwork is impaired. Ninety percent of all glaucomas are primary chronic open-angle glaucomas. This is increasingly prevalent after 40 years of age. Treatment options include parasympathomimetics (to induce sustained contraction of the ciliary muscle and pupillary sphincter), prostaglandin analogues (to improve aqueous drainage), and beta-adrenergic agonists (to decrease production of aqueous humor).

**Fig. 6.44 Normal drainage of aqueous humor**
The aqueous humor (approximately 0.3 mL per eye) is an important determinant of the intraocular pressure. It is produced by the non-pigmented ciliary epithelium of the ciliary processes in the *posterior* chamber (approximately 0.15 mL/hour) and passes through the pupil into the *anterior* chamber of the eye. The aqueous humor seeps through the spaces of the trabecular meshwork (Fontana spaces) in the chamber angle and enters the canal of Schlemm (venous sinus of the sclera), through which it drains to the episcleral veins. The draining aqueous humor flows toward the chamber angle along a pressure gradient (intraocular pressure = 15 mm Hg, pressure in the episcleral veins = 9 mm Hg) and must surmount a physiological resistance at two sites:

• *Pupillary resistance* (between the iris and lens)
• *Trabecular resistance* (narrow spaces in the trabecular meshwork)

Approximately 85% of the aqueous humor flows through the trabecular meshwork into the canal of Schlemm. Only 15% drains through the uveoscleral vascular system into the vortical veins (uveoscleral drainage route).

# Eye: Retina

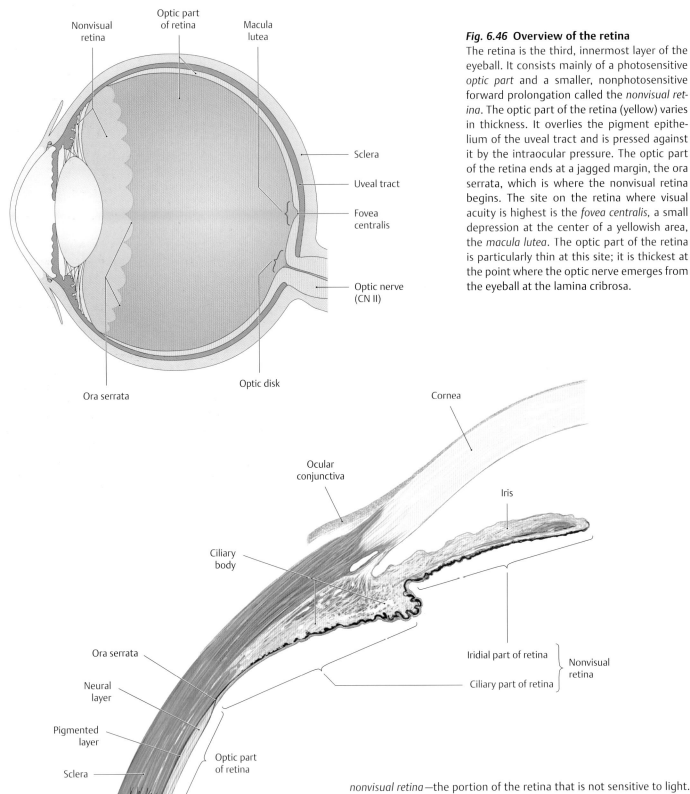

**Fig. 6.46 Overview of the retina**
The retina is the third, innermost layer of the eyeball. It consists mainly of a photosensitive *optic part* and a smaller, nonphotosensitive forward prolongation called the *nonvisual retina*. The optic part of the retina (yellow) varies in thickness. It overlies the pigment epithelium of the uveal tract and is pressed against it by the intraocular pressure. The optic part of the retina ends at a jagged margin, the ora serrata, which is where the nonvisual retina begins. The site on the retina where visual acuity is highest is the *fovea centralis*, a small depression at the center of a yellowish area, the *macula lutea*. The optic part of the retina is particularly thin at this site; it is thickest at the point where the optic nerve emerges from the eyeball at the lamina cribrosa.

**Fig. 6.47 Parts of the retina**
The posterior surface of the iris bears a double layer of pigment epithelium, the *iridial part* of the retina. Just peripheral to it is the *ciliary part* of the retina, also formed by a *double* layer of epithelium (one of which is pigmented) and covering the posterior surface of the ciliary body. The iridial and ciliary parts of the retina together constitute the *nonvisual retina*—the portion of the retina that is not sensitive to light. The nonvisual retina ends at a jagged line, the ora serrata, where the light-sensitive *optic part* of the retina begins. Consistent with the development of the retina from the embryonic optic cup, two layers can be distinguished within the optic part:

- An outer layer nearer the sclera: the *pigmented layer*, consisting of a single layer of pigmented retinal epithelium.
- An inner layer nearer the vitreous body: the *neural layer*, comprising a system of receptor cells, interneurons, and ganglion cells.

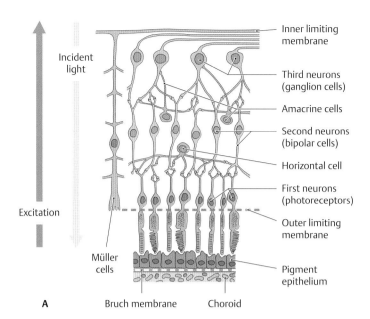

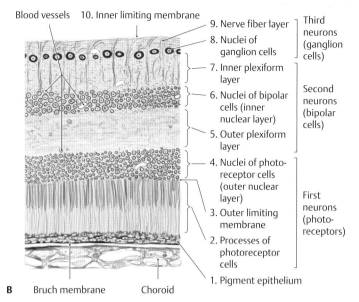

## Fig. 6.48 Structure of the retina

**A** Retinal neurons of the visual pathway. **B** Anatomical layers of the retina. Light passes through all the layers of the retina to be received by the photoreceptors on the outermost surface of the retina. Sensory information is then transmitted via three retinal neurons of the visual pathway to the optic disk:

- First neurons (pink): Photoreceptor cells (light-sensitive sensory cells) that transform light stimuli (photons) into electrochemical signals. The two types of photoreceptors are rods and cones, named for the shape of their receptor segment. The retina contains 100 million to 125 million rods, which are responsible for twilight and night vision, but only about 6 million to 7 million cones. Different cones are specialized for the perception of red, green, and blue. The processes and nuclei of the first neurons compose anatomical layers 2 to 4 (see **B**).
- Second neurons (yellow): Bipolar cells that receive impulses from the photoreceptors and relay them to the ganglion cells. These neurons compose anatomical layers 5 to 7.

- Third neurons (green): Retinal ganglion cells whose axons converge at the optic disk to form the optic nerve (CN II) and reach the lateral geniculate and superior colliculus. These neurons compose anatomical layers 8 to 10. There are approximately 1 million retinal ganglion axons per eye.

*Support cells:* Müller cells (blue) are glial cells that span the neural layer radially from the inner to the outer limiting membranes, creating a supporting framework for the neurons. In addition to the vertical connections, horizontal and amacrine cells (gray) function as interneurons that establish lateral connections. Impulses transmitted by the receptor cells are thereby processed and organized within the retina (signal convergence).

*Pigment epithelium:* The outer layer of the retina (the pigment epithelium, brown) is attached to the Bruch membrane, which contains elastic fibers and collagen fibrils and mediates the exchange of substances between the adjacent choroid (choriocapillaris) and the photoreceptor cells. *Note:* The photoreceptors are in contact with the pigment epithelium but are not attached to it. The retina may become detached (if untreated, this leads to blindness).

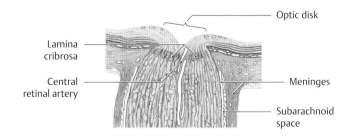

## Fig. 6.49 Optic disk ("blind spot") and lamina cribrosa

The unmyelinated axons of the third neurons (retinal ganglion cells) pass to a collecting point at the posterior pole of the eye. There they unite to form the optic nerve and leave the retina through numerous perforations in the sclera (lamina cribrosa). (*Note:* The optic disk has no photoreceptors and is therefore the physiological blind spot.) In the optic nerve, these axons are myelinated by oligodendrocytes. The optic nerve (CN II) is an extension of the diencephalon and therefore has all the coverings of the brain (dura mater, arachnoid, and pia mater). It is surrounded by a subarachnoid space that contains cerebrospinal fluid (CSF) and communicates with the subarachnoid spaces of the brain and spinal cord.

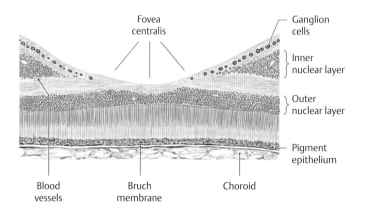

## Fig. 6.50 Macula lutea and fovea centralis

Temporal to the optic disk is the macula lutea. At its center is a funnel-shaped depression approximately 1.5 mm in diameter, the fovea centralis, which is the site of maximum visual acuity. At this site the inner retinal layers are heaped toward the margin of the depression, so that the cells of the photoreceptors (just cones, no rods) are directly exposed to the incident light. This arrangement significantly reduces scattering of the light rays.

# Visual System (I): Overview & Geniculate Part

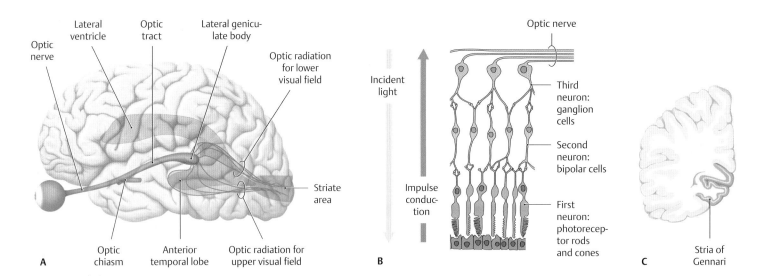

| | | | |
|---|---|---|---|
| **A** | Optic chiasm | Anterior temporal lobe | Optic radiation for upper visual field |

**B**

**C** Stria of Gennari

**Fig. 6.51 Overview of the visual pathway**

Left lateral view. The visual pathway extends from the eye, an anterior prolongation of the diencephalon, back to the occipital pole. Thus, it encompasses almost the entire longitudinal axis of the brain. The principal stations are as follows:

**Retina:** The first three neurons of the visual pathway (**B**):

- First neuron: photoreceptor rods and cones, located on the deep retinal surface opposite the direction of the incoming light ("inversion of the retina").
- Second neuron: bipolar cells.
- Third neuron: ganglion cells whose axons are collected to form the optic nerve.

**Optic nerve (CN II), optic chiasm, and optic tract:** This neural portion of the visual pathway is part of the central nervous system and is surrounded by meninges. Thus, the optic nerve is actually a tract rather than a true nerve. The optic nerves join below the base of the diencephalon to form the optic chiasm, which then divides into the two optic tracts. Each of these tracts divides in turn into a lateral and medial root.

**Lateral geniculate body:** Ninety percent of the axons of the third neuron (= 90% of the optic nerve fibers) terminate in the lateral geniculate body on neurons that project to the striate area (visual cortex, see below). This is the *geniculate part of the visual pathway.* It is concerned with *conscious* visual perception and is conveyed by the lateral root of the optic tract. The remaining 10% of the third-neuron axons in the visual pathway do not terminate in the lateral geniculate body. This is the *nongeniculate part of the visual pathway* (medial root, see **Fig. 6.56**), and its signals are not consciously perceived.

**Optic radiation and visual cortex (striate area):** The optic radiation begins in the lateral geniculate body, forms a band that winds around the inferior and posterior horns of the lateral ventricles, and terminates in the visual cortex or striate area (= Brodmann area 17). Located in the occipital lobe, the visual cortex can be grossly identified by a prominent stripe of white matter in the otherwise gray cerebral cortex (the stria of Gennari, see **C**). This white stripe runs parallel to the brain surface and is shown in the inset, where the gray matter of the visual cortex is shaded light red.

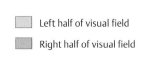

☐ Left half of visual field

☐ Right half of visual field

**Fig. 6.52 Representation of each visual field in the contralateral visual cortex**

Superior view. The light rays in the *nasal* part of each visual field are projected to the *temporal* half of the retina, and those from the *temporal* part are projected to the nasal half. Because of this arrangement, the left half of the visual field projects to the visual cortex of the right occipital pole, and the right half projects to the visual cortex of the left occipital pole. For clarity, each visual field in the diagram is divided into two halves. *Note:* The axonal fibers from the nasal half of each retina cross to the opposite side at the optic chiasm and then travel with the uncrossed fibers from the temporal half of each retina.

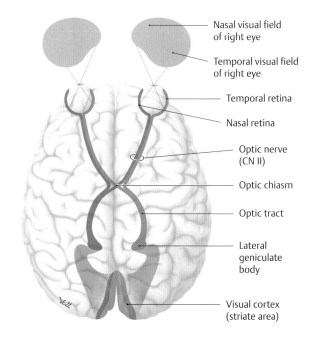

Nasal visual field of right eye

Temporal visual field of right eye

Temporal retina

Nasal retina

Optic nerve (CN II)

Optic chiasm

Optic tract

Lateral geniculate body

Visual cortex (striate area)

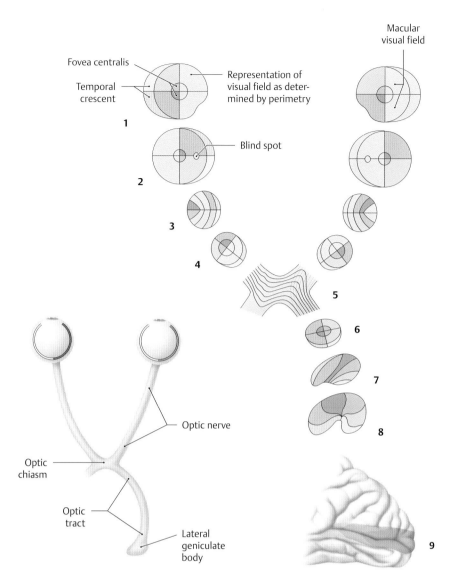

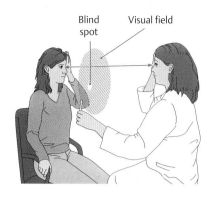

**Fig. 6.54 Informal visual field examination with the confrontation test**

The visual field examination is an essential step in the examination of lesions of the visual pathway (see **Fig. 6.55**). The **confrontation test** is an *informal* test in which the examiner (with an intact visual field) and the patient sit face-to-face, cover one eye, and each fixes their gaze on the other's open eye, creating identical visual axes. The examiner then moves his or her index finger from the outer edge of the visual field toward the center until the patient signals that he or she can see the finger. With this test the examiner can make a gross assessment as to the presence and approximate location of a possible visual field defect. The *precise* location and extent of a visual field defect can be determined by **perimetry**, in which points of light replace the examiner's finger. The results of the test are entered in charts that resemble the small diagrams in **Fig. 6.53**.

**Fig. 6.53 Geniculate part of visual pathway: topographic organization**

The visual field is divided into four quadrants: upper temporal, upper nasal, lower nasal, and lower temporal. The lower nasal quadrant is indented by the nose. The representation of this subdivision is continued into the visual cortex. *Note:* Only the left visual hemifield (blue) is shown here (compare to **Fig. 6.52**).

1 **Visual hemifield:** Each visual hemifield is divided into three zones (indicated by color shading):

- Fovea centralis: The smallest and darkest zone is at the center of the visual field. It corresponds to the fovea centralis, the point of maximum visual acuity on the retina. The fovea centralis has a high receptor density; accordingly, a great many axons pass centrally from its receptors. It is therefore represented by a disproportionately large area in the visual cortex.
- Macular visual field: The largest zone in the visual hemisphere; it also contains the blind spot.
- Temporal crescent: The temporal, monocular part of the visual field. This corresponds to more peripheral portions of the retina that contain fewer receptors and therefore fewer axons, resulting in a smaller representational area in the visual cortex.

2 **Retinal projection:** All light that reaches the retina must pass through the narrow pupil, which functions like the aperture of a camera. Up/down and nasal/temporal are therefore reversed when the image is projected on the retina.

**3,4 Optic nerve:** In the distal part of the optic nerve, the fibers that represent the macular visual field initially occupy a lateral position (**3**), then move increasingly toward the center of the nerve (**4**).

5 **Optic chiasm:** While traversing the optic chiasm, the fibers of the nasal retina of the optic nerve cross the midline to the opposite side.

6 **Start of the optic tract:** Fibers from the corresponding halves of the retinas unite (e.g., right halves of the left and right retinas in the right optic tract). The impulses from the left visual field (right retinal half) will therefore terminate in the right striate area.

7 **End of the optic tract:** Fibers are collected to form a wedge before entering the lateral geniculate body.

8 **Lateral geniculate body:** Macular fibers occupy almost half of the wedge. After the fibers are relayed to the fourth neuron, they project to the posterior end of the occipital pole (= visual cortex).

9 **Visual cortex:** There exists a point-to-point (retinotopic) correlation between the number of axons in the retina and the number of axons in the visual cortex (e.g., the central part of the visual field is represented by the largest area in the visual cortex, due to the large number of axons concentrated in the fovea centralis). The central lower half of the visual field is represented by a large area on the occipital pole above the calcarine sulcus; the central upper half of the visual field is represented below the sulcus.

# Visual System (II): Lesions & Nongeniculate Part

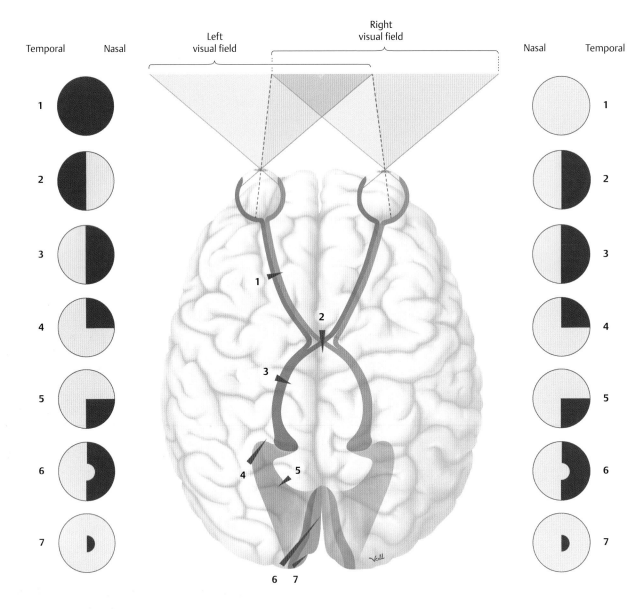

**Fig. 6.55 Visual field defects and lesions of the visual pathway**
Circles represent the perceived visual disturbances (scotomas, or areas of darkness) in the left and right eyes. These characteristic visual field defects (anopias) result from lesions at specific sites along the visual pathway. Lesion sites are illustrated in the left visual pathway as red wedges. The nature of the visual field defect often points to the location of the lesion. *Note:* Lesions past the optic chiasm will all be homonymous (same visual field in both eyes).

**1** Unilateral optic nerve lesion: Blindness (amaurosis) in the affected eye.
**2** Lesion of optic chiasm: Bitemporal hemianopia (think of a horse wearing blinders). Only fibers from the nasal portions of the retina (representing the temporal visual field) cross in the optic chiasm.
**3** Unilateral optic tract lesion: Contralateral homonymous hemianopia. The lesion interrupts fibers from the temporal portion of the retina on the ipsilateral side and nasal portions of the retina on the contralateral side. The patient therefore has visual impairment of the same visual hemisphere in both eyes.

**4** Unilateral lesion of the optic radiation in the anterior temporal lobe: Contralateral upper quadrantanopia ("pie in the sky" deficit). Lesions in the anterior temporal lobe affect only those fibers winding under the inferior horn of the lateral ventricle (see **Fig. 6.51**). These fibers represent only the upper half of the visual field (in this case the nasal portion).
**5** Unilateral lesion of the optic radiation in the parietal lobe: Contralateral lower quadrantanopia. Fibers from the lower half of the visual field course superior to the lateral ventricle in the parietal lobe.
**6** Occipital lobe lesion: Homonymous hemianopia. The lesion affects the optic radiations from both the upper and lower visual fields. However, as the optic radiation fans out widely before entering the visual cortex, foveal vision is often spared. These lesions are most commonly due to intracerebral hemorrhage; the visual field defects vary considerably with the size of the hemorrhage.
**7** Occipital pole lesion (confined to cortical area): Homonymous hemianopic central scotoma. The cortical areas of the occipital pole represent the macula.

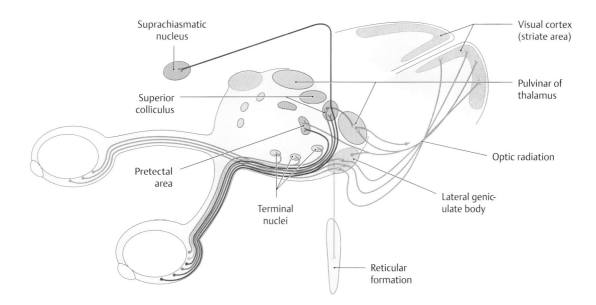

### Fig. 6.56 Nongeniculate part of the visual pathway

Approximately 10% of the axons of the optic nerve do not terminate on neurons in the lateral geniculate body for projection to the visual cortex. They continue along the medial root of the optic tract, forming the *nongeniculate part* of the visual pathway. The information from these fibers is not processed at a conscious level but plays an important role in the unconscious regulation of various vision-related processes and in visually mediated reflexes (e.g., the afferent limb of the pupillary light reflex). Axons from the nongeniculate part of the visual pathway terminate in the following regions:

- Axons to the superior colliculus transmit kinetic information that is necessary for tracking moving objects by unconscious eye and head movements (retinotectal system).
- Axons to the pretectal area transmit afferents for pupillary responses and accommodation reflexes (retinopretectal system). Subdivision

into specific nuclei has not yet been accomplished in humans, and so the term "area" is used.

- Axons to the suprachiasmatic nucleus of the hypothalamus influence circadian rhythms.
- Axons to the thalamic nuclei (optic tract) in the tegmentum of the mesencephalon and to the vestibular nuclei transmit afferent fibers for optokinetic nystagmus (= jerky, physiological eye movements during the tracking of fast-moving objects). This has also been called the "accessory visual system."
- Axons to the pulvinar of the thalamus form the visual association cortex for oculomotor function (neurons are relayed in the superior colliculus).
- Axons to the parvocellular nucleus of the reticular formation function during arousal.

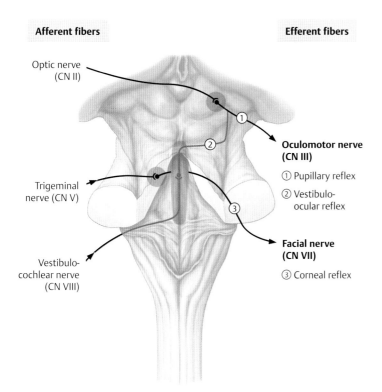

### Fig. 6.57 Brainstem reflexes

Brainstem reflexes are important in the examination of comatose patients. Loss of all brainstem reflexes is considered evidence of brain death. Three of these reflexes are described below:

**Pupillary reflex:** The pupillary reflex relies on the nongeniculate parts of the visual pathway (see **Fig. 6.59**). The afferent fibers for this reflex come from the optic nerve, which is an extension of the diencephalon. The efferents for the pupillary reflex come from the accessory nucleus of the oculomotor nerve (CN III), which is located in the brainstem. Loss of the pupillary reflex may signify a lesion of the diencephalon (interbrain) or mesencephalon (midbrain).

**Vestibulo-ocular reflex:** Irrigating the ear canal with cold water in a normal individual evokes nystagmus that beats toward the opposite side (afferent fibers are conveyed in the vestibulocochlear nerve [CN VIII], efferent fibers in the oculomotor nerve [CN III]). When the vestibulo-ocular reflex is absent in a comatose patient, it is considered a poor sign because this reflex is the most reliable clinical test of brainstem function.

**Corneal reflex:** This reflex is not mediated by the visual pathway. The afferent fibers for the reflex (elicited by stimulation of the cornea, as by touching it with a sterile cotton wisp) are conveyed in the trigeminal nerve (CN V) and the efferent fibers (contraction of the orbicularis oculi in response to corneal irritation) in the facial nerve (CN VII). The relay center for the corneal reflex is located in the pontine region of the brainstem.

# Visual System (III): Reflexes

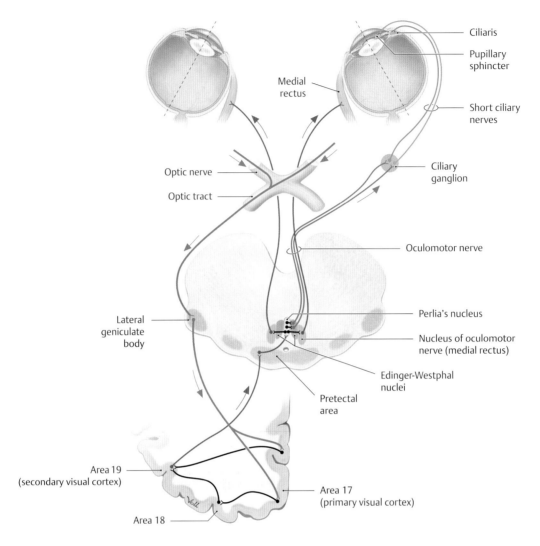

***Fig. 6.58* Pathways for convergence and accommodation**
When the distance between the eyes and an object decreases, three processes must occur in order to produce a sharp, three-dimensional visual impression (the first two are simultaneous):

1. Convergence (red): The visual axes of the eyes move closer together. The two medial rectus muscles contract to move the ocular axis medially. This keeps the image of the approaching object on the fovea centralis.
2. Accommodation: The lenses adjust their focal length. The curvature of the lens is increased to keep the image of the object sharply focused on the retina. The ciliary muscle contracts, which relaxes the tension on the lenticular fibers. The intrinsic pressure of the lens then causes it to assume a more rounded shape. (*Note:* The lens is flattened by the contraction of the lenticular fibers, which are attached to the ciliary muscle.)
3. Pupillary constriction: The pupil is constricted by the pupillary sphincter to increase visual acuity.

Convergence and accommodation may be conscious (fixing the gaze on a near object) or unconscious (fixing the gaze on an approaching automobile).
**Pathways:** The pathways can be broken into three components:

1. Geniculate visual pathway (purple): Axons of the first neurons (photoreceptors) and second neurons (bipolar cells) relay sensory information to the third neurons (retinal ganglion cells), which course in the optic nerve (CN II) to the lateral geniculate body. There they syn-

apse with the fourth neuron, whose axons project to the primary visual cortex (area 17).
2. Visual cortexes to cranial nerve nuclei: Interneurons (black) connect the primary (area 17) and secondary (area 19) visual cortexes. Synaptic relays (red) connect area 19 to the pretectal area and ultimately Perlia's nucleus (yellow), located between the two Edinger-Westphal (visceral oculomotor) nuclei (green).
3. Cranial nerves: At Perlia's nucleus, the pathway for convergence diverges with the pathways for accommodation and pupillary constriction:

   • Convergence: Neurons relay impulses to the somatomotor nucleus of the oculomotor nerve, whose axons pass directly to the medial rectus muscle via the oculomotor nerve (CN III).
   • Accommodation and pupillary constriction: Neurons relay impulses to the Edinger-Westphal nucleus, whose preganglionic parasympathetic axons project to the ciliary ganglion. After synapsing in the ciliary ganglion, the postganglionic axons pass either to the ciliary muscle (accommodation) or the pupillary sphincter (pupillary constriction) via the short ciliary nerves.

*Note:* The pupillary sphincter light response is abolished in tertiary syphilis, while accommodation (ciliary muscle) and convergence (medial rectus) are preserved. This phenomenon, called an Argyll Robertson pupil, indicates that the connections to the ciliary and pupillary sphincter muscles are mediated by different tracts, although the anatomy of these tracts is not yet fully understood.

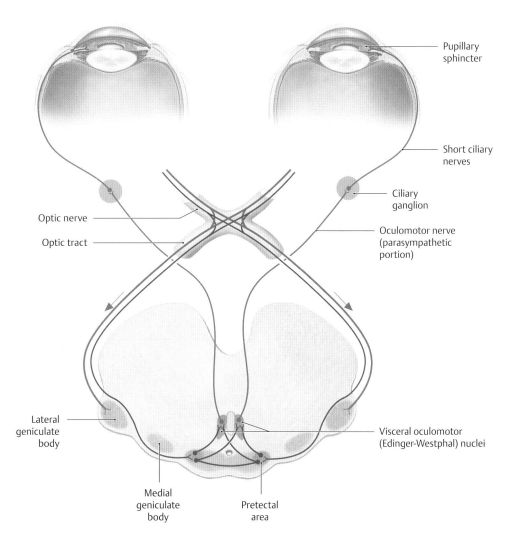

Pupillary
sphincter

Short ciliary
nerves

Ciliary
ganglion

Oculomotor nerve
(parasympathetic
portion)

Optic nerve

Optic tract

Visceral oculomotor
(Edinger-Westphal) nuclei

Lateral
geniculate
body

Medial
geniculate
body

Pretectal
area

*Fig. 6.59* **Pupillary light reflex**
The pupillary light reflex enables the eye to adapt to varying levels of brightness. When a large amount of light enters the eye (e.g., beam of a headlight), the pupil constricts to protect the photoreceptors in the retina; when the light fades, the pupil dilates. This reflexive pathway takes place without conscious input via the nongeniculate part of the visual pathway. The reflex can be broken into components:

1. Afferent limb: The first (photoreceptor) and second (bipolar) neurons relay sensory information to the third (retinal ganglion) neurons, which combine to form the optic nerve (CN II). Most third neurons (purple) synapse at the lateral geniculate body (geniculate part of the visual pathway). The third neurons responsible for the light reflex (blue) synapse at the pretectal area in the medial root of the optic tract (nongeniculate part of the visual pathway). Fourth neurons from the pretectal area pass to the parasympathetic Edinger-Westphal nuclei. *Note:* Because both nuclei are innervated, a consensual light response can occur (contraction of one pupil will cause contraction of the other).
2. Efferent limb: Fifth neurons from the Edinger-Westphal nuclei (preganglionic parasympathetic neurons) synapse in the ciliary ganglion. Sixth neurons (postganglionic parasympathetic neurons) pass to the pupillary sphincter via the short ciliary nerves.

**Loss of light response:** Because fourth neurons from the pretectal area pass to both Edinger-Westphal nuclei, a consensual light response can occur (contraction of one pupil will cause contraction of the other). The light response must therefore be tested both directly and indirectly:

- Direct light response: Tested by covering both eyes of the conscious, cooperative patient and then uncovering one eye. After a short latency period, the pupil of the light-exposed eye will contract.
- Indirect light response: Tested by placing the examiner's hand on the bridge of the patient's nose, shading one eye from the beam of a flashlight while shining it into the other eye. The object is to test whether shining the light into one eye will cause the pupil of the shaded eye to contract as well (consensual light response).

Lesions can occur all along the pathway for the pupillary light reflex. The direct and indirect light responses can be used to determine the level:

- Unilateral optic nerve lesion: This produces blindness on the affected side. If the patient is unconscious or uncooperative, the light responses can determine the lesion, as the afferent limb of the pupillary light reflex is lost. Affected side: No direct light response and no consensual light response on the opposite side. Unaffected side: Direct light response and consensual light response on the opposite (affected) side. Because the efferent limb of the reflex is not mediated by the optic nerve, the functional afferent limb can bypass the impaired afferent limb.
- Lesion of the parasympathetic Edinger-Westphal nucleus or the ciliary ganglion: The efferent limb of the pupillary light reflex is lost. Affected side: No direct or indirect pupillary light response on the opposite side. Unaffected side: Direct light response, no indirect light response on the opposite (affected) side.
- Lesion of the optic radiation or visual cortex (geniculate part of the visual pathway): Intact pupillary reflex (direct and indirect light response on both sides).

# Visual System (IV): Coordination of Eye Movement

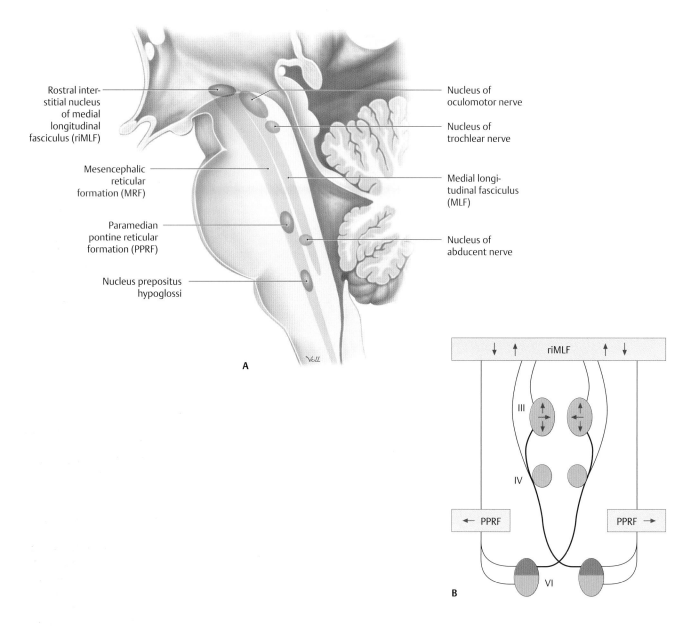

**Fig. 6.60 Oculomotor nuclei and connections in the brainstem**
**A** Midsagittal section viewed from left side. **B** Circuit diagram showing the supranuclear organization of eye movements.
The extraocular muscles receive motor innervation from the oculomotor (CN III), trochlear (CN IV), and abducent (CN VI) nerves. The concerted movement of the extraocular muscles allows for shifting of gaze, the swift movement of the visual axis toward the intended target. These rapid, precise, "ballistic" eye movements are called *saccades*. They are preprogrammed and, once initiated, cannot be altered until the end of the saccadic movement. The nuclei of CN III, IV, and VI (red) are involved in these saccadic movements. They are interconnected for this purpose by the medial longitudinal fasciculus (MLF, blue). Because these complex movements involve all the extraocular muscles and their associated nerves, the activity of the nuclei must be coordinated at a higher, or supranuclear, level. For example, gazing to the right requires four concerted movements:

- Contract right lateral rectus (CN VI nucleus activated)
- Relax right medial rectus (CN III nucleus inhibited)
- Relax left lateral rectus (CN VI nucleus inhibited)
- Contract left medial rectus (CN III nucleus activated)

These conjugate eye movements are coordinated by premotor nuclei (purple) in the mesencephalic reticular formation (green). Horizontal gaze movements are programmed in the nuclear region of the paramedian pontine reticular formation (PPRF). Vertical gaze movements are programmed in the rostral interstitial nucleus of the medial longitudinal fasciculus (riMLF). Both gaze centers establish bilateral connections with the nuclei of CN III, IV, and VI. The tonic signals for maintaining the new eye position originate from the nucleus prepositus hypoglossi.

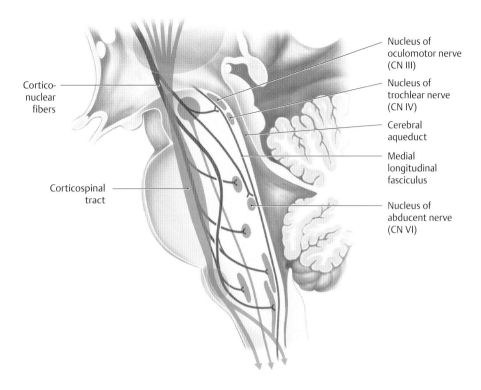

Cortico-nuclear fibers

Corticospinal tract

Nucleus of oculomotor nerve (CN III)

Nucleus of trochlear nerve (CN IV)

Cerebral aqueduct

Medial longitudinal fasciculus

Nucleus of abducent nerve (CN VI)

**Fig. 6.61 Course of the MLF in the brainstem**
Midsagittal section viewed from the left side. The MLF runs anterior to the cerebral aqueduct on both sides and continues from the mesencephalon to the cervical spinal cord. It transmits fibers for the coordination of conjugate eye movements. A lesion of the MLF results in internuclear ophthalmoplegia (see **Fig. 6.62**).

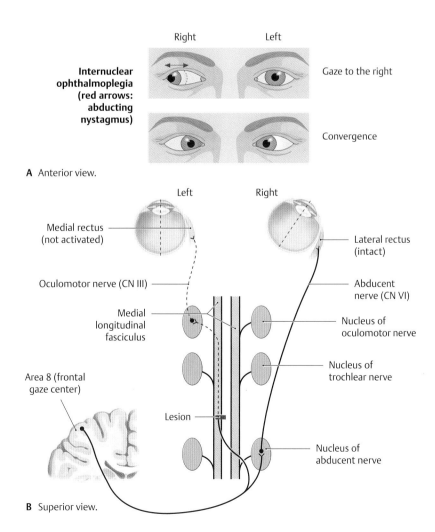

Right    Left

**Internuclear ophthalmoplegia (red arrows: abducting nystagmus)**

Gaze to the right

Convergence

**A** Anterior view.

Left    Right

Medial rectus (not activated)

Oculomotor nerve (CN III)

Medial longitudinal fasciculus

Area 8 (frontal gaze center)

Lesion

Lateral rectus (intact)

Abducent nerve (CN VI)

Nucleus of oculomotor nerve

Nucleus of trochlear nerve

Nucleus of abducent nerve

**B** Superior view.

**Fig. 6.62 Internuclear ophthalmoplegia**
The MLF interconnects the oculomotor nuclei and also connects them with the opposite side. When this "information highway" is interrupted, internuclear ophthalmoplegia develops. This type of lesion most commonly occurs between the nuclei of the abducent and the oculomotor nerves. It may be unilateral or bilateral. Typical causes are multiple sclerosis and diminished blood flow. The lesion is manifested by the loss of conjugate eye movements. With a lesion of the left MLF, as shown here, the left medial rectus muscle is no longer activated during gaze to the right. The eye cannot be moved *inward* on the side of the lesion (loss of the medial rectus), and the opposite eye goes into an abducting nystagmus (lateral rectus is intact and innervated by the abducent nerve). Reflex movements such as convergence are not impaired, as there is no peripheral or nuclear lesion, and this reaction is not mediated by the MLF.

**141**

# Nose: Nasal Skeleton

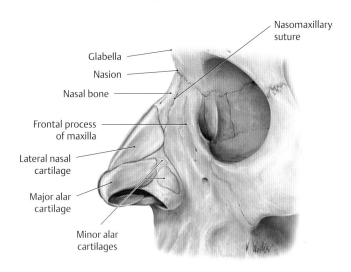

**Fig. 7.1 Skeleton of the external nose**
Left lateral view. The skeleton of the nose is composed of bone, cartilage, and connective tissue. Its upper portion is bony and frequently involved in midfacial fractures, whereas its lower, distal portion is cartilaginous and therefore more elastic and less susceptible to injury. The proximal lower portion of the nostrils (alae) is composed of connective tissue with small embedded pieces of cartilage. The lateral nasal cartilage is a winglike lateral expansion of the cartilaginous part of the nasal septum rather than a separate piece of cartilage.

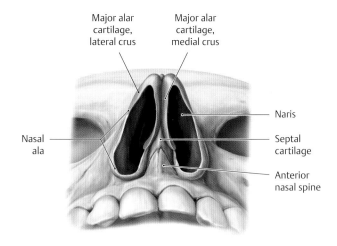

**Fig. 7.2 Nasal cartilage**
Inferior view. Viewed from below, each of the major alar cartilages is seen to consist of a medial and lateral crus. This view also displays the two nares, which open into the nasal cavities. The right and left nasal cavities are separated by the nasal septum, whose inferior cartilaginous portion is just visible in the diagram.

*9 bones make up the Nasopharynx*

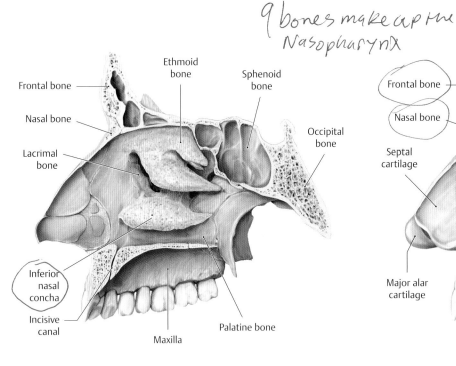

**Fig. 7.3 Bones of the lateral wall of the right nasal cavity**
Left lateral view. The lateral wall of the right nasal cavity is formed by six bones: the maxilla, nasal bone, ethmoid bone, inferior nasal concha, palatine bone, and sphenoid bone. Of the nasal concha, only the inferior is a separate bone; the middle and superior conchae are parts of the ethmoid bone.

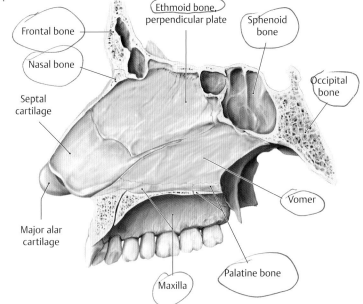

**Fig. 7.4 Bones of the nasal septum**
Parasagittal section. The nasal septum is formed by six bones. The ethmoid and vomer bones are the major components of the septum. The sphenoid bone, palatine bone, maxilla, and nasal bone (roof of the septum) contribute only small bony projections to the nasal septum.

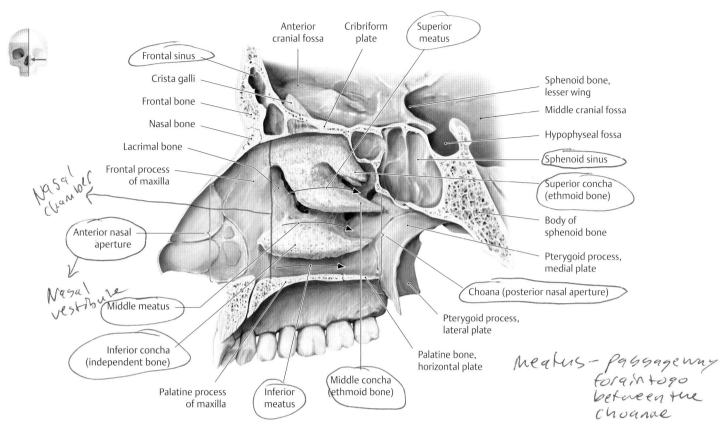

**Fig. 7.5 Lateral wall of the right nasal cavity**

Medial view. Air enters the bony nasal cavity through the anterior nasal aperture and travels through the three nasal passages: the superior meatus, middle meatus, and inferior meatus, which are the spaces infero-lateral to the superior, middle, and inferior conchae, respectively. Air leaves the nose through the choanae (posterior nasal apertures), entering the nasopharynx.

*Handwritten notes: Nasal chamber; Nasal vestibule; Meatus- passageway for air to go between the choanae*

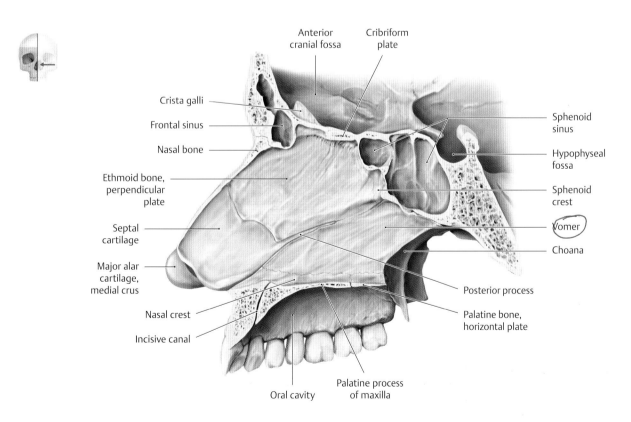

**Fig. 7.6 Nasal septum**

Parasagittal section viewed from the left side. The left lateral wall of the nasal cavity has been removed with the adjacent bones. The nasal septum consists of an anterior septal cartilage and a posterior bony part composed of several bones. The posterior process of the carti-laginous septum extends deep into the bony septum. Deviations of the nasal septum are common and may involve the cartilaginous part of the septum, the bony part, or both. Cases in which the septal deviation is sufficient to cause obstruction of nasal breathing can be surgically corrected.

**143**

# Nose: Paranasal Sinuses

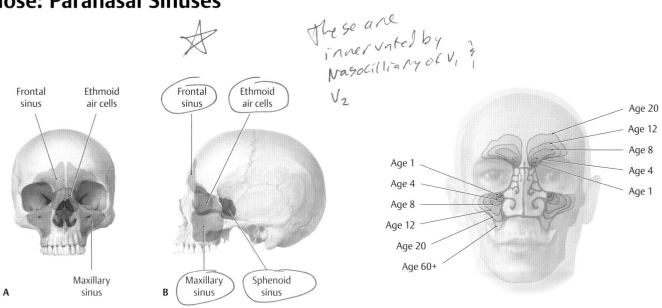

*handwritten: These are innervated by Nasocilliary of V₁ & V₂*

**Fig. 7.7 Projection of the paranasal sinuses onto the skull**
**A** Anterior view. **B** Lateral view.
The paranasal sinuses are air-filled cavities that reduce the weight of the skull. They are subject to inflammation that may cause pain over the affected sinus (e.g., frontal headache due to frontal sinusitis). Knowing the location and sensory supply of the sinuses is helpful in making the correct diagnosis.

**Fig. 7.8 Pneumatization of the maxillary and frontal sinuses**
Anterior view. The frontal and maxillary sinuses develop gradually during the course of cranial growth (pneumatization), unlike the ethmoid air cells, which are already pneumatized at birth. As a result, sinusitis in children is most likely to involve the ethmoid air cells (with risk of orbital penetration: red, swollen eye).

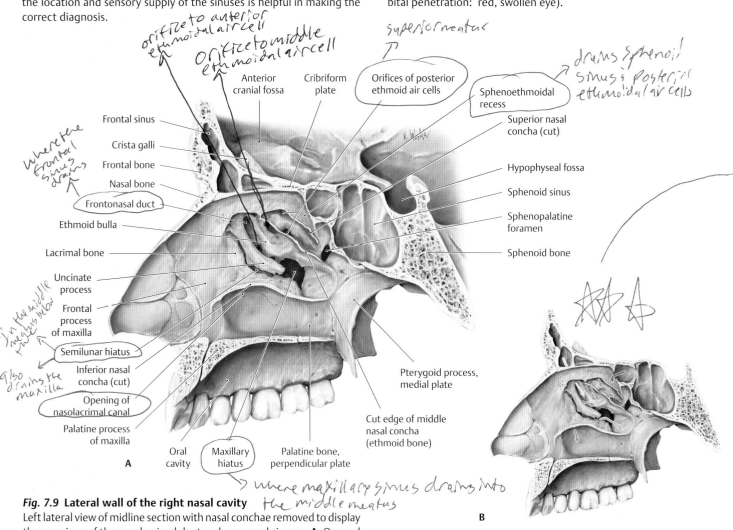

*handwritten annotations: orifice to anterior ethmoidal air cell; orifice to middle ethmoidal air cell; superior meatus; drains Sphenoid Sinus & Posterior ethmoidal air cells; where the frontal sinus drains; In the middle meatus; also drains the maxilla; where maxillary sinus drains into the middle meatus*

**Fig. 7.9 Lateral wall of the right nasal cavity**
Left lateral view of midline section with nasal conchae removed to display the openings of the nasolacrimal duct and paranasal sinuses. **A** Opened nasal wall. **B** Drainage of the paranasal sinuses. See **Table 7.1**.

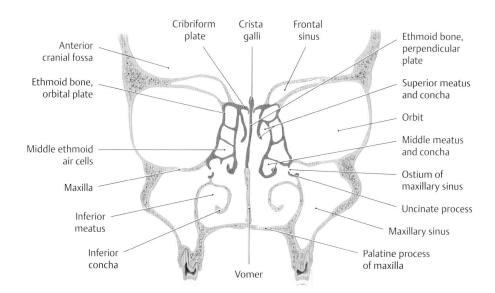

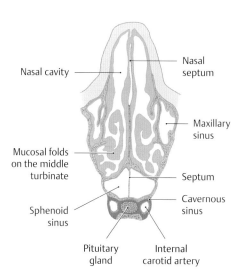

**Fig. 7.10 Bony structure of the paranasal sinuses**

Anterior view. The central structure of the *paranasal sinuses* is the ethmoid bone (red). Its cribriform plate forms a portion of the anterior skull base. The frontal and maxillary sinuses are grouped around the ethmoid bone. The inferior, middle, and superior meatuses of the nasal cavity are bounded by the accordingly named conchae. The bony ostium of the maxillary sinus opens into the middle meatus, lateral to the middle concha. Below the middle concha and above the maxillary sinus ostium is the ethmoid bulla, which contains the middle ethmoid air cells. At its anterior margin is a bony hook, the uncinate process, which bounds the maxillary sinus ostium anteriorly. The middle concha is a useful landmark in surgical procedures on the maxillary sinus and anterior ethmoid. The lateral wall separating the ethmoid bone from the orbit is the paper-thin orbital plate (= lamina papyracea). Inflammatory processes and tumors may penetrate this thin plate in either direction. *Note:* The maxilla forms the floor of the orbit and roof of the maxillary sinus. In addition, roots of the maxillary dentition may project into the maxillary sinus.

**Fig. 7.11 Nasal cavity and paranasal sinuses**

Transverse section viewed from above. The mucosal surface anatomy has been left intact to show how narrow the nasal passages are. Even relatively mild swelling of the mucosa may obstruct the nasal cavity, impeding aeration of the paranasal sinuses.

The pituitary gland, located behind the sphenoid sinus in the hypophyseal fossa, is accessible via transnasal surgical procedures.

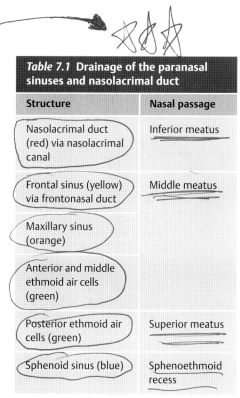

| Table 7.1 Drainage of the paranasal sinuses and nasolacrimal duct | |
|---|---|
| **Structure** | **Nasal passage** |
| Nasolacrimal duct (red) via nasolacrimal canal | Inferior meatus |
| Frontal sinus (yellow) via frontonasal duct | Middle meatus |
| Maxillary sinus (orange) | |
| Anterior and middle ethmoid air cells (green) | |
| Posterior ethmoid air cells (green) | Superior meatus |
| Sphenoid sinus (blue) | Sphenoethmoid recess |

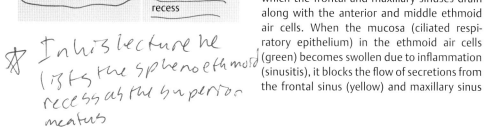

*In his lecture he lists the sphenoethmoid recess as the superior meatus*

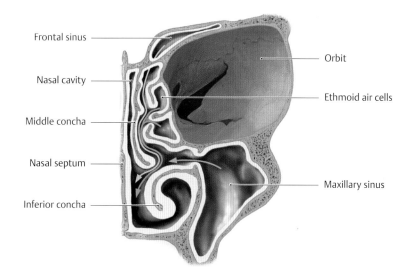

**Fig. 7.12 Osteomeatal unit (complex)**

Coronal section. The osteomeatal unit (complex) is that part of the middle meatus into which the frontal and maxillary sinuses drain along with the anterior and middle ethmoid air cells. When the mucosa (ciliated respiratory epithelium) in the ethmoid air cells (green) becomes swollen due to inflammation (sinusitis), it blocks the flow of secretions from the frontal sinus (yellow) and maxillary sinus (orange) in the osteomeatal unit (red). Because of this blockage, microorganisms also become trapped in the other sinuses, where they may incite an inflammation. Thus, whereas the anatomical focus of the disease lies in the ethmoid air cells, inflammatory symptoms are also manifested in the frontal and maxillary sinuses. In patients with *chronic sinusitis*, the narrow sites can be surgically widened to establish an effective drainage route.

**145**

# Nasal Cavity

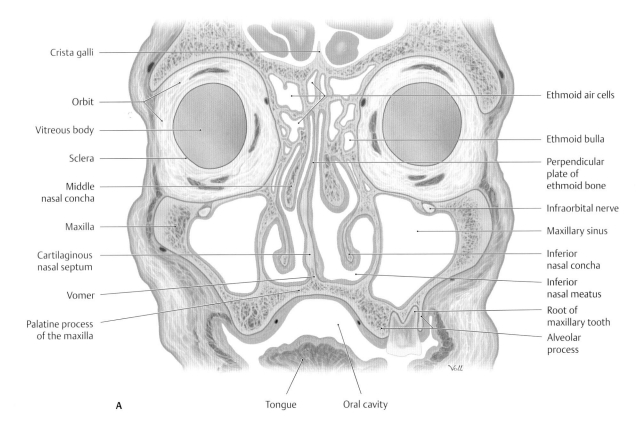

Crista galli

Orbit

Vitreous body

Sclera

Middle
nasal concha

Maxilla

Cartilaginous
nasal septum

Vomer

Palatine process
of the maxilla

Ethmoid air cells

Ethmoid bulla

Perpendicular
plate of
ethmoid bone

Infraorbital nerve

Maxillary sinus

Inferior
nasal concha

Inferior
nasal meatus

Root of
maxillary tooth

Alveolar
process

**A**    Tongue    Oral cavity

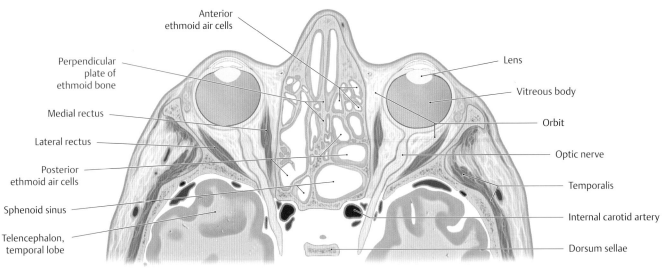

Anterior
ethmoid air cells

Perpendicular
plate of
ethmoid bone

Medial rectus

Lateral rectus

Posterior
ethmoid air cells

Sphenoid sinus

Telencephalon,
temporal lobe

Lens

Vitreous body

Orbit

Optic nerve

Temporalis

Internal carotid artery

Dorsum sellae

**B**

### Fig. 7.13 Overview of the nose and paranasal sinuses

**A** Coronal section, anterior view. **B** Transverse section, superior view.
The nasal cavities and paranasal sinuses are arranged in pairs. The left
and right nasal cavities are separated by the nasal septum and have an
approximately triangular shape. Below the base of the triangle is the
oral cavity. Note the relations of the infraorbital nerve and maxillary
dentition to the maxillary sinus. The following paired paranasal sinuses
are shown in the drawings:

- Frontal sinus
- Ethmoid air cells (ethmoid sinus*)
- Maxillary sinus
- Sphenoid sinus

The interior of each sinus is lined with ciliated respiratory epithelium
(see p. 150).

*The term *ethmoid sinus* has been dropped from the latest anatomical nomenclature, although it is still widely used by medical practitioners.

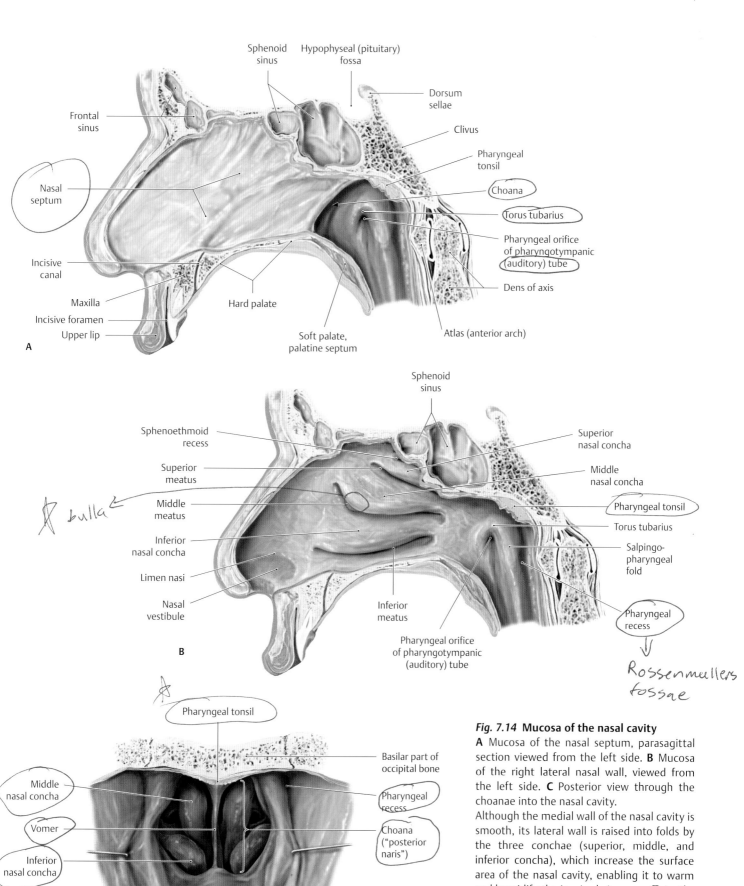

**A** Mucosa of the nasal septum, parasagittal section viewed from the left side.

Labels in A:
- Sphenoid sinus
- Hypophyseal (pituitary) fossa
- Dorsum sellae
- Clivus
- Pharyngeal tonsil
- Choana
- Torus tubarius
- Pharyngeal orifice of pharyngotympanic (auditory) tube
- Dens of axis
- Atlas (anterior arch)
- Soft palate, palatine septum
- Hard palate
- Maxilla
- Incisive foramen
- Upper lip
- Incisive canal
- Nasal septum
- Frontal sinus

Labels in B:
- Sphenoid sinus
- Superior nasal concha
- Middle nasal concha
- Pharyngeal tonsil
- Torus tubarius
- Salpingo-pharyngeal fold
- Pharyngeal recess
- Pharyngeal orifice of pharyngotympanic (auditory) tube
- Inferior meatus
- Nasal vestibule
- Limen nasi
- Inferior nasal concha
- Middle meatus
- Superior meatus
- Sphenoethmoid recess

*handwritten:* bulla

*handwritten:* Rossenmullers fossae

Labels in C:
- Pharyngeal tonsil
- Basilar part of occipital bone
- Pharyngeal recess
- Choana ("posterior naris")
- Palato-pharyngeal arch
- Uvula
- Palatine tonsil
- Epiglottis
- Tongue base with lingual tonsil
- Soft palate
- Inferior nasal concha
- Vomer
- Middle nasal concha

**Fig. 7.14 Mucosa of the nasal cavity**
**A** Mucosa of the nasal septum, parasagittal section viewed from the left side. **B** Mucosa of the right lateral nasal wall, viewed from the left side. **C** Posterior view through the choanae into the nasal cavity.
Although the medial wall of the nasal cavity is smooth, its lateral wall is raised into folds by the three conchae (superior, middle, and inferior concha), which increase the surface area of the nasal cavity, enabling it to warm and humidify the inspired air more efficiently. They also create turbulence, mixing olfactory stimulants (see p. 148 for olfactory nerve). The choanae (posterior nasal apertures) (**C**) are the posterior openings by which the nasal cavity communicates with the nasopharynx. Note the close proximity of the choanae to the pharyngotympanic (auditory) tube and pharyngeal tonsil.

**147**

# Nasal Cavity: Neurovascular Supply

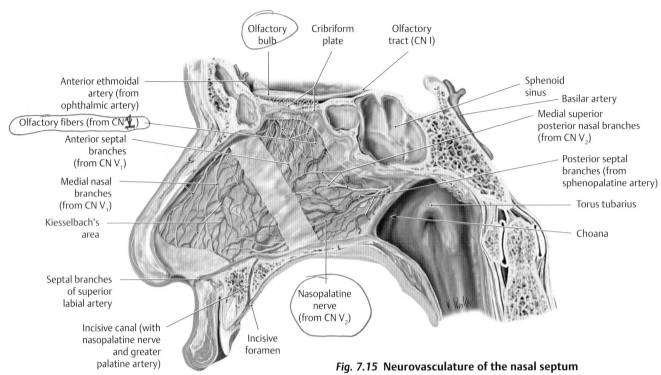

Olfactory bulb

Cribriform plate

Olfactory tract (CN I)

Anterior ethmoidal artery (from ophthalmic artery)

Olfactory fibers (from CN I)

Anterior septal branches (from CN V₁)

Medial nasal branches (from CN V₁)

Kiesselbach's area

Septal branches of superior labial artery

Incisive canal (with nasopalatine nerve and greater palatine artery)

Incisive foramen

Nasopalatine nerve (from CN V₂)

Sphenoid sinus

Basilar artery

Medial superior posterior nasal branches (from CN V₂)

Posterior septal branches (from sphenopalatine artery)

Torus tubarius

Choana

**Fig. 7.15 Neurovasculature of the nasal septum**
Parasagittal section, left lateral view. The nasal septum is supplied anterosuperiorly by CN V₁ and posteroinferiorly by CN V₂. It receives blood primarily from branches of the ophthalmic and maxillary arteries, with contribution from the facial artery (septal branches of the superior labial artery).

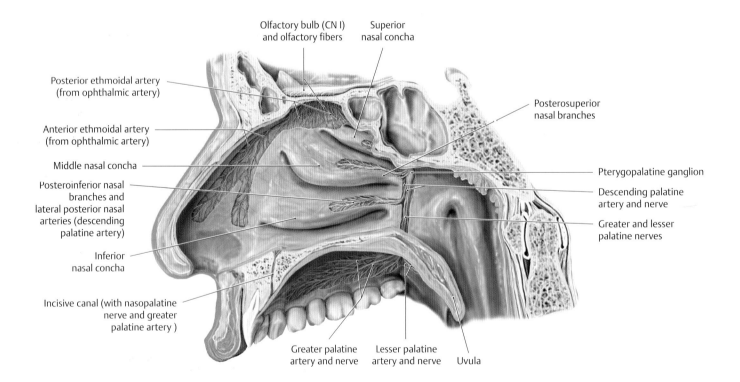

Olfactory bulb (CN I) and olfactory fibers

Superior nasal concha

Posterior ethmoidal artery (from ophthalmic artery)

Anterior ethmoidal artery (from ophthalmic artery)

Middle nasal concha

Posteroinferior nasal branches and lateral posterior nasal arteries (descending palatine artery)

Inferior nasal concha

Incisive canal (with nasopalatine nerve and greater palatine artery )

Posterosuperior nasal branches

Pterygopalatine ganglion

Descending palatine artery and nerve

Greater and lesser palatine nerves

Greater palatine artery and nerve

Lesser palatine artery and nerve

Uvula

**Fig. 7.16 Neurovasculature of the lateral nasal wall**
Left medial view of right lateral nasal wall. The pterygopalatine ganglion (located in the pterygopalatine fossa but exposed here) is an important relay in the parasympathetic nervous system. The CN V₂ nerve fibers passing through it pass to the small nasal glands of the nasal conchae, along with palatine glands. The anterosuperior portion of the lateral nasal wall is supplied by branches of the ophthalmic artery and CN V₁. *Note:* Olfactory fibers (CN I) pass through the cribriform plate to the olfactory mucosa at the level of the superior concha.

*Note:* The ophthalmic artery arises from the internal carotid artery and travels with the optic nerve (CN II), entering the orbit via the optic canal. Within the orbit it gives off the ethmoidal branches, which enter the nasal cavity via the ethmoid bone.

### Fig. 7.17 Arteries of the nasal septum

Left lateral view. The vessels of the nasal septum arise from branches of the external and internal carotid arteries. The anterior part of the septum contains a highly vascularized area called Kiesselbach's area, which is supplied by vessels from both major arteries. This area is the most common site of significant nosebleed due to anastomoses.

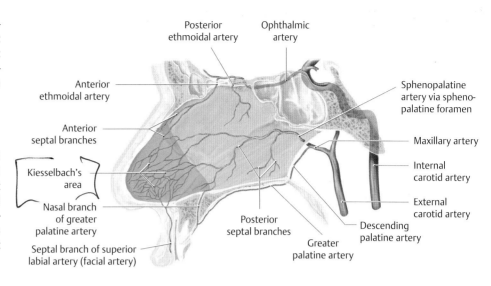

### Fig. 7.18 Nerves of the nasal septum

Left mesial view of lateral septum. The nasal septum receives its general sensory innervation from branches of the trigeminal nerve (CN V). The anterosuperior part of the septum is supplied by branches of the ophthalmic division (CN V₁) and the rest by branches of the maxillary division (CN V₂). Bundles of olfactory nerve fibers (CN I) arise from receptors in the olfactory mucosa on the superior part of the septum, pass through the cribriform plate, and enter the olfactory bulb.

*internal from anterior ethmoid*

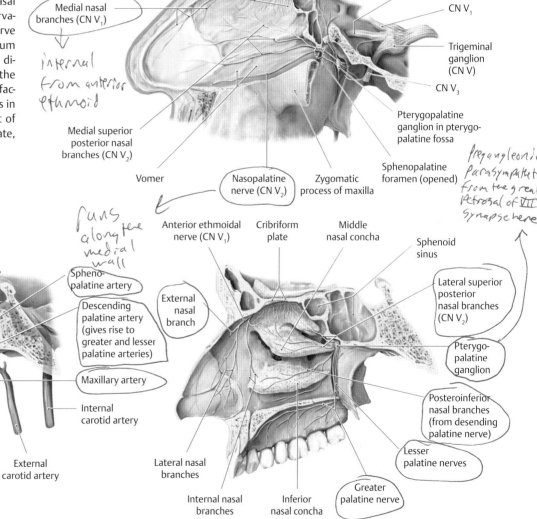

*runs along the medial wall*

*Preganglionic Parasympathetics from the greater Petrosal of VII synapse here*

### Fig. 7.19 Arteries of the right lateral nasal wall

Left mesial view of lateral nasal wall. The nasal wall is supplied primarily by branches of the ophthalmic artery (anterosuperiorly) and maxillary artery (posteroinferiorly), with contributions from the facial artery (alar branches of the lateral nasal artery).

### Fig. 7.20 Nerves of the right lateral nasal wall

Left mesial view of lateral nasal wall. The nasal wall derives its sensory innervation from branches of the ophthalmic division (CN V₁) and the maxillary division (CN V₂). Receptor neurons in the olfactory mucosa send their axons in the olfactory nerve (CN I) to the olfactory bulb.

*✳✳✳ Nerves I, V₁, V₂, & VII are involved y the Nasopharynx*

**149**

# Nose & Paranasal Sinuses: Histology & Clinical Anatomy

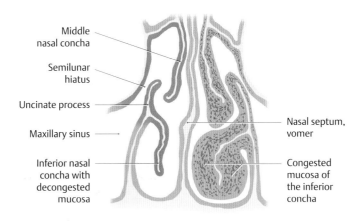

**Fig. 7.21 Functional states of the nasal mucosa**
Coronal section, anterior view. The function of the nasal mucosa is to warm and humidify the inspired air and mix olfactory stimulants. This is accomplished by an increase of blood flow through the mucosa, placing it in a congested (swollen) state. The mucous membranes are not simultaneously congested on both sides, but undergo a normal cycle of congestion and decongestion that lasts approximately six hours (the right side is decongested in the drawing). Examination of the nasal cavity can be facilitated by first administering a decongestant to shrink the mucosa.

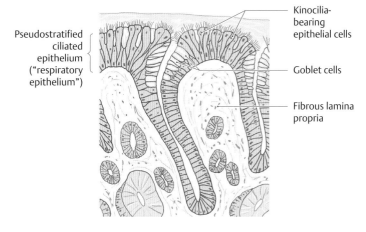

**Fig. 7.22 Histology of the nasal mucosa**
The surface of the pseudostratified respiratory epithelium of the nasal mucosa consists of kinocilia-bearing cells and goblet cells, which secrete their mucus into a watery film on the epithelial surface. Serous and seromucous glands are embedded in the connective tissue and also release secretions into the superficial fluid film. The directional fluid flow produced by the cilia is an important component of the non-specific immune response. If coordinated beating of the cilia is impaired, the patient will suffer chronic recurring infections of the respiratory tract.

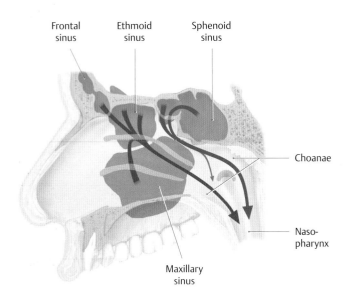

**Fig. 7.23 Normal drainage of secretions from the paranasal sinus**
Left lateral view. The beating cilia propel the mucous blanket over the cilia and through the choana into the nasopharynx, where it is swallowed.

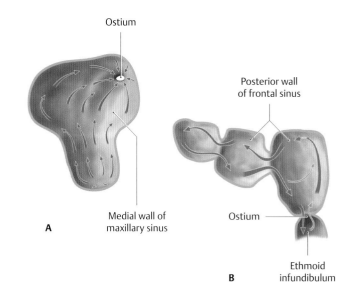

**Fig. 7.24 Ciliary beating and fluid flow in the right maxillary and frontal sinuses**
Schematic coronal sections of the right maxillary sinus (**A**) and frontal sinus (**B**), anterior view.
Beating of the cilia produces a flow of fluid in the paranasal sinuses that is always directed toward the sinus ostium. This clears the sinus of particles and microorganisms that are trapped in the mucous layer. If the ostium is obstructed due to swelling of the mucosa, inflammation may develop in the affected sinus (*sinusitis*). This occurs most commonly in the osteomeatal complex of the middle meatus.

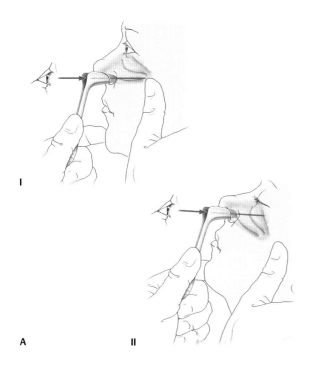

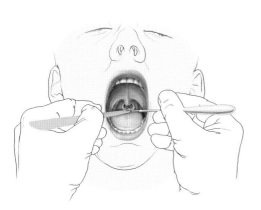

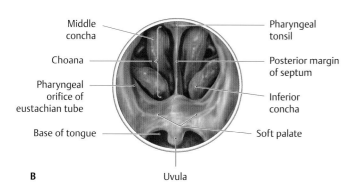

**Fig. 7.25 Anterior and posterior rhinoscopy**

**A Anterior rhinoscopy** is a procedure for inspection of the nasal cavity. Two different positions (I, II) are used to ensure that all of the anterior nasal cavity is examined.

**B** In **posterior rhinoscopy**, the choanae and pharyngeal tonsil are accessible to clinical examination. The rhinoscope can be angled and rotated to demonstrate the structures shown in the composite image. Today the rhinoscope is frequently replaced by an endoscope.

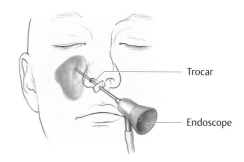

**Fig. 7.26 Endoscopy of the maxillary sinus**

Anterior view. The maxillary sinus is not accessible to direct inspection and must therefore be examined with an endoscope. To enter the maxillary sinus, the examiner pierces the thin bony wall below the inferior concha with a trocar and advances the endoscope through the opening. The scope can then be angled and rotated to inspect all of the mucosal surfaces.

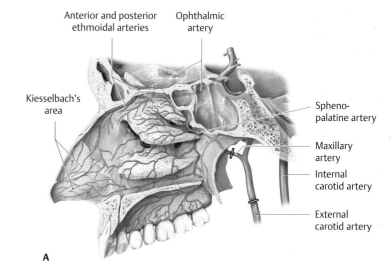

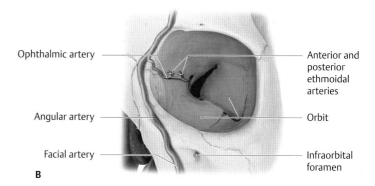

**Fig. 7.27 Sites of potential arterial ligation for the treatment of severe nosebleed**

If a severe nosebleed cannot be controlled with ordinary intranasal packing, it may be necessary to ligate relatively large arterial vessels. The following arteries may be ligated due to the rich aterial anastomoses in the blood supply to the nasal cavity:

- Maxillary artery or sphenopalatine artery (**A**)
- Both ethmoidal arteries in the orbit (**B**)

**151**

# Olfactory System (Smell)

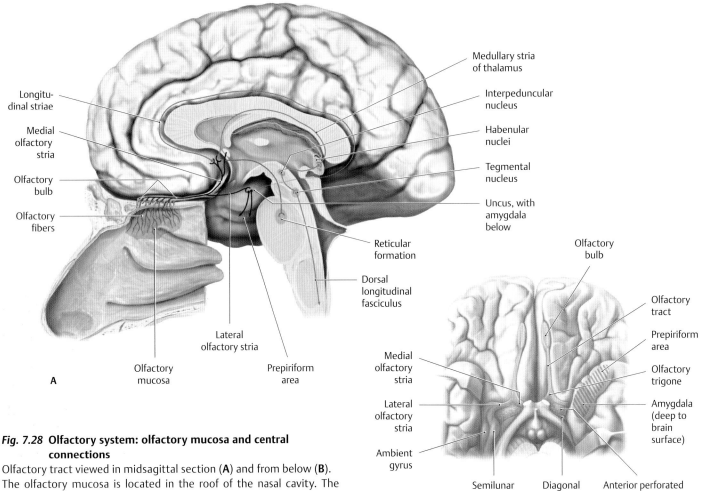

**Fig. 7.28 Olfactory system: olfactory mucosa and central connections**

Olfactory tract viewed in midsagittal section (**A**) and from below (**B**). The olfactory mucosa is located in the roof of the nasal cavity. The olfactory cells (= primary sensory cells) are bipolar neurons. Their peripheral receptor-bearing processes terminate in the epithelium of the nasal mucosa, and their central processes pass to the olfactory bulb. The olfactory bulb, where the second neurons of the olfactory pathway (mitral and tufted cells) are located, is considered an extension of the telencephalon. The axons of these second neurons pass centrally as the *olfactory tract.* In front of the anterior perforated substance, the olfactory tract widens to form the olfactory trigone and splits into the lateral and medial olfactory striae.

- Some of the axons of the olfactory tract run in the **lateral olfactory stria** to the olfactory centers: the amygdala, semilunar gyrus, and ambient gyrus. The prepiriform area (Brodmann area 28) is considered to be the primary olfactory cortex in the strict sense. It contains the third neurons of the olfactory pathway. *Note:* The prepiriform area is shaded in **B**, lying at the junction of the basal side of the frontal lobe and the medial side of the temporal lobe.
- Other axons of the olfactory tract run in the **medial olfactory stria** to nuclei in the septal (subcallosal) area, which is part of the limbic system, and to the olfactory tubercle, a small elevation in the anterior perforated substance.
- Yet other axons of the olfactory tract terminate in the **anterior olfactory nucleus,** where the fibers that cross to the opposite side branch off and are relayed. This nucleus is located in the olfactory trigone, which lies between the two olfactory striae and in front of the anterior perforated substance.

*Note:* None of these three tracts are routed through the thalamus. Thus, the olfactory system is the only sensory system that is not relayed in the thalamus before reaching the cortex. There is, however, an indirect route from the primary olfactory cortex to the neocortex passing through the thalamus and terminating in the basal forebrain. The olfactory signals are further analyzed in these basal portions of the forebrain (not shown).

The olfactory system is linked to other brain areas well beyond the primary olfactory cortical areas, with the result that olfactory stimuli can evoke complex emotional and behavioral responses. Noxious smells induce nausea, and appetizing smells evoke watering of the mouth. Presumably these sensations are processed by the hypothalamus, thalamus, and limbic system via connections established mainly by the medial forebrain bundle and the medullary striae of the thalamus. The medial forebrain bundle distributes axons to the following structures:

- Hypothalamic nuclei
- Reticular formation
- Salivatory nuclei
- Dorsal vagal nucleus

The axons that run in the medullary striae of the thalamus terminate in the habenular nuclei. This tract also continues to the brainstem, where it stimulates salivation in response to smell.

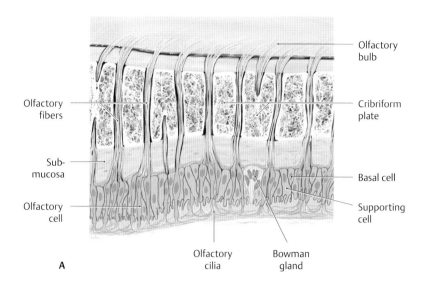

Olfactory bulb

Cribriform plate

Basal cell

Supporting cell

Olfactory fibers

Sub-mucosa

Olfactory cell

Olfactory cilia

Bowman gland

A

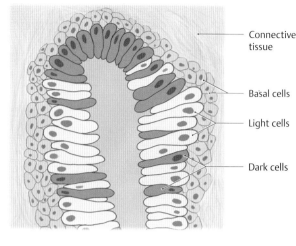

Connective tissue

Basal cells

Light cells

Dark cells

C

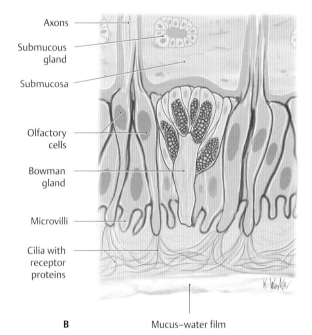

Axons

Submucous gland

Submucosa

Olfactory cells

Bowman gland

Microvilli

Cilia with receptor proteins

B

Mucus–water film

### Fig. 7.29 Olfactory mucosa and vomeronasal (Jacobson's) organ (VNO)

The **olfactory mucosa** occupies an area of approximately 2 cm² on the roof of each nasal cavity, and $10^7$ primary sensory cells are concentrated in each of these areas (**A**). At the molecular level, the olfactory receptor proteins are located in the cilia of the sensory cells (**B**). Each sensory cell has only one specialized receptor protein that mediates signal transduction when an odorant molecule binds to it. Although humans are microsmatic, having a sense of smell that is feeble compared with other mammals, the olfactory receptor proteins still make up 2% of the human genome. This underscores the importance of olfaction in humans. The primary olfactory sensory cells have a life span of approximately 60 days and regenerate from the basal cells (lifelong division of neurons). The bundled central processes (axons) from hundreds of olfactory cells form olfactory fibers (**A**) that pass through the cribriform plate of the ethmoid bone and terminate in the *olfactory bulb*, which lies above the cribriform plate. The VNO (**C**) is located on both sides of the anterior nasal septum. It is an accessory olfactory organ and is generally considered vestigial in adult humans. However, it responds to steroids and evokes subconscious reactions in subjects (possibly influences the choice of a mate). Mate selection in many animal species is known to be mediated by olfactory impulses that are perceived in the VNO.

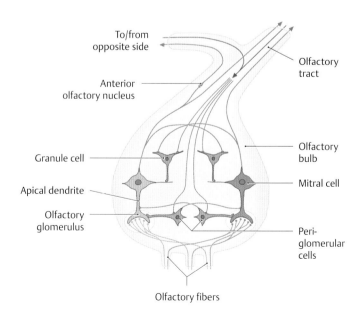

To/from opposite side

Anterior olfactory nucleus

Granule cell

Apical dendrite

Olfactory glomerulus

Olfactory fibers

Olfactory tract

Olfactory bulb

Mitral cell

Peri-glomerular cells

### Fig. 7.30 Synaptic patterns in an olfactory bulb

Specialized neurons in the olfactory bulb, called mitral cells, form apical dendrites that receive synaptic contact from the axons of thousands of primary sensory cells. The dendrite plus the synapses make up the *olfactory glomeruli*. Axons from sensory cells with the same receptor protein form glomeruli with only one or a small number of mitral cells. The basal axons of the mitral cells form the olfactory tract. The axons that run in the olfactory tract project primarily to the olfactory cortex but are also distributed to other nuclei in the central nervous system. The axon collaterals of the mitral cells pass to granule cells: both granule cells and periglomerular cells inhibit the activity of the mitral cells, causing less sensory information to reach higher centers. These inhibitory processes are believed to heighten olfactory contrast, which aids in the more accurate perception of smells. The tufted cells, which also project to the primary olfactory cortex, are not shown.

# Temporal Bone

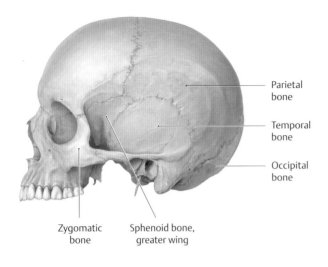

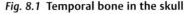

## Fig. 8.1 Temporal bone in the skull

Left lateral view. The temporal bone is a major component of the base of the skull. It forms the capsule for the auditory and vestibular apparatus and bears the articular fossa of the temporomandibular joint (TMJ).

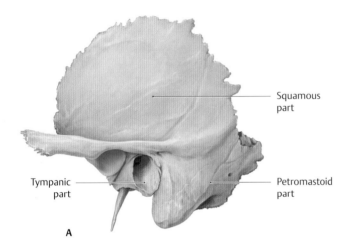

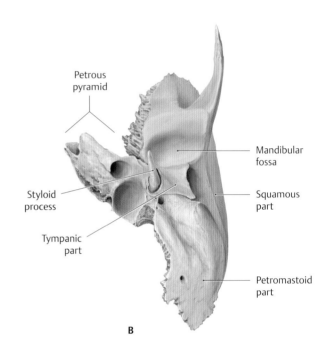

## Fig. 8.2 Parts of the left temporal bone

**A** Left lateral view. **B** Inferior view.

The temporal bone develops from four centers that fuse to form a single bone:

- The squamous part, or temporal squama (light green), bears the articular fossa of the TMJ (mandibular fossa).

- The petromastoid part, or petrous bone (pale green), contains the auditory and vestibular apparatus.
- The tympanic part (darker green) forms large portions of the external auditory canal.
- The styloid part (styloid process) develops from cartilage derived from the second branchial arch. It is a site of muscle attachment.

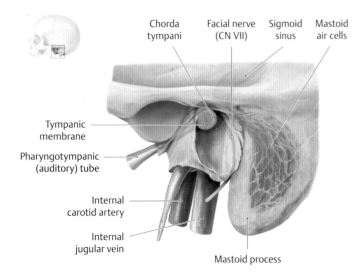

## Fig. 8.3 Clinically important relations in the temporal bone

Left lateral view with projected structures. The petrous part of the temporal bone contains the tympanic cavity of the middle ear (see **Fig. 8.15**). The middle ear communicates with the nasopharynx via the pharyngotympanic (auditory) tube. During chronic suppurative otitis media, an inflammation of the middle ear, pathogenic bacteria from the nasopharynx may spread to the tympanic cavity and then to surrounding structures. Bacterial spread upward (through the roof of the tympanic cavity into the middle cranial fossa) may incite meningitis or a cerebral abscess of the temporal lobe. Invasion of the mastoid air cells may cause mastoiditis; invasion of the sigmoid sinus may cause sinus thrombosis. Passage into the facial nerve canal may cause facial paralysis. Bacteria may even pass through the mastoid air cells and into the overlying cerebrospinal fluid (CSF) spaces.

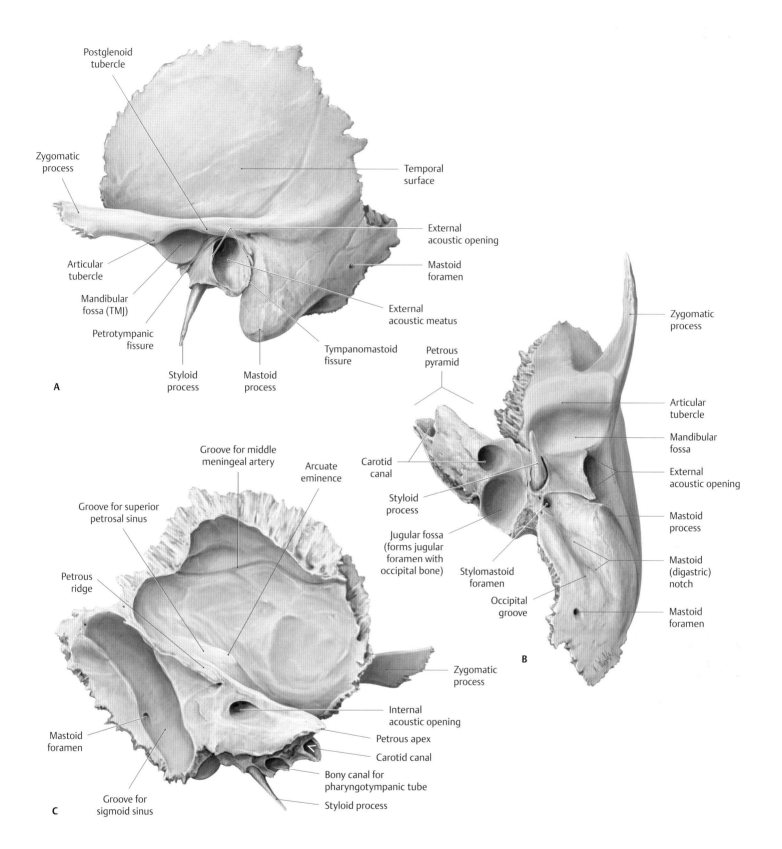

**Fig. 8.4 Left temporal bone**

**A Lateral view.** The mandibular fossa articulates with the head of the mandible via an articular disk (TMJ). The external acoustic meatus is the opening of the external auditory canal, which communicates with the tympanic cavity (middle ear) within the petrous part via the intervening tympanic membrane. The mastoid part contains a mastoid foramen that conducts an emissary vein from the scalp to the sigmoid sinus (see **C**). The chorda tympani and anterior tympanic artery pass through the medial part of the petrotympanic fissure to enter the tympanic cavity.

**B Inferior view.** The facial nerve (CN VII) emerges from the base of the skull via the stylomastoid foramen. The jugular fossa of the tem-

poral bone combines with the jugular process of the occipital bone to form the jugular foramen (containing the jugular bulb proximal to the internal jugular vein).

**C Medial view.** The internal acoustic meatus conveys the facial (CN VII) and vestibulocochlear (CN VIII) nerves, along with the labyrinthine artery and vein. *Note:* The arcuate eminence marks the position of the anterior semicircular canal. A bony canal within the petrous part of the temporal bone connects the pharyngotympanic (auditory) tube to the nasopharynx (see **Fig. 8.5**). The petrous pyramid separates the posterior and middle cranial fossa.

**155**

# Ear: Overview & External Ear

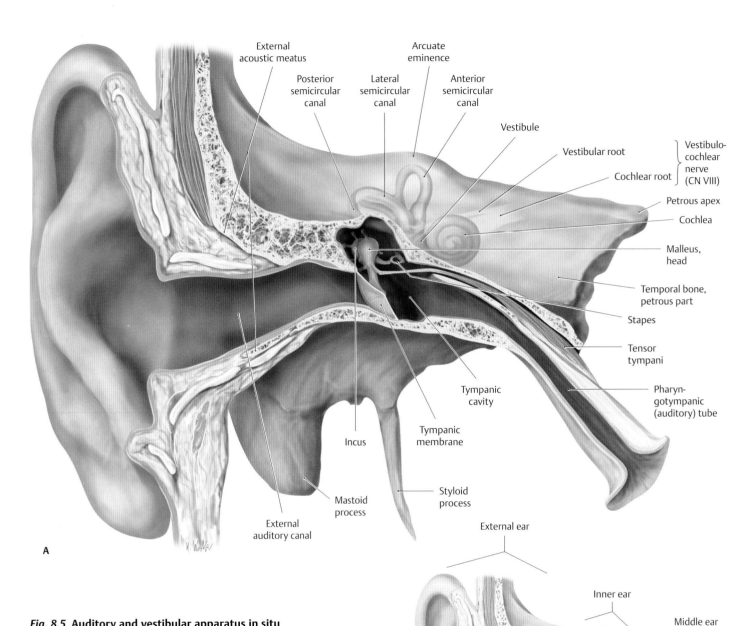

**Fig. 8.5 Auditory and vestibular apparatus in situ**
**A** Coronal section through the right ear, anterior view. **B** Auditory apparatus: external ear (yellow), middle ear (blue), and inner ear (green). The auditory and vestibular apparatus are located deep in the petrous part of the temporal bone. The **auditory apparatus** consists of the external ear, middle ear, and inner ear. Sound waves are captured by the auricle and travel through the external auditory canal to the tympanic membrane (the lateral boundary of the middle ear). The sound waves set the tympanic membrane into motion, and these mechanical vibrations are transmitted by the chain of auditory ossicles in the middle ear to the oval window, which leads into the inner ear. The ossicular chain induces vibrations in the membrane covering the oval window, and these in turn cause a fluid column in the inner ear to vibrate, setting receptor cells in motion. The transformation of sound waves into electrical impulses takes place in the inner ear, which is the actual organ of hearing. The external ear and middle ear, on the other hand, constitute the *sound conduction apparatus*. The organ of balance is the **vestibular apparatus**, which is also located in the auditory apparatus. It contains the *semicircular canals* for the perception of angular acceleration (rotational head movements) and the *saccule* and *utricle* for the perception of linear acceleration. Diseases of the vestibular apparatus produce dizziness (vertigo).

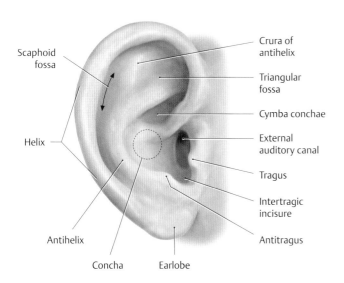

### Fig. 8.6 Right auricle

The auricle of the ear encloses a cartilaginous framework (auricular cartilage) that forms a funnel-shaped receptor for acoustic vibrations.

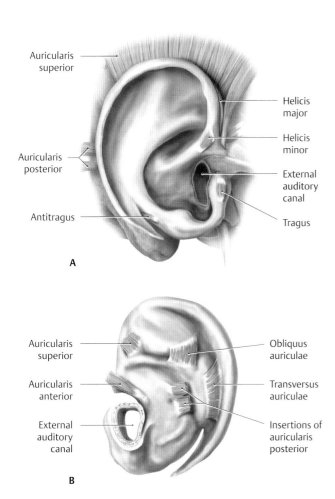

### Fig. 8.7 Cartilage and muscles of the auricle

**A** Lateral view of the external surface. **B** Medial view of the posterior surface of the right ear.

The skin (removed here) is closely applied to the elastic cartilage of the auricle (light blue). The muscles of the ear are classified as muscles of facial expression and, like the other members of this group, are supplied by the facial nerve (CN VII). Prominent in other mammals, the auricular muscles are vestigial in humans, with no significant function.

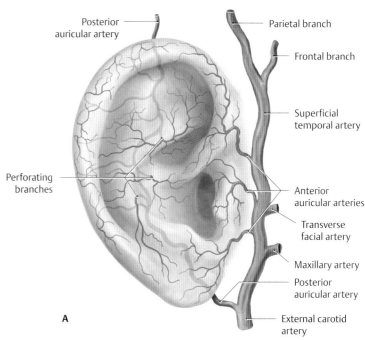

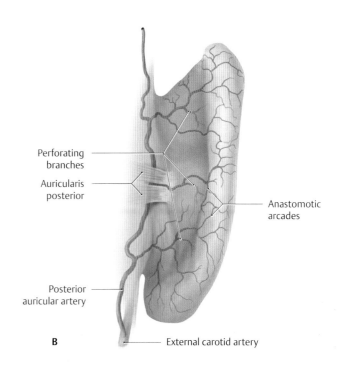

### Fig. 8.8 Arterial supply of the auricle

Lateral view (**A**) and posterior view (**B**) of right auricle.

The proximal and medial portions of the laterally directed anterior surface of the ear are supplied by the anterior auricular arteries, which arise from the superficial temporal artery. The other parts of the auricle are supplied by branches of the posterior auricular artery, which arises from the external carotid artery. These vessels are linked by extensive anastomoses, so operations on the external ear are unlikely to compromise the auricular blood supply. The copious blood flow through the auricle contributes to temperature regulation: dilation of the vessels helps dissipate heat through the skin. The lack of insulating fat predisposes the ear to frostbite, which is particularly common in the upper third of the auricle. The auricular arteries have corresponding veins that drain to the superficial temporal vein.

**157**

# External Ear

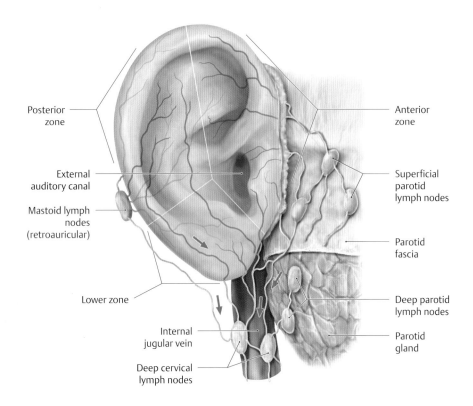

Posterior zone

External auditory canal

Mastoid lymph nodes (retroauricular)

Lower zone

Internal jugular vein

Deep cervical lymph nodes

Anterior zone

Superficial parotid lymph nodes

Parotid fascia

Deep parotid lymph nodes

Parotid gland

**Fig. 8.9 Auricle and external auditory canal: lymphatic drainage**
Right ear, oblique lateral view. The lymphatic drainage of the ear is divided into three zones, all of which drain directly or indirectly into the deep cervical lymph nodes along the internal jugular vein. The lower zone drains directly into the deep cervical lymph nodes. The anterior zone first drains into the parotid lymph nodes, the posterior zone into the mastoid lymph nodes.

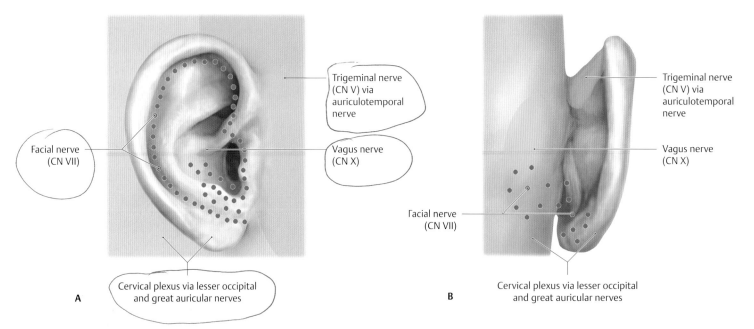

Trigeminal nerve (CN V) via auriculotemporal nerve

Facial nerve (CN VII)

Vagus nerve (CN X)

Cervical plexus via lesser occipital and great auricular nerves

**A**

Trigeminal nerve (CN V) via auriculotemporal nerve

Vagus nerve (CN X)

Facial nerve (CN VII)

Cervical plexus via lesser occipital and great auricular nerves

**B**

**Fig. 8.10 Sensory innervation of the auricle**
Right ear, lateral view (**A**) and posterior view (**B**). The auricular region has a complex nerve supply because, developmentally, it is located at the boundary between the cranial nerves (pharyngeal arch nerves) and branches of the cervical plexus. Three cranial nerves contribute to the innervation of the auricle:

- Trigeminal nerve (CN V)
- Facial nerve (CN VII; the skin area that receives sensory innervation from the facial nerve is not precisely known)
- Vagus nerve (CN X)

Two branches of the **cervical plexus** are involved:
- Lesser occipital nerve (C 2)
- Great auricular nerve (C 2, C 3)

*Note:* Because the vagus nerve contributes to the innervation of the external auditory canal (auricular branch, see below), mechanical cleaning of the ear canal (by inserting an aural speculum or by irrigating the ear) may evoke coughing and nausea. The auricular branch of the vagus nerve passes through the mastoid canaliculus and through a space between the mastoid process and the tympanic part of the temporal bone (tympanomastoid fissure, see p. 155) to the external ear and external auditory canal.

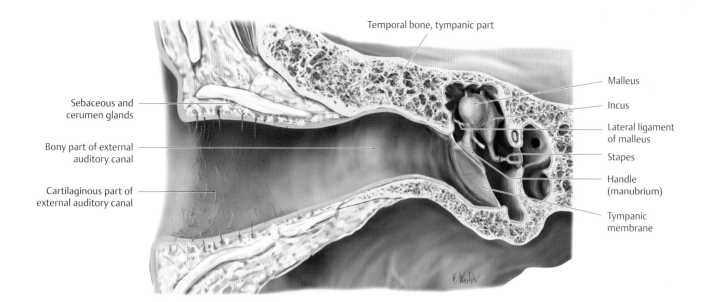

**Fig. 8.11 External auditory canal, tympanic membrane, and tympanic cavity**

Right ear, coronal section, anterior view. The tympanic membrane (eardrum) separates the external auditory canal from the tympanic cavity of the middle ear. The external auditory canal is an S-shaped tunnel that is approximately 3 cm long with an average diameter of 0.6 cm. The outer third of the ear canal is cartilaginous. The inner two thirds of the canal are osseous, the wall being formed by the tympanic part of the temporal bone. The cartilaginous part in particular bears numerous sebaceous and cerumen glands beneath the keratinized stratified squamous epithelium. The cerumen glands produce a watery secretion that combines with the sebum and sloughed epithelial cells to form a protective barrier (cerumen, "earwax") that screens out foreign bodies and keeps the epithelium from drying out. If the cerumen absorbs water (e.g., after swimming), it may obstruct the ear canal (cerumen impaction), temporarily causing a partial loss of hearing.

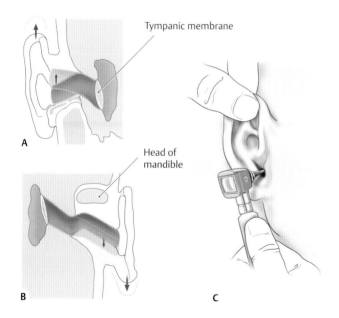

**Fig. 8.12 Curvature of the external auditory canal**

Right ear, anterior view (**A**) and transverse section (**B**).

The external auditory canal is most curved in its cartilaginous portion. When the tympanic membrane is inspected with an otoscope, the auricle should be pulled backward and upward in order to straighten the cartilaginous part of the ear canal so that the speculum of the otoscope can be introduced (**C**).

Note the proximity of the cartilaginous anterior wall of the external auditory canal to the TMJ. This allows the examiner to palpate movements of the mandibular head by inserting the small finger into the outer part of the ear canal.

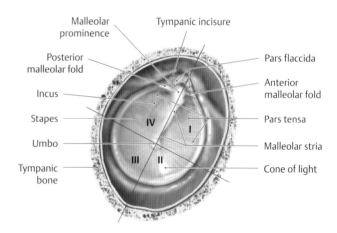

**Fig. 8.13 Tympanic membrane**

Right tympanic membrane, lateral view. The healthy tympanic membrane has a pearly gray color and an oval shape with an average surface area of approximately 75 mm². It consists of a lax portion, the *pars flaccida* (Shrapnell membrane), and a larger taut portion, the *pars tensa*, which is drawn inward at its center to form the umbo ("navel"). The umbo marks the lower tip of the handle (manubrium) of the malleus, which is attached to the tympanic membrane all along its length. It is visible through the pars tensa as a light-colored streak (malleolar stria). The tympanic membrane is divided into four quadrants in a clockwise direction: anterosuperior (I), anteroinferior (II), posteroinferior (III), posterosuperior (!V). The boundary lines of the quadrants are the malleolar stria and a line intersecting it perpendicularly at the umbo. The quadrants of the tympanic membrane are clinically important because they are used in describing the location of lesions. A triangular area of reflected light can be seen in the anteroinferior quadrant of a normal tympanic membrane. The location of this "cone of light" is helpful in evaluating the tension of the tympanic membrane.

# Middle Ear (I): Tympanic Cavity & Pharyngotympanic Tube

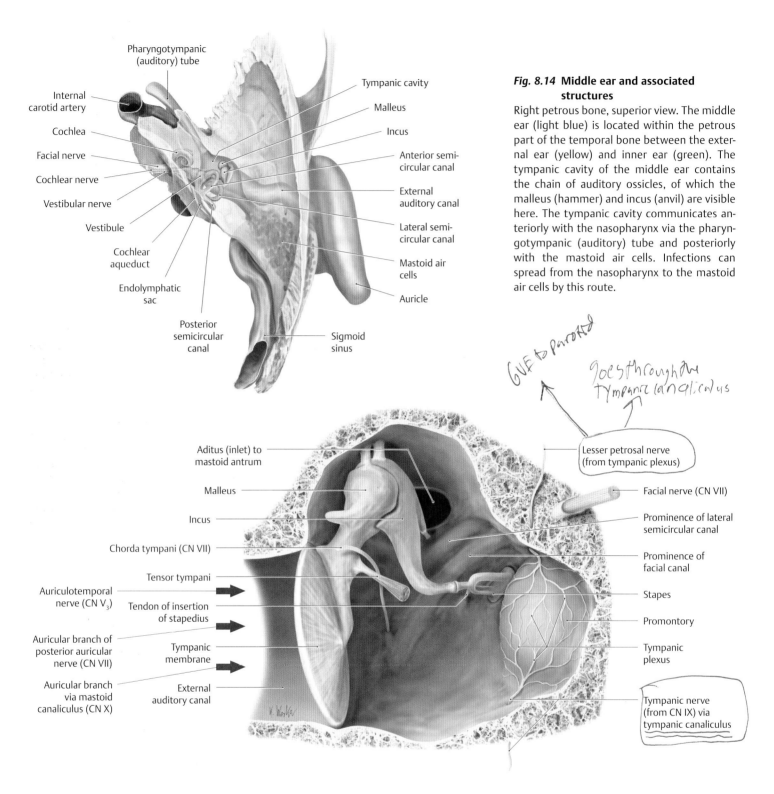

Labels for upper figure:
- Pharyngotympanic (auditory) tube
- Internal carotid artery
- Cochlea
- Facial nerve
- Cochlear nerve
- Vestibular nerve
- Vestibule
- Cochlear aqueduct
- Endolymphatic sac
- Posterior semicircular canal
- Tympanic cavity
- Malleus
- Incus
- Anterior semicircular canal
- External auditory canal
- Lateral semicircular canal
- Mastoid air cells
- Auricle
- Sigmoid sinus

**Fig. 8.14 Middle ear and associated structures**

Right petrous bone, superior view. The middle ear (light blue) is located within the petrous part of the temporal bone between the external ear (yellow) and inner ear (green). The tympanic cavity of the middle ear contains the chain of auditory ossicles, of which the malleus (hammer) and incus (anvil) are visible here. The tympanic cavity communicates anteriorly with the nasopharynx via the pharyngotympanic (auditory) tube and posteriorly with the mastoid air cells. Infections can spread from the nasopharynx to the mastoid air cells by this route.

Handwritten annotations: GVE to parotid; goes through the Tympanic canaliculus

Labels for lower figure:
- Aditus (inlet) to mastoid antrum
- Malleus
- Incus
- Chorda tympani (CN VII)
- Tensor tympani
- Auriculotemporal nerve (CN V₃)
- Tendon of insertion of stapedius
- Auricular branch of posterior auricular nerve (CN VII)
- Tympanic membrane
- Auricular branch via mastoid canaliculus (CN X)
- External auditory canal
- Lesser petrosal nerve (from tympanic plexus)
- Facial nerve (CN VII)
- Prominence of lateral semicircular canal
- Prominence of facial canal
- Stapes
- Promontory
- Tympanic plexus
- Tympanic nerve (from CN IX) via tympanic canaliculus

**Fig. 8.15 Walls of the tympanic cavity**

Anterior view with the anterior wall removed. The tympanic cavity is a slightly oblique space that is bounded by six walls:

- Lateral (membranous) wall: boundary with the external ear; formed largely by the tympanic membrane.
- Medial (labyrinthine) wall: boundary with the inner ear; formed largely by the promontory, or the bony eminence, overlying the basal turn of the cochlea.
- Inferior (jugular) wall: forms the floor of the tympanic cavity and borders on the bulb of the jugular vein.

- Posterior (mastoid) wall: borders on the air cells of the mastoid process, communicating with the cells through the aditus (inlet) of the mastoid antrum.
- Superior (tegmental) wall: forms the roof of the tympanic cavity.
- Anterior (carotid) wall (removed here): includes the opening to the pharyngotympanic (auditory) tube and borders on the carotid canal.

The lateral side of the tympanic membrane is innervated by three cranial nerves: CN V (auriculotemporal nerve [branch of CN V₃]), CN VII (posterior auricular nerve; pathway uncertain), and CN X (auricular branch). The medial side of the tympanic membrane is innervated by CN IX (tympanic branch).

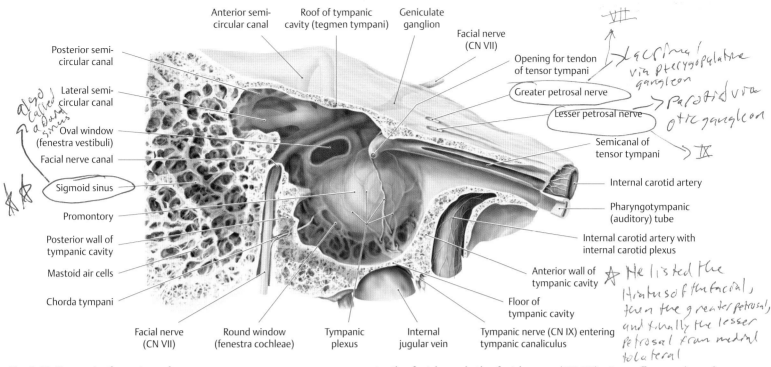

Posterior semi-circular canal

Lateral semi-circular canal

Oval window (fenestra vestibuli)

Facial nerve canal

Sigmoid sinus

Promontory

Posterior wall of tympanic cavity

Mastoid air cells

Chorda tympani

Anterior semi-circular canal

Roof of tympanic cavity (tegmen tympani)

Geniculate ganglion

Facial nerve (CN VII)

Opening for tendon of tensor tympani

Greater petrosal nerve

Lesser petrosal nerve

Semicanal of tensor tympani

Internal carotid artery

Pharyngotympanic (auditory) tube

Internal carotid artery with internal carotid plexus

Anterior wall of tympanic cavity

Floor of tympanic cavity

Tympanic nerve (CN IX) entering tympanic canaliculus

Facial nerve (CN VII)

Round window (fenestra cochleae)

Tympanic plexus

Internal jugular vein

*[handwritten notes: also called a bony sinus; ** ; VII → lacrimal via pterygopalatine ganglion → parotid via otic ganglion → IX; ★ He listed the Hiatus of the facial, then the greater petrosal, and finally the lesser petrosal from medial to lateral]*

**Fig. 8.16 Nerves in the petrous bone**

Oblique sagittal section showing the medial wall of the tympanic cavity (see **Fig. 8.15**). The tympanic nerve branches from CN IX as it passes through the jugular foramen, and conveys sensory and preganglionic parasympathetic fibers into the tympanic cavity by passing through the tympanic canaliculus. The fibers from the tympanic plexus provide sensory innervation to the tympanic cavity (including the medial surface of the tympanic membrane), mastoid air cells, and part of the pharyngotympanic tube. *Note:* The lateral surface of the tympanic membrane receives sensory innervation from branches of CN V$_3$, CN VII, and CN X (see **Fig. 8.15**).

The preganglionic parasympathetic fibers of the tympanic nerve are reformed from the tympanic plexus as the lesser petrosal nerve. These fibers synapse in the otic ganglion; the postganglionic parasympathetic fibers travel with the auriculotemporal nerve (a branch of CN V$_3$) to supply the parotid gland.

In the facial canal, the facial nerve (CN VII) gives off a number of branches: the greater petrosal nerve, the nerve to the stapedius, the chorda tympani, and an auricular branch. The greater petrosal nerve and the chorda tympani both carry taste fibers and preganglionic parasympathetic fibers. The greater petrosal nerve joins with the deep petrosal nerve (postganglionic sympathetic) to form the nerve of the pterygoid canal (vidian nerve). The preganglionic parasympathetic fibers in the nerve of the pterygoid canal synapse at the pterygopalatine ganglion. The postganglionic parasympathetic fibers are then distributed by branches of the maxillary nerve to the lacrimal gland, palatine glands, superior labial glands, and mucosa of the paranasal sinuses and nasal cavity. The preganglionic parasympathetic fibers of the chorda tympani synapse at the submandibular ganglion, and the postganglionic fibers are distributed to the submandibular and sublingual glands.

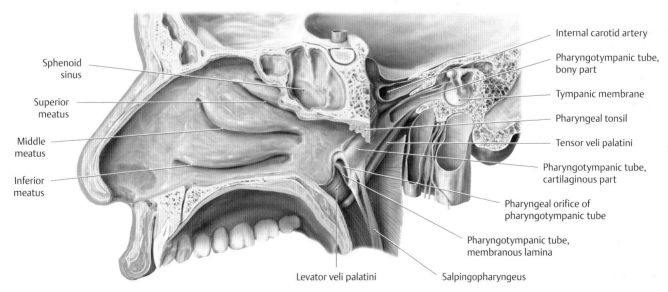

Sphenoid sinus

Superior meatus

Middle meatus

Inferior meatus

Internal carotid artery

Pharyngotympanic tube, bony part

Tympanic membrane

Pharyngeal tonsil

Tensor veli palatini

Pharyngotympanic tube, cartilaginous part

Pharyngeal orifice of pharyngotympanic tube

Pharyngotympanic tube, membranous lamina

Levator veli palatini

Salpingopharyngeus

**Fig. 8.17 Pharyngotympanic (auditory) tube**

Medial view of right nasal cavity. The pharyngotympanic tube creates an open channel between the middle ear and nasopharynx. Air passing through the tube serves to equalize the air pressure on the two sides of the tympanic membrane. This equalization is essential for maintaining normal tympanic membrane mobility, necessary for normal hearing. One third of the tube is bony (in the petrous bone). The cartilaginous two thirds continue toward the nasopharynx, expanding to form a

hook (hamulus) that is attached to a membranous lamina. The fibers of the tensor veli palatini arise from this lamina; when they tense the soft palate (during swallowing), these fibers open the pharyngotympanic tube. The tube is also opened by the salpingopharyngeus and levator veli palatini. The tube is lined with ciliated respiratory epithelium: the cilia beat toward the pharynx, inhibiting the passage of microorganisms into the middle ear.

**161**

# Middle Ear (II): Auditory Ossicles & Tympanic Cavity

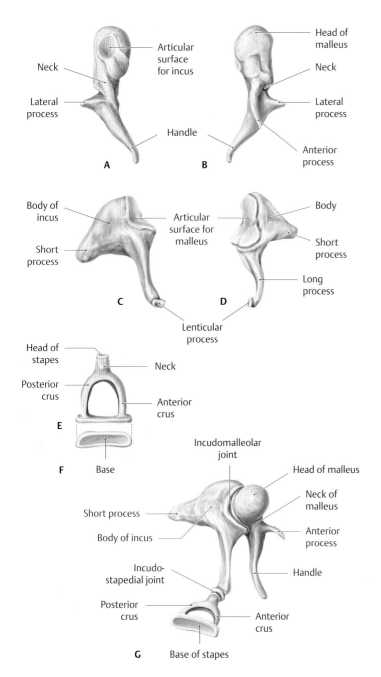

**Fig. 8.18 Auditory ossicles**
Auditory ossicles of the left ear. The ossicular chain (**G**) of the middle ear establishes an articular connection between the tympanic membrane and the oval window. It consists of three small bones:

- Malleus ("hammer"): **A** Posterior view. **B** Anterior view.
- Incus ("anvil"): **C** Medial view. **D** Anterolateral view.
- Stapes ("stirrup"): **E** Superior view. **F** Medial view.

Note the synovial joint articulations between the malleus and incus (incudomalleolar joint) and the incus and stapes (incudostapedial joint).

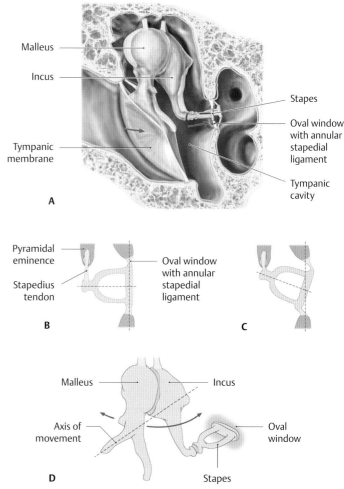

**Fig. 8.19 Function of the ossicular chain**
Anterior view.

**A** Sound waves (periodic pressure fluctuations in the air) set the tympanic membrane into vibration. The ossicular chain transmits the vibrations of the tympanic membrane (and thus the sound waves) to the oval window, which in turn communicates them to an aqueous medium (perilymph). Although sound waves encounter very little resistance in air, they encounter considerably higher impedance when they reach the fluid interface of the inner ear. The sound waves must therefore be amplified ("impedance matching"). The difference in surface area between the tympanic membrane and oval window increases the sound pressure by a factor of 17. This is augmented by the 1.3-fold mechanical advantage of the lever action of the ossicular chain. Thus, in passing from the tympanic membrane to the inner ear, the sound pressure is amplified by a factor of 22. If the ossicular chain fails to transform the sound pressure between the tympanic membrane and stapes base (footplate), the patient will experience conductive hearing loss of magnitude approximately 20 dB.

**B,C** Sound waves impinging on the tympanic membrane induce motion in the ossicular chain, causing a tilting movement of the stapes (**B** normal position, **C** tilted position). The movements of the stapes base against the membrane of the oval window (stapedial membrane) induce corresponding waves in the fluid column in the inner ear.

**D** The movements of the ossicular chain are essentially rocking movements (the dashed line indicates the axis of the movements, the arrows indicate their direction). Two muscles affect the mobility of the ossicular chain: the tensor tympani and the stapedius (see **Fig. 8.20**).

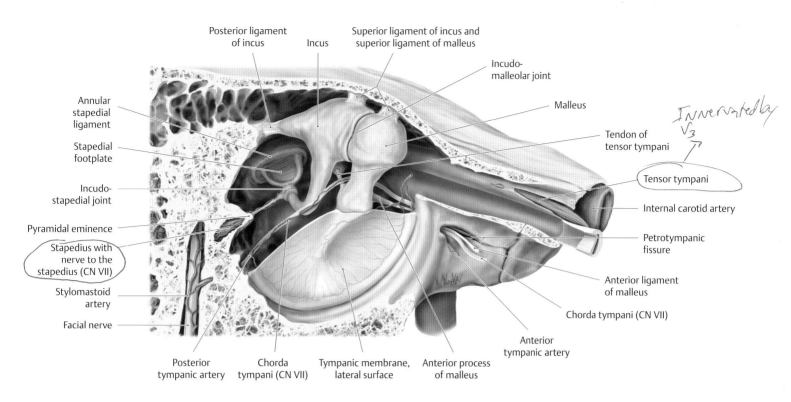

Posterior ligament of incus
Incus
Superior ligament of incus and superior ligament of malleus
Incudo-malleolar joint
Malleus
Annular stapedial ligament
Tendon of tensor tympani
Stapedial footplate
*Innervated by V₃*
Tensor tympani
Incudo-stapedial joint
Internal carotid artery
Pyramidal eminence
Petrotympanic fissure
Stapedius with nerve to the stapedius (CN VII)
Stylomastoid artery
Anterior ligament of malleus
Facial nerve
Chorda tympani (CN VII)
Posterior tympanic artery
Chorda tympani (CN VII)
Tympanic membrane, lateral surface
Anterior process of malleus
Anterior tympanic artery

**Fig. 8.20 Ossicular chain in the tympanic cavity**

Lateral view of the right ear. The joints and their stabilizing ligaments can be seen with the two muscles of the middle ear—the stapedius and tensor tympani. The *stapedius* (innervated by the stapedial branch of the facial nerve) inserts on the stapes. When it contracts, it stiffens the sound conduction apparatus and dampens sound transmission to the inner ear. This filtering function is believed to be particularly important at high sound frequencies ("high-pass filter"). When sound is transmitted into the middle ear through a probe placed in the external ear canal, one can measure the action of the stapedius (stapedius reflex test) by measuring the change in acoustic impedance (i.e., the amplification of the sound waves). Contraction of the *tensor tympani* (innervated by the trigeminal nerve via the medial pterygoid nerve) stiffens the tympanic membrane, thereby reducing the transmission of sound. Both muscles undergo a reflex contraction in response to loud acoustic stimuli. *Note:* The chorda tympani passes through the middle ear without a bony covering (making it susceptible to injury during otological surgery).

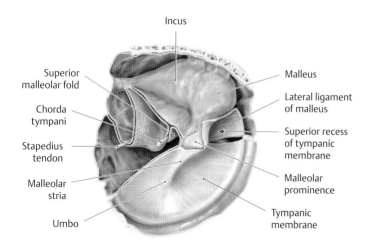

Incus
Superior malleolar fold
Malleus
Chorda tympani
Lateral ligament of malleus
Stapedius tendon
Superior recess of tympanic membrane
Malleolar stria
Malleolar prominence
Umbo
Tympanic membrane

**Fig. 8.21 Mucosal lining of the tympanic cavity**

Posterolateral view with the tympanic membrane partially removed. The tympanic cavity and the structures it contains (ossicular chain, tendons, nerves) are covered with mucosa. The epithelium consists mainly of a simple squamous type, with areas of ciliated columnar cells and goblet cells. Because the tympanic cavity communicates directly with the respiratory tract (nasopharynx) through the pharyngotympanic tube, it can also be interpreted as a specialized paranasal sinus. Like the sinuses, it is susceptible to frequent infections (otitis media).

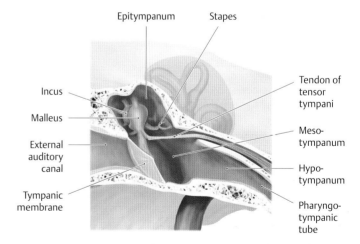

Epitympanum
Stapes
Incus
Malleus
External auditory canal
Tympanic membrane
Tendon of tensor tympani
Meso-tympanum
Hypo-tympanum
Pharyngo-tympanic tube

**Fig. 8.22 Clinically important levels of the tympanic cavity**

The tympanic cavity is divided into three levels in relation to the tympanic membrane:

- Epitympanum (epitympanic recess, attic) above the tympanic membrane
- Mesotympanum medial to the tympanic membrane
- Hypotympanum (hypotympanic recess) below the tympanic membrane

The epitympanum communicates with the mastoid air cells, and the hypotympanum communicates with the pharyngotympanic tube.

**163**

# Inner Ear

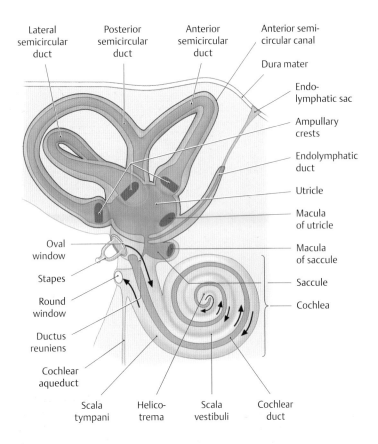

**Fig. 8.23 Inner ear**

The inner ear, embedded within the petrous part of the temporal bone, is formed by a membranous labyrinth, which floats within a similarly shaped bony labyrinth, loosely attached by connective tissue fibers. **Membranous labyrinth (blue):** The membranous labyrinth is filled with endolymph. This endolymphatic space (blue) communicates with the endolymphatic sac, an epidural pouch on the posterior surface of the petrous bone via the endolymphatic duct. *Note:* The auditory and vestibular endolymphatic spaces are connected by the ductus reuniens. **Bony labyrinth (beige):** The bony labyrinth is filled with perilymph. This perilymphatic space (beige) is connected to the subarachnoid space by the cochlear aqueduct (perilymphatic duct), which ends at the posterior surface of the petrous part of the temporal bone, inferior to the internal acoustic meatus.

The inner ear contains the auditory apparatus (hearing) and the vestibular apparatus (balance). **Auditory apparatus** (see pp. 170–171): The sensory epithelium of the auditory apparatus (organ of Corti) is found in the cochlea. The cochlea consists of the membranous cochlear duct and bony cochlear labyrinth. **Vestibular apparatus** (see pp. 174–175): The sensory epithelium of the vestibular apparatus is found in the saccule, the utricle, and the three membranous semicircular ducts. The saccule and utricle are enclosed in the bony vestibule, and the ducts are enclosed in bony semicircular canals.

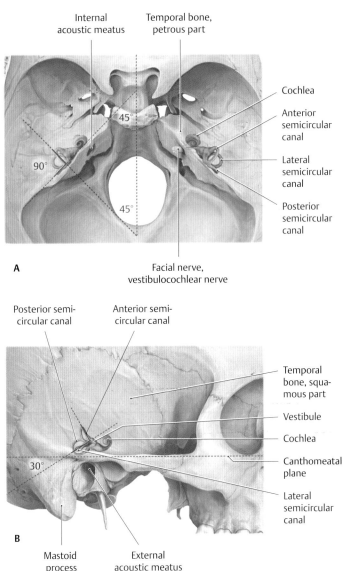

**Fig. 8.24 Projection of the inner ear onto the bony skull**

**A** Superior view of the petrous part of the temporal bone. **B** Right lateral view of the squamous part of the temporal bone.

The apex of the cochlea is directed anteriorly and laterally—not upward as one might intuitively expect. The bony semicircular canals are oriented at an approximately 45-degree angle to the cardinal body planes (coronal, transverse, and sagittal). It is important to know this arrangement when interpreting thin-slice CT scans of the petrous bone. *Note:* The location of the semicircular canals is of clinical importance in thermal function tests of the vestibular apparatus. The lateral (horizontal) semicircular canal is directed 30 degrees forward and upward. If the head of the *supine* patient is elevated by 30 degrees, the horizontal semicircular canal will assume a vertical alignment. Because warm fluids tend to rise, irrigating the auditory canal with warm (44°C) or cool (30°C) water (relative to the normal body temperature) can induce a thermal current in the endolymph of the semicircular canal, causing the patient to manifest vestibular nystagmus (jerky eye movements, vestibulo-ocular reflex). Because head movements always stimulate both vestibular apparatuses, caloric testing is the only method of *separately* testing the function of each vestibular apparatus (important in the diagnosis of unexplained vertigo).

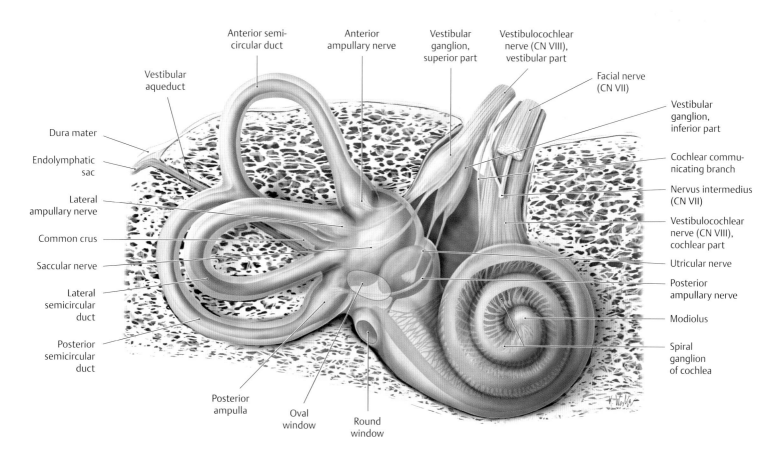

**Fig. 8.25 Innervation of the membranous labyrinth**
Right ear, anterior view. Afferent impulses from the vestibular and auditory membranous labyrinths are relayed via dentritic processes to cell bodies in the *vestibular* and *spiral ganglia*, respectively. The central processes of the vestibular and spiral ganglia form the vestibular and cochlear parts of the vestibulocochlear nerve (CN VIII), respectively. CN VIII relays afferent impulses to the brainstem through the internal acoustic meatus and cerebellopontine angle. *Vestibular ganglion:* The cell bodies of afferent neurons (bipolar ganglion cells) in the superior part of the vestibular ganglion receive afferent impulses from the anterior and lateral semicircular canals and the saccule; cell bodies in the inferior part receive afferent impulses from the posterior semicircular canal and utricle. *Spiral ganglia:* Located in the central bony core of the cochlea (modiolus), the cell bodies of bipolar ganglion cells in the spiral ganglia receive afferent impulses from the auditory apparatus via their dentritic processes.

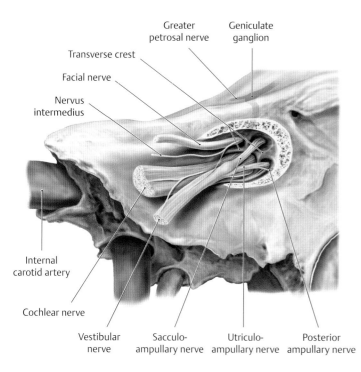

**Fig. 8.26 Cranial nerves in the right internal acoustic meatus**
Posterior oblique view of the fundus of the internal acoustic meatus. The approximately 1 cm-long internal auditory canal begins at the internal acoustic meatus on the posterior wall of the petrous bone. It contains:

- Vestibulocochlear nerve (CN VIII) with its cochlear and vestibular parts
- Facial nerve (CN VII), along with its parasympathetic and taste fibers (nervus intermedius)
- Labyrinthine artery and vein (not shown)

Given the close proximity of the vestibulocochlear nerve and facial nerve in the bony canal, a tumor of the vestibulocochlear nerve (*acoustic neuroma*) may exert pressure on the facial nerve, leading to peripheral facial paralysis. Acoustic neuroma is a benign tumor that originates from the Schwann cells of vestibular fibers, so it would be more accurate to call it a *vestibular schwannoma*. Tumor growth always begins in the internal auditory canal; as the tumor enlarges, it may grow into the cerebellopontine angle. Acute, unilateral inner ear dysfunction with hearing loss (sudden sensorineural hearing loss), often accompanied by tinnitus, typically reflects an underlying vascular disturbance (vasospasm of the labyrinthine artery causing decreased blood flow).

**165**

# Arteries & Veins of the Ear

The structures of the external and middle ear are supplied primarily by branches of the external carotid artery. (*Note:* The caroticotympanic arteries arise from the internal carotid artery.) The inner ear is supplied by the labyrinthine artery, which arises from the basilar artery. Venous drainage of the auricle is to the superficial temporal vein (via auricular veins), whereas drainage of the external ear is to the external jugular and maxillary veins and the pterygoid plexus. The veins of the tympanic cavity drain to the pterygoid plexus and superior petrosal sinus; the inner ear drains to the labyrinthine vein, which empties into the superior petrosal or transverse sinuses.

**Table 8.1** Arteries of the ear

| Artery | Origin | Distribution |
|---|---|---|
| Caroticotympanic aa. | Internal carotid a. | Pharyngotympanic (auditory) tube and anterior wall of tympanic cavity |
| Stylomastoid a. | Posterior auricular a. or occipital a. | Tympanic cavity, mastoid air cells and antrum, stapedius muscle, stapes |
| Inferior tympanic a. | Ascending pharyngeal a. | Medial wall of tympanic cavity, promontory |
| Deep auricular a. | Maxillary a. | External surface of tympanic membrane |
| Posterior tympanic a. | Stylomastoid a. | Chorda tympani, tympanic membrane, malleus |
| Superior tympanic a. | Middle meningeal a. | Tensor tympani, roof of tympanic cavity, stapes |
| Anterior tympanic a. | Maxillary a. | Tympanic membrane, mastoid antrum, malleus, incus |
| Tubal a. | Ascending pharyngeal a. | Pharyngotympanic tube and anterior tympanic cavity |
| Tympanic branches | A. of pterygoid canal | Tympanic cavity and pharyngotympanic tube |
| (Superficial) petrosal a. | Middle meningeal a. | Facial n. in facial canal and tympanic cavity |

*Note:* The arteries supplying the tympanic cavity and its contents form a rich arterial anastomotic network within the middle ear. The venous drainage of the middle ear is primarily into the pterygoid plexus of veins located in the infratemporal fossa or into dural venous sinuses.

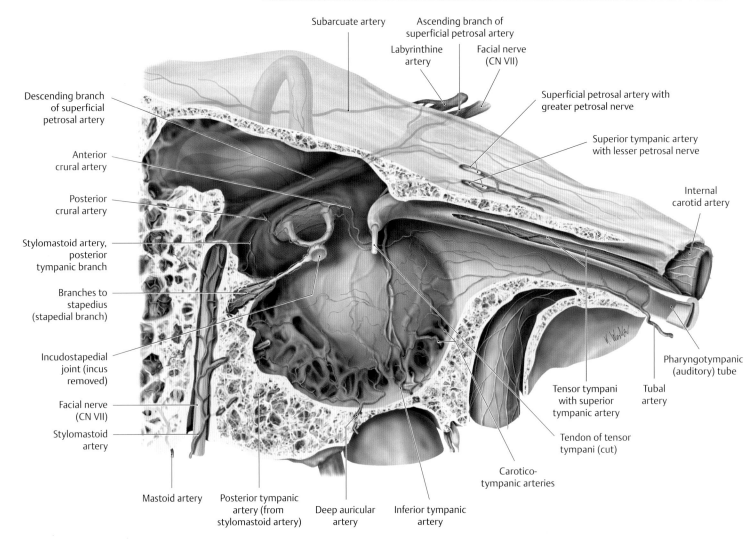

**Fig. 8.27 Arteries of the tympanic cavity and mastoid air cells**
Right petrous bone, anterior view. The malleus, incus, chorda tympani, and anterior tympanic artery have been removed (see **Fig. 8.28**).

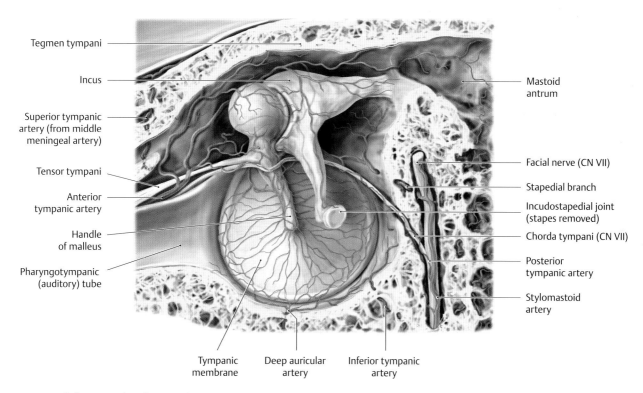

Tegmen tympani

Incus

Superior tympanic artery (from middle meningeal artery)

Tensor tympani

Anterior tympanic artery

Handle of malleus

Pharyngotympanic (auditory) tube

Mastoid antrum

Facial nerve (CN VII)

Stapedial branch

Incudostapedial joint (stapes removed)

Chorda tympani (CN VII)

Posterior tympanic artery

Stylomastoid artery

Tympanic membrane

Deep auricular artery

Inferior tympanic artery

**Fig. 8.28 Arteries of the ossicular chain and tympanic membrane**
Medial view of the right tympanic membrane. This region receives most of its blood supply from the anterior tympanic artery. With inflammation of the tympanic membrane, the arteries may become so dilated that their course in the tympanic membrane can be seen, as illustrated here.

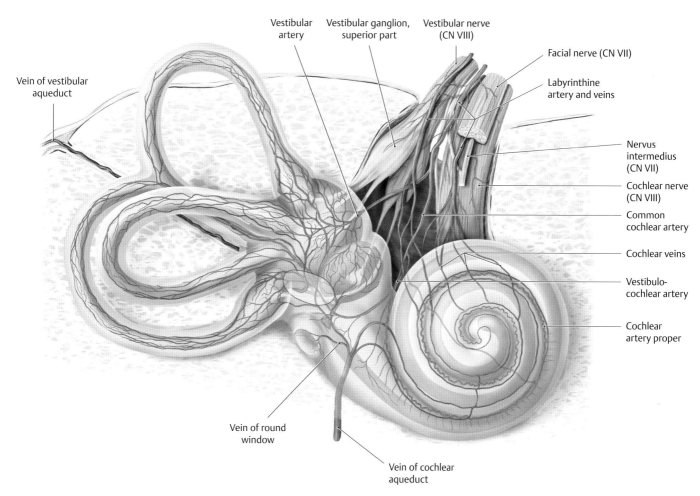

Vestibular artery

Vestibular ganglion, superior part

Vestibular nerve (CN VIII)

Facial nerve (CN VII)

Labyrinthine artery and veins

Vein of vestibular aqueduct

Nervus intermedius (CN VII)

Cochlear nerve (CN VIII)

Common cochlear artery

Cochlear veins

Vestibulo-cochlear artery

Cochlear artery proper

Vein of round window

Vein of cochlear aqueduct

**Fig. 8.29 Arteries and veins of the inner ear**
Right anterior view. The labyrinth receives its arterial blood supply from the labyrinthine (internal auditory) artery, which generally arises directly from the basilar artery, but may arise from the anterior inferior cerebellar artery. Venous blood drains to the labyrinthine vein and into the inferior petrosal sinus or the transverse sinuses.

**167**

# Vestibulocochlear Nerve (CN VIII)

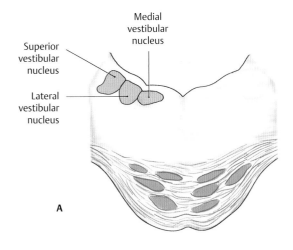

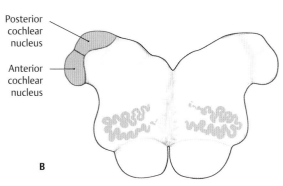

**Fig. 8.30 Nuclei of the vestibulocochlear nerve (CN VIII)**
Cross sections through the upper medulla oblongata.

**A Vestibular nuclei.** Four nuclear complexes are distinguished:

- Superior vestibular nucleus (of Bechterew)
- Lateral vestibular nucleus (of Deiters)
- Medial vestibular nucleus (of Schwalbe)
- Inferior vestibular nucleus (of Roller): does not appear in a cross section at this level

Most of the axons from the vestibular ganglion terminate in these four nuclei, but a smaller number pass directly through the inferior cerebellar peduncle into the cerebellum. The vestibular nuclei appear as eminences on the floor of the rhomboid fossa.

**B Cochlear nuclei.** Two nuclear complexes are distinguished:

- Anterior cochlear nucleus
- Posterior cochlear nucleus

Both nuclei are located lateral to the vestibular nuclei.
*Note:* The nuclei of CN VIII extend from the pons into the medulla oblongata.

---

| Table 8.2 Vestibulocochlear nerve (CN VIII): overview |
| --- |

**Fibers:** Special somatic afferent fibers (yellow)

**Structure and function:** CN VIII consists anatomically and functionally of two components:
- Vestibular root: Transmits impulses from the vestibular apparatus.
- Cochlear root: Transmits impulses from the auditory apparatus.
These roots are surrounded by a common connective tissue sheath. They pass from the inner ear through the internal acoustic meatus to the cerebellopontine angle, where they enter the brain.

**Nuclei and distribution:**
- Vestibular root: The vestibular ganglion contains bipolar ganglion cells whose central processes pass to the four vestibular nuclei on the floor of the rhomboid fossa of the medulla oblongata. Their peripheral processes begin at the sensory cells of the semicircular canals, saccule, and utricle.
- Cochlear root: The spiral ganglion contains bipolar ganglion cells whose central processes pass to the two cochlear nuclei, which are lateral to the vestibular nuclei in the rhomboid fossa. Their peripheral processes begin at the hair cells of the organ of Corti.

**Lesions:** Every thorough physical examination should include a rapid assessment of both nerve components (hearing and balance tests).
- Vestibular root lesion: Dizziness.
- Cochlear root lesion: Hearing loss (ranging to deafness).

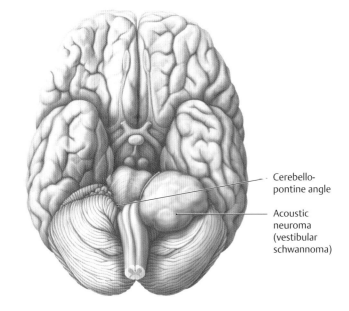

**Fig. 8.31 Acoustic neuroma in the cerebellopontine angle**
Acoustic neuromas (more accurately, vestibular schwannomas) are benign tumors of the cerebellopontine angle arising from the Schwann cells of the vestibular root of CN VIII. As they grow, they compress and displace the adjacent structures and cause slowly progressive hearing loss and gait ataxia. Large tumors can impair the egress of CSF from the fourth ventricle, causing hydrocephalus and symptomatic intracranial hypertension (vomiting, impairment of consciousness).

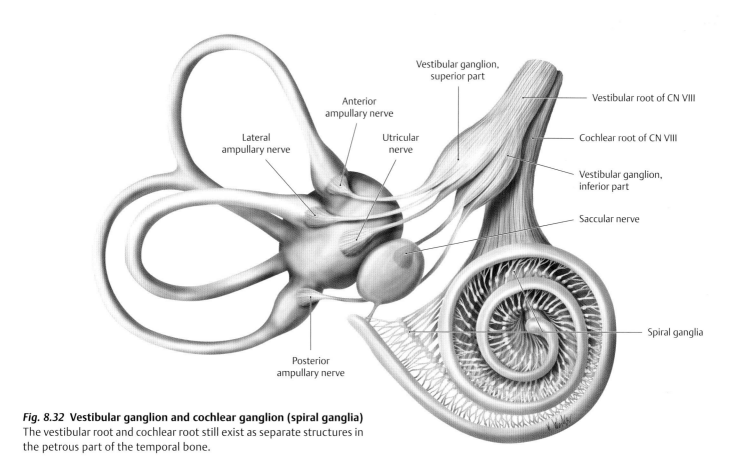

**Fig. 8.32 Vestibular ganglion and cochlear ganglion (spiral ganglia)**
The vestibular root and cochlear root still exist as separate structures in the petrous part of the temporal bone.

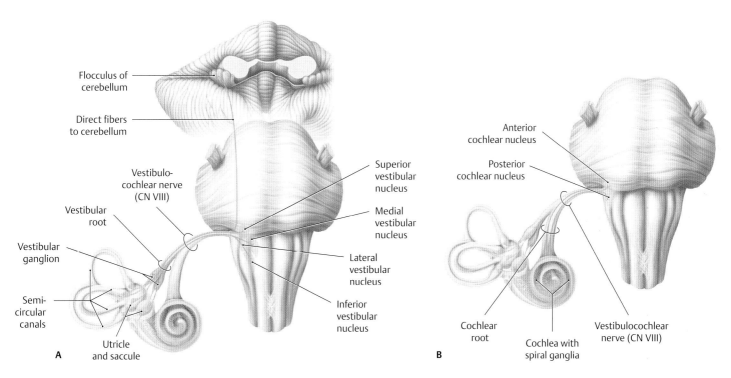

**Fig. 8.33 Nuclei of the vestibulocochlear nerve in the brainstem**
Anterior view of the medulla oblongata and pons.

**A Vestibular part:** The vestibular ganglion contains bipolar sensory cells whose peripheral (dendritic) processes pass to the semicircular canals, saccule, and utricle. Their axons travel as the vestibular root to the four vestibular nuclei on the floor of the rhomboid fossa. The vestibular organ processes information concerning orientation in space. An acute lesion of the vestibular organ is manifested clinically by dizziness (vertigo).

**B Cochlear part:** The spiral ganglia form a band of nerve cells that follows the course of the bony core of the cochlea. It contains bipolar sensory cells whose peripheral (dendritic) processes pass to the hair cells of the organ of Corti. Their central processes unite on the floor of the internal auditory canal to form the cochlear root and are distributed to the two nuclei that are posterior to the vestibular nuclei.

**169**

# Auditory Apparatus

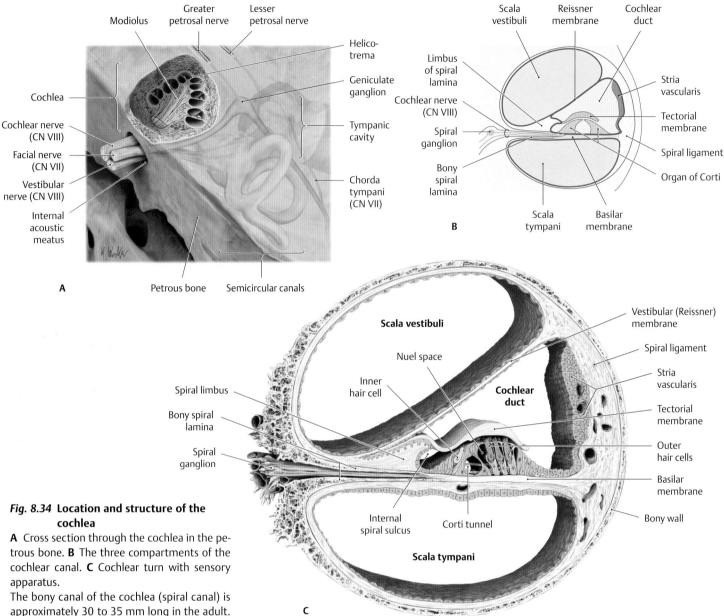

**Fig. 8.34 Location and structure of the cochlea**

**A** Cross section through the cochlea in the petrous bone. **B** The three compartments of the cochlear canal. **C** Cochlear turn with sensory apparatus.

The bony canal of the cochlea (spiral canal) is approximately 30 to 35 mm long in the adult. It makes two and a half turns around its bony axis, the *modiolus,* which is permeated by branched cavities and contains the spiral ganglion (perikarya of the afferent neurons). The base of the cochlea is directed toward the internal acoustic meatus (**A**). A cross section through the cochlear canal displays three membranous compartments arranged in three levels (**B**). The upper and lower compartments, the *scala vestibuli* and *scala tympani,* each contain perilymph; the middle level, the *cochlear duct* (scala media), contains endolymph. The perilymphatic spaces are interconnected at the apex by the *helicotrema,* and the endolymphatic space ends blindly at the apex. The cochlear duct, which is triangular in cross section, is separated from the scala vestibuli by the *vestibular Reissner membrane* and from the scala tympani by the *basilar membrane.* The basilar membrane represents a bony projection of the modiolus (*spiral lamina*) and

widens steadily from the base of the cochlea to the apex. High frequencies (up to 20,000 Hz) are perceived by the narrow portions of the basilar membrane, whereas low frequencies (down to about 200 Hz) are perceived by its broader portions (*tonotopic organization*). The basilar membrane and bony spiral lamina thus form the floor of the cochlear duct, upon which the actual organ of hearing, the organ of Corti, is located. This organ consists of a system of sensory cells and supporting cells covered by an acellular gelatinous flap, the *tectorial membrane.* The sensory cells (inner and outer hair cells) are the receptors of the organ of Corti (**C**). These cells bear approximately 50 to 100 stereocilia, and on their apical surface synapse on their basal side with the endings of afferent and efferent neurons. They

have the ability to transform mechanical energy into electrochemical potentials. A magnified cross-sectional view of a cochlear turn (**C**) also reveals the *stria vascularis,* a layer of vascularized epithelium in which the endolymph is formed. This endolymph fills the membranous labyrinth (appearing here as the cochlear duct, which is part of the labyrinth). The organ of Corti is located on the basilar membrane. It transforms the energy of the acoustic traveling wave into electrical impulses, which are then carried to the brain by the cochlear nerve. The principal cell of signal transduction is the inner hair cell. The function of the basilar membrane is to transmit acoustic waves to the inner hair cell, which transforms them into impulses that are received and relayed by the cochlear ganglion.

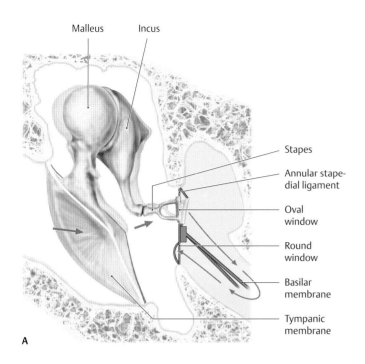

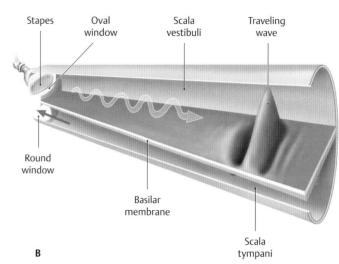

**Fig. 8.35 Sound conduction during hearing**

**A Sound conduction from the middle ear to the inner ear:** Sound waves in the air deflect the tympanic membrane, whose vibrations are conducted by the ossicular chain to the oval window. The sound pressure induces motion of the oval window membrane, whose vibrations are, in turn, transmitted through the perilymph to the basilar membrane of the inner ear (see **B**). The round window equalizes pressures between the middle and inner ear.

**B Formation of a traveling wave in the cochlea:** The sound wave begins at the oval window and travels up the scala vestibuli to the apex of the cochlea ("traveling wave"). The amplitude of the traveling wave gradually increases as a function of the sound frequency and reaches a maximum value at particular sites (shown greatly exaggerated in the drawing). These are the sites where the receptors of the organ of Corti are stimulated and signal transduction occurs. To understand this process, one must first grasp the structure of the organ of Corti (the actual organ of hearing), which is depicted in **Fig. 8.36**.

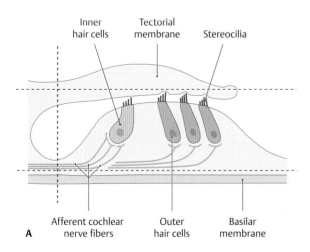

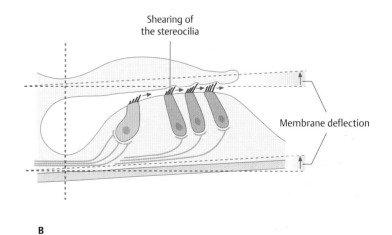

**Fig. 8.36 Organ of Corti at rest (A) and deflected by a traveling wave (B)**

The traveling wave is generated by vibrations of the oval window membrane. At each site that is associated with a particular sound frequency, the traveling wave causes a maximum deflection of the basilar membrane and thus of the tectorial membrane, setting up shearing movements between the two membranes. These shearing movements cause the stereocilia on the *outer* hair cells to bend. In response, the hair cells actively change their length, thereby increasing the local amplitude of the traveling wave. This additionally bends the stereocilia of the *inner* hair cells, stimulating the release of glutamate at their basal pole. The release of this substance generates an excitatory potential on the afferent nerve fibers, which is transmitted to the brain.

# Auditory Pathway

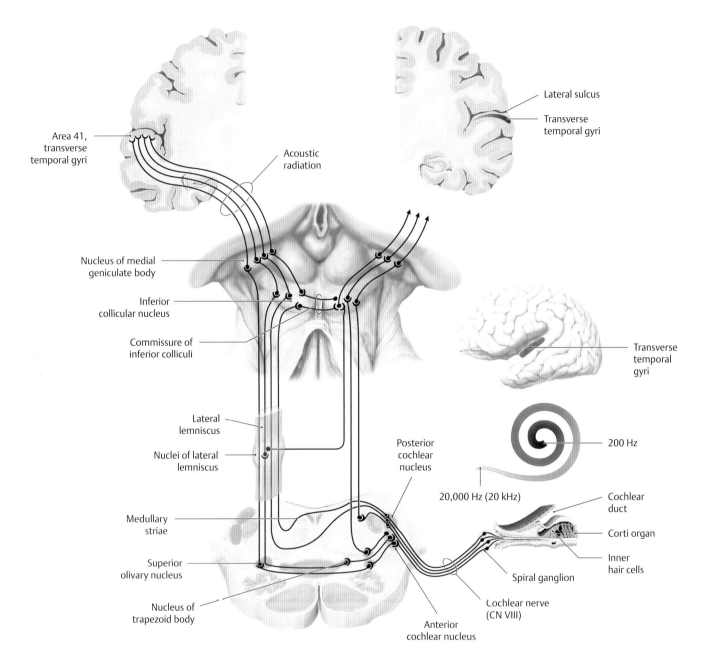

**Fig. 8.37 Afferent auditory pathway of the left ear**

The receptors of the auditory pathway are the inner hair cells of the organ of Corti. Because they lack neural processes, they are called *secondary sensory cells.* They are located in the cochlear duct of the basilar membrane and are studded with stereocilia, which are exposed to shearing forces from the tectorial membrane in response to a traveling wave. This causes bowing of the stereocilia (see **Fig. 8.36**). These bowing movements act as a stimulus to evoke cascades of neural signals. Dendritic processes of the bipolar neurons in the spiral ganglion pick up the stimulus. The bipolar neurons then transmit impulses via their axons, which are collected to form the cochlear nerve, to the anterior and posterior cochlear nuclei. In these nuclei the signals are relayed to the second neuron of the auditory pathway. Information from the cochlear nuclei is then transmitted via four to six nuclei to the primary auditory cortex, where the auditory information is consciously perceived (analogous to the visual cortex). The primary auditory cortex is located in the transverse temporal gyri (Heschl gyri, Brodmann area 41). The auditory pathway thus contains the following key stations:

- Inner hair cells in the organ of Corti
- Spiral ganglion
- Anterior and posterior cochlear nuclei
- Nucleus of the trapezoid body and superior olivary nucleus
- Nucleus of the lateral lemniscus
- Inferior collicular nucleus
- Nucleus of the medial geniculate body
- Primary auditory cortex in the temporal lobe (transverse temporal gyri = Heschl gyri or Brodmann area 41)

The individual parts of the cochlea are correlated with specific areas in the auditory cortex and its relay stations. This is known as the *tonotopic organization of the auditory pathway.* This organizational principle is similar to that in the visual pathway. Binaural processing of the auditory information (= stereo hearing) first occurs at the level of the superior olivary nucleus. At all further stages of the auditory pathway there are also interconnections between the right and left sides of the auditory pathway (for clarity, these are not shown here). A cochlea that has ceased to function can sometimes be replaced with a cochlear implant.

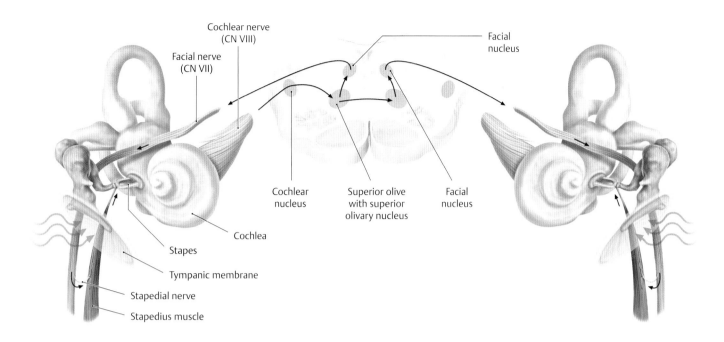

### Fig. 8.38 The stapedius reflex

When the volume of an acoustic signal reaches a certain threshold, the stapedius reflex triggers a contraction of the stapedius muscle. This reflex can be utilized to test hearing without the patient's cooperation ("objective" auditory testing). The test is done by introducing a sonic probe into the ear canal and presenting a test noise to the tympanic membrane. When the noise volume reaches a certain threshold, it evokes the stapedius reflex, and the tympanic membrane stiffens. The change in the resistance of the tympanic membrane is then measured and recorded. The *afferent* limb of this reflex is in the cochlear nerve. Information is conveyed to the facial nucleus on each side by way of the superior olivary nucleus. The *efferent* limb of this reflex is formed by branchiomotor (visceromotor) fibers of the facial nerve.

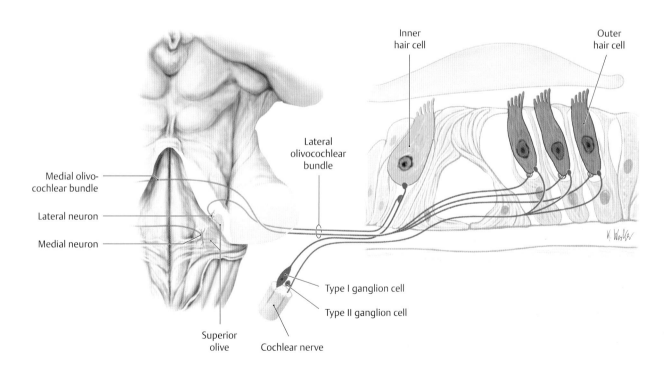

### Fig. 8.39 Efferent fibers from the olive to the Corti organ

Besides the afferent fibers from the organ of Corti, which form the vestibulocochlear nerve, there are also efferent fibers (red) that pass to the organ of Corti in the inner ear and are concerned with the active preprocessing of sound ("cochlear amplifier") and acoustic protection. The efferent fibers arise from neurons that are located in either the lateral or medial part of the superior olive and project from there to the cochlea (lateral or medial olivocochlear bundle). The fibers of the lateral neurons pass *uncrossed* to the dendrites of the *inner* hair cells, whereas the fibers of the medial neurons *cross* to the opposite side and terminate at the base of the *outer* hair cells, whose activity they influence. When stimulated, the outer hair cells can actively amplify the traveling wave. This increases the sensitivity of the inner hair cells (the actual receptor cells). The activity of the efferents from the olive can be recorded as otoacoustic emissions (OAE). This test can be used to screen for hearing abnormalities in newborns.

# Vestibular Apparatus

### Fig. 8.40 Structure of the vestibular apparatus

The vestibular apparatus is the organ of balance. It consists of the membranous semicircular ducts, which contain sensory ridges (ampullary crests) in their dilated portions (ampullae), and of the saccule and utricle with their macular organs. The sensory organs in the semicircular ducts respond to angular acceleration; the macular organs, which have an approximately vertical and horizontal orientation, respond to horizontal (utricular macula) and vertical (saccular macula) linear acceleration, as well as to gravitational forces.

### Fig. 8.41 Structure of the ampulla and ampullary crest

Cross section through the ampulla of a semicircular canal. Each canal has a bulbous expansion at one end (ampulla) that is traversed by a connective tissue ridge with sensory epithelium (ampullary crest). Extending above the ampullary crest is a gelatinous cupula, which is attached to the roof of the ampulla. Each of the sensory cells of the ampullary crest (approximately 7000 in all) bears on its apical pole one long kinocilium and approximately 80 shorter stereocilia, which project into the cupula. When the head is rotated in the plane of a particular semicircular canal, the inertial lag of the endolymph causes a deflection of the cupula, which in turn causes a bowing of the stereocilia. The sensory cells are either depolarized (excitation) or hyperpolarized (inhibition), depending on the direction of ciliary displacement.

### Fig. 8.42 Structure of the utricular and saccular maculae

The maculae are thickened oval areas in the epithelial lining of the utricle and saccule, each averaging 2 mm in diameter and containing arrays of sensory and supporting cells. Like the sensory cells of the ampullary crest, the sensory cells of the macular organs bear specialized stereocilia, which project into an otolithic membrane. The latter consists of a gelatinous layer, similar to the cupula, but it has calcium carbonate crystals or otoliths (*statoliths*) embedded in its surface. With their high specific gravity, these crystals exert traction on the gelatinous mass in response to linear acceleration, and this induces shearing movements of the cilia. The sensory cells are either depolarized or hyperpolarized by the movement, depending on the orientation of the cilia. There are two distinct categories of vestibular hair cells (type I and type II); type I cells (light red) are goblet shaped.

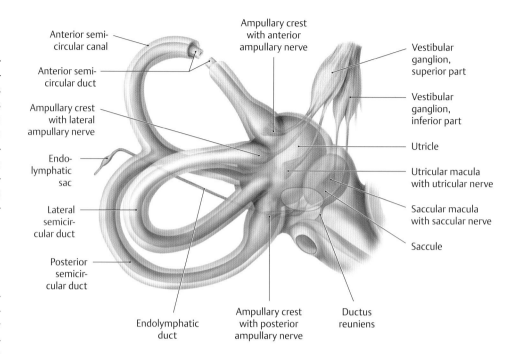

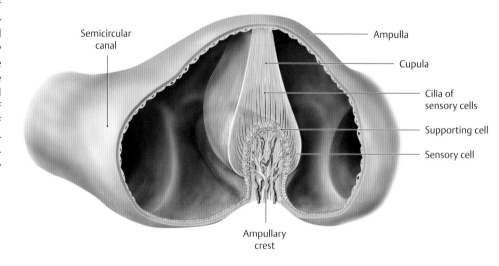

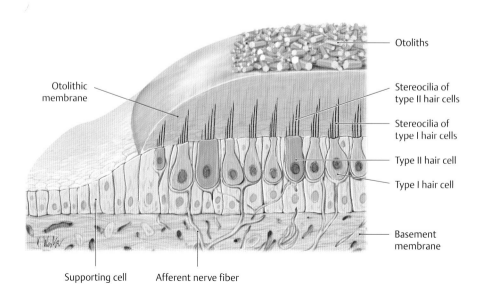

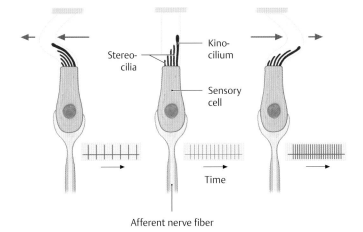

Afferent nerve fiber

### Fig. 8.43 Stimulus transduction in the vestibular sensory cells

Each of the sensory cells of the maculae and ampullary crest bears on its apical surface one long kinocilium and approximately 80 stereocilia of graduated lengths, forming an array that resembles a pipe organ. This arrangement results in a polar differentiation of the sensory cells. The cilia are straight while in a resting state. When the stereocilia are deflected toward the kinocilium, the sensory cell depolarizes, and the frequency of action potentials (discharge rate of impulses) is increased (right side of diagram). When the stereocilia are deflected away from the kinocilium, the cell hyperpolarizes, and the discharge rate is decreased (left side of diagram). This mechanism regulates the release of the transmitter glutamate at the basal pole of the sensory cell, thereby controlling the activation of the afferent nerve fiber (depolarization stimulates glutamate release, and hyperpolarization inhibits it). In this way the brain receives information on the magnitude and direction of movements and changes of position.

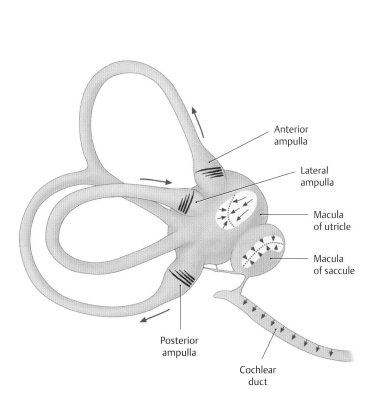

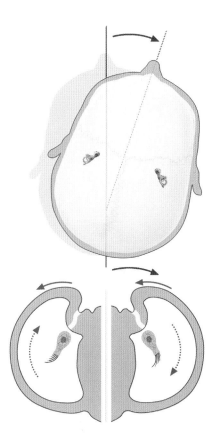

### Fig. 8.44 Specialized orientations of the stereocilia in the vestibular apparatus (ampullary crest and maculae)

Because the stimulation of the sensory cells by deflection of the stereocilia *away from* or *toward* the kinocilium is what initiates signal transduction, the spatial orientation of the cilia must be specialized to ensure that every position in space and every movement of the head stimulates or inhibits certain receptors. The ciliary arrangement shown here ensures that every direction in space will correlate with the maximum sensitivity of a particular receptor field. The arrows indicate the polarity of the cilia (i.e., each of the arrowheads points in the direction of the kinocilium in that particular field).

Note that the sensory cells show an opposite, reciprocal arrangement in the sensory fields of the utricle and saccule.

### Fig. 8.45 Interaction of contralateral semicircular canals during head rotation

When the head rotates to the right (red arrow), the endolymph flows to the left because of its inertial mass (solid blue arrow, taking the head as the reference point). Owing to the alignment of the stereocilia, the left and right semicircular canals are stimulated in opposite fashion. On the right side, the stereocilia are deflected toward the kinocilium (dotted arrow; the discharge rate increases). On the left side, the stereocilia are deflected away from the kinocilium (dotted arrow; the discharge rate decreases). This arrangement heightens the sensitivity to stimuli by increasing the stimulus contrast between the two sides. In other words, the difference between the decreased firing rate on one side and the increased firing rate on the other side enhances the perception of the kinetic stimulus.

# Vestibular System

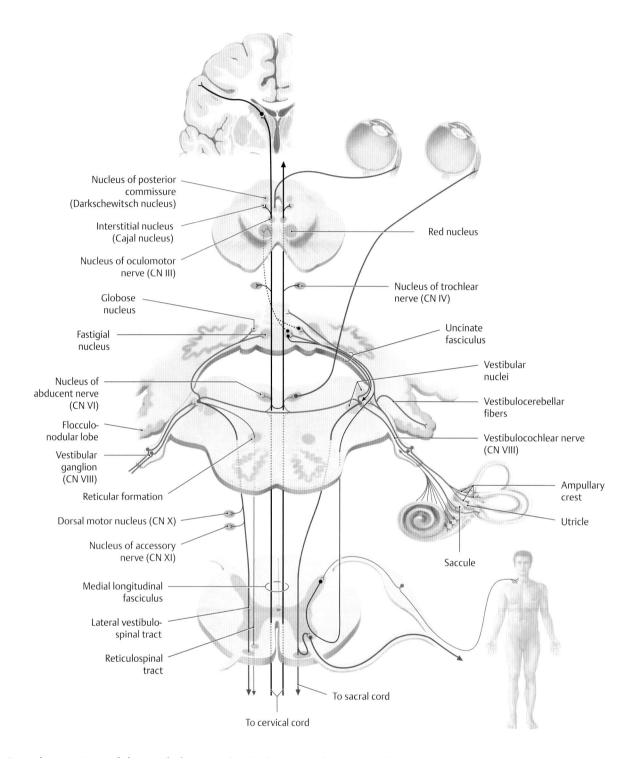

**Fig. 8.46 Central connections of the vestibular nerve (CN VIII)**
Three systems are involved in the regulation of human balance:

- Vestibular system
- Proprioceptive system
- Visual system

The peripheral receptors of the *vestibular system* are located in the membranous labyrinth, which consists of the utricle and saccule and the ampullae of the three semicircular ducts. The maculae of the utricle and saccule respond to linear acceleration, and the semicircular duct organs in the ampullary crests respond to angular (rotational) acceleration. Like the hair cells of the inner ear, the receptors of the vestibular system are *secondary* sensory cells. The basal portions of the secondary sensory cells are surrounded by dendritic processes of bipo-

lar neurons. Their perikarya are located in the vestibular ganglion. The axons from these neurons form the vestibular nerve and terminate in the four vestibular nuclei. Besides input from the vestibular apparatus, these nuclei also receive sensory input (see **Fig. 8.47**). The vestibular nuclei show a topographical organization (see **Fig. 8.48**) and distribute their efferent fibers to three targets:

- Motor neurons in the spinal cord via the lateral vestibulospinal tract. These motor neurons help to maintain an upright stance, mainly by increasing the tone of extensor muscles.
- Flocculonodular lobe of the cerebellum (archicerebellum) via vestibulocerebellar fibers.
- Ipsilateral and contralateral oculomotor nuclei via the ascending part of the medial longitudinal fasciculus.

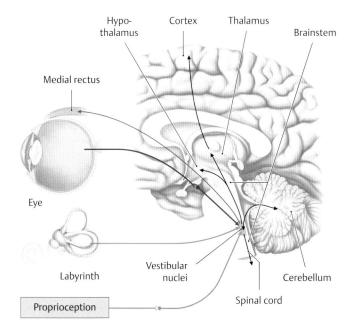

**Fig. 8.47 Role of the vestibular nuclei in the maintenance of balance**

The vestibular nuclei receive afferent input from the vestibular system, proprioceptive system (position sense, muscles, and joints), and visual system. They then distribute efferent fibers to nuclei that control the motor systems important for balance. These nuclei are located in the:

- Spinal cord (motor support)
- Cerebellum (fine control of motor function)
- Brainstem (oculomotor nuclei for oculomotor function)

Efferents from the vestibular nuclei are also distributed to the following regions:

- Thalamus and cortex (spatial sense)
- Hypothalamus (autonomic regulation: vomiting in response to vertigo)

*Note:* Acute failure of the vestibular system is manifested by rotary vertigo.

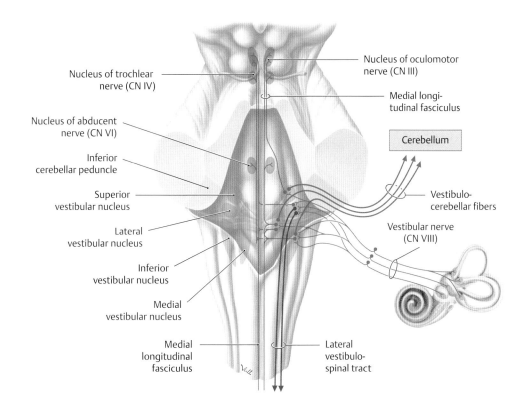

**Fig. 8.48 Vestibular nuclei: topographic organization and central connections**

Four nuclei are distinguished:

- Superior vestibular nucleus (of Bechterew)
- Lateral vestibular nucleus (of Deiters)
- Medial vestibular nucleus (of Schwalbe)
- Inferior vestibular nucleus (of Roller)

The vestibular system has a topographic organization:

- Afferent fibers of the saccular macula terminate in the inferior vestibular nucleus and lateral vestibular nucleus.
- Afferent fibers of the utricular macula terminate in the medial part of the inferior vestibular nucleus, the lateral part of the medial vestibular nucleus, and the lateral vestibular nucleus.

- Afferent fibers from the ampullary crests of the semicircular canals terminate in the superior vestibular nucleus, the upper part of the inferior vestibular nucleus, and the lateral vestibular nucleus.

The efferent fibers from the lateral vestibular nucleus pass to the lateral vestibulospinal tract. This tract extends to the sacral part of the spinal cord, its axons terminating on motor neurons. Functionally, it is concerned with keeping the body upright, chiefly by increasing the tone of the extensor muscles. The vestibulocerebellar fibers from the other three nuclei act through the cerebellum to modulate muscular tone. All four vestibular nuclei distribute ipsilateral and contralateral axons via the medial longitudinal fasciculus to the three motor nuclei of the nerves to the extraocular muscles (i.e., the nuclei of the oculomotor [CN III], trochlear [CN IV], and abducent [CN VI] nerves).

**177**

# Oral Cavity: Overview

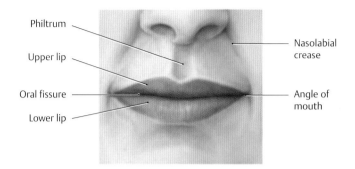

Philtrum

Upper lip

Oral fissure

Lower lip

Nasolabial crease

Angle of mouth

### *Fig. 9.1* **Lips and labial creases**

Anterior view. The upper and lower lips meet at the angle of the mouth. The oral fissure opens into the oral cavity. Changes in the lips noted on visual inspection may yield important diagnostic clues: Blue lips (cyanosis) suggest a disease of the heart, lung, or both, and deep nasolabial creases may reflect chronic diseases of the digestive tract.

### *Fig. 9.2* **Oral cavity**

Anterior view. The dental arches (with the alveolar processes of the maxilla and mandible) subdivide the oral cavity into two parts:

- Oral vestibule: portion outside the dental arches, bounded on one side by the lips/cheek and on the other by the dental arches.
- Oral cavity proper: region within the dental arches, bounded posteriorly by the palatoglossal arch.

The oral cavity is lined by oral mucosa, which is divided into lining, masticatory, and gingival mucosa. The mucosal lining consists of nonkeratinized, stratified squamous epithelium that is moistened by secretions from the salivary glands. The keratinized, stratified squamous epithelium of the skin blends with the nonkeratinized, stratified squamous epithelium of the oral cavity at the vermilion border of the lip. The masticatory mucosa is orthokeratinized to withstand masticatory stress. The gingiva that supports the teeth is keratinized.

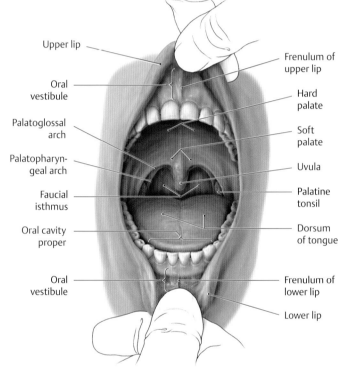

Upper lip

Oral vestibule

Palatoglossal arch

Palatopharyngeal arch

Faucial isthmus

Oral cavity proper

Oral vestibule

Frenulum of upper lip

Hard palate

Soft palate

Uvula

Palatine tonsil

Dorsum of tongue

Frenulum of lower lip

Lower lip

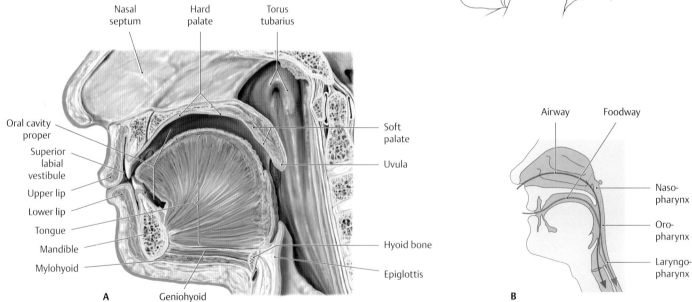

Nasal septum

Hard palate

Torus tubarius

Oral cavity proper

Superior labial vestibule

Upper lip

Lower lip

Tongue

Mandible

Mylohyoid

**A**

Geniohyoid

Soft palate

Uvula

Hyoid bone

Epiglottis

Airway

Foodway

Nasopharynx

Oropharynx

Laryngopharynx

**B**

### *Fig. 9.3* **Organization and boundaries of the oral cavity**

Midsagittal section, left lateral view. The oral cavity is located below the nasal cavity and anterior to the pharynx. The inferior boundary of the oral cavity proper is formed by mylohyoid muscle. The roof of the oral cavity is formed by the hard palate in its anterior two thirds and by the soft palate (velum) in its posterior third. The uvula hangs from the soft palate between the oral cavity and pharynx. The midportion of the pharynx (oropharynx) is the area in which the airway and foodway intersect (**B**).

### *Fig. 9.4* **Maxillary and mandibular arches**

**A** Maxilla. Inferior view.
**B** Mandible. Superior view.

There are three basic types of teeth—incisiform (incisors), caniniform (canines), and molariform (premolars and molars) — that perform cutting, piercing, and grinding actions, respectively. Each half of the maxilla and mandible contains the following sets of teeth:

- Anterior teeth: two incisors and one canine tooth.
- Posterior (postcanine) teeth: two premolars and three molars.

Each tooth is given an identification code to describe the specific location of dental lesions such as caries (see p. 180).

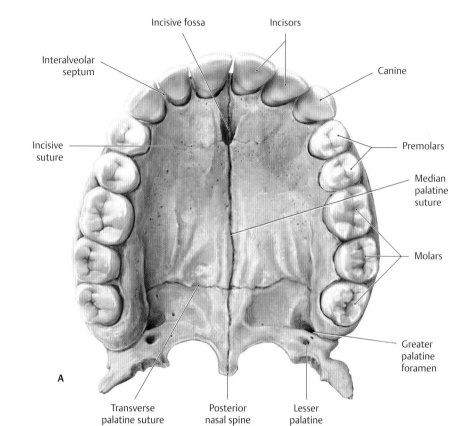

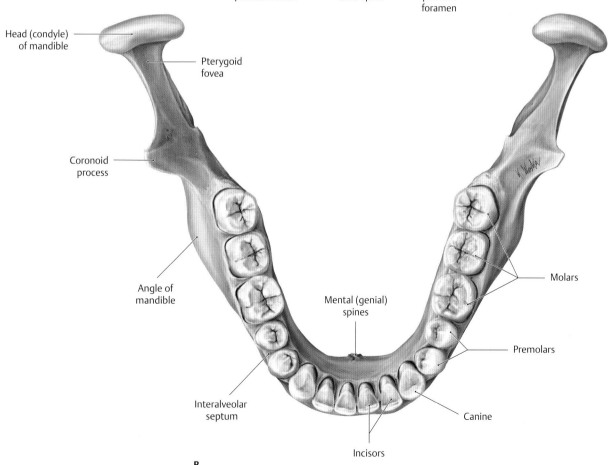

179

# Permanent Teeth

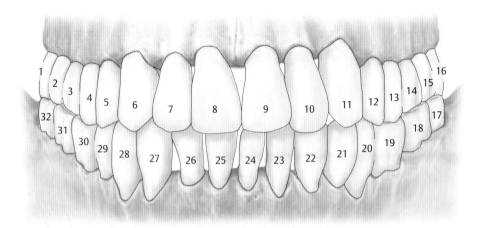

**Fig. 9.5 Coding the permanent teeth**

In the United States, the permanent teeth are numbered sequentially, not assigned to quadrants. Progressing in a clockwise fashion (from the perspective of the viewer), the teeth of the upper arc are numbered 1 to 16, and those of the lower are considered 17 to 32. *Note:* The third upper molar (wisdom tooth) on the patient's right is considered 1.

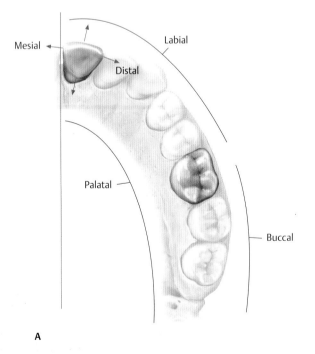

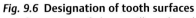

A

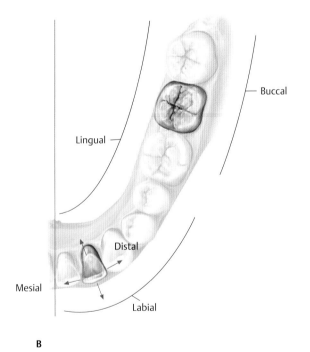

B

**Fig. 9.6 Designation of tooth surfaces**

**A** Inferior view of the maxillary dental arch. **B** Superior view of the mandibular dental arch. The *mesial* and *distal* tooth surfaces are those closest to and farthest from the midline, respectively. The term *labial* is used for incisors and canine teeth, and *buccal* is used for premolar and molar teeth. *Palatal* denotes the inside surface of maxillary teeth, and *lingual* denotes the inside surface of mandibular teeth. These designations are used to describe the precise location of small carious lesions.

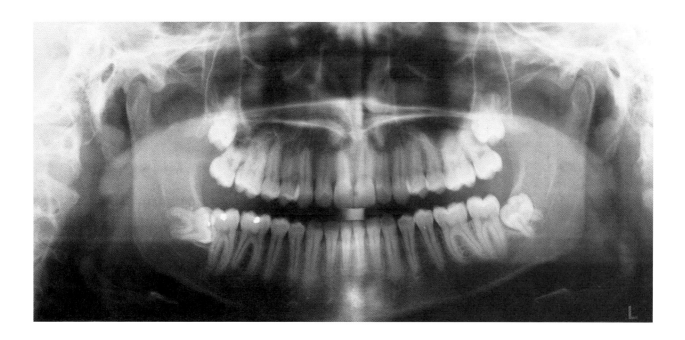

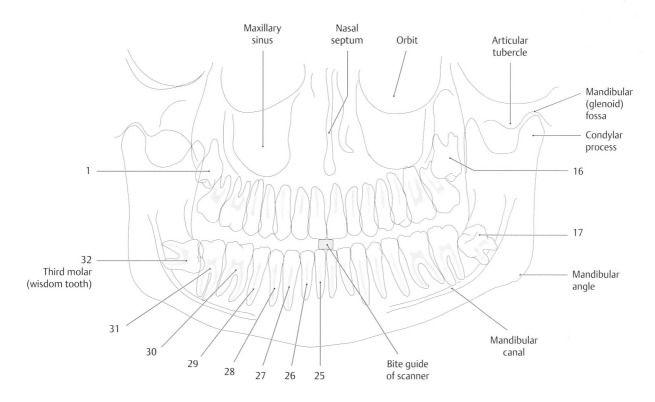

**Fig. 9.7 Dental panoramic tomogram**

The dental panoramic tomogram (DPT) is a survey radiograph that allows a preliminary assessment of the temporomandibular joints, maxillary sinuses, maxilla, mandible, and dental status (carious lesions, location of the wisdom teeth). It is based on the principle of conventional tomography in which the x-ray tube and film are moved about the plane of interest to blur out the shadows of structures outside the sectional plane. The plane of interest in the DPT is shaped like a parabola, conforming to the shape of the jaws. In the case shown here, all four wisdom teeth (third molars) should be extracted: teeth 1, 16, and 17 are not fully erupted, and tooth 32 is horizontally impacted (cannot erupt). If the DPT raises suspicion of caries or root disease, it should be followed with spot radiographs so that specific regions of interest can be evaluated at higher resolution.

(Tomogram courtesy of Prof. Dr. U. J. Rother, director of the Department of Diagnostic Radiology, Center for Dentistry and Oromaxillofacial Surgery, Eppendorf University Medical Center, Hamburg, Germany.)

*Note:* The upper incisors are broader than the lower incisors, leading to a "cusp-and-fissure" type of occlusion (see p. 183).

**181**

# Structure of the Teeth

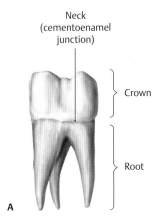

**A**

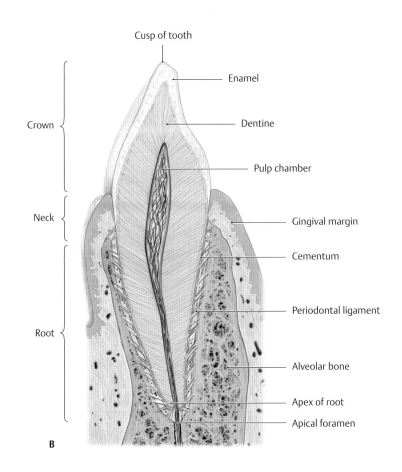

**B**

**Fig. 9.8 Parts of the tooth**

**A** Individual tooth (mandibular molar). **B** Cross section of a tooth (mandibular incisor). The teeth consist of an enamel-covered crown that meets the cementum-covered roots at the neck (cervical margin). The body of the tooth is primarily dentine.

| *Table 9.1* **Structures of the tooth** | |
|---|---|
| **Protective coverings:** These hard, avascular layers of tissue protect the underlying body of the tooth. They meet at the cervical margin (neck, cementoenamel junction). | **Enamel:** Hard, translucent covering of the crown of the tooth. Maximum thickness (2.5 mm) occurs over the cusps. The enamel covering meets the cementum at the neck (cervical margin, cementoenamel junction). Failure to do so exposes the underlying dentine, which has extremely sensitive pain responses. |
| | **Cementum:** Bonelike covering of the dental roots, lacking neurovascular structures. |
| **Body of the tooth:** The tooth is primarily composed of dentine, which is supported by the vascularized dental pulp. | **Dentine:** Tough tissue composing the majority of the body of the tooth. It consists of extensive networks of tubules (intratubular dentine) surrounded by peritubular dentine. The tubules connect the underlying dental pulp to the overlying tissue. Exposed dentine is extremely sensitive due to extensive innervation via the dental pulp. |
| | **Dental pulp:** Located in the pulp chamber, the dental pulp is a well-vascularized layer of loose connective tissue. Neurovascular structures enter the apical foramen at the apex of the root. The dental pulp receives sympathetic innervation from the superior cervical ganglion and sensory innervation from the trigeminal ganglion (CN V). |
| **Periodontium:** The tooth is anchored and supported by the periodontium, which consists of several tissue types. *Note:* The cementum is also considered part of the periodontium. | **Periodontal ligament:** Dense connective tissue fibers that connect the cementum of the roots in the osseous socket to the alveolar bone. |
| | **Alveolar bone** (alveolar processes of maxilla and mandible)**:** The portion of the maxilla or mandible in which the dental roots are embedded are considered the alveolar processes (the more proximal portion of the bones are considered the body). |
| | **Gingiva:** The attached gingivae bind the alveolar periosteum to the teeth; the free gingiva composes the 1 mm tissue radius surrounding the neck of the tooth. A mucosogingival line marks the boundary between the keratinized gingivae of the mandibular arch and the nonkeratinized lingual mucosa. The palatal mucosa is masticatory (orthokeratinized), so no visual distinction can be made with the gingiva of the maxillary arch. Third molars (wisdom teeth) often erupt through the mucosogingival line. The oral mucosa cannot support the tooth, and food can become trapped in the regions lacking attached gingiva. |

### *Fig. 9.9* Periodontium

The tooth is anchored in the alveolus by a special type of syndesmosis (gomphosis). The periodontium, the all-encompassing term for the tissues that collectively invest and support the tooth, consists of:

- Cementum
- Periodontal ligament
- Alveolar wall of alveolar bone
- Gingiva

The Sharpey fibers are collagenous fibers that pass obliquely downward from the alveolar bone and insert into the cementum of the tooth. This downward obliquity of the fibers transforms masticatory pressures on the dental arch into tensile stresses acting on the fibers and anchored bone (pressure would otherwise lead to bone atrophy).

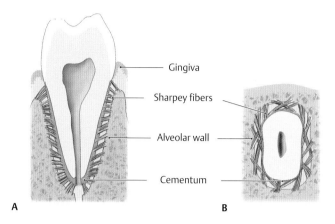

A    B

### *Fig. 9.10* Connective tissue fibers in the gingiva

Many of the tough collagenous fiber bundles in the connective tissue core of the gingiva above the alveolar bone are arranged in a screwlike pattern around the tooth, further strengthening its attachment.

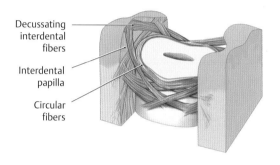

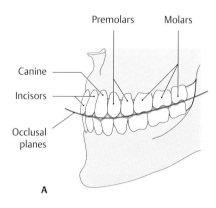

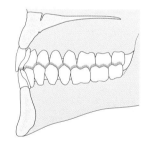

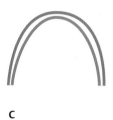

A    B    C

### *Fig. 9.11* Occlusal plane and dental arches

**A Occlusal plane.** The maxilla and mandible present a symmetrical arrangement of teeth. The occlusal plane (formed when the mouth is closed) often forms a superiorly open arch (von Spee curve, red).

**B Cusp-and-fissure dentition.** With the mouth closed (occlusal position), the maxillary teeth are apposed to their mandibular counterparts. They are offset relative to one another so that the cusps of one tooth fit into the fissures of the two opposing teeth (cusp-and-fissure dentition, blue). Because of this arrangement, every tooth comes into contact with two opposing teeth. This offset results from the slightly greater width of the maxillary incisors.

**C Dental arches.** The teeth of the maxilla (green) and mandible (blue) are arranged in superior and inferior arches. The superior dental arch forms a semi-ellipse, and the inferior arch is shaped like a parabola.

# Incisors, Canines & Premolars

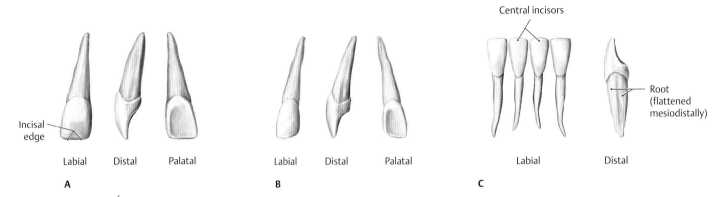

*Fig. 9.12* **Incisors**
**A** Central maxillary incisor (9). **B** Lateral maxillary incisor (10).
**C** Mandibular incisors (23–26).

### Table 9.2 Incisors and canines

| Tooth | | Crown | Surfaces | Root(s) |
|---|---|---|---|---|
| **Incisors:** The incisors have a sharp-edged crown for biting off bits of food. The palatal surface often bears a blind pit (foramen cecum), a site of predilection for dental caries. The maxillary incisors are considerably larger than the mandibular incisors. This results in cusp-and-fissure dentition (see **Fig. 9.11**). | | | | |
| Maxillary | Central incisor (8, 9); see **Fig. 9.12A** | Roughly trapezoidal in the labial view; contains an incisal edge with 3 tubercles (mamelons) | *Labial:* Convex *Palatal:* Concavoconvex | 1 rounded root |
| | Lateral incisor (7, 10); see **Fig. 9.12B** | | | |
| Mandibular | Central incisor (25, 24); see **Fig. 9.12C** | | *Labial:* Convex *Lingual:* Concavoconvex | 1 root, slightly flattened |
| | Lateral incisor (26, 23) see **Fig. 9.12C** | | | |
| **Canines:** These teeth (also known as cuspids or eyeteeth) are developed for piercing and gripping food. The crown is thicker mesially than distally and has greater curvature (arrow, **Fig. 9.13A**). | | | | |
| Maxillary (upper) canine (6, 11); see **Fig. 9.13A** | | Roughly trapezoidal with 1 labial cusp | *Labial:* Convex *Palatal:* Concavoconvex | 1 root, the longest of the teeth (note: mandibular canines are occasionally bifid) |
| Mandibular (lower) canine (27, 22); see **Fig. 9.13B** | | | *Labial:* Convex *Lingual:* Concavoconvex | |

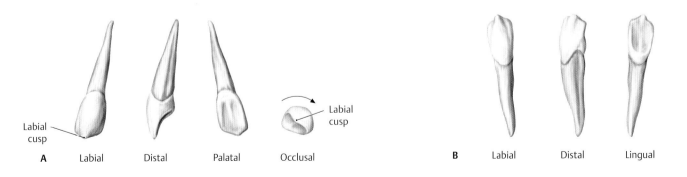

*Fig. 9.13* **Canines (cuspids)**
**A** Maxillary canine (11). **B** Mandibular canine (22).

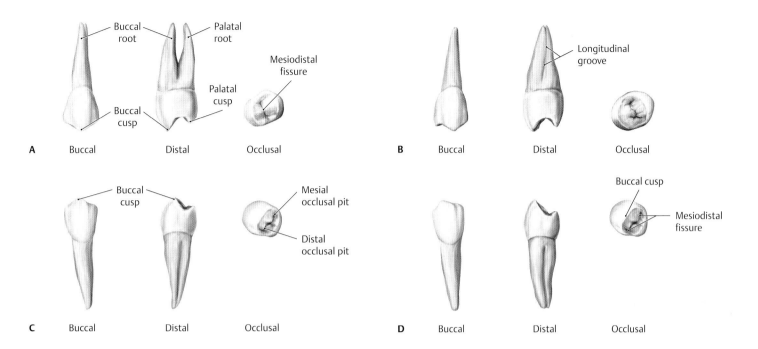

*Fig. 9.14* **Premolars (bicuspids)**
**A** First maxillary premolar (12). **B** Second maxillary premolar (13).
**C** First mandibular premolar (21). **D** Second mandibular premolar (20).

### Table 9.3 Premolars

The premolars represent a transitional form between the incisors and molars. Like the molars, they have cusps and fissures, indicating that their primary function is the grinding of food rather than biting or tearing.

| Tooth | Crown | | Surfaces | Root(s) |
|---|---|---|---|---|
| Maxillary | 1st premolar (5, 12); see **Fig. 9.14A** | 2 cusps (1 buccal, 1 palatal, separated by a mesodistal fissure) | *Buccal, distal, palatal/lingual, and mesial:* All convex, slightly flattened. The mesial surface often bears a small pit that is difficult to clean and vulnerable to caries. | The only premolar with 2 roots (1 buccal, 1 palatal) |
| | 2nd premolar (4, 13); see **Fig. 9.14B** | | | 1 root divided by a longitudinal groove and containing 2 root canals |
| Mandibular | 1st premolar (28, 21); see **Fig. 9.14C** | 2 cusps (1 tall buccal cusp connected to 1 smaller lingual cusp); the ridge between the cusps creates a mesial and a distal occlusal pit | *Occlusal:* The occlusal surfaces of the maxillary premolars tend to be more oval (less circular or square) than the mandibular premolars. | 1 root (occasionally bifid) |
| | 2nd premolar (29, 20); see **Fig. 9.14D** | 3 cusps (1 tall buccal cusp separated from 2 smaller lingual cusps by a mesiodistal fissure) | | 1 root |

# Molars

**Table 9.4  Molars**

Most of the molars have three roots to withstand the greater masticatory pressures in the molar region. Because the molars crush and grind food, they have a crown with a plateau. The fissures between the cusps are a frequent site of caries formation in adolescents. *Note:* The roots of the third molars (wisdom teeth, which erupt after 16 years of age, if at all) are commonly fused together, particularly in the upper third molar. The mandibular third molars erupt anterosuperiorly, and the maxillary third molars erupt posteroinferiorly. Impactions are therefore most common in mandibular wisdom teeth.

| Tooth | | Crown | Surfaces | Root(s) |
|---|---|---|---|---|
| Maxillary | 1st molar (3, 14); see **Fig. 9.15A** | 4 cusps (1 at each corner of its occlusal surface); a ridge connects the mesiopalatal and distobuccal cusps | *Buccal, distal, palatal/lingual, and mesial:* All convex, slightly flattened. | 3 roots (2 buccal and 1 palatal) |
| | 2nd molar (2, 15); see **Fig. 9.16A** | 4 cusps (though the distopalatal cusp is often small or absent) | *Occlusal:* Rhomboid | 3 roots (2 buccal and 1 palatal), occasionally fused |
| | 3rd molar (wisdom tooth, 1, 16); see **Fig. 9.17A** | 3 cusps (no distopalatal) | | 3 roots (2 buccal and 1 palatal), often fused |
| Mandibular | 1st molar (30, 19); see **Fig. 9.15B** | 5 cusps (3 buccal and 2 lingual), all of which are separated by fissures | *Buccal, distal, palatal/lingual, and mesial:* All convex, slightly flattened. | 2 roots (1 mesial and 1 distal); widely spaced |
| | 2nd molar (31, 18); see **Fig. 9.16B** | 4 cusps (2 buccal and 2 lingual) | *Occlusal:* Rectangular | 2 roots (1 mesial and 1 distal) |
| | 3rd molar (wisdom tooth, 32, 17); see **Fig. 9.17B** | May resemble either the 1st or 2nd molar | | 2 roots, often fused |

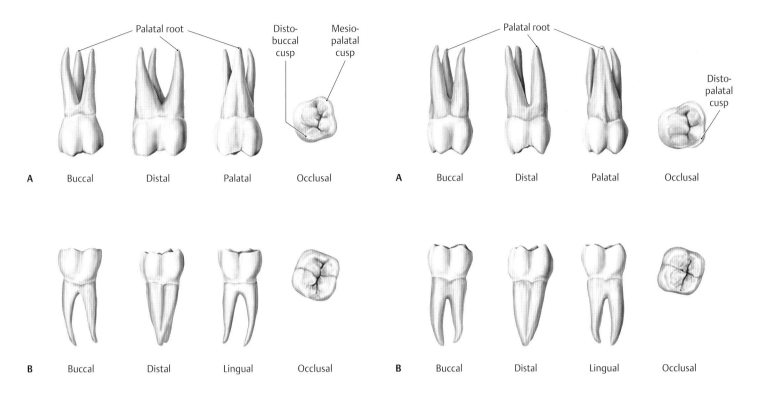

*Fig. 9.15* **First molars**
**A** Maxillary first molar (14). **B** Mandibular first molar (19). *Note:* The term *lingual* is used for the mandibular teeth, the term *palatal* for the maxillary.

*Fig. 9.16* **Second molars**
**A** Maxillary second molar (15). **B** Mandibular second molar (18).

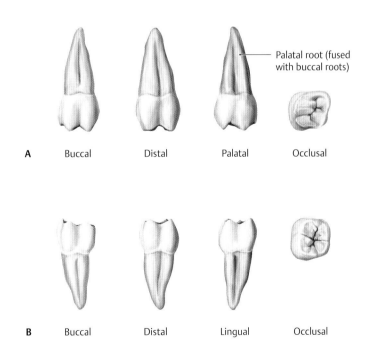

*Fig. 9.17* **Third molars (wisdom teeth)**
**A** Maxillary third molar (16). **B** Mandibular third molar (17).

# Deciduous Teeth

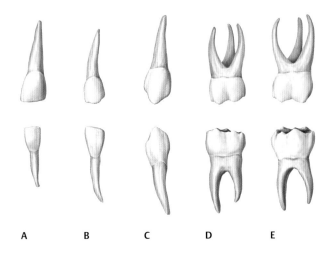

A    B    C    D    E

**Fig. 9.18 Deciduous teeth**
Left side. The deciduous dentition (baby teeth) consists of only 20 teeth. Each of the four quadrants contains the following teeth:

**A** Central incisor (first incisor). **B** Lateral incisor (second incisor). **C** Canine (cuspid). **D** First molar (6-yr molar). **E** Second molar (12-yr molar).

To distinguish the deciduous teeth from the permanent teeth, they are coded with letters. The upper arch is labeled A to J, the lower is labeled K to T.

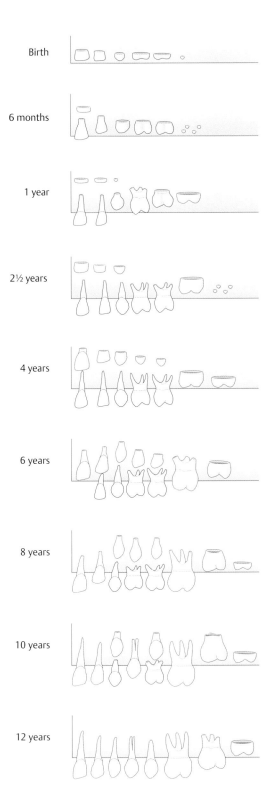

**Fig. 9.19 Eruption pattern of the deciduous and permanent teeth**
Left maxillary teeth. Deciduous teeth (black), permanent teeth (red). Eruption times can be used to diagnose growth delays in children.

| Table 9.5 Eruption of the teeth | | | |
|---|---|---|---|
| The eruptions of the deciduous and permanent teeth are called the first and second dentitions, respectively. Types of teeth are ordered by the time of eruption; individual teeth are listed from left to right (viewer's perspective). | | | |
| **Type of tooth** | **Tooth** | | **Time of eruption** |
| **First dentition (deciduous teeth)** | | | |
| Central incisor | E, F | P, O | 6–8 months |
| Lateral incisor | D, G | Q, N | 8–12 months |
| First molar | B, I | S, L | 12–16 months |
| Canine | C, H | R, M | 15–20 months |
| Second molar | A, J | T, K | 20–40 months |
| **Second dentition (permanent teeth)** | | | |
| First molar | 3, 14 | 30, 19 | 6–8 years ("6-yr molar") |
| Central incisor | 8, 9 | 25, 24 | 6–9 years |
| Lateral incisor | 7, 10 | 26, 23 | 7–10 years |
| First premolar | 5, 12 | 28, 21 | 9–13 years |
| Canine | 6, 11 | 27, 22 | 9–14 years |
| Second premolar | 4, 13 | 29, 20 | 11–14 years |
| Second molar | 2, 15 | 31, 18 | 10–14 years ("12-yr molar") |
| Third molar | 1, 16 | 32, 17 | 16–30 years ("wisdom tooth") |

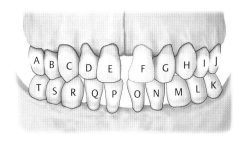

**Fig. 9.20 Coding the deciduous teeth**
The upper right molar is considered A. The lettering then proceeds clockwise along the upper arc and back across the lower.

**Fig. 9.21 Dentition of a 6-year-old child**
Anterior (**A,B**) and left lateral (**C,D**) views of maxillary (**A,C**) and mandibular (**B,D**) teeth. The anterior bony plate over the roots of the deciduous teeth has been removed to display the underlying permanent tooth buds (blue). At 6 years of age, all the deciduous teeth have erupted and are still present, along with the first permanent tooth, the first molar.

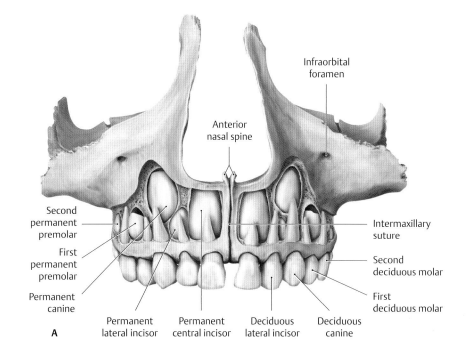

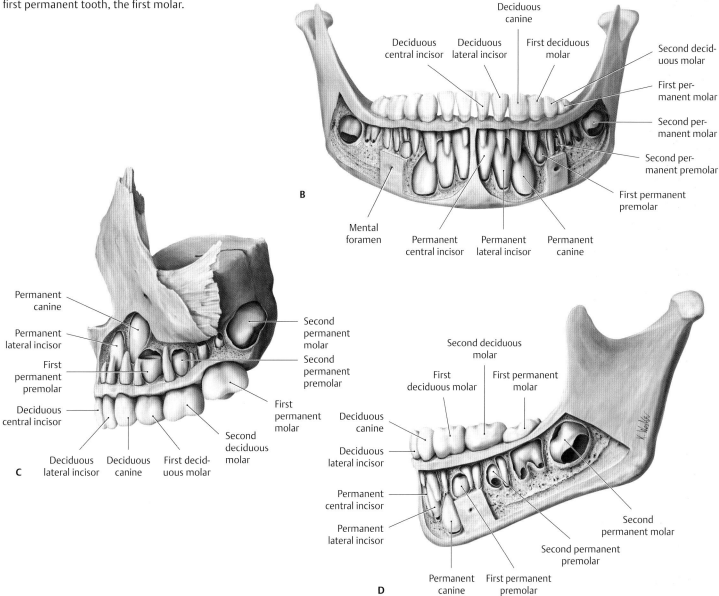

**189**

# Hard Palate

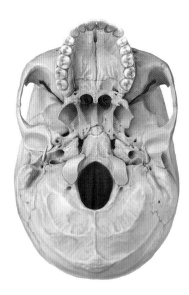

**Fig. 9.22 Hard palate in the skull base**
Inferior view.

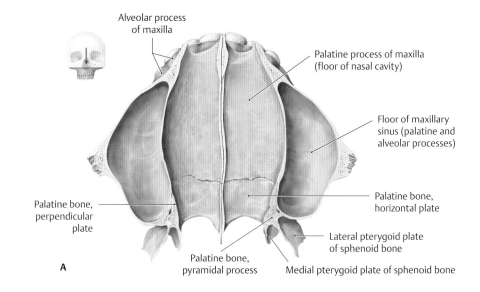

Alveolar process of maxilla

Palatine process of maxilla (floor of nasal cavity)

Floor of maxillary sinus (palatine and alveolar processes)

Palatine bone, horizontal plate

Lateral pterygoid plate of sphenoid bone

Medial pterygoid plate of sphenoid bone

Palatine bone, pyramidal process

Palatine bone, perpendicular plate

**A**

**Fig. 9.23 Bones of the hard palate**

**A,C Superior view.** The upper part of the maxilla is removed. The floor of the nasal cavity (**A**) and the roof of the oral cavity (**B**) are formed by the union of the palatine processes of two maxillary bones with the horizontal plates of two palatine bones. Cleft palate results from a failed fusion of the palatine processes at the median palatine suture.

**B,D Inferior view.** The nasal cavity communicates with the nasopharynx via the choanae, which begin at the posterior border of the hard palate. The two nasal cavities communicate with the oral cavity via the incisive canals (**D**), which combine and emerge at the incisive foramen (**E**).

**C,E Oblique posterior view.** This view illustrates the close anatomical relationship between the oral and nasal cavities. *Note:* The pyramidal process of the palatine bone is integrated into the lateral plate of the pterygoid process of the sphenoid bone. The palatine margin of the vomer articulates with the hard palate along the nasal crest.

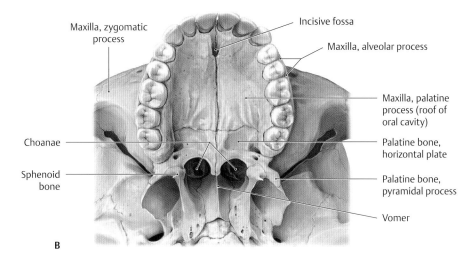

Maxilla, zygomatic process

Incisive fossa

Maxilla, alveolar process

Maxilla, palatine process (roof of oral cavity)

Palatine bone, horizontal plate

Palatine bone, pyramidal process

Vomer

Choanae

Sphenoid bone

**B**

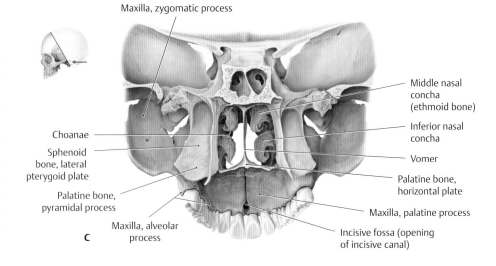

Maxilla, zygomatic process

Middle nasal concha (ethmoid bone)

Inferior nasal concha

Vomer

Palatine bone, horizontal plate

Maxilla, palatine process

Incisive fossa (opening of incisive canal)

Choanae

Sphenoid bone, lateral pterygoid plate

Palatine bone, pyramidal process

Maxilla, alveolar process

**C**

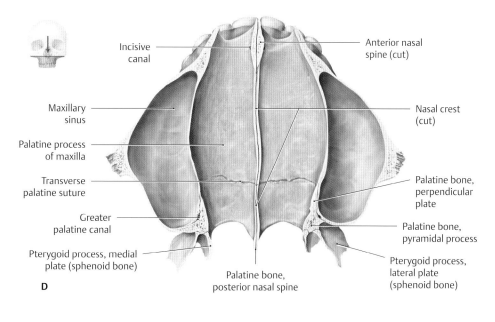

Incisive canal

Anterior nasal spine (cut)

Maxillary sinus

Nasal crest (cut)

Palatine process of maxilla

Transverse palatine suture

Palatine bone, perpendicular plate

Greater palatine canal

Palatine bone, pyramidal process

Pterygoid process, medial plate (sphenoid bone)

Pterygoid process, lateral plate (sphenoid bone)

Palatine bone, posterior nasal spine

**D**

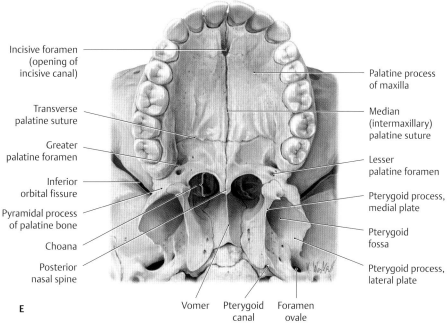

Incisive foramen (opening of incisive canal)

Palatine process of maxilla

Transverse palatine suture

Median (intermaxillary) palatine suture

Greater palatine foramen

Lesser palatine foramen

Inferior orbital fissure

Pterygoid process, medial plate

Pyramidal process of palatine bone

Pterygoid fossa

Choana

Posterior nasal spine

Pterygoid process, lateral plate

Vomer    Pterygoid canal    Foramen ovale

**E**

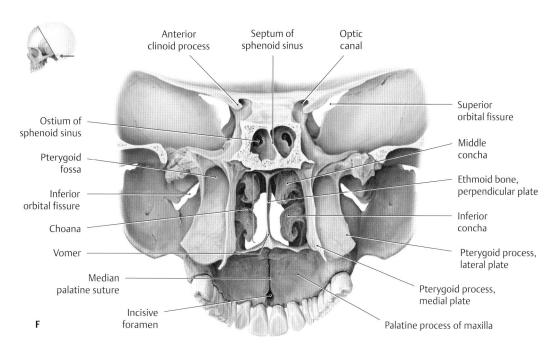

Anterior clinoid process

Septum of sphenoid sinus

Optic canal

Ostium of sphenoid sinus

Superior orbital fissure

Pterygoid fossa

Middle concha

Inferior orbital fissure

Ethmoid bone, perpendicular plate

Choana

Inferior concha

Vomer

Pterygoid process, lateral plate

Median palatine suture

Pterygoid process, medial plate

Incisive foramen

Palatine process of maxilla

**F**

# Mandible & Hyoid Bone

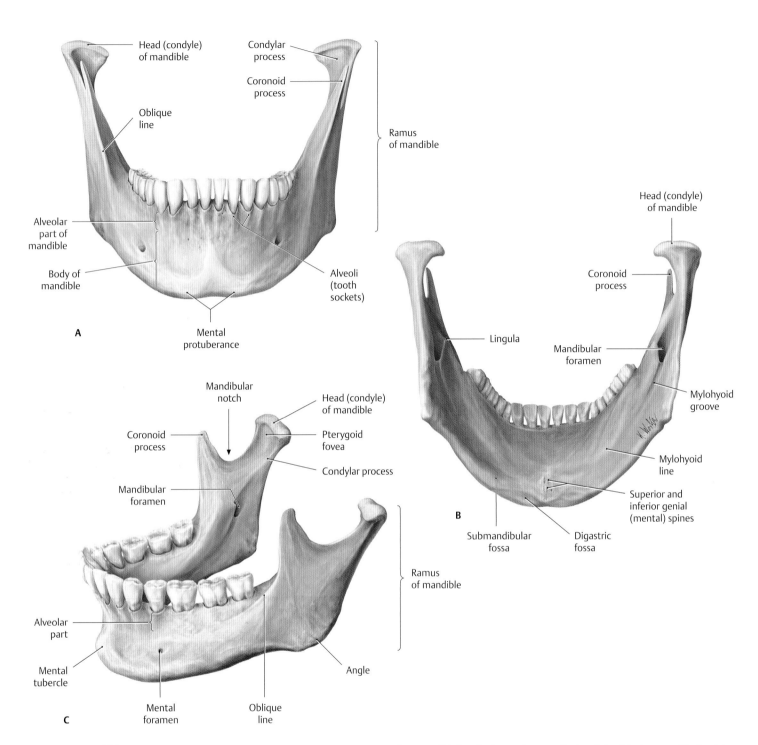

**Fig. 9.24 Mandible**
**A** Anterior view. **B** Posterior view. **C** Oblique left lateral view. The mandibular teeth are embedded in the alveolar processes of the mandible that run along the superior border of the body of the mandible. The vertical ramus joins the body of the mandible at the mandibular angle. The ramus contains a coronoid process (site of attachment of the temporalis) and a condylar process that are separated by the mandibular notch. The convex surface of the condylar process (the head of the mandible) articulates via an articular disk with the mandibular (glenoid) fossa of the temporal bone at the temporomandibular joint (see p. 194). The depression on the anteromedial side of the condylar process (pterygoid fovea) is a site of attachment of the lateral pterygoid. The inferior alveolar nerve (a branch of CN V$_3$) enters the mandibular foramen and runs through the mandibular canal in the body of the mandible, exiting the mental foramen as the mental nerve.

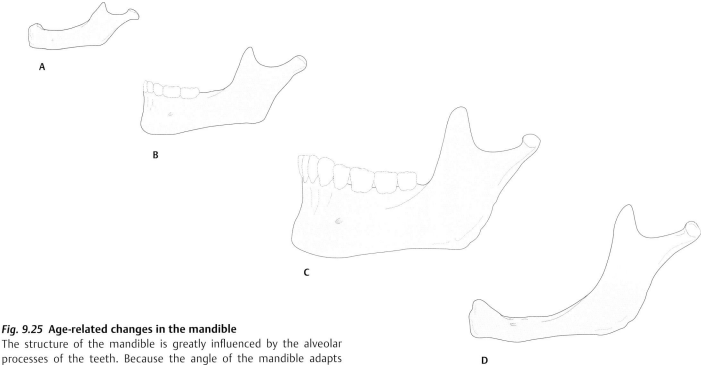

***Fig. 9.25*** **Age-related changes in the mandible**

The structure of the mandible is greatly influenced by the alveolar processes of the teeth. Because the angle of the mandible adapts to changes in the alveolar process, the angle between the body and ramus also varies with age-related changes in the dentition. The angle measures approximately 150 degrees at birth, and approximately 120 to 130 degrees in adults, decreasing to 140 degrees in the edentulous mandible of old age.

**A  At birth** the mandible is without teeth, and the alveolar part has not yet formed.
**B  In children** the mandible bears the deciduous teeth. The alveolar part is still relatively poorly developed because the deciduous teeth are considerably smaller than the permanent teeth.

**C  In adults** the mandible bears the permanent teeth, and the alveolar part of the bone is fully developed.
**D  Old age** is characterized by an edentulous mandible with resorption of the alveolar process.

*Note:* The resorption of the alveolar process with advanced age leads to a change in the position of the mental foramen (which is normally located below the second premolar tooth, as in **C**). This change must be taken into account in surgery or dissections involving the mental nerve.

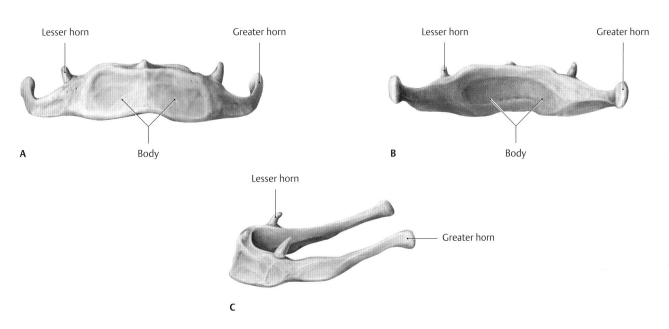

***Fig. 9.26*** **Hyoid bone**

**A** Anterior view. **B** Posterior view. **C** Oblique left lateral view. The hyoid bone is suspended by muscles and ligaments between the oral floor and the larynx. The greater horn and body of the hyoid bone are palpable in the neck. The physiological movement of the hyoid bone can be palpated during swallowing.

# Temporomandibular Joint (TMJ)

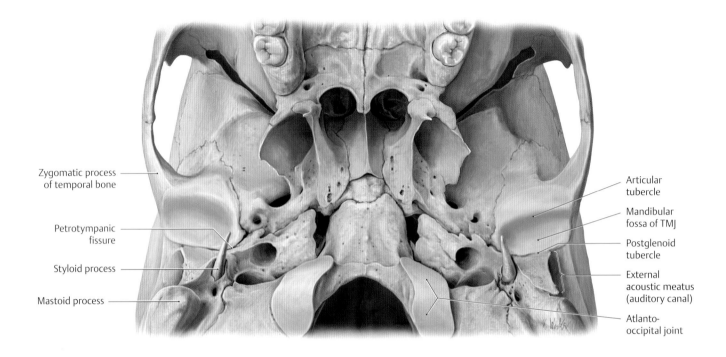

**Fig. 9.27 Mandibular fossa of the TMJ**
Inferior view of skull base. The head (condyle) of the mandible articulates with the mandibular fossa of the temporal bone via an articular disk. The mandibular fossa is a depression in the squamous part of the temporal bone, bounded by an articular tubercle and a postglenoid tubercle. Unlike other articular surfaces, the mandibular fossa is covered by fibrocartilage, not hyaline cartilage. As a result, it is not as clearly delineated on the skull (compare to the atlanto-occipital joints). The external auditory canal lies just posterior to the mandibular fossa. Trauma to the mandible may damage the auditory canal.

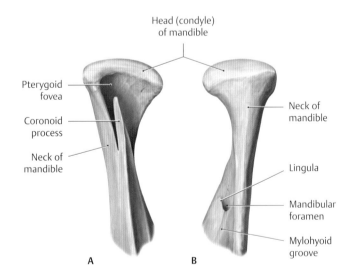

**Fig. 9.28 Head of the mandible in the TMJ**
**A** Anterior view. **B** Posterior view. The head (condyle) of the mandible is markedly smaller than the mandibular fossa and has a cylindrical shape. Both factors increase the mobility of the mandibular head, allowing rotational movements about a vertical axis.

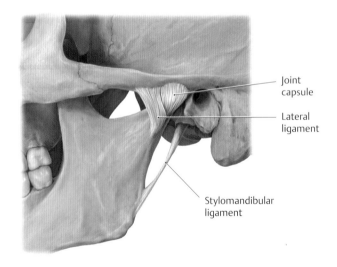

**Fig. 9.29 Ligaments of the lateral TMJ**
Left lateral view. The TMJ is surrounded by a relatively lax capsule that permits physiological dislocation during jaw opening. The joint is stabilized by three ligaments: lateral, stylomandibular, and sphenomandibular (see also **Fig. 9.30**). The strongest of these ligaments is the lateral ligament, which stretches over and blends with the joint capsule.

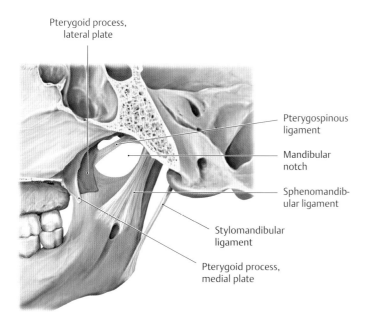

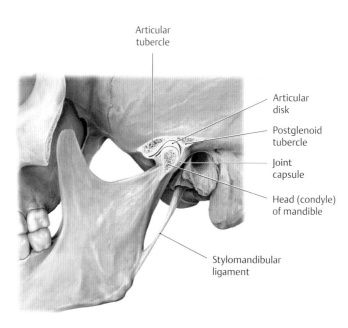

**Fig. 9.30 Ligaments of the medial TMJ**
Left medial view. Note the sphenomandibular ligament. The variable pterygospinous ligament is also present.

**Fig. 9.31 Opened TMJ**
Left lateral view. The TMJ capsule begins at the articular tubercle and extends posteriorly to the petrotympanic fissure (see **Fig. 9.27**). Interposed between the mandibular head and fossa is the fibrocartilaginous articular disk, which is attached to the joint capsule on all sides.

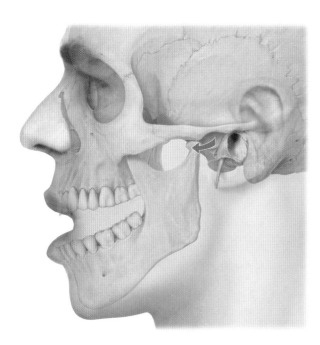

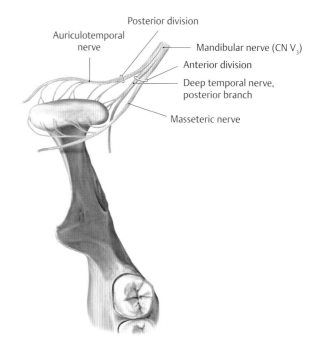

**Fig. 9.32 Dislocation of the TMJ**
The head of the mandible may slide past the articular tubercle when the mouth is opened, dislocating the TMJ. This may result from heavy yawning or a blow to the opened mandible. When the joint dislocates, the mandible becomes locked in a protruded position and can no longer be closed. This condition is easily diagnosed clinically and is reduced by pressing on the mandibular row of teeth.

**Fig. 9.33 Sensory innervation of the TMJ capsule**
Superior view. The TMJ capsule is supplied by articular branches arising from three nerves from the mandibular division of the trigeminal nerve (CN V$_3$):

- Auriculotemporal nerve
- Deep temporal nerve, posterior branch
- Masseteric nerve

# Temporomandibular Joint (TMJ): Biomechanics

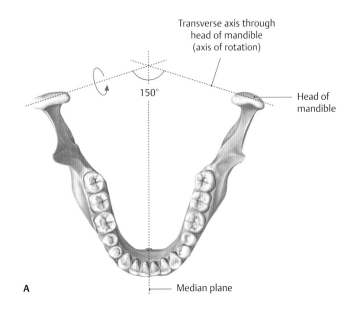

**A** Median plane

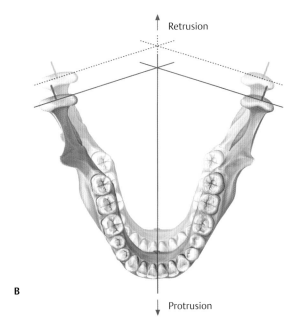

**B**

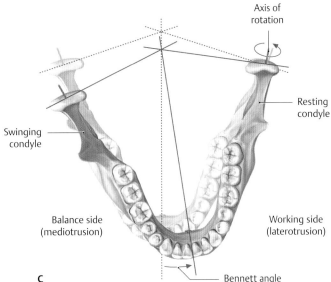

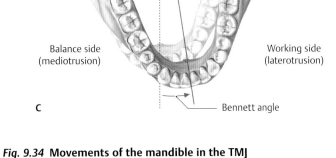

**C**

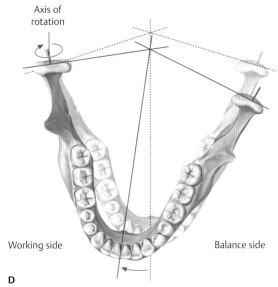

**D**

**Fig. 9.34 Movements of the mandible in the TMJ**
Superior view. Most of the movements in the TMJ are complex motions that have three main components:

- Rotation (opening and closing the mouth)
- Translation (protrusion and retrusion of the mandible)
- Grinding movements during mastication

**A Rotation.** The axis for joint rotation runs transversely through both heads of the mandible. The two axes intersect at an angle of approximately 150 degrees (range of 110 to 180 degrees between individuals). During this movement the TMJ acts as a hinge joint (abduction/depression and adduction/elevation of the mandible). In humans, pure rotation in the TMJ usually occurs only during sleep with the mouth slightly open (aperture angle up to approximately 15 degrees). When the mouth is opened past 15 degrees, rotation is combined with translation (gliding) of the mandibular head.

**B Translation.** In this movement the mandible is advanced (protruded) and retracted (retruded). The axes for this movement are parallel to the median axes through the center of the mandibular heads.

**C Grinding movements in the left TMJ.** In describing these lateral movements, a distinction is made between the "resting condyle" and the "swinging condyle." The resting condyle on the left working side rotates about an almost vertical axis through the head of the mandible (also a rotational axis), whereas the swinging condyle on the right balance side swings forward and inward in a translational movement. The lateral excursion of the mandible is measured in degrees and is called the Bennett angle. During this movement the mandible moves in laterotrusion on the working side and in mediotrusion on the balance side.

**D Grinding movements in the right TMJ.** Here, the right TMJ is the working side. The right resting condyle rotates about an almost vertical axis, and the left condyle on the balance side swings forward and inward.

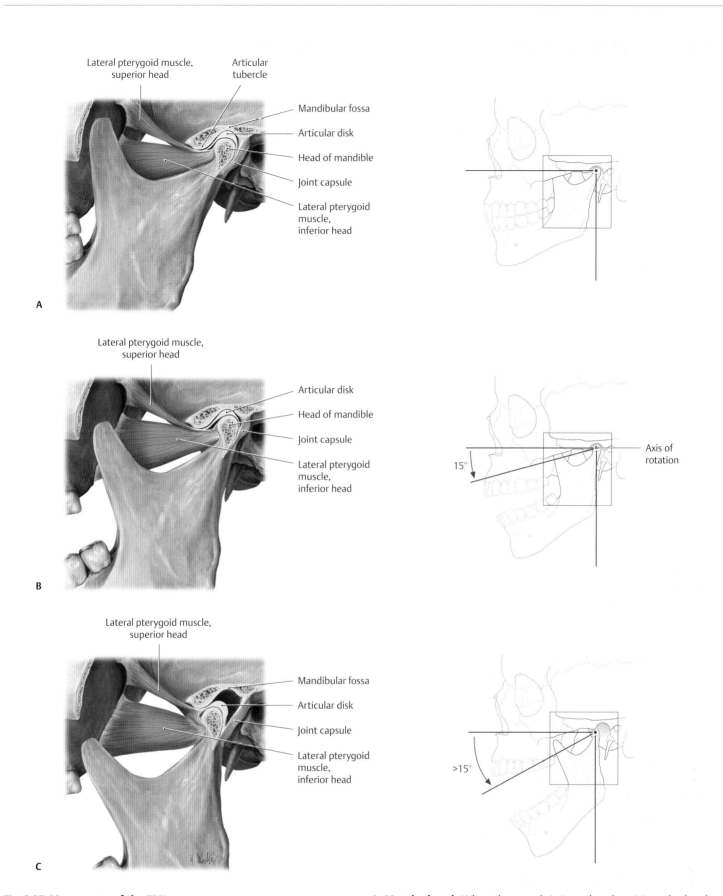

**Fig. 9.35 Movements of the TMJ**

Left lateral view. Each drawing shows the left TMJ, including the articular disk and capsule and the lateral pterygoid muscle. Each schematic diagram at right shows the corresponding axis of joint movement. The muscle, capsule, and disk form a functionally coordinated musculo-disco-capsular system and work closely together when the mouth is opened and closed. *Note:* The space between the muscle heads is greatly exaggerated for clarity.

**A Mouth closed.** When the mouth is in a closed position, the head of the mandible rests against the mandibular fossa of the temporal bone with the intervening articular disk.

**B Mouth opened to 15 degrees.** Up to 15 degrees of abduction, the head of the mandible remains in the mandibular fossa.

**C Mouth opened past 15 degrees.** At this point the head of the mandible glides forward onto the articular tubercle. The joint axis that runs transversely through the mandibular head is shifted forward. The articular disk is pulled forward by the superior part of the lateral pterygoid muscle, and the head of the mandible is drawn forward by the inferior part of that muscle.

**197**

# Muscles of Mastication: Overview

The muscles of mastication are derived from the first branchial arch and are located at various depths in the parotid and infratemporal regions of the face. They attach to the mandible and receive their motor innervation from the mandibular division of the trigeminal nerve (CN V$_3$). The muscles of the oral floor (mylohyoid and geniohyoid) are found on pp. 178, 203.

**Table 9.6** Masseter and temporalis muscles

| Muscle | | Origin | Insertion | Innervation* | Action |
|---|---|---|---|---|---|
| Masseter | ① Superficial head | Zygomatic bone (maxillary process) and zygomatic arch (lateral aspect of anterior ⅔) | Mandibular angle and ramus (lower posterior lateral surface) | Masseteric n. (anterior division of CN V$_3$) | Elevates mandible; also assists in protraction, retraction, and side-to-side motion |
| | Middle head | Zygomatic arch (medial aspect of anterior ⅔) | Mandibular ramus (central part) | | |
| | ② Deep head | Zygomatic arch (deep surface of posterior ⅓) | Mandibular ramus (upper portion) and lateral side of coronoid process | | |
| Temporalis | ③ Superficial head | Temporal fascia | Coronoid process of mandible (apex and medial and anterior surfaces) | Deep temporal nn. (anterior division of CN V$_3$) | *Vertical (anterior) fibers:* Elevate mandible *Horizontal (posterior) fibers:* Retract (retrude) mandible *Unilateral:* Lateral movement of mandible (chewing) |
| | ④ Deep head | Temporal fossa (inferior temporal line) | | | |

*The muscles of mastication are innervated by motor branches of the mandibular nerve (CN V$_3$), the 3rd division of the trigeminal nerve (CN V).

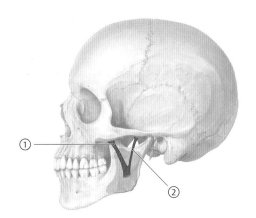

**Fig. 9.36** Masseter

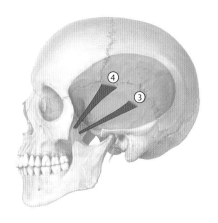

**Fig. 9.37** Temporalis

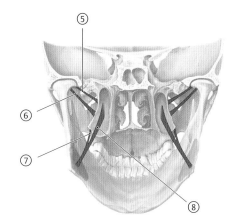

**Fig. 9.38** Pterygoids

**Table 9.7** Lateral and medial pterygoid muscles

| Muscle | | Origin | Insertion | Innervation | Action |
|---|---|---|---|---|---|
| Lateral pterygoid | ⑤ Superior head | Greater wing of sphenoid bone (infratemporal crest) | Mandible (pterygoid fovea) and temporomandibular joint (articular disk) | Mandibular n. (CN V$_3$) via lateral pterygoid n. (from anterior division of CN V$_3$) | *Bilateral:* Protrudes mandible (pulls articular disk forward) *Unilateral:* Lateral movements of mandible (chewing) |
| | ⑥ Inferior head | Lateral pterygoid plate (lateral surface) | Mandible (pterygoid fovea and condylar process) | | |
| Medial pterygoid | ⑦ Superficial head | Maxilla (maxillary tuberosity) and palatine bone (pyramidal process) | Pterygoid tuberosity on medial surface of the mandibular angle | Mandibular n. (CN V$_3$) via medial pterygoid n. (from trunk of CN V$_3$) | Raises (adducts) mandible |
| | ⑧ Deep head | Medial surface of lateral pterygoid plate and pterygoid fossa | | | |

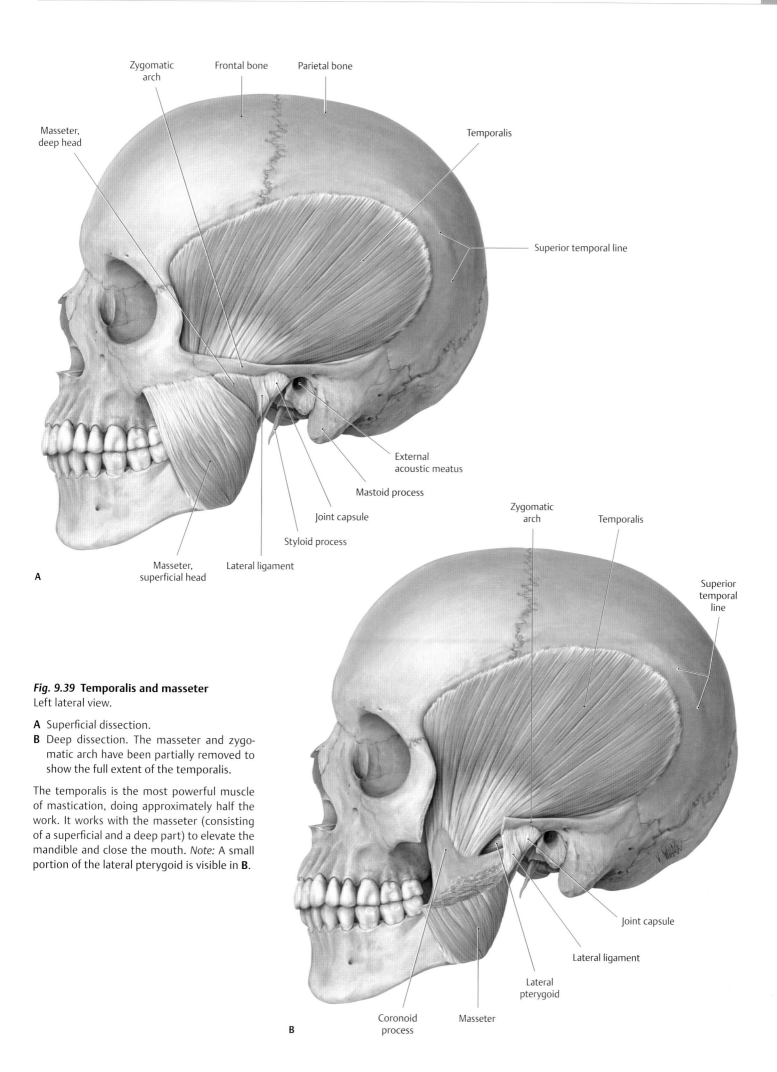

**Fig. 9.39 Temporalis and masseter**
Left lateral view.

**A** Superficial dissection.
**B** Deep dissection. The masseter and zygomatic arch have been partially removed to show the full extent of the temporalis.

The temporalis is the most powerful muscle of mastication, doing approximately half the work. It works with the masseter (consisting of a superficial and a deep part) to elevate the mandible and close the mouth. *Note:* A small portion of the lateral pterygoid is visible in **B**.

**199**

# Muscles of Mastication: Deep Muscles

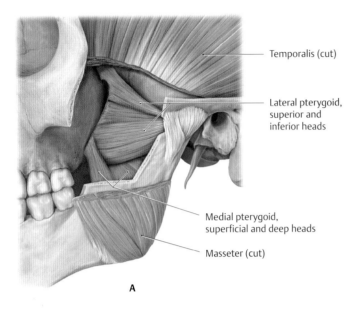

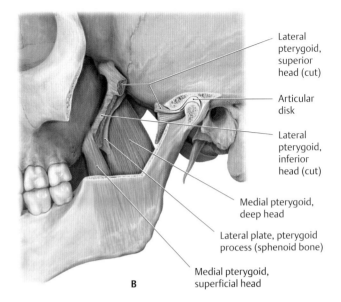

**Fig. 9.40 Lateral and medial pterygoid muscles**

Left lateral views.

A The coronoid process of the mandible has been removed here along with the lower part of the temporalis so that both pterygoid muscles can be seen.

B Here the temporalis has been completely removed, and the superior and inferior heads of the lateral pterygoid have been windowed. The *lateral* pterygoid initiates mouth opening, which is then continued by the digastric and the suprahyoid muscles, along with gravity.

With the temporomandibular joint opened, we can see that fibers from the lateral pterygoid blend with the articular disk. The lateral pterygoid functions as the guide muscle of the temporomandibular joint. Because both its superior and inferior heads are active during all movements, its actions are more complex than those of the other muscles of mastication. The *medial* pterygoid runs almost perpendicular to the lateral pterygoid and contributes to the formation of a muscular sling, along with the masseter, that partially encompasses the mandible (see **Fig. 9.41**).

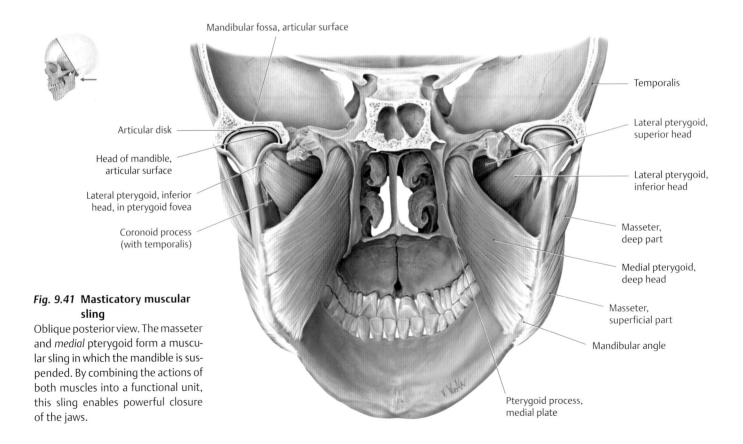

**Fig. 9.41 Masticatory muscular sling**

Oblique posterior view. The masseter and *medial* pterygoid form a muscular sling in which the mandible is suspended. By combining the actions of both muscles into a functional unit, this sling enables powerful closure of the jaws.

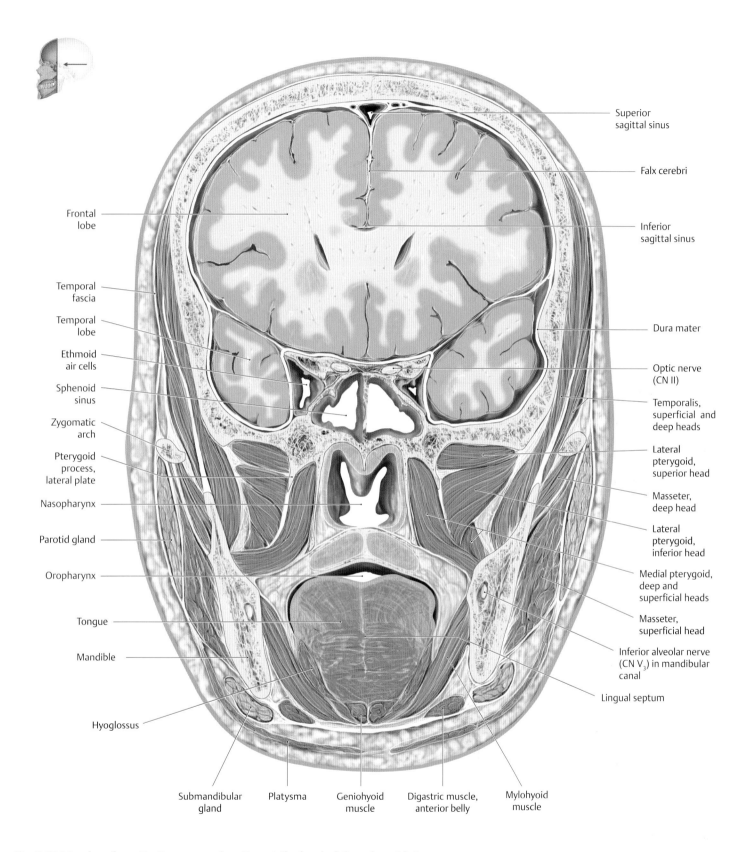

Superior
sagittal sinus

Falx cerebri

Frontal
lobe

Inferior
sagittal sinus

Temporal
fascia

Temporal
lobe

Dura mater

Ethmoid
air cells

Optic nerve
(CN II)

Sphenoid
sinus

Temporalis,
superficial and
deep heads

Zygomatic
arch

Lateral
pterygoid,
superior head

Pterygoid
process,
lateral plate

Masseter,
deep head

Nasopharynx

Lateral
pterygoid,
inferior head

Parotid gland

Medial pterygoid,
deep and
superficial heads

Oropharynx

Masseter,
superficial head

Tongue

Inferior alveolar nerve
(CN V$_3$) in mandibular
canal

Mandible

Lingual septum

Hyoglossus

Submandibular
gland

Platysma

Geniohyoid
muscle

Digastric muscle,
anterior belly

Mylohyoid
muscle

**Fig. 9.42 Muscles of mastication, coronal section at the level of the sphenoid sinus**
Posterior view.

**201**

# Suprahyoid Muscles

The suprahyoid and infrahyoid muscles attach to the hyoid bone inferiorly and superiorly, respectively. The infrahyoid muscles depress the hyoid during phonation and swallowing. They are discussed with the suprahyoid muscles and larynx in the neck (see p. 255).

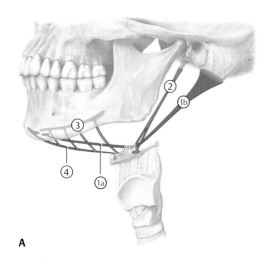

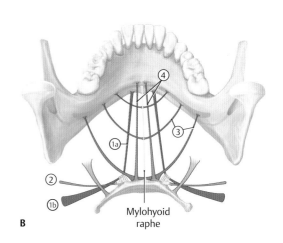

Mylohyoid
raphe

B

A

*Fig. 9.43* **Suprahyoid muscles: schematic**
**A** Left lateral view. **B** Superior view.

| Table 9.8 Suprahyoid muscles | | | | | |
|---|---|---|---|---|---|
| **Muscle** | | **Origin** | **Insertion** | **Innervation** | **Action** |
| **Suprahyoid muscles:** The suprahyoid muscles are also considered accessory muscles of mastication. | | | | | |
| Digastric | ① Anterior belly | Mandible (digastric fossa) | Hyoid bone (body) — Via an intermediate tendon with a fibrous loop | Mylohyoid n. (from CN V₃) | Elevates hyoid bone (during swallowing); assists in depressing mandible |
| | ① Posterior belly | Temporal bone (mastoid notch, medial to mastoid process) | | Facial n. (CN VII) | |
| ② Stylohyoid | | Temporal bone (styloid process) | Via a split tendon | | |
| ③ Mylohyoid | | Mandible (mylohyoid line) | Via median tendon of insertion (mylohyoid raphe) | Mylohyoid n. (from CN V₃) | Tightens and elevates oral floor; draws hyoid bone forward (during swallowing); assists in opening mandible and moving it side to side (mastication) |
| ④ Geniohyoid | | Mandible (inferior genial [mental] spine) | Body of hyoid bone | Ventral ramus of C1 | Draws hyoid bone forward (during swallowing); assists in opening mandible |

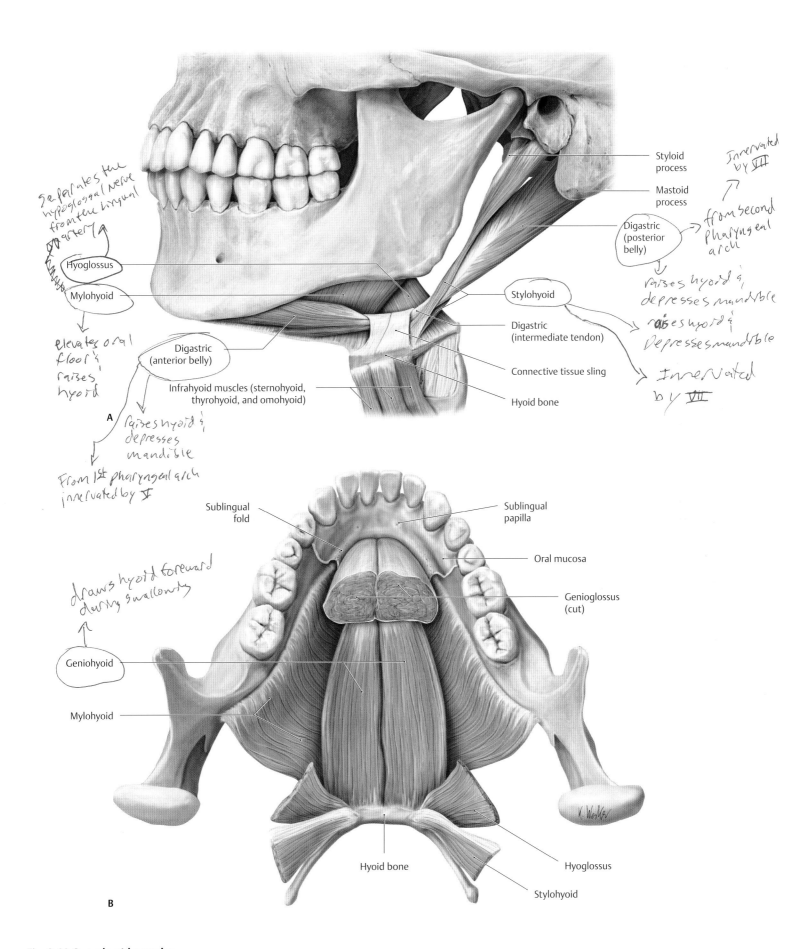

*Separates the hypoglossal nerve from the lingual artery*

Hyoglossus

Mylohyoid

*elevates oral floor & raises hyoid*

Digastric (anterior belly)

Infrahyoid muscles (sternohyoid, thyrohyoid, and omohyoid)

A

*raises hyoid & depresses mandible*

*From 1st pharyngeal arch innervated by V*

Styloid process

Mastoid process

Digastric (posterior belly)

Stylohyoid

Digastric (intermediate tendon)

Connective tissue sling

Hyoid bone

*Innervated by VII*

*from second pharyngeal arch*

*raises hyoid & depresses mandible*

*raises hyoid & depresses mandible*

*Innervated by VII*

Sublingual fold

Sublingual papilla

Oral mucosa

Genioglossus (cut)

*draws hyoid forward during swallowing*

Geniohyoid

Mylohyoid

Hyoid bone

Hyoglossus

Stylohyoid

B

***Fig. 9.44 Suprahyoid muscles***
**A** Left lateral view. **B** Superior view.

# Lingual Muscles

There are two sets of lingual muscles: extrinsic and intrinsic. The extrinsic muscles, which are attached to specific bony sites outside the tongue, move the tongue as a whole. The intrinsic muscles, which have no attachments to skeletal structures, alter the shape of the tongue. With the exception of the palatoglossus, the lingual muscles are supplied by the hypoglossal nerve (CN XII).

| Muscle | Origin | Insertion | Innervation | Action |
|---|---|---|---|---|
| **Table 9.9** Muscles of the tongue | | | | |
| **Extrinsic lingual muscles** | | | | |
| Genioglossus | Mandible (superior genial [mental] spine via an intermediate tendon); more posteriorly the two genioglossi are separated by the lingual septum | Inferior fibers: Hyoid body (anterosuperior surface) | Hypoglossal n. (CN XII) | Protrusion of the tongue |
| | | Intermediate fibers: Posterior tongue | | *Bilaterally:* Makes dorsum concave |
| | | Superior fibers: Ventral surface of tongue (mix with intrinsic muscles) | | *Unilaterally:* Deviation to opposite side |
| Hyoglossus | Hyoid bone (greater cornu and anterior body) | Lateral tongue, between styloglossus and inferior longitudinal muscle | | Depresses the tongue |
| Styloglossus | Styloid process of temporal bone (anterolateral aspect of apex) and stylomandibular ligament | Longitudinal part: Dorsolateral tongue (mix with inferior longitudinal muscle) | | Superior and posterior movement of the tongue |
| | | Oblique part: Mix with fibers of the hyoglossus | | |
| Palatoglossus | Palatine aponeurosis (oral surface) | Lateral tongue to dorsum and fibers of the transverse muscle | Vagus n. (CN X) via the pharyngeal plexus | Elevates the root of the tongue; closes the oropharyngeal isthmus by contracting the palatoglossal arch |
| **Intrinsic lingual muscles** | | | | |
| Superior longitudinal muscle | Thin layer of muscle inferior to the dorsal mucosa; fibers run anterolaterally from the epiglottis and median lingual septum | | Hypoglossal n. (CN XII) | Shortens tongue; makes dorsum concave (pulls apex and lateral margin upward) |
| Inferior longitudinal muscle | Thin layer of muscle superior to the genioglossus and hyoglossus; fibers run anteriorly from the root to the apex of the tongue | | | Shortens tongue; makes dorsum convex (pulls apex down) |
| Transverse muscle | Fibers run laterally from the lingual septum to the lateral tongue | | | Narrows tongue; elongates tongue |
| Vertical muscle | In the anterior tongue, fibers run inferiorly from the dorsum of the tongue to its ventral surface | | | Widens and flattens tongue |

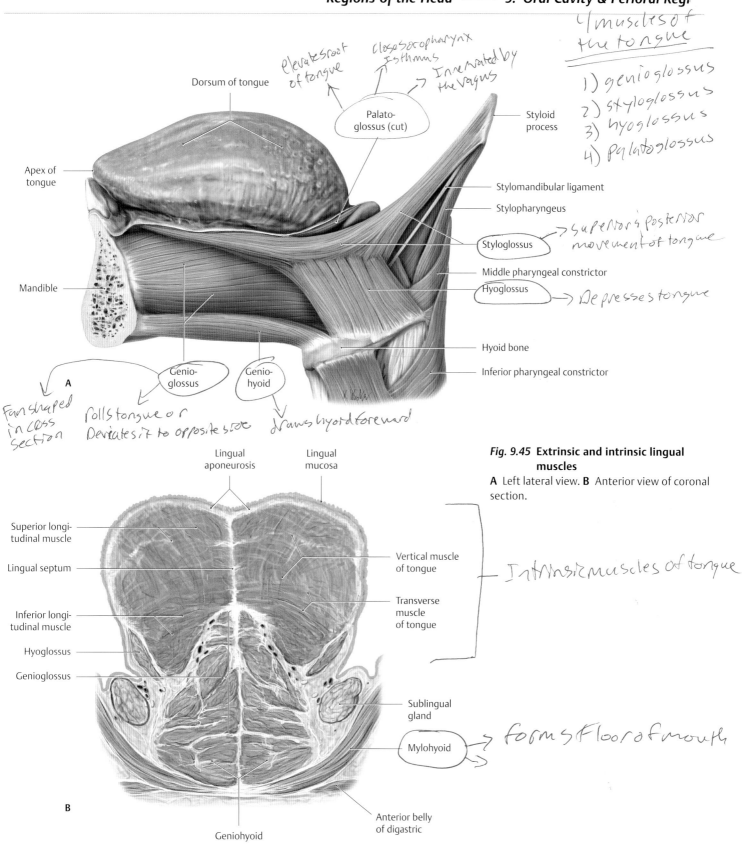

*Handwritten annotations:*

4 muscles of the tongue
1) genioglossus
2) styloglossus
3) hyoglossus
4) palatoglossus

elevates root of tongue

closes oropharynx isthmus → innervated by the vagus

Palato-glossus (cut)

Dorsum of tongue

Apex of tongue

Mandible

Styloid process

Stylomandibular ligament

Stylopharyngeus

Styloglossus → superior & posterior movement of tongue

Middle pharyngeal constrictor

Hyoglossus → Depresses tongue

Hyoid bone

Inferior pharyngeal constrictor

A — Fan shaped in cross section

Genio-glossus — rolls tongue or Deviates it to opposite side

Genio-hyoid — draws hyoid forward

Lingual aponeurosis

Lingual mucosa

Superior longi-tudinal muscle

Lingual septum

Inferior longi-tudinal muscle

Hyoglossus

Genioglossus

Vertical muscle of tongue

Transverse muscle of tongue

Intrinsic muscles of tongue

Sublingual gland

Mylohyoid → forms floor of mouth

B

Geniohyoid

Anterior belly of digastric

**Fig. 9.45 Extrinsic and intrinsic lingual muscles**
**A** Left lateral view. **B** Anterior view of coronal section.

**Fig. 9.46 Unilateral hypoglossal nerve palsy**
Active protrusion of the tongue with an intact hypoglossal nerve (**A**) and with a unilateral hypoglossal nerve lesion (**B**).
When the hypoglossal nerve is damaged on one side, the genioglossus muscle is paralyzed on the affected side. As a result, the healthy (inner-vated) genioglossus on the opposite side dominates the tongue across the midline toward the affected side. When the tongue is protruded, therefore, it deviates *toward* the paralyzed side.

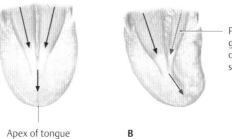

Paralyzed genioglossus on affected side

**A** Apex of tongue   **B**

# Lingual Mucosa

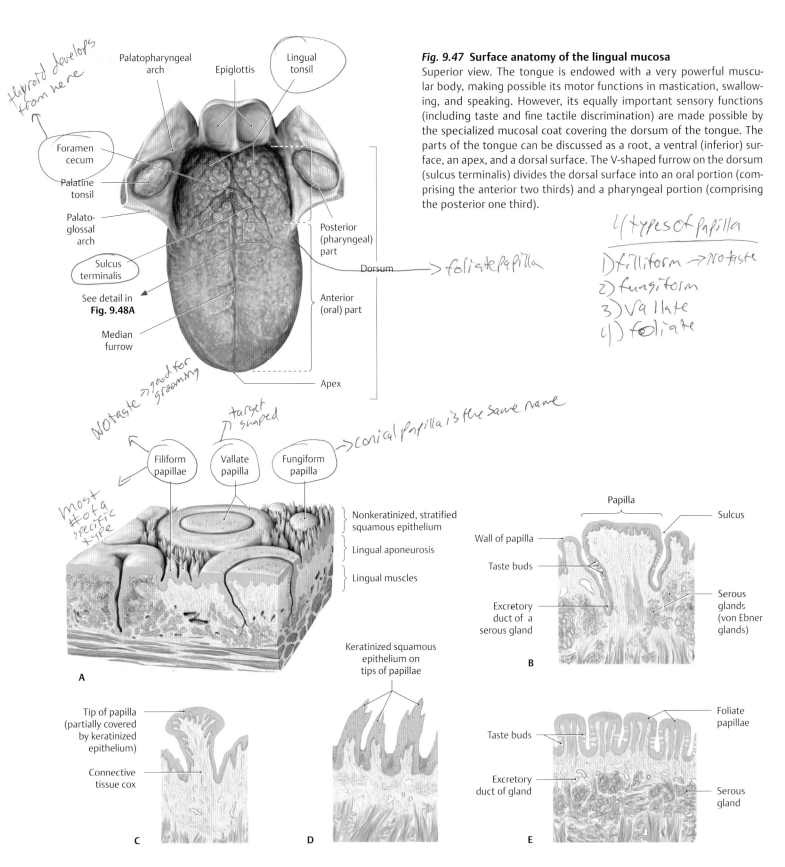

*Handwritten annotations:*
- Hyoid develops from here
- 4 types of papilla
  1) filiform → no taste
  2) fungiform
  3) vallate
  4) foliate
- → foliate papilla
- No taste → good for grooming
- target shaped
- conical papilla is the same name
- most # of a specific type

**Fig. 9.47 Surface anatomy of the lingual mucosa**
Superior view. The tongue is endowed with a very powerful muscular body, making possible its motor functions in mastication, swallowing, and speaking. However, its equally important sensory functions (including taste and fine tactile discrimination) are made possible by the specialized mucosal coat covering the dorsum of the tongue. The parts of the tongue can be discussed as a root, a ventral (inferior) surface, an apex, and a dorsal surface. The V-shaped furrow on the dorsum (sulcus terminalis) divides the dorsal surface into an oral portion (comprising the anterior two thirds) and a pharyngeal portion (comprising the posterior one third).

Labels in figure (top): Palatopharyngeal arch, Epiglottis, Lingual tonsil, Foramen cecum, Palatine tonsil, Palatoglossal arch, Sulcus terminalis, See detail in Fig. 9.48A, Median furrow, Posterior (pharyngeal) part, Dorsum, Anterior (oral) part, Apex

Labels in figure (bottom): Filiform papillae, Vallate papilla, Fungiform papilla, Nonkeratinized, stratified squamous epithelium, Lingual aponeurosis, Lingual muscles, Tip of papilla (partially covered by keratinized epithelium), Connective tissue cox, A, Keratinized squamous epithelium on tips of papillae, C, D, Papilla, Wall of papilla, Taste buds, Excretory duct of a serous gland, Sulcus, Serous glands (von Ebner glands), B, Taste buds, Excretory duct of gland, Foliate papillae, Serous gland, E

**Fig. 9.48 Papillae of the tongue**
The mucosa of the anterior dorsum is composed of numerous papillae (**A**), and the connective tissue between the mucosal surface and musculature contains many small salivary glands. The papillae are divided into four morphologically distinct types (see **Table 9.10**):

- Circumvallate (**B**): Encircled and containing taste buds.
- Fungiform (**C**): Mushroom-shaped and containing mechanical and thermal receptors and taste buds.
- Filiform (**D**): Thread-shaped and sensitive to tactile stimuli (the only lingual papillae without taste buds).
- Foliate (**E**): Containing taste buds.

| Table 9.10 Regions and structures of the tongue | |
|---|---|
| **Region** | **Structures** |
| **Anterior (oral, presulcal) portion of the tongue** | |
| The anterior ⅔ of the tongue contains the apex and the majority of the dorsum. It is tethered to the oral floor by the lingual frenulum.<br>• **Mucosa:**<br>  ◦ Dorsal lingual mucosa: This portion (with no underlying submucosa) contains numerous papillae.<br>  ◦ Ventral mucosa: Covered with the same smooth (nonkeratinized, stratified squamous epithelial) mucosa that lines the oral floor and gums.<br>• **Innervation:** The anterior portion is derived from the first (mandibular) arch and is therefore innervated by the lingual nerve, a branch of the mandibular nerve (CN V$_3$). | **Median furrow (midline septum):** The furrow running anteriorly down the midline of the tongue; this corresponds to the position of the lingual septum. *Note:* Muscle fibers do not cross the lingual septum.<br><br>**Papillae (Fig. 9.48A):** The dorsal mucosa, which has no submucosa, is covered with nipplelike projections (papillae) that increase the surface area of the tongue. There are four types, all of which occur in the presulcal but not postsulcal portion of the tongue.<br>• Circumvallate (**Fig. 9.48B**): Encircled by a wall and containing abundant taste buds.<br>• Fungiform (**Fig. 9.48C**): Mushroom-shaped papillae located on the lateral margin of the posterior oral portion near the palatoglossal arches. These have mechanical receptors, thermal receptors, and taste buds.<br>• Filiform (**Fig. 9.48D**): Thread-shaped papillae that are sensitive to tactile stimuli. These are the only papillae that do not contain taste buds.<br>• Foliate (**Fig. 9.48E**): Located near the sulcus terminalis, these contain numerous taste buds. |
| **Sulcus terminalis** | |
| The sulcus terminalis is the V-shaped furrow that divides the tongue functionally and anatomically into an anterior and a posterior portion. | **Foramen cecum:** The embryonic remnant of the passage of the thyroid gland that migrates from the dorsum of the tongue during development. The foramen cecum is located at the convergence of the sulci terminalis. |
| **Posterior (pharyngeal, postsulcal) portion of the tongue** | |
| The base of the tongue is located posterior to the palatoglossal arches and sulcus terminalis.<br>• **Mucosa:** The same mucosa that lines the palatine tonsils, pharyngeal walls, and epiglottis. The pharyngeal portion of the tongue does not contain papillae.<br>• **Innervation:** The posterior portion is innervated by the glossopharyngeal nerve (CN IX). | **Lingual tonsils:** The submucosa of the posterior portion contains embedded lymph nodes known as the lingual tonsils, which create the uneven surface of the posterior portion.<br><br>**Oropharynx:** The region posterior to the palatoglossal arch. The oropharynx, which contains the palatine tonsils, communicates with the oral cavity via the oropharyngeal isthmus (defined by the palatoglossal arches). |
| **Glossoepiglottic folds and epiglottic valleculae:** The (nonkeratinized, stratified squamous) mucosal covering of the posterior tongue and pharyngeal walls is reflected onto the anterior aspect of the epiglottis, forming one median and two lateral glossoepiglottic folds. The median glossoepiglottic fold is flanked by two depressions, the epiglottic valleculae. | |

**207**

# Pharynx & Tonsils

***Fig. 9.49 Waldeyer's ring***
Posterior view of the opened pharynx. Waldeyer's ring is composed of immunocompetent lymphatic tissue (tonsils and lymph follicles). The tonsils are "immunological sentinels" surrounding the passageways from the mouth and nasal cavity to the pharynx. The lymph follicles are distributed over all of the epithelium, showing marked regional variations. Waldeyer's ring consists of the following structures:

- Unpaired pharyngeal tonsil on the roof of the pharynx
- Paired palatine tonsils in the oropharynx
- Lingual tonsil, the lymph nodes embedded in the postsulcal portion of the tongue
- Paired tubal tonsils (tonsillae tubariae), which may be thought of as lateral extensions of the pharyngeal tonsil
- Paired lateral bands in the salpingopharyngeal fold

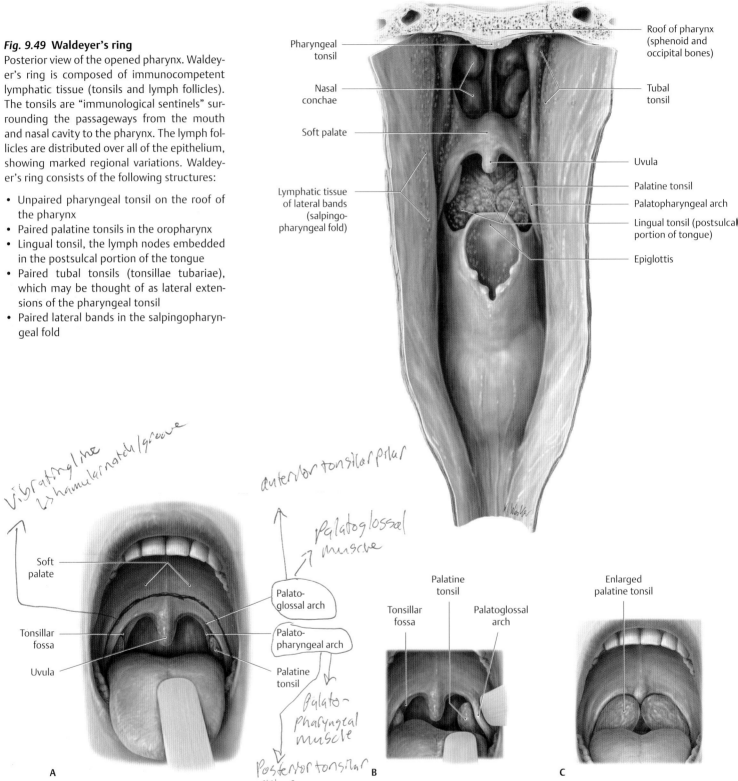

Pharyngeal tonsil

Nasal conchae

Soft palate

Lymphatic tissue of lateral bands (salpingo-pharyngeal fold)

Roof of pharynx (sphenoid and occipital bones)

Tubal tonsil

Uvula

Palatine tonsil

Palatopharyngeal arch

Lingual tonsil (postsulcal portion of tongue)

Epiglottis

*[Handwritten annotations: Vibrating line — is hamular notch/groove; anterior tonsilar pilar; palatoglossal muscle; palato-pharyngeal muscle; Posterior tonsilar pilar]*

Soft palate

Tonsillar fossa

Uvula

Palato-glossal arch

Palato-pharyngeal arch

Palatine tonsil

**A**

Palatine tonsil

Tonsillar fossa

Palatoglossal arch

**B**

Enlarged palatine tonsil

**C**

***Fig. 9.50 Palatine tonsils: location and abnormal enlargement***
Anterior view of the oral cavity. The palatine tonsils occupy a shallow recess on each side, the tonsillar fossa, which is located between the anterior and posterior pillars (palatoglossal arch and palatopharyngeal arch). The palatine tonsil is examined clinically by placing a tongue depressor on the anterior pillar and displacing the tonsil from its fossa while a second instrument depresses the tongue (**B**). Severe enlargement of the palatine tonsil (due to viral or bacterial infection, as in tonsillitis) may significantly narrow the outlet of the oral cavity, causing difficulty in swallowing (dysphagia, **C**).

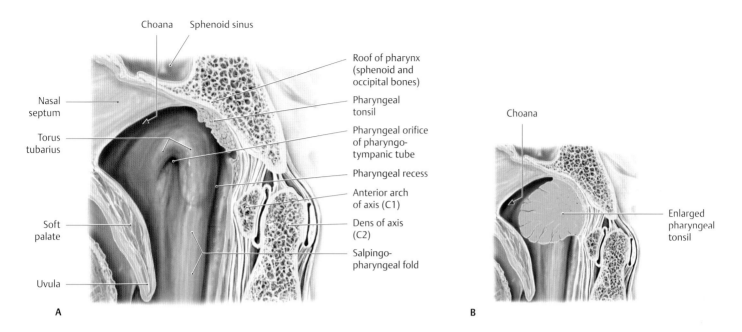

**A**  **B**

**Fig. 9.51 Pharyngeal tonsil: location and abnormal enlargement**
Sagittal section through the roof of the pharynx. Located on the roof
of the pharynx, the unpaired pharyngeal tonsil can be examined by
means of posterior rhinoscopy. It is particularly well developed in
(small) children and begins to regress at 6 or 7 years of age. An enlarged pharyngeal tonsil is very common in preschool-aged children
(**B**). (Chronic recurrent nasopharyngeal infections at this age often

evoke a heightened immune response in the lymphatic tissue, causing "adenoids" or "polyps.") The enlarged pharyngeal tonsil blocks the
choanae, obstructing the nasal airway and forcing the child to breathe
through the mouth. Because the mouth is then constantly open during
respiration at rest, an experienced examiner can quickly diagnose the
adenoidal condition by visual inspection.

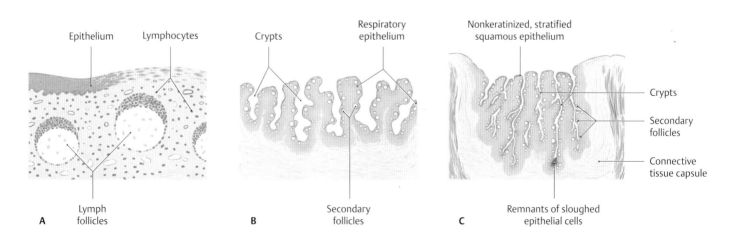

**A**  **B**  **C**

**Fig. 9.52 Histology of the lymphatic tissue of the oral cavity and
pharynx**
Because of the close anatomical relationship between the epithelium
and lymphatic tissue, the lymphatic tissue of Waldeyer's ring is also
designated lymphoepithelial tissue.

**A Lymphoepithelial tissue.** Lymphatic tissue, both organized and
diffusely distributed, is found in the lamina propria of all mucous
membranes and is known as mucosa-associated lymphatic tissue
(MALT). The epithelium acquires a looser texture, with abundant
lymphocytes and macrophages. Besides the well-defined tonsils,
smaller collections of lymph follicles may be found in the lateral

bands (salpingopharyngeal folds). They extend almost vertically
from the lateral wall to the posterior wall of the oropharynx and
nasopharynx.

**B Pharyngeal tonsil.** The mucosal surface of the pharyngeal tonsil is
raised into ridges that greatly increase its surface area. The ridges
and intervening crypts are lined by ciliated respiratory epithelium.

**C Palatine tonsil.** The surface area of the palatine tonsil is increased
by deep depressions in the mucosal surface (creating an active surface area as large as 300 cm²). The mucosa is covered by nonkeratinized, stratified squamous epithelium.

**209**

# Pharynx: Divisions & Contents

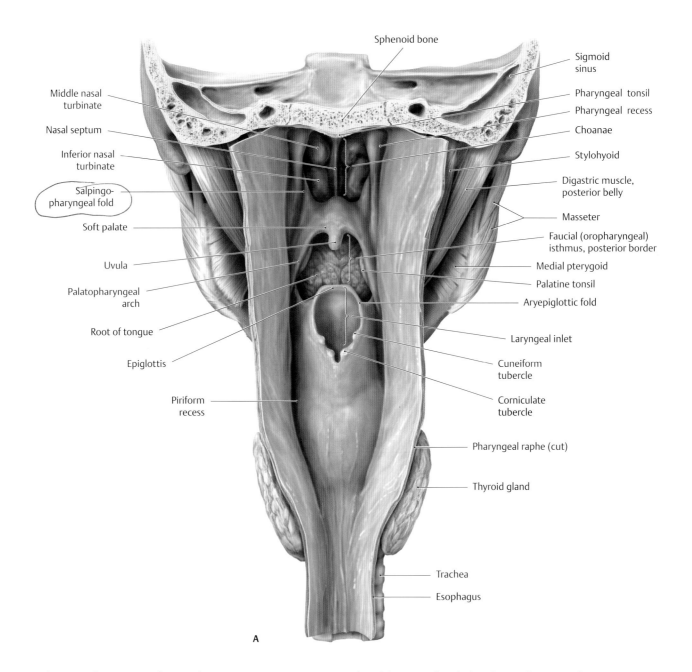

Sphenoid bone

Sigmoid sinus

Middle nasal turbinate

Pharyngeal tonsil

Pharyngeal recess

Nasal septum

Choanae

Inferior nasal turbinate

Stylohyoid

Salpingo-pharyngeal fold

Digastric muscle, posterior belly

Soft palate

Masseter

Faucial (oropharyngeal) isthmus, posterior border

Uvula

Medial pterygoid

Palatine tonsil

Palatopharyngeal arch

Aryepiglottic fold

Root of tongue

Laryngeal inlet

Epiglottis

Cuneiform tubercle

Piriform recess

Corniculate tubercle

Pharyngeal raphe (cut)

Thyroid gland

Trachea

Esophagus

A

**Fig. 9.53 Pharyngeal mucosa and musculature**
Posterior view. **A** Mucosal lining. **B** Internal musculature. The muscular posterior wall of the pharynx has been divided along the midline (pharyngeal raphe) and spread open to demonstrate its mucosal anatomy.

**Table 9.11 Levels of the pharynx**

The anterior portion of the muscular pharyngeal tube communicates with three cavities (nasal, oral, and laryngeal). The three anterior openings divide the pharynx into three parts with corresponding vertebral levels.

| Region | Level | Description | Communications | |
|---|---|---|---|---|
| Nasopharynx (Epipharynx) | C1 | Upper portion, lying between the roof (formed by sphenoid and occipital bones) and the soft palate | Nasal cavity | Via choanae |
| | | | Tympanic cavity | Via pharyngotympanic tube |
| Oropharynx (Mesopharynx) | C2–C3 | Middle portion, lying between the uvula and the epiglottis | Oral cavity | Via oropharyngeal isthmus (formed by the palatoglossal arch) |
| Laryngopharynx (Hypopharynx) | C4–C6 | Lower portion, lying between the epiglottis and the inferior border of the cricoid cartilage | Larynx | Via laryngeal inlet |
| | | | Esophagus | Via cricopharyngeus (pharyngeal sphincter) |

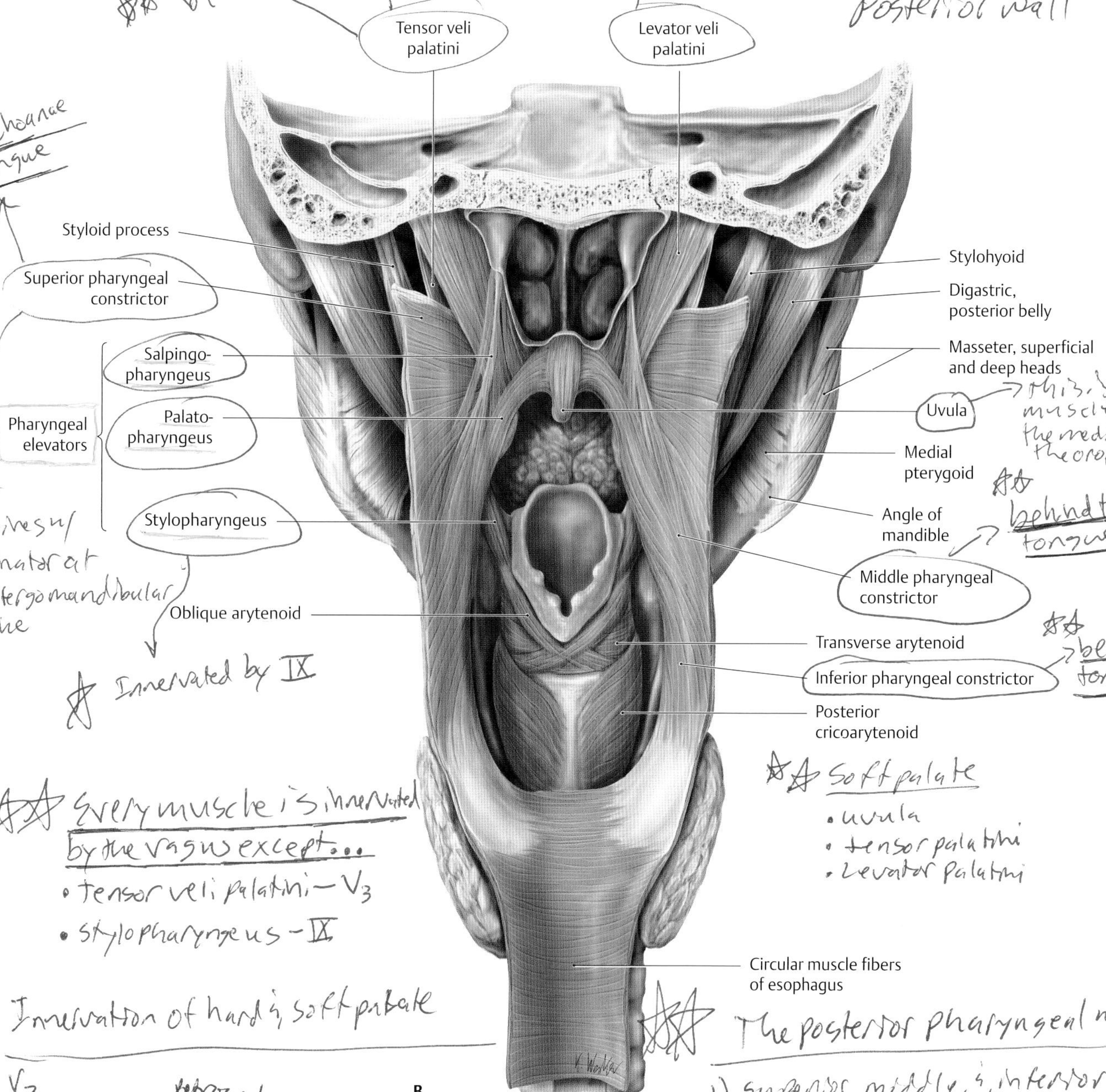

*Flattens soft palate &
separates naso from oral
pharynx*

*Pulls soft palate up
" "*

*⋆ ⋆⋆ muscles of the
posterior wall*

*⋆⋆ Innervated
by V₃*

Tensor veli
palatini

Levator veli
palatini

*⋆
from choana
to tongue*

Styloid process

Superior pharyngeal
constrictor

Stylohyoid

Digastric,
posterior belly

Masseter, superficial
and deep heads

*⋆ this sits own
muscle & takes up
the median portion of
the oropharynx*

Salpingo-
pharyngeus

Palato-
pharyngeus

Pharyngeal
elevators

Uvula

Medial
pterygoid

Angle of
mandible

*⋆⋆ behind the
tongue*

*combines w/
buccinator at
the pterygomandibular
Raphe*

Stylopharyngeus

Middle pharyngeal
constrictor

Oblique arytenoid

*⋆ Innervated by IX*

Transverse arytenoid

Inferior pharyngeal constrictor

*⋆⋆ below the
tongue*

Posterior
cricoarytenoid

*⋆⋆ Soft palate
• uvula
• tensor palatini
• levator palatini*

*⋆⋆⋆ Every muscle is innervated
by the vagus except...
• tensor veli palatini — V₃
• stylopharyngeus — IX*

*⋆ Innervation of hard & soft palate*

*• V₃
• VII - greater petrosal ~~lesser petrosal components~~
• pharyngeal plexus - XI, X*

Circular muscle fibers
of esophagus

B

*⋆⋆ The posterior pharyngeal wall
1) superior, middle, & inferior pharyngeal
constrictors
2) pharyngeal elevators
• salpingopharyngeus
• palatopharyngeus
• stylopharyngeus
If it has the
word
"pharyngeus"
it has an
elevator*

V. Wedlar

### Fig. 9.54 Posterior rhinoscopy

The nasopharynx can be visually inspected by posterior rhinoscopy.

**A** Technique of holding the tongue blade and mirror. The angulation
of the mirror is continually adjusted to permit complete inspection
of the nasopharynx.

**B** Composite posterior rhinoscopic image acquired at various mirror
angles. The pharyngotympanic (auditory) tube orifice and pharyngeal tonsil can be identified.

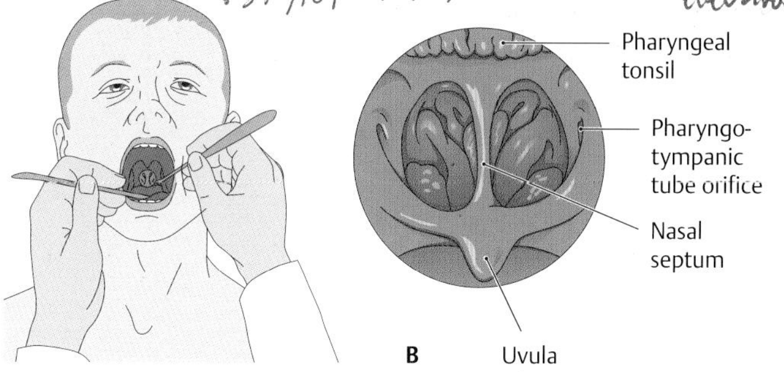

Pharyngeal
tonsil

Pharyngo-
tympanic
tube orifice

Nasal
septum

A

B Uvula

**211**

# Muscles of the Soft Palate & Pharynx

The soft palate is the aponeurotic and muscular region hanging from the hard palate at the posterior portion of the oral cavity. It separates the nasopharynx from the oropharynx. During swallowing, it can be tensed to further restrict the communication between the cavities. The palato-glossus restricts the communication between the oral cavity and phar-

ynx. The pharyngeal muscles elevate and constrict the pharynx (see **Table 9.12**, **Table 9.13**, and **Fig. 9.56**). Though several muscles originate on the pharyngotympanic (auditory) tube, only the tensor veli palatini plays a significant role in its opening.

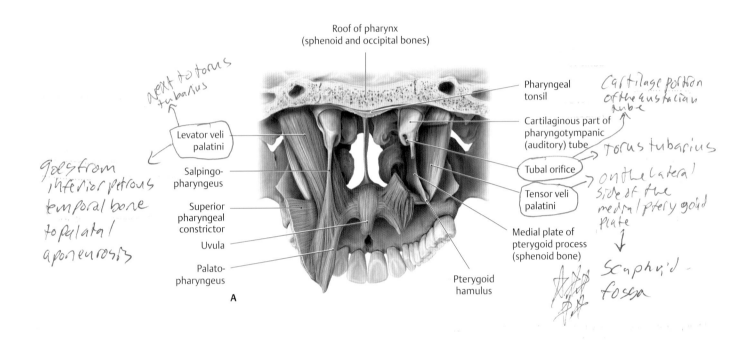

*Handwritten annotations (left):*
next to torus tubarius

goes from inferior petrous temporal bone to palatal aponeurosis

*Handwritten annotations (right):*
Cartilage portion of the eustacian tube

torus tubarius

on the lateral side of the medial pterygoid plate

Scaphoid fossa

*Labels (A):*
Roof of pharynx (sphenoid and occipital bones)
Pharyngeal tonsil
Cartilaginous part of pharyngotympanic (auditory) tube
Levator veli palatini
Tubal orifice
Salpingo-pharyngeus
Tensor veli palatini
Superior pharyngeal constrictor
Medial plate of pterygoid process (sphenoid bone)
Uvula
Palato-pharyngeus
Pterygoid hamulus

**A**

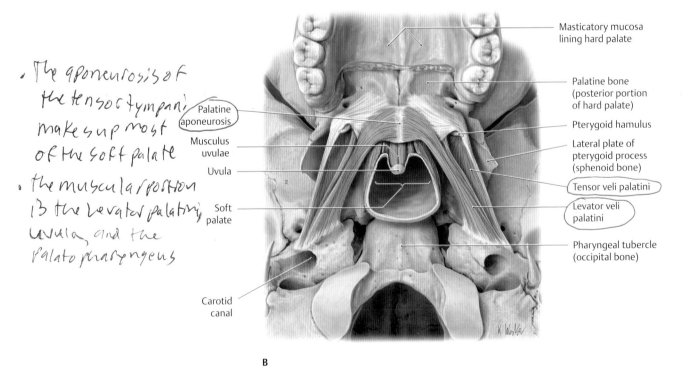

*Handwritten annotations (left):*
. The aponeurosis of the tensor tympani makes up most of the soft palate

. the muscular portion is the Levator palatini, uvula, and the Palatopharyngeus

*Labels (B):*
Masticatory mucosa lining hard palate
Palatine aponeurosis
Palatine bone (posterior portion of hard palate)
Musculus uvulae
Pterygoid hamulus
Uvula
Lateral plate of pterygoid process (sphenoid bone)
Soft palate
Tensor veli palatini
Levator veli palatini
Carotid canal
Pharyngeal tubercle (occipital bone)

**B**

***Fig. 9.55*** **Muscles of the soft palate and pharyngotympanic tube**
**A** Posterior view. **B** Inferior view.

**Table 9.12** **Muscles of the soft palate and pharyngeal elevators**

| Muscle | Origin | Insertion | Innervation | Action |
|---|---|---|---|---|
| Tensor veli palatini | Sphenoid bone (scaphoid fossa of pterygoid process and medial aspect of the spine); it is connected to the anterolateral membranous wall of the pharyngotympanic (auditory) tube | Palatine aponeurosis and palatine bone (horizontal plate) via a tendon that is redirected medially by the pterygoid hamulus | N. to medial pterygoid (CN $V_3$) | *Bilaterally:* Tenses anterior portion of the soft palate and flattens its arch, separating the nasopharynx from the oropharynx. Opens pharyngotympanic (auditory) tube. *Unilaterally:* Deviates soft palate laterally. |
| Levator veli palatini | Vaginal process and petrous part of temporal bone (via a tendon, anterior to the carotid canal); it is connected to the inferior portion of the cartilaginous pharyngotympanic tube | Palatine aponeurosis (the two levators combine to form a muscular sling) | Vagus n. (CN X) via pharyngeal plexus | *Bilaterally:* Pulls the posterior portion of the soft palate superoposteriorly, separating the nasopharynx from the oropharynx. |
| Musculus uvulae | Palatine bone (posterior nasal spine) and palatine aponeurosis (superior surface) | Mucosa of the uvula | | Pulls the uvula posterosuperiorly, separating the nasopharynx from the oropharynx. |
| Palatoglossus (palatoglossal arch) | Palatine aponeurosis (oral surface) | Lateral tongue to dorsum or intrinsic transverse muscle | | Pulls the root of the tongue superiorly and approximates the palatoglossal arch, separating the oral cavity from the oropharynx. |
| Palatopharyngeus (palatopharyngeal arch) | Palatine aponeurosis (superior surface) and posterior border of palatine bone | Thyroid cartilage (posterior border) or lateral pharynx | | *Bilaterally:* Elevates the pharynx anteromedially. |
| Salpingopharyngeus | Cartilaginous pharyngotympanic tube (inferior surface) | Along salpingopharyngeal fold to palatopharyngeus | | *Bilaterally:* Elevates the pharynx; may also open the pharyngotympanic tube. |
| Stylopharyngeus | Styloid process (medial surface of base) | Lateral pharynx, mixing with pharyngeal constrictors, palatopharyngeus, and thyroid cartilage (posterior border) | Glossopharyngeal n. (CN IX) | *Bilaterally:* Elevates the pharynx and larynx. |

**Table 9.13** **Pharyngeal constrictors**

| Muscle | | Origin | Insertion | Innervation | Action |
|---|---|---|---|---|---|
| Superior pharyngeal constrictor | Pterygopharyngeus | Pterygoid hamulus (occasionally to the medial pterygoid plate) | Occipital bone (pharyngeal tubercle of basilar part, via median pharyngeal raphe) | Vagus n. (CN X) via pharyngeal plexus | Constricts the upper pharynx |
| | Buccopharyngeus | Pterygomandibular raphe | | | |
| | Mylopharyngeus | Mylohyoid line of mandible | | | |
| | Glossopharyngeus | Lateral tongue | | | |
| Middle pharyngeal constrictor | Chondropharyngeus | Hyoid (lesser cornu) and stylohyoid ligament | | | Constricts the middle pharynx |
| | Ceratopharyngeus | Hyoid (greater cornu) | | | |
| Inferior pharyngeal constrictor | Thyropharyngeus | Thyroid lamina and hyoid bone (inferior cornu) | | | Constricts the lower pharynx |
| | Cricopharyngeus | Cricoid cartilage (lateral margin) | | Recurrent laryngeal n. (CN X) and/or external laryngeal n. | Sphincter at intersection of laryngopharynx and esophagus |

# Muscles of the Pharynx

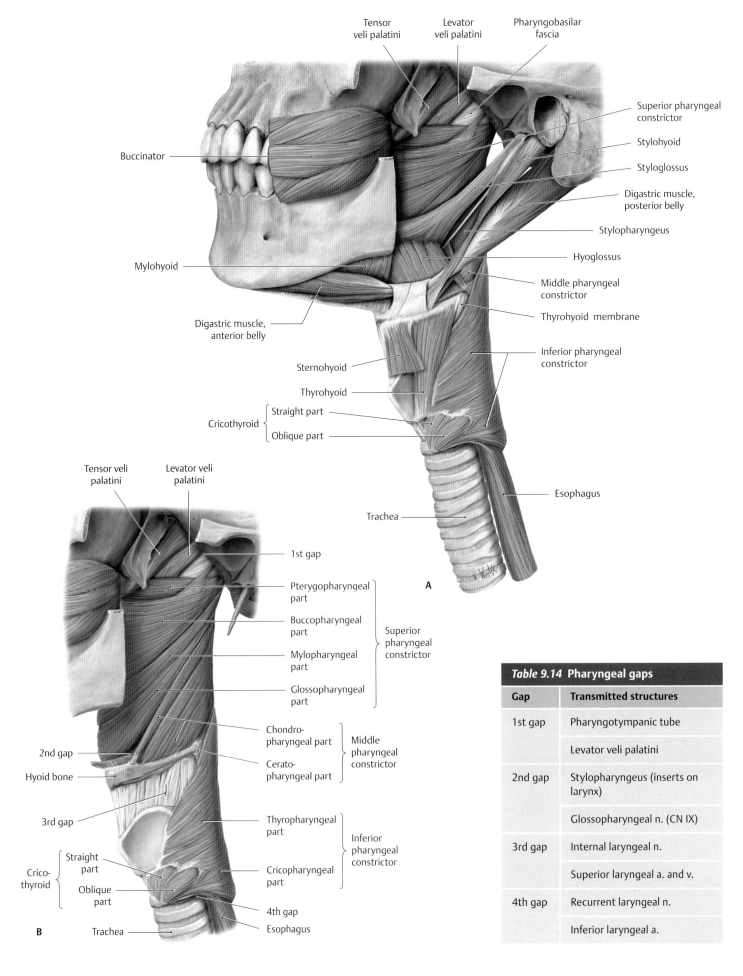

| Table 9.14 Pharyngeal gaps | |
|---|---|
| **Gap** | **Transmitted structures** |
| 1st gap | Pharyngotympanic tube |
| | Levator veli palatini |
| 2nd gap | Stylopharyngeus (inserts on larynx) |
| | Glossopharyngeal n. (CN IX) |
| 3rd gap | Internal laryngeal n. |
| | Superior laryngeal a. and v. |
| 4th gap | Recurrent laryngeal n. |
| | Inferior laryngeal a. |

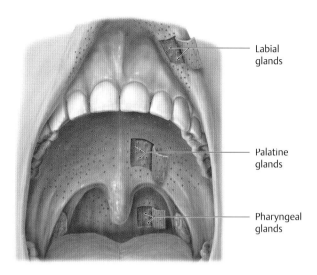

**Fig. 9.63 Minor salivary glands**
In addition to the three major paired glands, 700 to 1000 minor glands secrete saliva into the oral cavity. They produce only 5 to 8 percent of the total output, but this amount suffices to keep the mouth moist when the major salivary glands are not functioning.

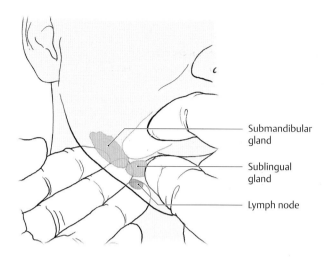

**Fig. 9.64 Bimanual examination of the salivary glands**
The two salivary glands of the mandible, the submandibular gland and sublingual gland, and the adjacent lymph nodes are grouped around the mobile oral floor and therefore must be palpated against resistance. This is done with bimanual examination.

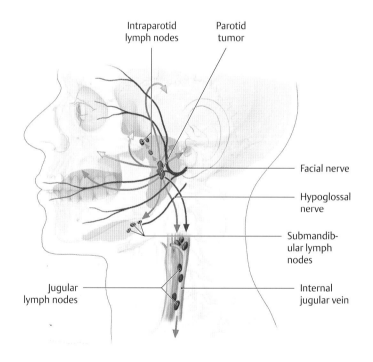

**Fig. 9.65 Spread of malignant parotid tumors**
Malignant tumors of the parotid gland may invade surrounding structures directly (white arrowheads) or indirectly via regional lymph nodes (red arrowheads). They may also spread systematically (metastasize) through the vascular system.

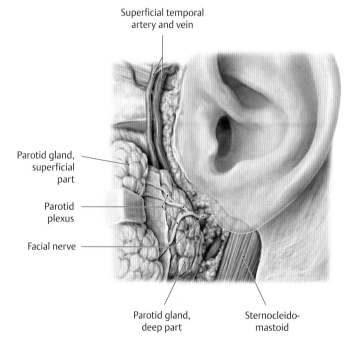

**Fig. 9.66 Intraglandular course of the facial nerve in the parotid gland**
The facial nerve divides into branches within the parotid gland and is vulnerable during the surgical removal of parotid tumors. To preserve the facial nerve during parotidectomy, it is first necessary to locate and identify the facial nerve trunk. The best landmark for locating the nerve trunk is the tip of the cartilaginous auditory canal.

**219**

# Neurovasculature of the Tongue

*☆ The Hypoglossal nerve runs on top of the hyoglossus*

*From anterior to posterior*
*1) Lingual Nerve → lingual starts superior & lateral*
*2) submandibular duct & ends inferior & medial to whastons ☆☆☆*
*3) hypoglossal - Lagest one → duct*
*4) glossopharyngeal - enters on the back of the tongue*

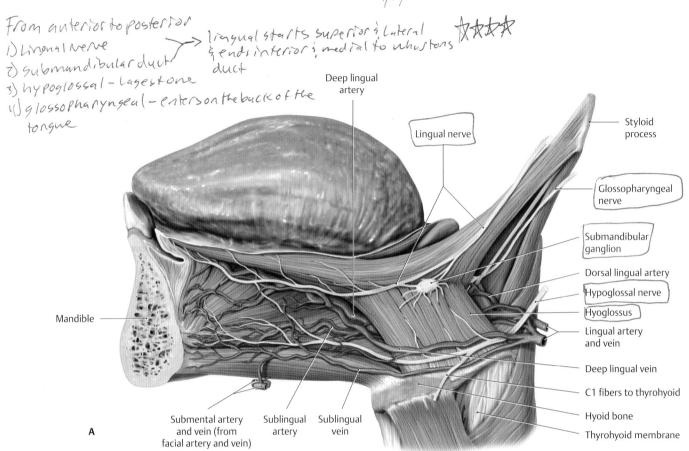

*Board question*
*↑ ☆☆☆*

## Fig. 9.67 Nerves and vessels of the tongue

**A** Left lateral view. **B** View of the inferior surface of the tongue.

The tongue is supplied by the *lingual artery* (from the maxillary artery), which divides into its terminal branches, the deep lingual artery and the sublingual artery. The lingual vein usually runs parallel to the artery but on the medial surface of the hyoglossus muscle and drains into the *internal jugular vein*. The anterior two thirds of the lingual mucosa receives its *somatosensory* innervation (sensitivity to thermal and tactile stimuli) from the *lingual nerve,* which is a branch of the trigeminal nerve's mandibular division (CN V₃). The lingual nerve transmits fibers from the chorda tympani of the facial nerve (CN VII), among them the afferent taste fibers for the anterior two thirds of the tongue. The chorda tympani also contains presynaptic, parasympathetic visceromotor axons that synapse in the submandibular ganglion, whose neurons in turn innervate the submandibular and sublingual glands. The palatoglossus receives its *somatomotor* innervation from the vagus nerve (CN X) via the pharyngeal plexus, the other lingual muscles from the hypoglossal nerve (CN XII).

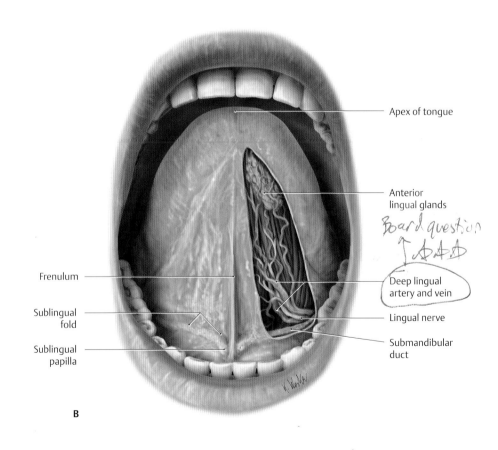

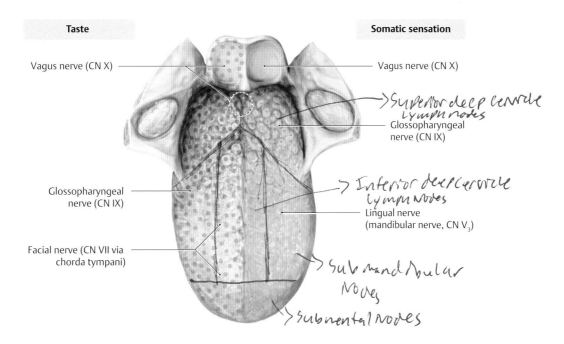

| Taste | Somatic sensation |

Vagus nerve (CN X)

Vagus nerve (CN X)

*Superior deep cervicle lymph nodes*

Glossopharyngeal nerve (CN IX)

*Inferior deep cervicle lymph Nodes*

Glossopharyngeal nerve (CN IX)

Lingual nerve (mandibular nerve, CN V₃)

Facial nerve (CN VII via chorda tympani)

*Submandibular Nodes*

*Submental Nodes*

**Fig. 9.68 Innervation of the tongue**
Anterior view. Left side: Somatosensory innervation. Right side: Taste innervation.
The posterior one third of the tongue (postsulcal part) primarily receives somatosensory and taste innervation from the glossopharyngeal nerve (CN IX), with additional taste sensation conveyed by the vagus nerve (CN X). The anterior two thirds of the tongue (presulcal part) receives its somatosensory innervation (e.g., touch, pain, and temperature) from the lingual nerve (branch of CN V₃) and its taste sensation from the chorda tympani branch of the facial nerve (CN VII). Disturbances of sensation in the presulcal tongue can therefore be used to determine facial or trigeminal nerve lesions.

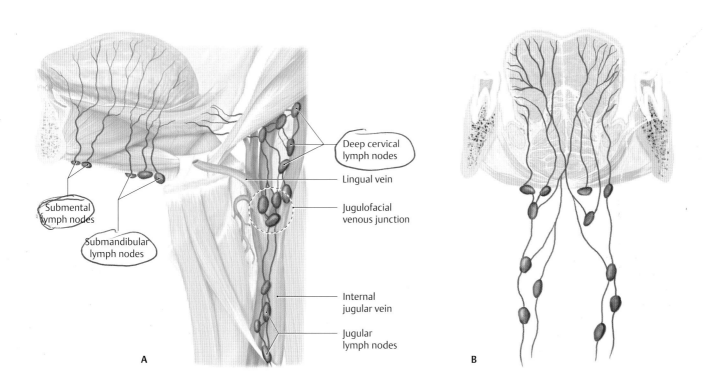

Deep cervical lymph nodes

Lingual vein

Submental lymph nodes

Jugulofacial venous junction

Submandibular lymph nodes

Internal jugular vein

Jugular lymph nodes

A

B

**Fig. 9.69 Lymphatic drainage of the tongue and oral floor**
**A** Left lateral view. **B** Anterior view.
The lymphatic drainage of the tongue and oral floor is mediated by submental and submandibular groups of lymph nodes that ultimately drain into the lymph nodes along the internal jugular vein (**A**, jugular lymph nodes). Because the lymph nodes receive drainage from both the ipsilateral and contralateral sides (**B**), tumor cells may become widely disseminated in this region (e.g., metastatic squamous cell carcinoma, especially on the lateral border of the tongue, frequently metastasizes to the opposite side).

**221**

# Gustatory System

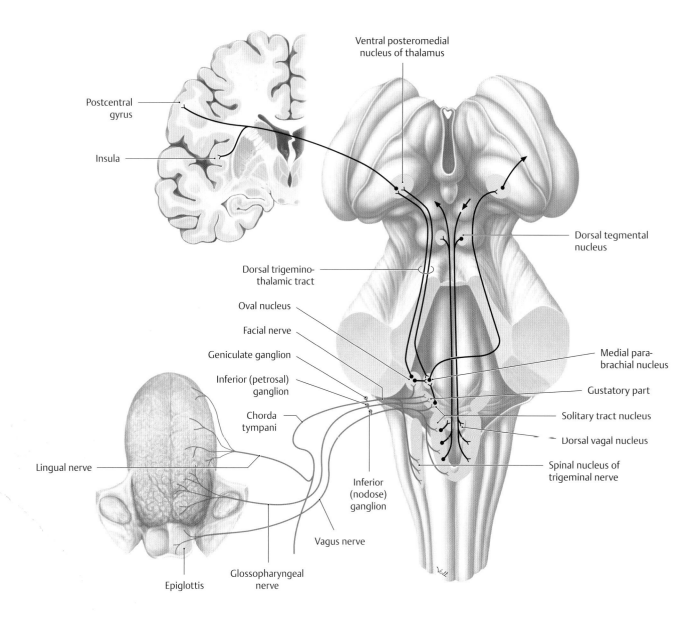

**Fig. 9.70 Gustatory pathway**

The receptors for the sense of taste are the taste buds of the tongue (see **Fig. 9.71**). Unlike other receptor cells, the receptor cells of the taste buds are specialized epithelial cells (secondary sensory cells, as they do not have an axon). When these epithelial cells are chemically stimulated, the base of the cells releases glutamate, which stimulates the peripheral processes of afferent cranial nerves. These different cranial nerves serve different areas of the tongue. It is rare, therefore, for a complete loss of taste (ageusia) to occur.

- The *anterior two thirds* of the tongue is supplied by the facial nerve (CN VII), the afferent fibers first passing in the lingual nerve (branch of the trigeminal nerve) and then in the chorda tympani to the geniculate ganglion of the facial nerve.
- The *posterior third of the tongue* and the *vallate papillae* are supplied by the glossopharyngeal nerve (CN IX). A small area on the posterior third of the tongue is also supplied by the vagus nerve (CN X).
- The *epiglottis* and *valleculae* are supplied by the vagus nerve (CN X).

Peripheral processes from pseudounipolar ganglion cells (which correspond to pseudounipolar spinal ganglion cells) terminate on the taste buds. The central portions of these processes convey taste information to the gustatory part of the nucleus of the solitary tract. Thus, they function as the first afferent neuron of the gustatory pathway. Their

perikarya are located in the geniculate ganglion for the facial nerve, in the inferior (petrosal) ganglion for the glossopharyngeal nerve, and in the inferior (nodose) ganglion for the vagus nerve. After synapsing in the gustatory part of the nucleus of the solitary tract, the axons from the second neuron are believed to terminate in the medial parabrachial nucleus, where they are relayed to the third neuron. Most of the axons from the third neuron cross to the opposite side and pass in the dorsal trigeminothalamic tract to the contralateral ventral posteromedial nucleus of the thalamus. Some of the axons travel uncrossed in the same structures. The fourth neurons of the gustatory pathway, located in the thalamus, project to the postcentral gyrus and insular cortex, where the fifth neuron is located. Collaterals from the first and second neurons of the gustatory afferent pathway are distributed to the superior and inferior salivatory nuclei. Afferent impulses in these fibers induce the secretion of saliva during eating ("salivary reflex"). The parasympathetic preganglionic fibers exit the brainstem via cranial nerves VII and IX (see the descriptions of these cranial nerves for details). Besides this purely gustatory pathway, spicy foods may also stimulate trigeminal fibers (not shown), which contribute to the sensation of taste. Finally, olfaction (the sense of smell), too, is a major component of the sense of taste as it is subjectively perceived: patients who cannot smell (anosmosia) report that their food tastes abnormally bland.

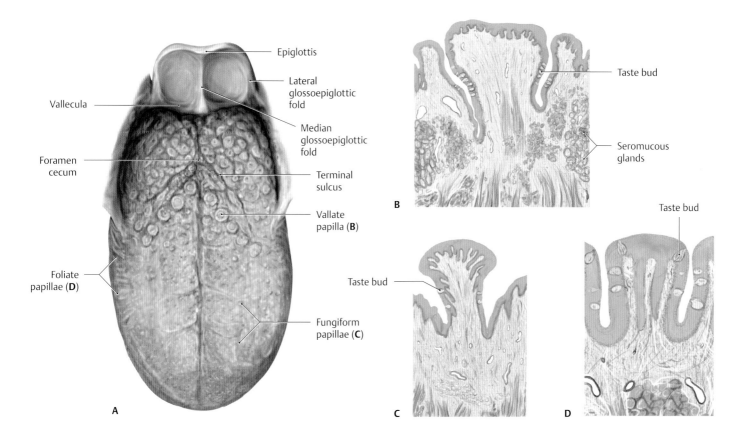

**Fig. 9.71 Organization of the taste receptors in the tongue**
The human tongue contains approximately 4600 taste buds in which the secondary sensory cells for taste perception are collected. The taste buds are embedded in the epithelium of the lingual mucosa and are located on the surface expansions of the lingual mucosa—the vallate papillae (principal site, **B**), the fungiform papillae (**C**), and the foliate papillae (**D**). Additionally, isolated taste buds are located in the mucous membranes of the soft palate and pharynx. The surrounding serous glands of the tongue (Ebner glands), which are most closely associated with the vallate papillae, constantly wash the taste buds clean to allow for new tasting. Humans can perceive five basic taste qualities: sweet, sour, salty, bitter, and a fifth "savory" quality, called umami, which is activated by glutamate (a taste enhancer).

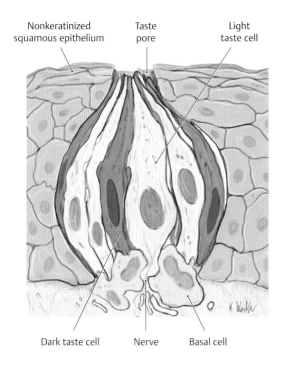

**Fig. 9.72 Microscopic structure of a taste bud**
Nerves induce the formation of taste buds in the oral mucosa. Axons of cranial nerves VII, IX, and X grow into the oral mucosa from the basal side and induce the epithelium to differentiate into the light and dark taste cells (= modified epithelial cells). Both types of taste cell have microvilli that extend to the gustatory pore. For sweet and salty, the taste cell is stimulated by hydrogen ions and other cations. The other taste qualities are mediated by receptor proteins to which the low-molecular-weight flavored substances bind (details may be found in textbooks of physiology). When the low-molecular-weight flavored substances bind to the receptor proteins, they induce signal transduction that causes the release of glutamate, which excites the peripheral processes of the pseudounipolar neurons of the three cranial nerve ganglia. The taste cells have a life span of approximately 12 days and regenerate from cells at the base of the taste buds, which differentiate into new taste cells.

*Note:* The old notion that particular areas of the tongue are sensitive to specific taste qualities has been found to be false.

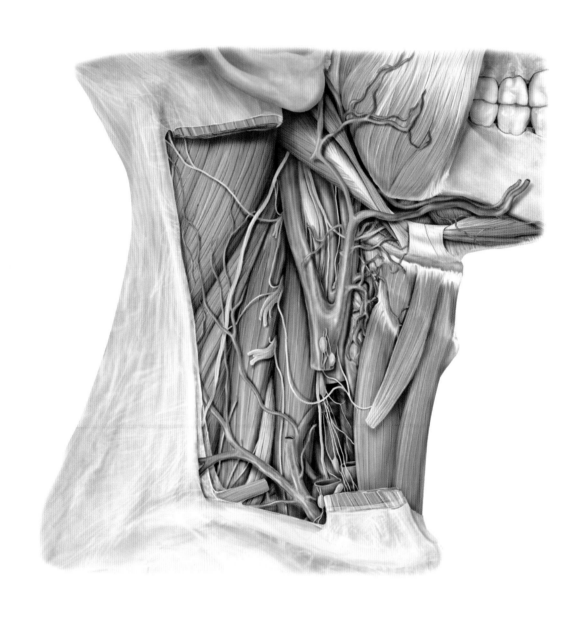

# Neck

# Vertebral Column & Vertebrae

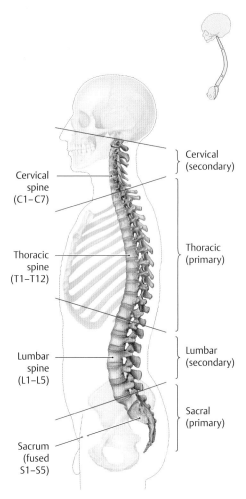

**Fig. 10.1 Spinal curvature**

Left lateral view. The spinal (vertebral) column is divided into four regions: the cervical, thoracic, lumbar, and sacral spines. In the neonate, all regions demonstrate an anteriorly concave curvature. This single concave curvature in the neonate is referred to as the primary curvature of the vertebral column.

During development, the cervical and lumbar regions of the vertebral column develop anteriorly convex curvatures. These changes are referred to as secondary curvatures. The cervical secondary curvature develops as infants begin to hold up their heads. The lumbar secondary curvatures are the result of upright bipedal locomotion.

Kyphosis is a pathological condition where the thoracic primary curvature is abnormally exaggerated (hunchback, rounded back). Lordosis is a pathological condition where the secondary curvatures are exaggerated. Lordosis may occur in either the cervical or lumbar regions (swayback) of the vertebral column. Differing from the abnormal development of primary and secondary curvatures, scoliosis is an abnormal lateral deviation of the vertebral column.

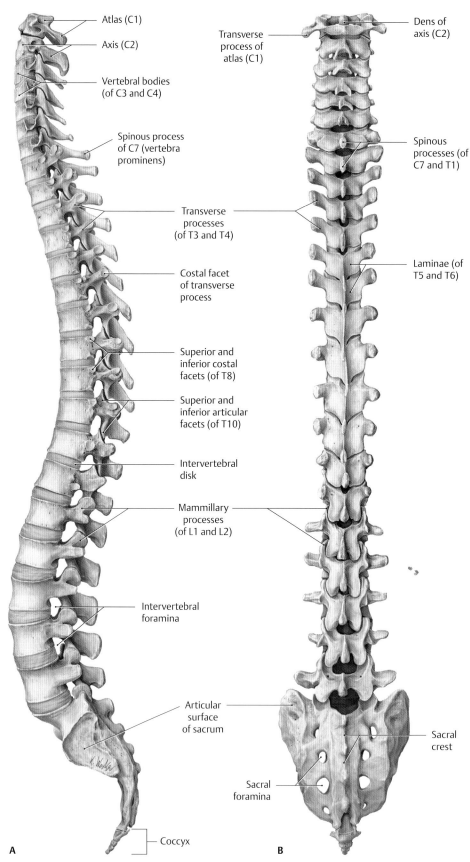

**Fig. 10.2 Vertebral column**

**A** Left lateral view. **B** Posterior view. The vertebral column is divided into four regions: cervical, thoracic, lumbar, and sacral. Each vertebra consists of a vertebral body and vertebral (neural) arch. The vertebral bodies (with intervening intervertebral disks) form the load-bearing component of the vertebral column. The vertebral (neural) arches enclose the vertebral canal, protecting the spinal cord.

### *Fig. 10.3* Structure of vertebrae

Left oblique posterosuperior view. Each vertebra consists of a load-bearing body and an arch that encloses the vertebral foramen. The arch is divided into the pedicle and lamina. Vertebrae have transverse and spinous processes that provide sites of attachment for muscles. Vertebrae articulate at facets on the superior and inferior articular processes. Thoracic vertebrae articulate with ribs at costal facets.

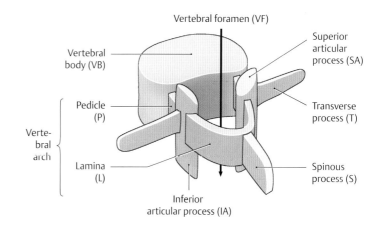

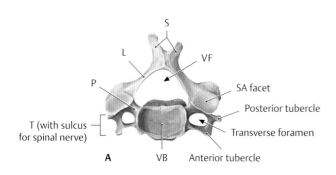

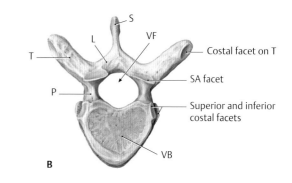

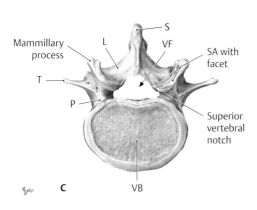

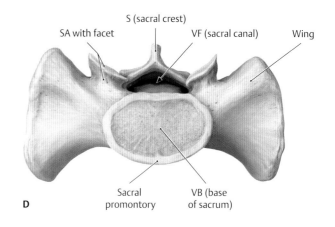

### *Fig. 10.4* Typical vertebrae

Superior view. **A** Cervical vertebra (C4). **B** Thoracic vertebra (T6). **C** Lumbar vertebra (L4). **D** Sacrum. The vertebral bodies increase in size cranially to caudally. See **Fig. 10.3** for abbreviation key.

### *Table 10.1* Structural elements of vertebrae

Each vertebra consists of a body and an arch that enclose the vertebral foramen. The types of vertebrae can be distinguished particularly easily by examining their transverse processes. The sacrum has structures that are analogous to the other vertebrae.

| Vertebrae | Body (VB) | Foramen (VF) | Transverse process (T) | Spinous process (S) |
|-----------|-----------|--------------|------------------------|---------------------|
| Cervical vertebrae C3–C7 | Small (kidney-shaped) | Large (triangular) | Transverse foramina | C3–C5: short<br>C7: long<br>C3–C6: bifid |
| Thoracic vertebrae T1–T12 | Medium (heart-shaped) with costal facets | Small (circular) | Costal facets | Long |
| Lumbar vertebrae L1–L5 | Large (kidney-shaped) | Medium (triangular) | Mammillary processes | Short and broad |
| Sacrum (fused S1–S5) | Large to small (decreases from base to apex) | Sacral canal (triangular) | Fused (forms wing of sacrum) | Short (median sacral crest) |

# Ligaments of the Vertebral Column

### Fig. 10.5 Ligaments of the vertebral column

The ligaments of the vertebral column bind the vertebrae to one another and enable the spine to withstand high mechanical loads and shearing stresses. The ligaments are divided into ligaments of the vertebral bodies and arches (**Table 10.2**).

**A** Ligaments of the vertebral column. Left lateral view of T11–L3 with T11 and T12 sectioned midsagittally.

**B** Ligaments of the vertebral body (anterior and posterior longitudinal ligaments, and intervertebral disk).

**C** Ligamenta flava.

**D** Interspinous ligaments and ligamenta flava.

**E** Complete ligaments of the vertebral column.

| Table 10.2 Ligaments of the vertebral column |
|---|
| **Vertebral body ligaments** |
| Anterior longitudinal ligament (along anterior surface of vertebral bodies) |
| Posterior longitudinal ligament (along posterior surface of vertebral bodies, i.e., anterior surface of vertebral canal) |
| Intervertebral disk (between adjacent vertebral bodies; the anulus fibrosus limits rotation, and the nucleus pulposus absorbs compressive forces) |
| **Vertebral (neural) arch ligaments** |
| Ligamenta flava (between laminae) |
| Interspinous ligaments (between spinous processes) |
| Supraspinous ligaments (along posterior border of spinous processes; in the cervical spine, the supraspinous ligament is broadened into the nuchal ligament) |
| Intertransverse ligaments (between transverse processes) |
| Facet joint capsules (enclose the articulation between the facets of the superior and inferior articular processes of adjacent vertebrae) |

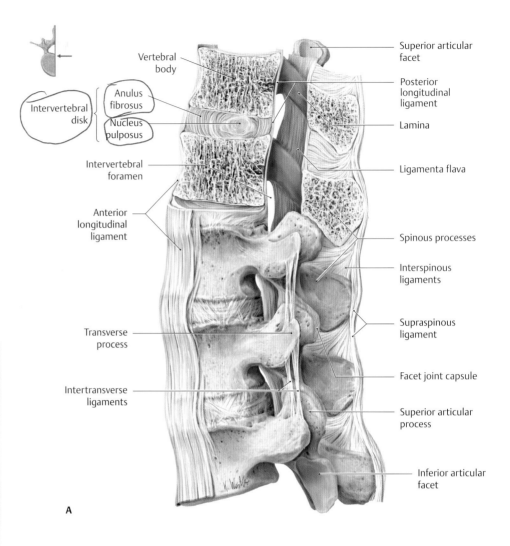

**A**

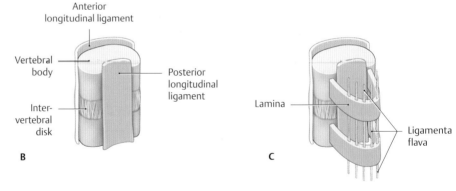

**B**   **C**

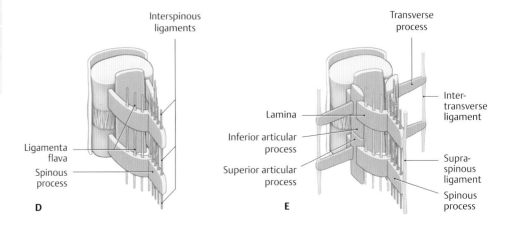

**D**   **E**

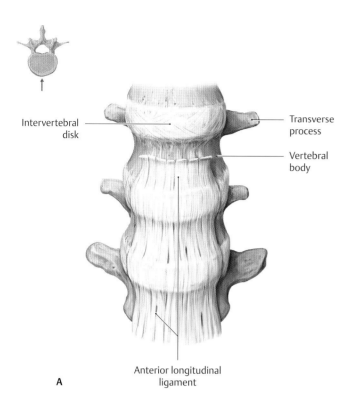

Intervertebral disk

Transverse process

Vertebral body

Anterior longitudinal ligament

**A**

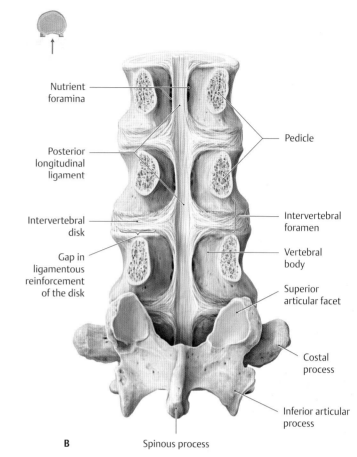

Nutrient foramina

Posterior longitudinal ligament

Intervertebral disk

Gap in ligamentous reinforcement of the disk

Pedicle

Intervertebral foramen

Vertebral body

Superior articular facet

Costal process

Inferior articular process

**B**  Spinous process

### Fig. 10.6 Individual ligaments of the vertebral column

The anterior and posterior longitudinal ligaments and ligamenta flava maintain the normal curvature of the spine.

**A**  Anterior longitudinal ligament. Anterior view. The anterior longitudinal ligament runs broadly on the anterior side of the vertebral bodies from the skull base to the sacrum. Its deep collagenous fibers bind adjacent vertebral bodies together (they are firmly attached to vertebral bodies and loosely attached to intervertebral disks). Its superficial fibers span multiple vertebrae.

**B**  Posterior longitudinal ligament. Posterior view with vertebral canal windowed (vertebral arches removed). The thinner posterior longitudinal ligament descends from the clivus along the posterior surface of the vertebral bodies, passing into the sacral canal. The ligament broadens at the level of the intervertebral disk (to which it is attached by tapered lateral extensions). It narrows again while passing the vertebral body (to which it is attached at the superior and inferior margins).

**C**  Ligamenta flava and intertransverse ligaments. Anterior view with vertebral canal windowed (vertebral bodies removed). The ligamentum flavum is a thick, powerful ligament that connects adjacent laminae and reinforces the wall of the vertebral canal posterior to the intervertebral foramina. The ligament consists mainly of elastic fibers that produce the characteristic yellow color. When the spinal column is erect, the ligamenta flava are tensed, stabilizing the spine in the sagittal plane. The ligamenta flava also limit forward flexion of the spine. *Note:* The tips of the transverse processes are connected by interspinous ligaments that limit the rocking movements of vertebrae upon one another.

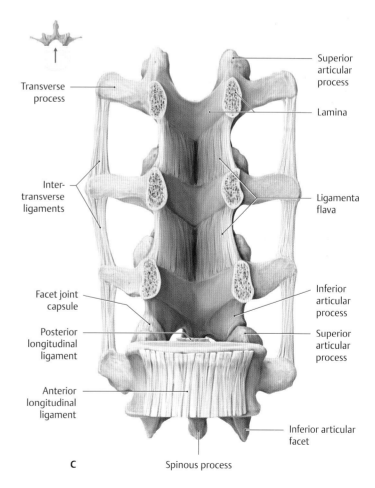

Transverse process

Inter-transverse ligaments

Facet joint capsule

Posterior longitudinal ligament

Anterior longitudinal ligament

Superior articular process

Lamina

Ligamenta flava

Inferior articular process

Superior articular process

Inferior articular facet

**C**  Spinous process

# Cervical Spine

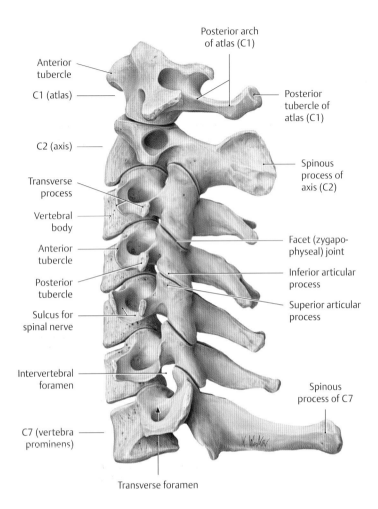

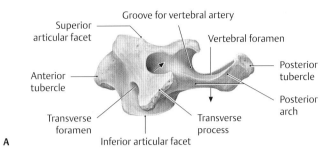

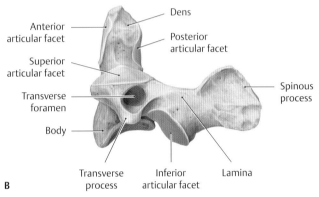

**Fig. 10.7 Cervical spine (C1–C7)**
Left lateral view. The cervical spine consists of seven vertebrae. C1 and C2 are atypical and are discussed individually.

**Typical cervical vertebrae (C3–C7):** Typical cervical vertebrae have relatively small, kidney-shaped bodies. The superior and inferior articular processes are broad and flat; their facets are flat and inclined at approximately 45 degrees from the horizontal. The vertebral arches enclose a large, triangular vertebral foramen. Spinal nerves emerge from the vertebral canal via the intervertebral foramina formed between the pedicles of adjacent vertebrae. The transverse processes of cervical vertebrae are furrowed to accommodate the emerging nerve (sulcus for spinal nerve). The transverse processes also consist of an anterior and a posterior portion that enclose a transverse foramen. The transverse foramina allow the vertebral artery to ascend to the base of the skull. The spinous processes of C3–C6 are short and bifid. The spinous process of C7 (vertebra prominens) is longer and thicker; it is the first spinous process that is palpable through the skin.
**Atlas (C1) and axis (C2):** The atlas and axis are specialized for bearing the weight of the head and allowing it to move in all directions. The body of the axis contains a vertical prominence (dens) around which the atlas turns. The atlas does not have a vertebral body: it consists of an anterior and a posterior arch that allow the head to rotate in the horizontal plane.

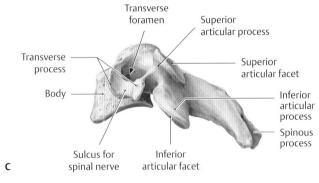

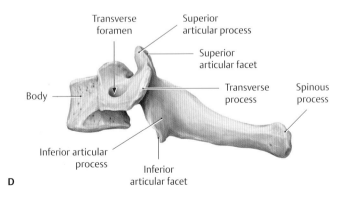

**Fig. 10.8 Left lateral view of cervical vertebrae**
**A** Atlas (C1). **B** Axis (C2). **C** Typical cervical vertebra (C4). **D** Vertebra prominens (C7).

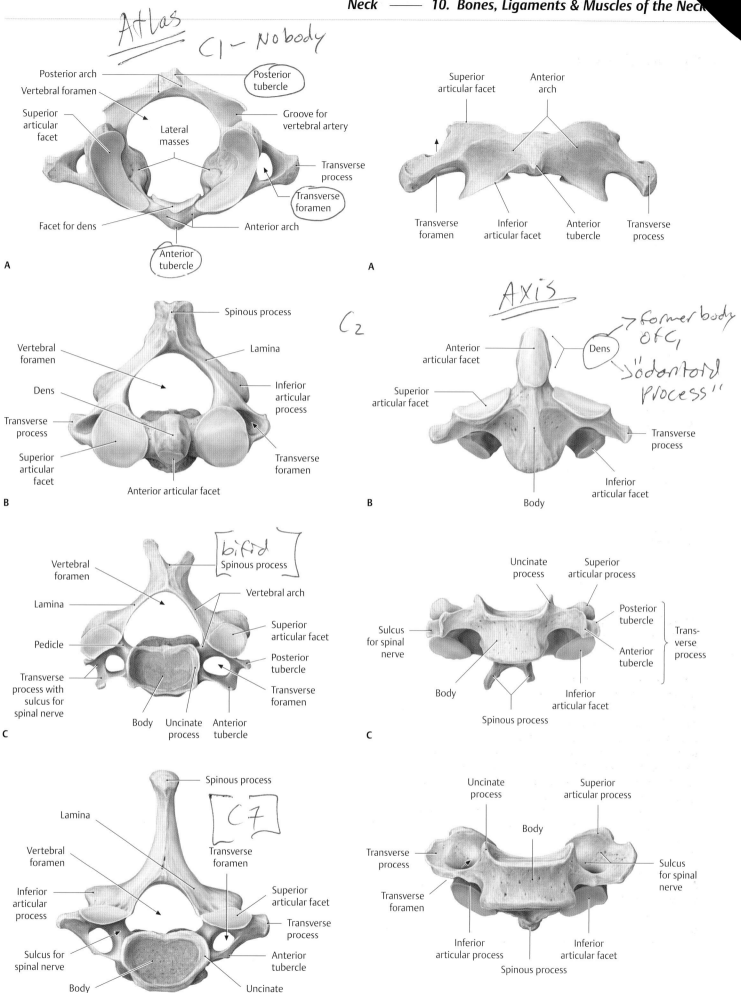

**Atlas** C1 — No body

**AXIS** C2

→ former body of C1

"odontoid Process"

bifid Spinous process

C7

*Fig. 10.9* **Superior view of cervical vertebrae**
**A** Atlas (C1). **B** Axis (C2). **C** Typical cervical vertebra (C4). **D** Vertebra prominens (C7).

*Fig. 10.10* **Anterior view of cervical vertebrae**
**A** Atlas (C1). **B** Axis (C2). **C** Typical cervical vertebra (C4). **D** Vertebra prominens (C7).

**231**

# Joints of the Cervical Spine

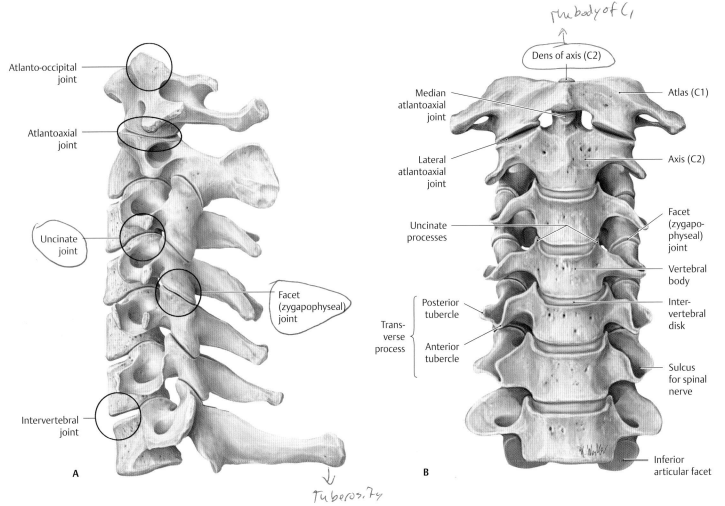

A

*Atlanto-occipital joint*

*Atlantoaxial joint*

*Uncinate joint*

*Facet (zygapophyseal) joint*

*Intervertebral joint*

*Tuberosity*

B

*the body of C1*

*Dens of axis (C2)*

*Median atlantoaxial joint*

*Lateral atlantoaxial joint*

*Uncinate processes*

*Transverse process*

*Posterior tubercle*

*Anterior tubercle*

*Atlas (C1)*

*Axis (C2)*

*Facet (zygapophyseal) joint*

*Vertebral body*

*Intervertebral disk*

*Sulcus for spinal nerve*

*Inferior articular facet*

### Fig. 10.11 Joints of the cervical spine

**A** Left lateral view. **B** Anterior view. **C** Radiograph of the cervical spine.

The cervical spine has five types of joints. Two joints (intervertebral and facet) are common to all regions of the spine, and three are specialized joints of the cervical spine.

**Joints of the vertebral column:** Adjacent vertebrae articulate at two points: vertebral bodies and articular processes. The bodies of adjacent vertebrae articulate at roughly horizontal intervertebral joints (via intervertebral disks). The articular processes of adjacent vertebrae articulate at facet (zygapophyseal) joints. In the cervical spine, the intervertebral joints are angled slightly anteroinferiorly, and the zygapophyseal joints are angled posteroinferiorly (roughly 45 degrees below horizontal).

**Joints of the cervical spine:** There are two types of joints that are particular to the cervical spine:

1. Uncovertebral joints: Upward protrusions of the lateral margins of cervical vertebral bodies form uncinate processes. These processes may articulate with the inferolateral margin of the adjacent superior vertebra, forming uncovertebral joints.
2. Craniovertebral joints: The atlas (C1) and axis (C2) are specialized to bear the weight of the head and facilitate movement in all directions. This is made possible by craniovertebral joints (see **Fig. 10.12**).

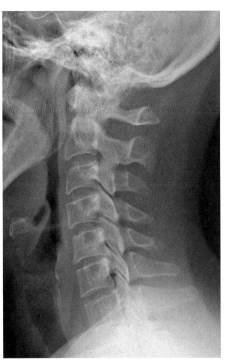

C

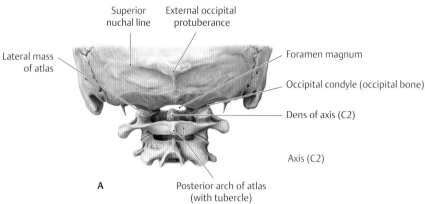

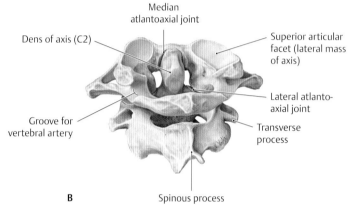

**Fig. 10.12 Craniovertebral joints**
**A** Posterior view. **B** Left oblique posterosuperior view.
There are five craniovertebral joints. The paired atlanto-occipital joints are articulations between the concave superior articular facets of the atlas (C1) and the convex occipital condyle of the occipital bone. These allow the head to rock back and forth in the sagittal plane. The atlanto-axial joints (two lateral and one medial) allow the atlas to rotate in the horizontal plane around the dens of the axis. The lateral atlantoaxial joints are the paired articulations between the inferior and superior articular facets of the atlas and axis, respectively. The median atlantoaxial joint is the unpaired articulation between the dens of the axis and the fovea of the atlas. *Note:* While only the atlanto-occipital joints are direct articulations between the cranium and vertebral column, the atlanto-axial joints are generally classified as craniovertebral joints as well.

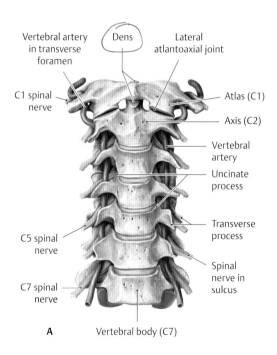

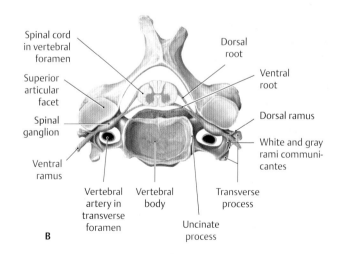

**Fig. 10.13 Neurovasculature of the cervical spine**
**A** Anterior view. **B** Superior view.
The transverse processes of the cervical vertebrae are extremely important in communicating neurovascular structures. Spinal nerves arise from the spinal cord in the vertebral canal. They exit via the intervertebral foramina formed by the pedicles of adjacent vertebrae. The transverse processes of cervical vertebrae contain grooves (sulci) through which the spinal nerves pass. The transverse processes also contain transverse foramina that allow the vertebral artery to ascend from the subclavian artery and enter the skull via the foramen magnum. Injury to the cervical spine can compress the neurovascular structures as they emerge and ascend from the vertebral column.

# Ligaments of the Cervical Spine

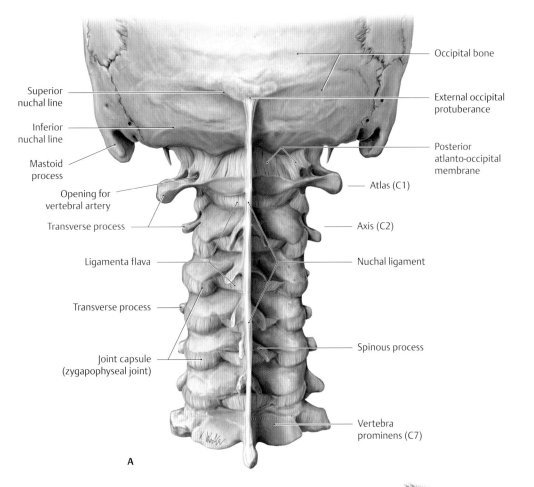

Occipital bone

External occipital protuberance

Posterior atlanto-occipital membrane

Atlas (C1)

Axis (C2)

Nuchal ligament

Spinous process

Vertebra prominens (C7)

Superior nuchal line

Inferior nuchal line

Mastoid process

Opening for vertebral artery

Transverse process

Ligamenta flava

Transverse process

Joint capsule (zygapophyseal joint)

**A**

*Fig. 10.14* **Ligaments of the cervical spine**
**A** Posterior view.
**B** Anterior view after removal of the anterior skull base.
**C** Midsagittal section, left lateral view. The nuchal ligament is the broadened, sagittally oriented part of the supraspinous ligament that extends from the vertebra prominens (C7) to the external occipital protuberance.

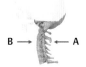

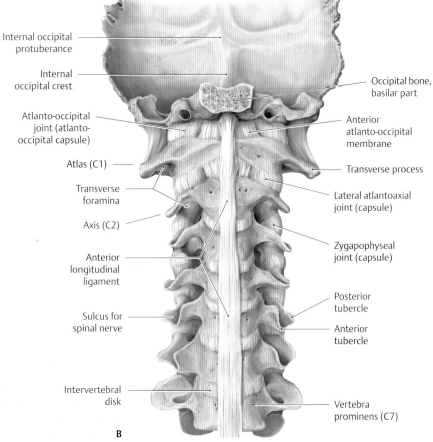

Internal occipital protuberance

Internal occipital crest

Atlanto-occipital joint (atlanto-occipital capsule)

Atlas (C1)

Transverse foramina

Axis (C2)

Anterior longitudinal ligament

Sulcus for spinal nerve

Intervertebral disk

Occipital bone, basilar part

Anterior atlanto-occipital membrane

Transverse process

Lateral atlantoaxial joint (capsule)

Zygapophyseal joint (capsule)

Posterior tubercle

Anterior tubercle

Vertebra prominens (C7)

**B**

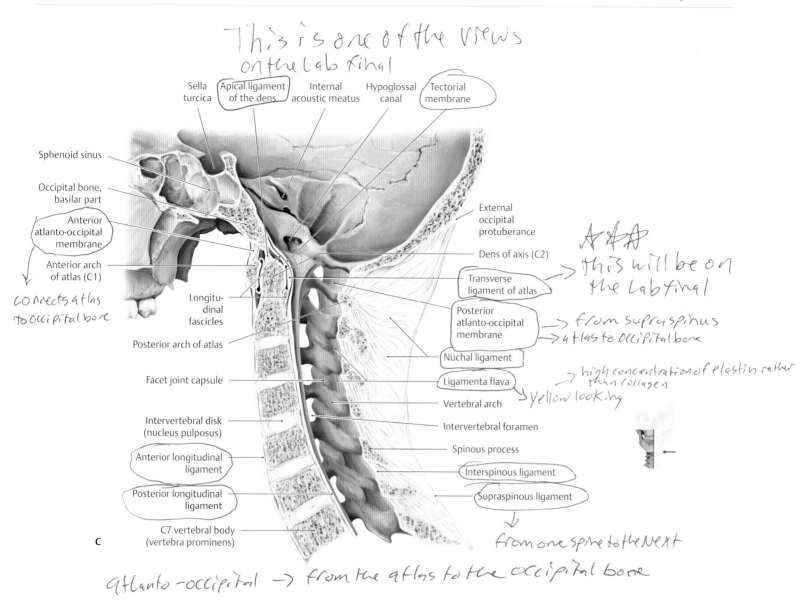

*This is one of the views on the Lab final*

Sella turcica

Apical ligament of the dens

Internal acoustic meatus

Hypoglossal canal

Tectorial membrane

Sphenoid sinus

Occipital bone, basilar part

Anterior atlanto-occipital membrane

*connects atlas to occipital bone*

Anterior arch of atlas (C1)

Longitudinal fascicles

Posterior arch of atlas

Facet joint capsule

Intervertebral disk (nucleus pulposus)

Anterior longitudinal ligament

Posterior longitudinal ligament

C7 vertebral body (vertebra prominens)

C

External occipital protuberance

Dens of axis (C2)

Transverse ligament of atlas

Posterior atlanto-occipital membrane

Nuchal ligament

Ligamenta flava

Vertebral arch

Intervertebral foramen

Spinous process

Interspinous ligament

Supraspinous ligament

*AAA This will be on the Lab final*

*→ from supraspinus*

*→ atlas to occipital bone*

*→ high concentration of elastin rather than collagen*

*→ yellow looking*

*→ from one spine to the next*

*atlanto-occipital → from the atlas to the occipital bone*

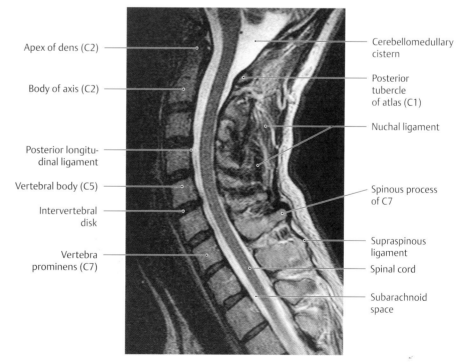

Apex of dens (C2)

Body of axis (C2)

Posterior longitudinal ligament

Vertebral body (C5)

Intervertebral disk

Vertebra prominens (C7)

Cerebellomedullary cistern

Posterior tubercle of atlas (C1)

Nuchal ligament

Spinous process of C7

Supraspinous ligament

Spinal cord

Subarachnoid space

**Fig. 10.15 Magnetic resonance image of the cervical spine**
Midsagittal section, left lateral view, T2-weighted TSE sequence.
(From Vahlensieck M, Reiser M. MRT des Bewegungsapparates. 2nd ed.
Stuttgart: Thieme; 2001.)

# Ligaments of the Craniovertebral Joints

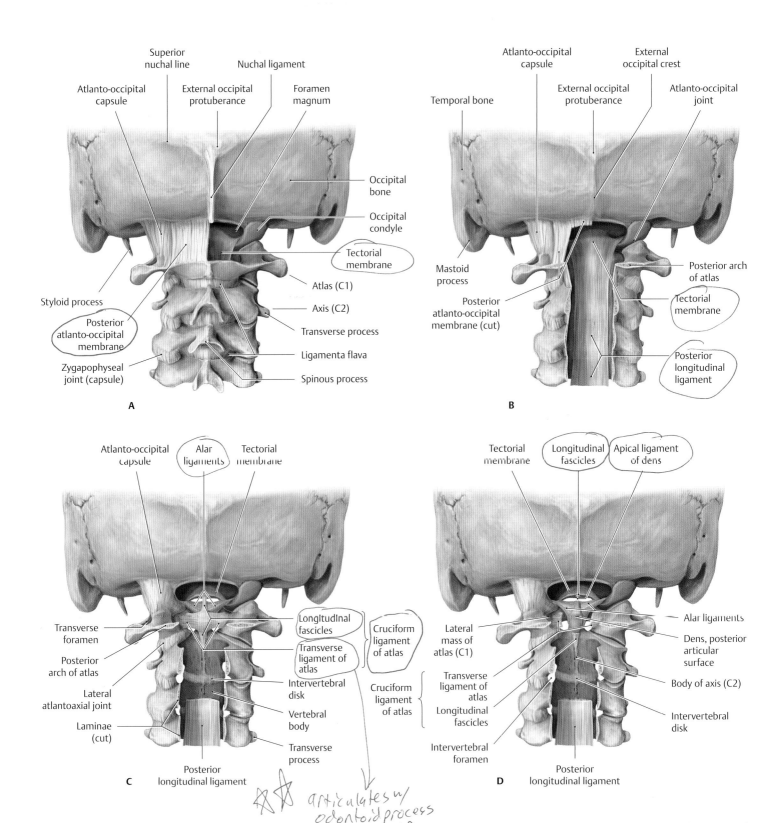

**Fig. 10.16 Ligaments of the craniovertebral joints and cervical spine**

Skull and upper cervical spine, posterior view.

*[handwritten notes: articulates w/ odontoid process on the posterior part]*

**A** The posterior atlanto-occipital membrane stretches from the posterior arch of the atlas to the posterior rim of the foramen magnum. This membrane has been removed on the right side.

**B** With the vertebral canal opened and the spinal cord removed, the tectorial membrane, a broadened expansion of the posterior longitudinal ligament, is seen to form the anterior boundary of the vertebral canal at the level of the craniovertebral joints.

**C** With the tectorial membrane removed, the cruciform ligament of the atlas can be seen. The transverse ligament of the atlas forms the thick horizontal bar of the cross, and the longitudinal fascicles form the thinner vertical bar.

**D** The transverse ligament of the atlas and longitudinal fascicles have been partially removed to demonstrate the paired alar ligaments, which extend from the lateral surfaces of the dens to the corresponding inner surfaces of the occipital condyles, and the unpaired apical ligament of the dens, which passes from the tip of the dens to the anterior rim of the foramen magnum.

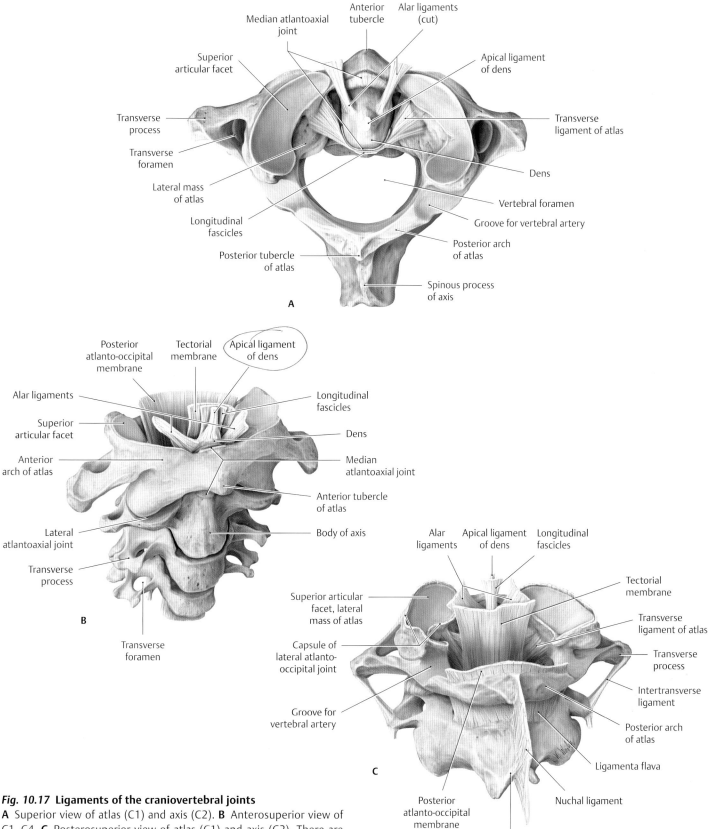

**Fig. 10.17 Ligaments of the craniovertebral joints**
**A** Superior view of atlas (C1) and axis (C2). **B** Anterosuperior view of
C1–C4. **C** Posterosuperior view of atlas (C1) and axis (C2). There are
five craniovertebral joints. The paired atlanto-occipital joints are articulations between the concave superior articular facets of the atlas and
the convex occipital condyles of the occipital bone. The joints are stabilized by the atlanto-occipital joint capsule and the posterior atlanto-
occipital membrane (the equivalent of the ligamenta flava). The paired
lateral atlantoaxial and unpaired median atlantoaxial joints allow the
atlas to rotate in the horizontal plane around the dens of the axis. They
are stabilized by the alar ligaments, the apical ligament of the dens,
and the cruciform ligament of the atlas (transverse ligament and longitudinal fascicles).

# Muscles of the Neck: Overview

*Fig. 10.18* **Sternocleidomastoid and trapezius**
**A** Sternocleidomastoid, right lateral view.
**B** Trapezius, posterior view.

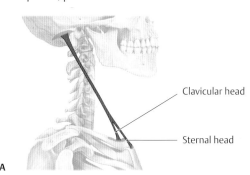

Clavicular head

Sternal head

**A**

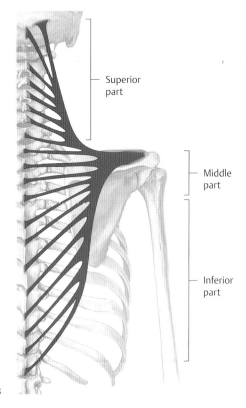

Superior part

Middle part

Inferior part

**B**

*Fig. 10.19* **Superficial neck muscles**
**A** Left lateral view. **B** Anterior view of sternocleidomastoid and trapezius. Unlike the rest of the neck muscles, the superficial neck muscles are located superficial to the deep cervical fascia.

**Platysma:** The platysma, like the muscles of facial expression, is not enveloped in its own fascial sheath, but is instead directly associated with (and in parts inserted into) the skin. (*Note:* It is innervated by the same nerve as the muscles of facial expression, the facial nerve.) The platysma is highly variable in size — its fibers may reach from the lower face to the upper thorax.

**Sternocleidomastoid and trapezius:** The trapezius lies between the investing and prevertebral layers of cervical fascia. The investing layer splits to enclose the sternocleidomastoid and the trapezius.

| *Table 10.3* Muscles of the neck | |
|---|---|
| The muscles of the neck lie at the intersection of the skull, vertebral column, and upper limb. They can therefore be classified in multiple ways based on location and function. In the pages that follow, the neck muscles are grouped as follows: | |
| **Superficial neck muscles** | |
| Muscles that lie superficial to the deep layer (lamina) of the deep cervical fascia and are innervated by the ventral rami of spinal nerves | p. 239 |
| **Posterior neck muscles (intrinsic back muscles)** | |
| Muscles that insert on the cervical spine and are innervated by the dorsal rami of spinal nerves | p. 240 |
| • Intrinsic back muscles (including nuchal muscles) | pp. 242, 243 |
|    ◦ Short nuchal/craniovertebral muscles | p. 245 |
| **Anterior neck muscles** | |
| Muscles that insert on the anterior cervical spine and are innervated by the ventral rami of spinal nerves | p. 252 |
| • Anterior vertebral (prevertebral) muscles | p. 253 |
| • Lateral vertebral muscles (scalenes) | p. 253 |
| Muscles that do not insert on the cervical spine | p. 254 |
| • Suprahyoid muscles | p. 255 |
| • Infrahyoid muscles | p. 255 |

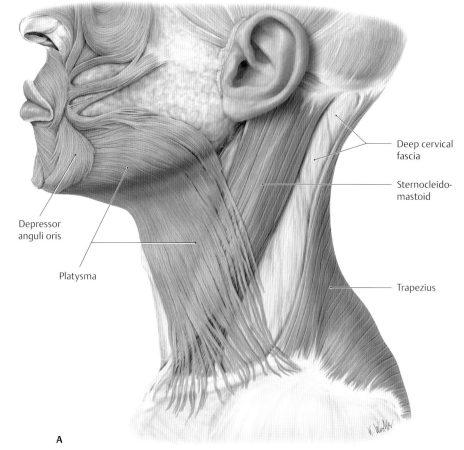

Deep cervical fascia

Sternocleidomastoid

Trapezius

Depressor anguli oris

Platysma

**A**

### Table 10.4 Superficial neck muscles

| Muscle | Origin | Insertion | Innervation | Action |
|---|---|---|---|---|
| Platysma | Mandible (inferior border); skin of lower face and angle of mouth | Skin over lower neck and superior and lateral thorax | Facial n. (CN VII), cervical branch | Depresses and wrinkles skin of lower face and mouth; tenses skin of neck; aids forced depression of mandible |
| Sternocleidomastoid | Occipital bone (superior nuchal line); temporal bone (mastoid process) | Sternal head: sternum (manubrium)<br><br>Clavicular head: clavicle (medial ⅓) | Accessory n. (CN IX), spinal part | *Unilateral:* Moves chin up and out (tilts occiput to same side and rotates face to opposite side)<br>*Bilateral:* Extends head; aids in respiration when head is fixed |
| Trapezius, superior fibers* | Occipital bone; C1–C7 spinous processes | Clavicle (lateral ⅓) | | Draws scapula obliquely upward; rotates glenoid cavity inferiorly |
| Rhomboid minor | Ligamentum nuchae (inferior part); spinous processes of C7–T1 vertebrae | Medial (vertebral) border of the scapula, superior to the intersection with the scapular spine | C4–C5 ventral rami (C5 fibers are from the dorsal scapular n.) | Scapular movements (e.g., retraction and rotation) |
| Levator scapulae | C1–C4 cervical vertebrae; posterior tubercles of transverse processes | Scapula, medial to superior angle | C3–C5 ventral rami (C5 fibers are from the dorsal scapular n.) | Scapular movements (e.g., elevation, retraction, and rotation) |
| Serratus posterior superior | Ligamentum nuchae (inferior part); spinous processes of C7–T3 vertebrae | Ribs 2–5 | Ventral rami of thoracic spinal nn. (intercostal nn.) | Postulated to be an accessory muscle of respiration; assists in elevating ribs |

*The middle and inferior parts are not described here.

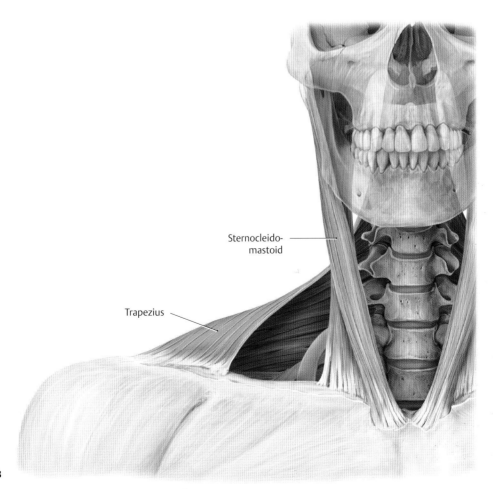

Sternocleido-
mastoid

Trapezius

B

239

# Muscles of the Neck & Back (I)

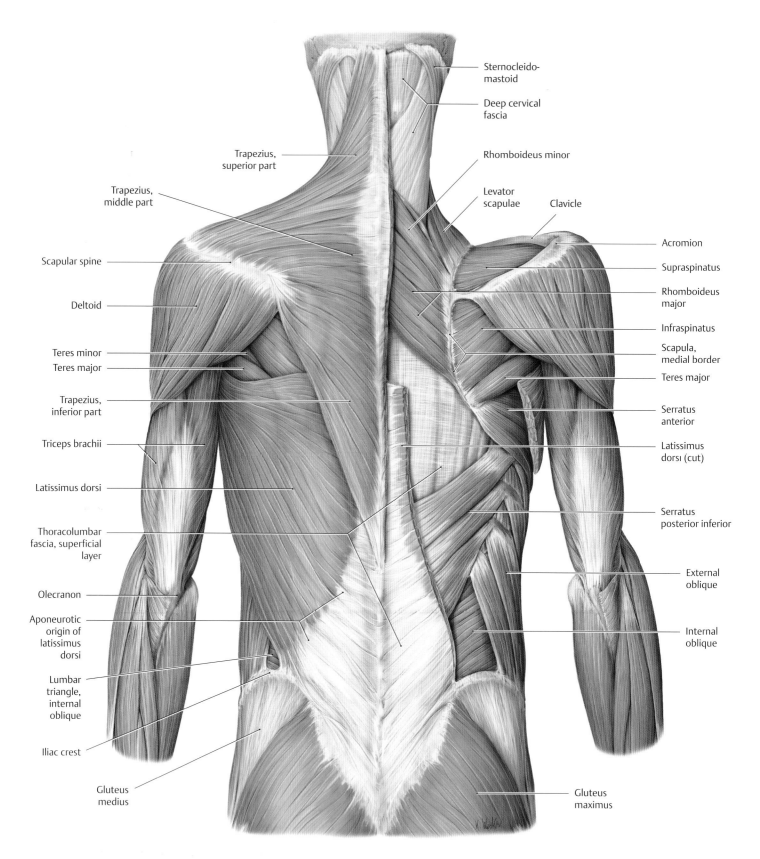

**Fig. 10.20 Muscles of the neck and back**

Posterior view with trapezius and latissimus dorsi cut on right side. The extrinsic back muscles lie superficial to the thoracolumbar and deep cervical fascia. They are muscles of the upper limb (derived from the limb buds) that have migrated to the back. The intrinsic back muscles lie within the thoracolumbar and deep cervical fascia. They are derived from epaxial muscle. Because of their different embryonic origins, the intrinsic back muscles are innervated by the dorsal rami of the spinal nerves, and the extrinsic back muscles are innervated by the ventral rami. *Note:* The trapezius and sternocleidomastoid are innervated by the accessory nerve (CN XI).

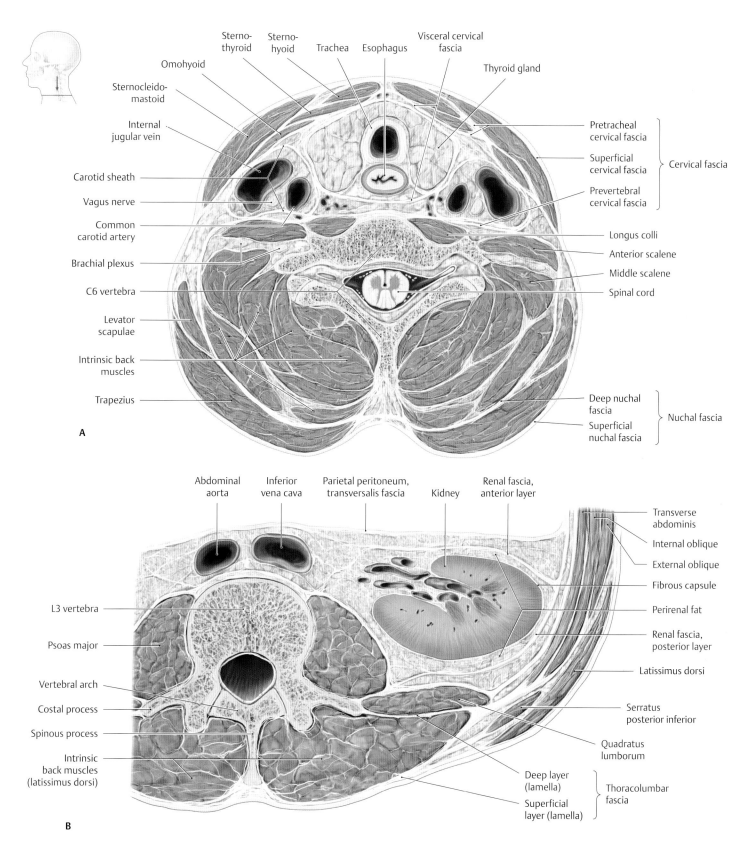

**Fig. 10.21 Fascial planes**

Transverse sections, superior view.

**A** Neck at the level of the C6 vertebra.

**B** Posterior trunk wall at the level of the L3 vertebra (with cauda equina removed from vertebral canal).

The muscles of the neck and back are separated by layers of deep fascia (see p. 242). The outermost layer, the deep investing cervical fascia, encloses all muscles with the exception of the platysma (this is located in the superficial fascia, not to be confused with the superficial

layer of the deep cervical fascia). The deep cervical fascia, located in the anterior neck, is continuous posteriorly with the nuchal fascia in the posterior neck. The superficial layer of the nuchal fascia is continuous inferiorly with the superficial layer (lamella) of the thoracolumbar fascia. The intrinsic muscles of the neck and back lie within the deep nuchal fascia, which is continuous with the prevertebral cervical fascia (anteriorly) and thoracolumbar fascia (inferiorly). The muscles and structures of the anterior neck are enclosed in individual fascial sheaths (i.e., the visceral fascia, pretracheal fascia, and carotid sheath).

# Muscles of the Neck & Back (II)

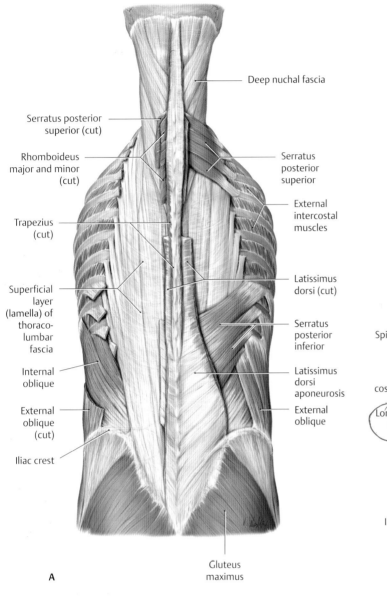

**A**

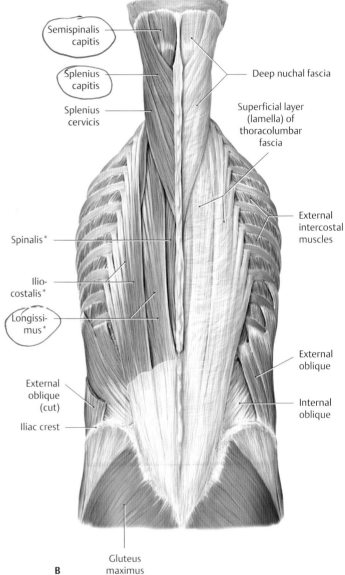

**B**

## Fig. 10.22 Extrinsic and intrinsic back muscles

Posterior view. These dissections demonstrate the distinction between the intrinsic back muscles and the surrounding extrinsic back muscles and trunk muscles. The intrinsic back muscles lie within the deep nuchal fascia, which is continuous inferiorly with the superficial layer (lamella) of the thoracolumbar fascia. They are derived from epaxial muscles and therefore innervated by the dorsal rami of spinal nerves (see p. 246). The muscles of the trunk are derived from hypaxial muscle and therefore innervated by the ventral rami of spinal nerves. The visible trunk muscles are the abdominal muscles (internal and external obliques) and the thoracic muscles (external intercostals).

**A** *Removed:* Extrinsic back muscles (with the exception of the serratus posterior and the aponeurotic origin of the latissimus dorsi on the right side).

**B** *Removed:* All extrinsic back muscles and portions of the fascial covering (deep nuchal and superficial layers [lamellae] of the thoracolumbar fasciae).

*The spinalis, iliocostalis, and longissimus are collectively known as the erector spinae.

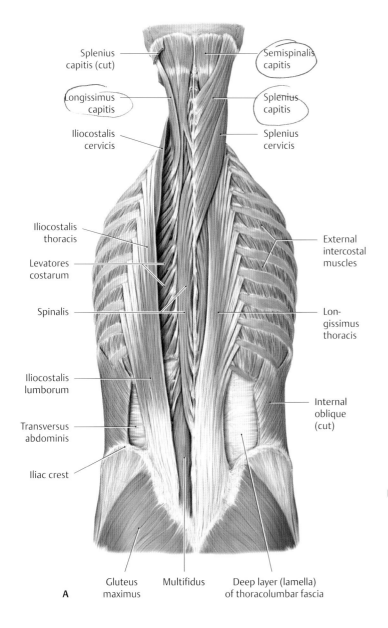

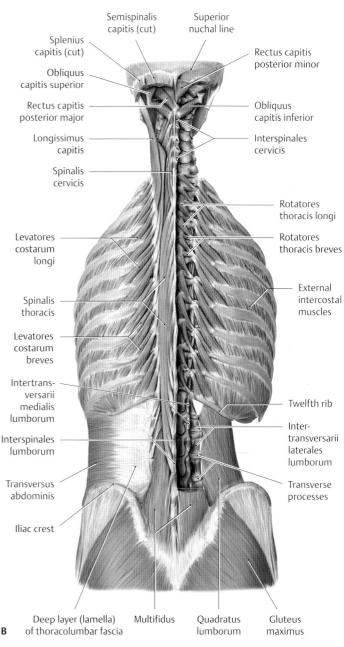

## Fig. 10.23 Intrinsic back muscles

Posterior view. These dissections reveal the layers of intrinsic back muscles. The iliocostalis, longissimus, and spinalis collectively form the erector spinae. They lie deep to the superficial layer (lamella) of the thoracolumbar fascia and cover the other intrinsic back muscles.

**A** *Removed on left side:* Longissimus (except cervical portion), splenii capitis and cervicis. *Removed on right side:* Iliocostalis. Note the deep layer (lamella) of the thoracolumbar fascia, which gives origin to the internal oblique and transversus abdominis.

**B** *Removed on left side:* Iliocostalis, longissimus, and internal oblique. *Removed on right side:* Erector spinae, multifidus, transversus abdominis, splenius capitis, and semispinalis capitis.

# Muscles of the Posterior Neck

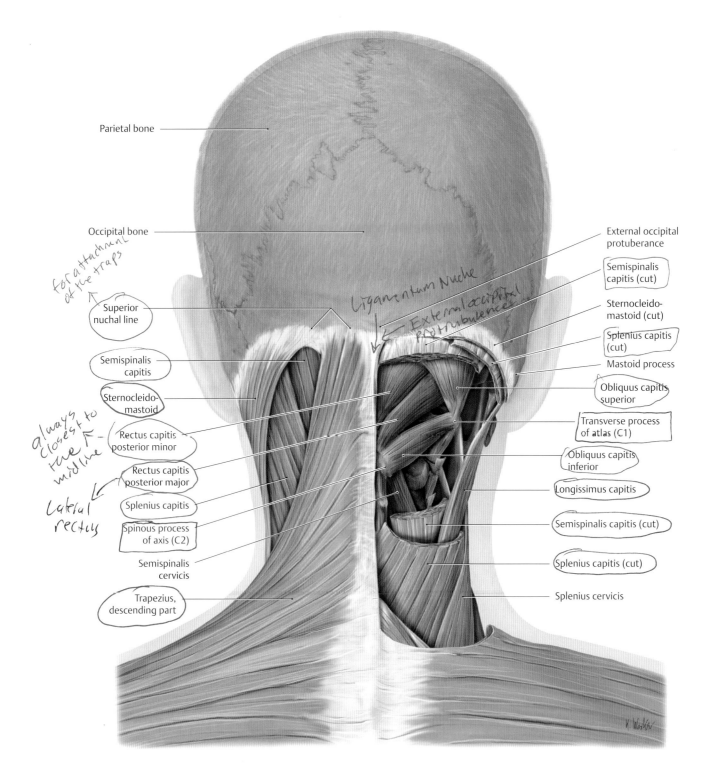

Parietal bone

Occipital bone

*for attachment of the traps*

Superior nuchal line

Semispinalis capitis

Sternocleido-mastoid

*always closest to the midline*

*Lateral rectus*

Rectus capitis posterior minor

Rectus capitis posterior major

Splenius capitis

Spinous process of axis (C2)

Semispinalis cervicis

Trapezius, descending part

*Ligamentum Nuchae*

*External occipital protruberances*

External occipital protuberance

Semispinalis capitis (cut)

Sternocleido-mastoid (cut)

Splenius capitis (cut)

Mastoid process

Obliquus capitis superior

Transverse process of atlas (C1)

Obliquus capitis inferior

Longissimus capitis

Semispinalis capitis (cut)

Splenius capitis (cut)

Splenius cervicis

**Fig. 10.24 Muscles in the nuchal region**
Posterior view of nuchal region. As the neck is at the intersection of the trunk, head, and upper limb, its muscles can be divided according to embryonic origin, function, or location. Those muscles (extrinsic and intrinsic) located in the posterior neck are often referred to as the nuchal muscles. The nuchal muscles are further divided into short nuchal muscles, which are intrinsic back muscles innervated by the dorsal rami of cervical spinal nerves. Based on location, the short nuchal muscles may also be referred to as suboccipital muscles. The anterior and posterior vertebral muscles collectively move the craniovertebral joints.

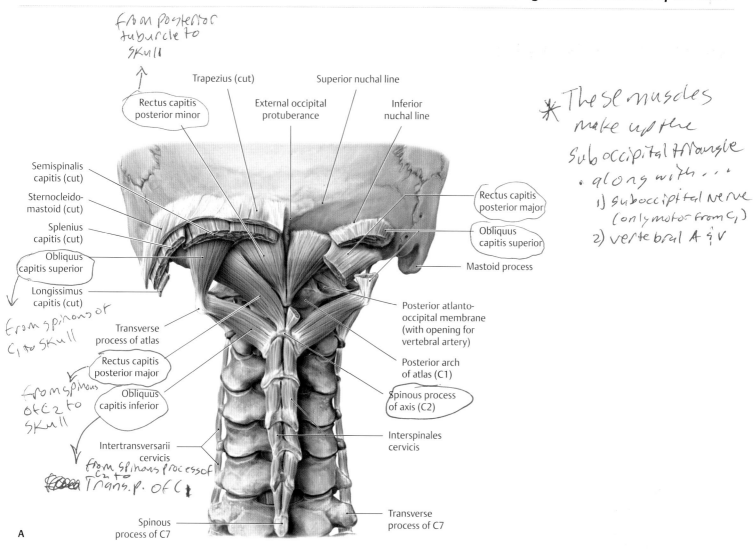

*(handwritten note, top left)* from posterior tubercle to skull

Rectus capitis posterior minor

Trapezius (cut)

External occipital protuberance

Superior nuchal line

Inferior nuchal line

Semispinalis capitis (cut)

Sternocleido-mastoid (cut)

Splenius capitis (cut)

Obliquus capitis superior

Longissimus capitis (cut)

*(handwritten note, left)* from spinous of C₁ to skull

Rectus capitis posterior major

Obliquus capitis superior

Mastoid process

Transverse process of atlas

Rectus capitis posterior major

*(handwritten note, left)* from spinous of C₂ to skull

Obliquus capitis inferior

Intertransversarii cervicis

*(handwritten note, left)* from spinous process of C₂ to Trans. p. of C₁

Spinous process of C7

Posterior atlanto-occipital membrane (with opening for vertebral artery)

Posterior arch of atlas (C1)

Spinous process of axis (C2)

Interspinales cervicis

Transverse process of C7

*(handwritten note, right)* ✱ These muscles make up the suboccipital triangle
• along with...
1) suboccipital nerve (only motor from C₁)
2) vertebral A & V

A

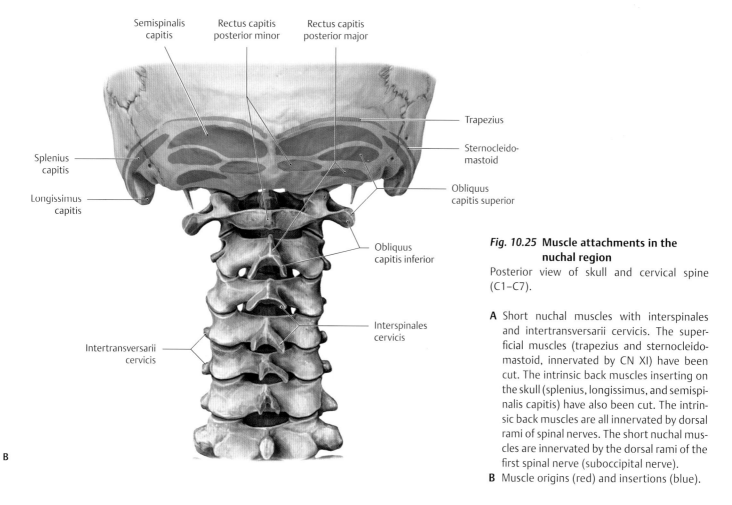

Semispinalis capitis

Rectus capitis posterior minor

Rectus capitis posterior major

Splenius capitis

Longissimus capitis

Intertransversarii cervicis

Trapezius

Sternocleido-mastoid

Obliquus capitis superior

Obliquus capitis inferior

Interspinales cervicis

B

**Fig. 10.25 Muscle attachments in the nuchal region**

Posterior view of skull and cervical spine (C1–C7).

**A** Short nuchal muscles with interspinales and intertransversarii cervicis. The superficial muscles (trapezius and sternocleidomastoid, innervated by CN XI) have been cut. The intrinsic back muscles inserting on the skull (splenius, longissimus, and semispinalis capitis) have also been cut. The intrinsic back muscles are all innervated by dorsal rami of spinal nerves. The short nuchal muscles are innervated by the dorsal rami of the first spinal nerve (suboccipital nerve).

**B** Muscle origins (red) and insertions (blue).

245

# Intrinsic Back Muscles (I): Erector Spinae & Interspinales

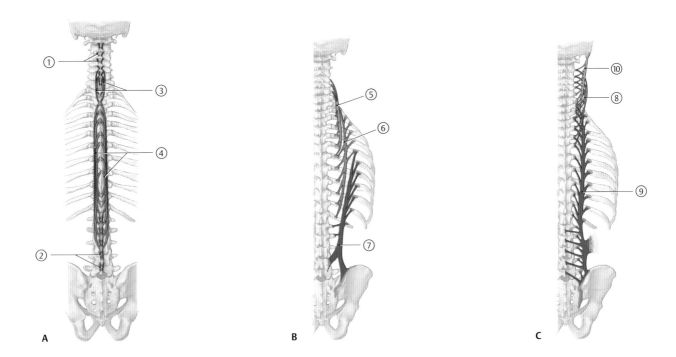

**Fig. 10.26 Interspinales and erector spinae**
**A** Interspinales and spinalis. **B** Iliocostalis. **C** Longissimus.

## Table 10.5 Erector spinae and interspinales

Like all intrinsic back muscles, these muscles are innervated by dorsal rami of spinal nerves. The erector spinae and interspinales are innervated by lateral branches of the dorsal rami. The longissimus is innervated by spinal nerves C1–L5, the iliocostalis by C8–L1.

| Muscle | | Origin | Insertion | Action |
|---|---|---|---|---|
| Interspinalis | ① I. cervicis | C1–C7 (between spinous processes of adjacent vertebrae) | | Extends cervical spine |
| | ② I. lumborum | L1–L5 (between spinous processes of adjacent vertebrae | | Extends lumbar spine |
| Spinalis* | ③ S. cervicis | C5–T2 (spinous processes) | C2–C5 (spinous processes) | *Bilateral:* Extends spine *Unilateral:* Bends laterally to same side |
| | ④ S. thoracis | T10–L3 (spinous processes, lateral surface) | T2–T8 (spinous processes, lateral surface) | |
| Iliocostalis* | ⑤ I. cervicis | 3rd–7th ribs | C4–C6 (transverse processes) | |
| | ⑥ I. thoracis | 7th–12th ribs | 1st–6th ribs | |
| | ⑦ I. lumborum | Sacrum; iliac crest; thoracolumbar fascia | 6th–12th ribs; deep thoracolumbar fascia; upper lumbar vertebrae (transverse processes) | |
| Longissimus* | ⑧ L. cervicis | T1–T6 (transverse processes) | C2–C5 (transverse processes) | |
| | ⑨ L. thoracis | Sacrum; iliac crest; L1–L5 (spinous processes); lower thoracic vertebrae (transverse processes) | 2nd–12th ribs; T1–L5 (transverse processes) | |
| | ⑩ L. capitis | T1–T3 (transverse processes); C4–C7 (transverse and articular processes) | Occipital bone (mastoid process) | *Bilateral:* Extends head *Unilateral:* Flexes and rotates head to same side |

*The spinalis, iliocostalis, and longissimus are collectively known as the erector spinae. *Note:* The iliocostalis and longissimus extend the entire spine. The spinalis acts only on the cervical and thoracic spines.

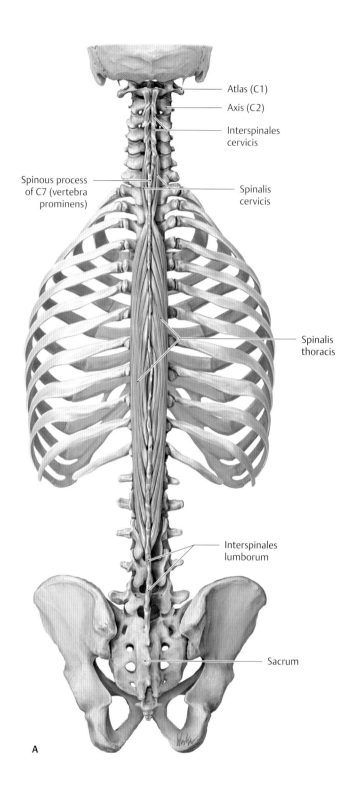

Atlas (C1)

Axis (C2)

Interspinales
cervicis

Spinous process
of C7 (vertebra
prominens)

Spinalis
cervicis

Spinalis
thoracis

Interspinales
lumborum

Sacrum

A

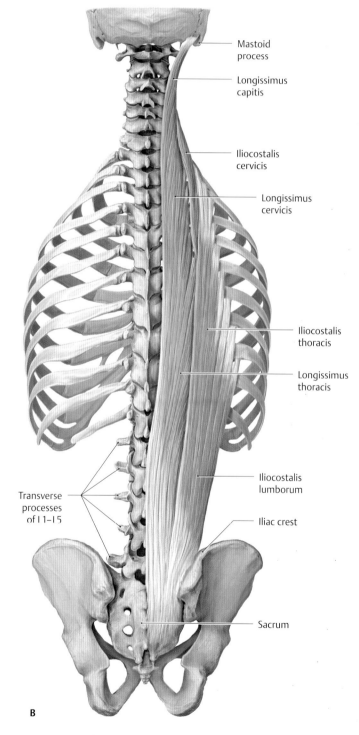

Mastoid
process

Longissimus
capitis

Iliocostalis
cervicis

Longissimus
cervicis

Iliocostalis
thoracis

Longissimus
thoracis

Iliocostalis
lumborum

Iliac crest

Transverse
processes
of L1–L5

Sacrum

B

*Fig. 10.27* **Interspinales and erector spinae muscles**
The spinalis, iliocostalis, and longissimus are collectively known as the
erector spinae.
**A** Interspinales and spinalis. **B** Iliocostalis and longissimus.

# Intrinsic Back Muscles (II)

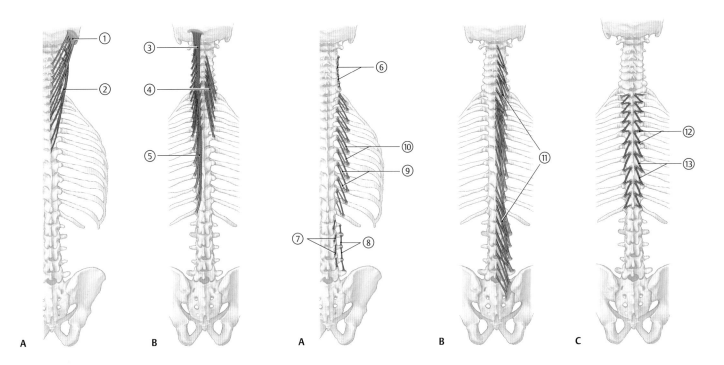

*Fig. 10.28* **Splenius and semispinalis**
A Splenius. **B** Semispinalis.

*Fig. 10.29* **Intertransversarii, levatores costarum, multifidus, and rotatores**
A Intertransversarii and levatores costarum. **B** Multifidus. **C** Rotatores.

| Table 10.6 Splenius, semispinalis, intertransversarii, levatores costarum, multifidus, and rotatores |||||
|---|---|---|---|---|
| All intrinsic back muscles are innervated by the dorsal rami of the spinal nerves. The splenius is innervated by spinal nerves C1–C6. |||||
| **Muscle** || **Origin** | **Insertion** | **Action** |
| Splenius | ① S. capitis | C3–T3 (spinous processes) | Occipital bone (lateral superior nuchal line; mastoid process) | *Bilateral:* Extends cervical spine and head<br>*Unilateral:* Flexes and rotates head to same side |
| | ② S. cervicis | T3–T6 (spinous processes) | C1–C2 (transverse processes) | |
| Semispinalis | ③ S. capitis | C2–C7 (transverse processes) | Occipital bone (between superior and inferior nuchal lines) | *Bilateral:* Extends spine and head (stabilizes craniovertebral joints)<br>*Unilateral:* Bends head and spine to same side, rotates to opposite side |
| | ④ S. cervicis | T1–T6 (transverse processes) | C2–C7 (spinous processes) | |
| | ⑤ S. thoracis | T6–T12 (transverse processes) | C6–T4 (spinous processes) | |
| Inter-transversarii | I. anteriores cervicis | C2–C7 (between anterior tubercles of adjacent vertebrae) || *Bilateral:* Stabilizes and extends spine<br>*Unilateral:* Bends spine laterally to same side |
| | ⑥ I. posteriores cervicis | C2–C7 (between posterior tubercles of adjacent vertebrae) || |
| | ⑦ I. mediales lumborum | L1–L5 (between mammillary processes of adjacent vertebrae) || |
| | ⑧ I. laterales lumborum | L1–L5 (between transverse processes of adjacent vertebrae) || |
| Levatores costarum | ⑨ L.c. breves | C7–T11 (transverse processes) | Costal angle of next lower rib | *Bilateral:* Extends thoracic spine<br>*Unilateral:* Bends thoracic spine to same side, rotates to opposite side |
| | ⑩ L.c. longi | | Costal angle of rib to vertebrae below | |
| ⑪ Multifidus || C2–sacrum (between transverse and spinous processes, skipping two to four vertebrae) || *Bilateral:* Extends spine<br>*Unilateral:* Flexes spine to same side, rotates to opposite side |
| Rotatores | ⑫ R. brevis | T1–T12 (between transverse and spinous processes of adjacent vertebrae) || *Bilateral:* Extends thoracic spine<br>*Unilateral:* Rotates spine to opposite side |
| | ⑬ R. longi | T1–T12 (between transverse and spinous processes, skipping one vertebra) || |

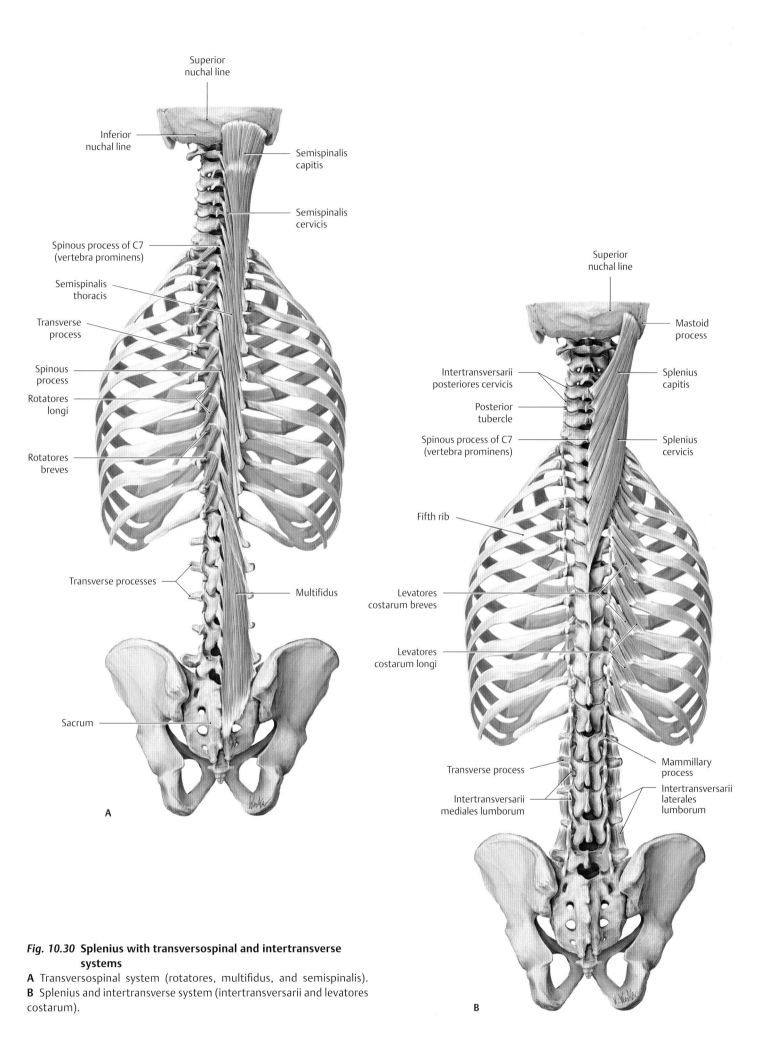

Superior
nuchal line

Inferior
nuchal line

Semispinalis
capitis

Semispinalis
cervicis

Spinous process of C7
(vertebra prominens)

Semispinalis
thoracis

Transverse
process

Spinous
process

Rotatores
longi

Rotatores
breves

Transverse processes

Multifidus

Sacrum

**A**

Superior
nuchal line

Intertransversarii
posteriores cervicis

Posterior
tubercle

Spinous process of C7
(vertebra prominens)

Fifth rib

Levatores
costarum breves

Levatores
costarum longi

Transverse process

Intertransversarii
mediales lumborum

Mastoid
process

Splenius
capitis

Splenius
cervicis

Mammillary
process

Intertransversarii
laterales
lumborum

**B**

*Fig. 10.30* **Splenius with transversospinal and intertransverse systems**
**A** Transversospinal system (rotatores, multifidus, and semispinalis).
**B** Splenius and intertransverse system (intertransversarii and levatores costarum).

# Intrinsic Back Muscles (III): Short Nuchal Muscles

### Fig. 10.31 Short nuchal muscles

Posterior view. The short nuchal muscles are intrinsic back muscles that are innervated by the dorsal ramus of the first spinal nerve (suboccipital nerve). These muscles contribute to the extension of the atlanto-occipital joint and rotation about the atlantoaxial joint.

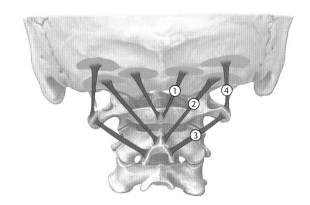

| Table 10.7 Short nuchal muscles | | | | | |
|---|---|---|---|---|---|
| **Muscle** | | **Origin** | **Insertion** | **Innervation** | **Action** |
| Rectii capitis posterioris | ① R.c.p. minor | C1 (posterior tubercle) | Inferior nuchal line (inner ⅓) | C1 spinal nerve (suboccipital n.), dorsal ramus | *Bilateral:* Extends head<br>*Unilateral:* Rotates head to same side |
| | ② R.c.p. major | C2 (spinous process) | Inferior nuchal line (middle ⅓) | | |
| Obliquii capitis | ③ O.c. inferior | C2 (spinous process) | C1 (transverse process) | | |
| | ④ O.c. superior | C1 (transverse process) | Above the insertion of the rectus capitis posterior major | | *Bilateral:* Extends head<br>*Unilateral:* Tilts head to same side; rotates head to opposite side |

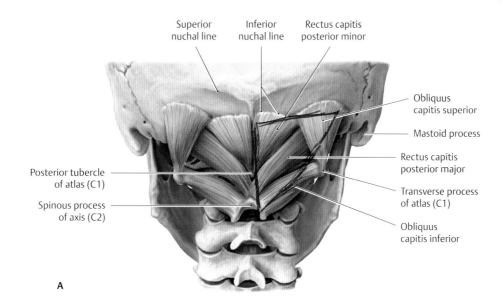

Superior nuchal line | Inferior nuchal line | Rectus capitis posterior minor

Obliquus capitis superior

Mastoid process

Posterior tubercle of atlas (C1)

Spinous process of axis (C2)

Rectus capitis posterior major

Transverse process of atlas (C1)

Obliquus capitis inferior

**A**

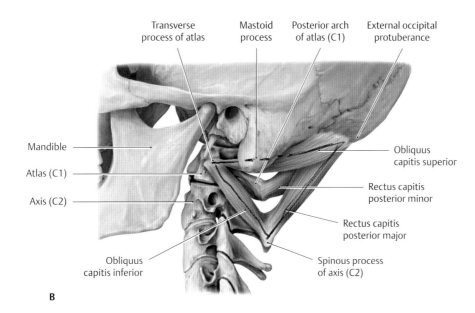

Transverse process of atlas | Mastoid process | Posterior arch of atlas (C1) | External occipital protuberance

Mandible

Atlas (C1)

Axis (C2)

Obliquus capitis superior

Rectus capitis posterior minor

Rectus capitis posterior major

Obliquus capitis inferior

Spinous process of axis (C2)

**B**

*Fig. 10.32* **Suboccipital muscles**
**A** Posterior view. **B** Left lateral view.
The suboccipital muscles collectively act on the craniovertebral joints. The suboccipital muscles are the rectus capitis posterior major, rectus capitis posterior minor, obliquus capitis inferior, and obliquus capitis superior. The dorsal ramus of the first cervical spinal nerve innervates all four suboccipital muscles. *Note:* The suboccipital triangle is located between the rectus capitis posterior major, the obliquus capitis superior, and the obliquus capitis inferior.

Suboccipital triangle has — the four Nuchal muscles
— Suboccipital N (motor only)
— vertebral A. & V.

# Prevertebral & Scalene Muscles

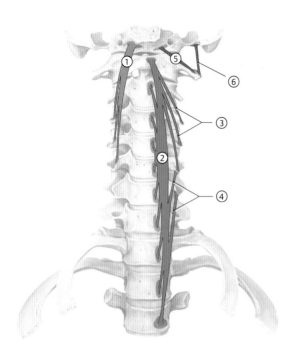

**Fig. 10.33 Prevertebral muscles**
Anterior view.

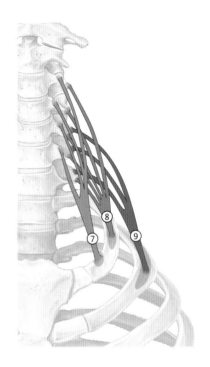

**Fig. 10.34 Scalene muscles**
Anterior view.

| Table 10.8 Prevertebral and scalene muscles | | | | |
|---|---|---|---|---|
| **Muscle** | | **Origin** | **Insertion** | **Innervation** | **Action** |
| ① Longus capitis | | C3–C6 (anterior tubercles) | Occipital bone, basilar part | Cervical plexus, direct branches (C1–C3) | *Bilateral:* Flexes head *Unilateral:* Tilts and slightly rotates head to same side |
| Longus colli | ② Vertical (intermediate) part | C5–T3 (anterior surfaces of vertebral bodies) | C2–C4 (anterior surfaces) | Cervical plexus, direct branches (C2–C6) | *Bilateral:* Flexes cervical spine *Unilateral:* Tilts and slightly rotates cervical spine to same side |
| | ③ Superior oblique part | C3–C5 (anterior tubercles) | C1 (anterior tubercle) | | |
| | ④ Inferior oblique part | T1–T3 (anterior surfaces of vertebral bodies) | C5–C6 (anterior tubercles) | | |
| Rectus capitis | ⑤ R.c. anterior | C1 (lateral mass) | Occipital bone (basilar part) | Ventral ramus of C1 spinal n. (suboccipital n.) | *Bilateral:* Flexion at atlanto-occipital joint *Unilateral:* Lateral flexion at atlanto-occipital joint |
| | ⑥ R.c. lateralis | C1 (transverse process) | Occipital bone (basilar part, lateral to occipital condyles) | | |
| Scalenes | ⑦ S. anterior | C3–C6 (anterior tubercles) | 1st rib (scalene tubercle) | Ventral rami of cervical spinal nn. | *With ribs mobile:* Inspiration (elevate upper ribs) *With ribs fixed:* Bend cervical spine to same side (unilateral contraction); flex cervical spine (bilateral contraction) |
| | ⑧ S. medius | C1 and C2 (transverse processes); C3–C7 (posterior tubercles) | 1st rib (posterior to groove for subclavian a.) | | |
| | ⑨ S. posterior | C5–C7 (posterior tubercles) | 2nd rib (outer surface) | | |

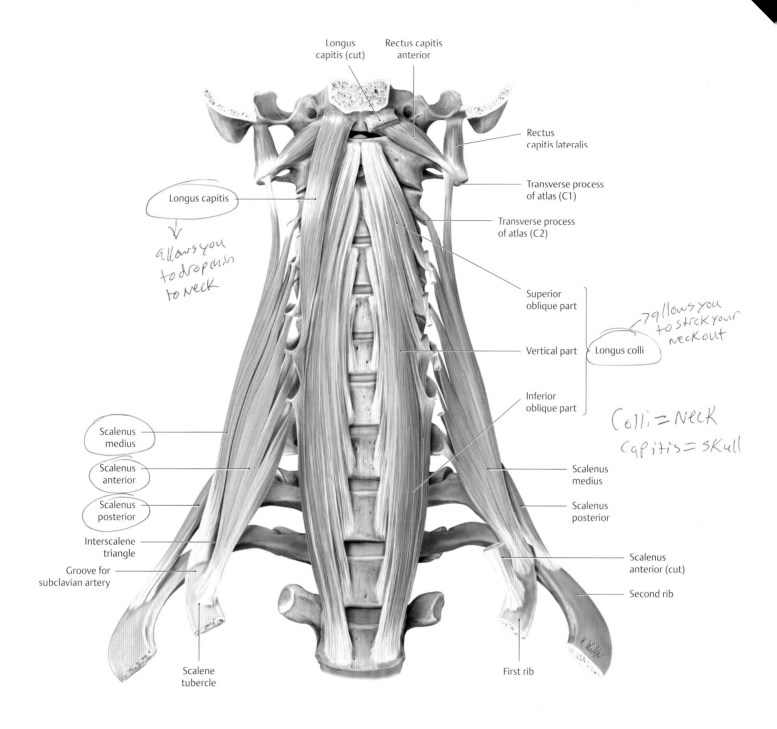

**Fig. 10.35 Anterior vertebral (prevertebral) and lateral vertebral muscles**

Anterior view. *Removed on left side:* Longus capitis and anterior scalene. The anterior vertebral muscles are the longus colli, longus capitis, rec-

tus capitis lateralis, and rectus capitis anterior. The lateral vertebral muscles are the anterior, middle, and posterior scalenes. The anterior and lateral vertebral muscles are innervated by the ventral rami of the cervical spinal nerves.

Labels in figure:
- Longus capitis (cut)
- Rectus capitis anterior
- Rectus capitis lateralis
- Transverse process of atlas (C1)
- Transverse process of atlas (C2)
- Superior oblique part
- Vertical part
- Longus colli
- Inferior oblique part
- Scalenus medius
- Scalenus posterior
- Scalenus anterior (cut)
- Second rib
- First rib
- Scalenus medius
- Scalenus anterior
- Scalenus posterior
- Interscalene triangle
- Groove for subclavian artery
- Scalene tubercle
- Longus capitis

Handwritten notes:
- Longus capitis → allows you to drop chin to neck
- Longus colli → allows you to stick your neck out
- Colli = Neck
- Capitis = skull

253

# Suprahyoid & Infrahyoid Muscles

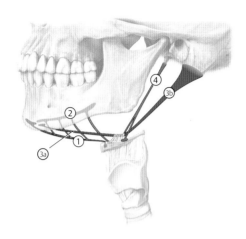

**Fig. 10.36 Suprahyoid muscles**
Left lateral view.

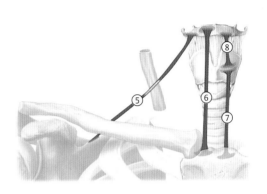

**Fig. 10.37 Infrahyoid muscles**
Anterior view.

| Table 10.9 Suprahyoid and infrahyoid muscles | | | | |
|---|---|---|---|---|
| **Muscle** | **Origin** | **Insertion** | **Innervation** | **Action** |
| ① Geniohyoid | Mandible (inferior genial spine) | Hyoid bone | Ventral ramus of C1 via CN XII** | Draws hyoid bone forward (during swallowing); assists in opening mandible |
| ② Mylohyoid | Mandible (mylohyoid line) | Hyoid bone (via median tendon of insertion, the mylohyoid raphe) | Mylohyoid n. (from CN V₃) | Tightens and elevates oral floor; draws hyoid bone forward (during swallowing); assists in opening mandible and moving it side to side (mastication) |
| ③ª Digastric, anterior belly | Mandible (digastric fossa) | Hyoid bone (via an intermediate tendon with a fibrous loop) | Facial n. (CN VII) | Elevates hyoid bone (during swallowing); assists in depressing mandible |
| ③ᵇ Digastric, posterior belly | Temporal bone (mastoid notch, medial to mastoid process) | | | |
| ④ Stylohyoid | Temporal bone (styloid process) | Hyoid bone (via a split tendon) | | |
| ⑤ Omohyoid, inferior belly | Scapula (superior border, medial to suprascapular notch) | Hyoid bone | Ansa cervicalis of cervical plexus (C1–C3) | Depresses (fixes) hyoid; draws larynx and hyoid down for phonation and terminal phases of swallowing* |
| ⑥ Sternohyoid | Manubrium and sternoclavicular joint (posterior surface) | | | |
| ⑦ Sternothyroid | Manubrium (posterior surface) | Thyroid cartilage (oblique line) | | |
| ⑧ Thyrohyoid | Thyroid cartilage (oblique line) | Hyoid bone | Ventral ramus of C1 via CN XII | Depresses and fixes hyoid; raises the larynx during swallowing |

*The omohyoid also tenses the cervical fascia (with an intermediate tendon). The intermediate tendon is attached to the clavicle, pulling the omohyoid into a more pronounced triangle.

**C1 ventral ramus fibers travel with the hypoglossal nerve for part of its pathway to target muscles.

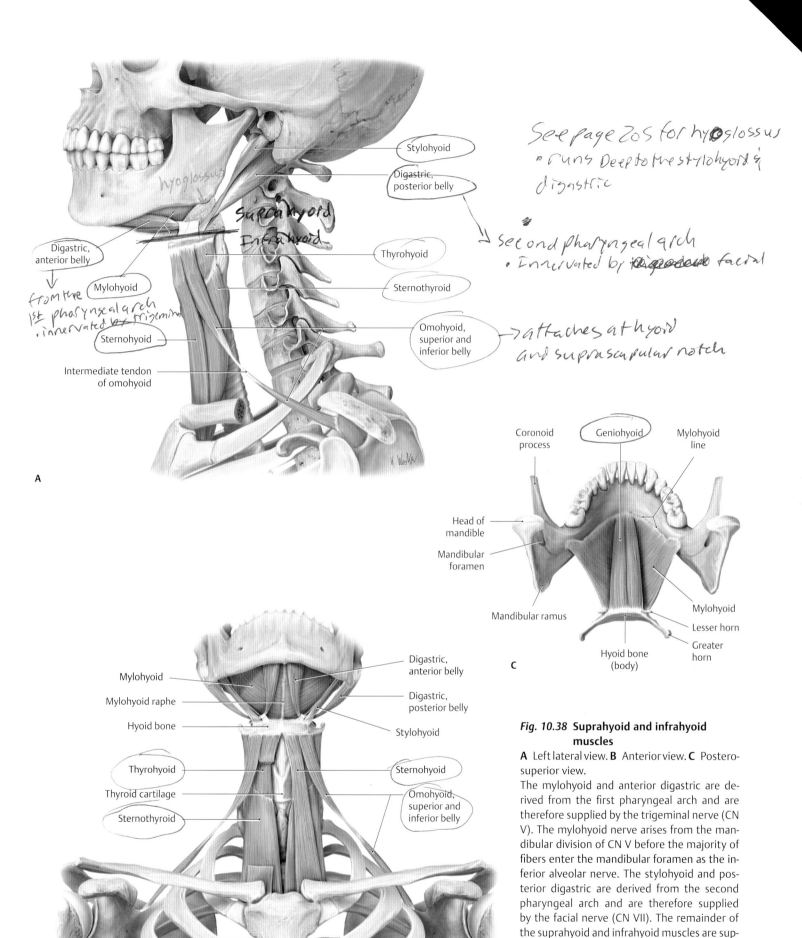

*Handwritten notes:*

See page 205 for hyoglossus
• runs Deep to the stylohyoid & digastric

→ second pharyngeal arch
• Innervated by ~~the second~~ facial

→ attaches at hyoid
and suprascapular notch

hyoglossus

Suprahyoid
Infrahyoid

from the
1st pharyngeal arch
• innervated by trigeminal

**A** (Left lateral view labels):
- Stylohyoid
- Digastric, posterior belly
- Thyrohyoid
- Sternothyroid
- Omohyoid, superior and inferior belly
- Digastric, anterior belly
- Mylohyoid
- Sternohyoid
- Intermediate tendon of omohyoid

**B** (Anterior view labels):
- Mylohyoid
- Mylohyoid raphe
- Hyoid bone
- Thyrohyoid
- Thyroid cartilage
- Sternothyroid
- Digastric, anterior belly
- Digastric, posterior belly
- Stylohyoid
- Sternohyoid
- Omohyoid, superior and inferior belly

**C** (Posterosuperior view labels):
- Coronoid process
- Geniohyoid
- Mylohyoid line
- Head of mandible
- Mandibular foramen
- Mandibular ramus
- Mylohyoid
- Lesser horn
- Greater horn
- Hyoid bone (body)

**Fig. 10.38 Suprahyoid and infrahyoid muscles**

**A** Left lateral view. **B** Anterior view. **C** Postero-superior view.

The mylohyoid and anterior digastric are derived from the first pharyngeal arch and are therefore supplied by the trigeminal nerve (CN V). The mylohyoid nerve arises from the mandibular division of CN V before the majority of fibers enter the mandibular foramen as the inferior alveolar nerve. The stylohyoid and posterior digastric are derived from the second pharyngeal arch and are therefore supplied by the facial nerve (CN VII). The remainder of the suprahyoid and infrahyoid muscles are supplied by the ventral rami of the cervical spinal nerves. Fibers from the ventral ramus of C1 travel with the hypoglossal nerve (CN XII) to the geniohyoid and thyrohyoid. Fibers from the ventral rami of C1–C3 combine to form the ansa cervicalis, which gives off branches to the omohyoid, sternohyoid, and sternothyroid.

**255**

# Larynx

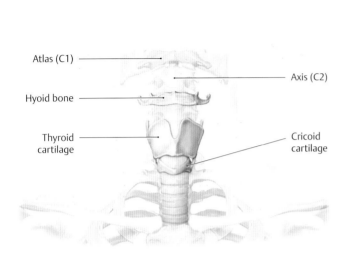

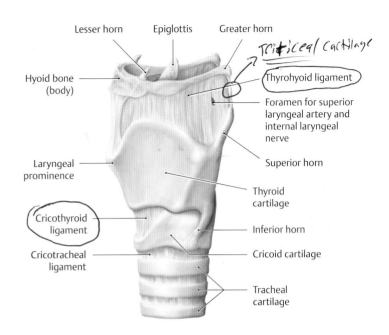

## Fig. 11.1 Location of the larynx

Anterior view. The bony structures of the neck have characteristic vertebral levels (shown for upright adult male):

- Hyoid bone: C3
- Thyroid cartilage (superior border): C4
- Laryngotracheal junction: C6–C7

These structures are a half vertebra higher in women and children. The thyroid cartilage is especially prominent in males, forming the laryngeal prominence ("Adam's apple").

## Fig. 11.2 Larynx: overview

Oblique left anterolateral view. The larynx consists of five cartilages: two external cartilages (thyroid and cricoid) and three internal cartilages (epiglottic, arytenoid, and corniculate). Elastic ligaments connect these cartilages to each other as well as to the trachea and hyoid bone. This allows laryngeal motion during swallowing. The thyroid, cricoid, and arytenoid cartilages are hyaline, and the epiglottis and corniculate cartilages are elastic fibrocartilage.

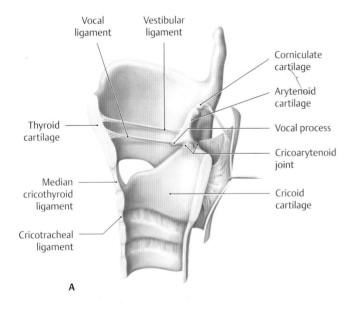

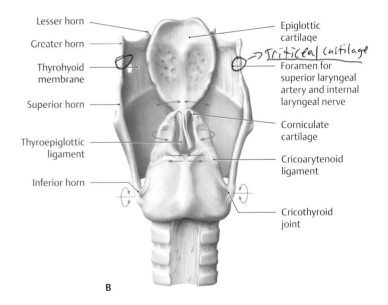

## Fig. 11.3 Laryngeal cartilages and ligaments

**A** Left medial view of sagittal section. **B** Posterior view. Arrows indicate movement in the various joints.

The large thyroid cartilage encloses most of the other cartilages. It articulates with the cricoid cartilage inferiorly at the paired crico-

thyroid joints, allowing it to tilt relative to the cricoid cartilage. The arytenoid cartilages move during phonation: their bases can translate or rotate relative to the cricoid cartilage at the cricoarytenoid joint.

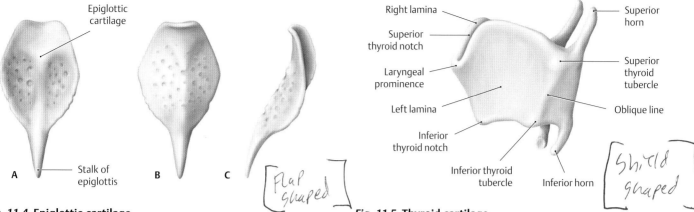

*Fig. 11.4* **Epiglottic cartilage**
**A** Laryngeal (posteroinferior) view. **B** Lingual (anterosuperior) view.
**C** Left lateral view.
The elastic epiglottic cartilage regulates the entrance of material into the larynx. During breathing, it is angled posterosuperiorly, allowing air to enter the larynx and trachea. During swallowing, the larynx is elevated relative to the hyoid bone. The epiglottis assumes a more horizontal position, preventing food from entering the airway.

*Fig. 11.5* **Thyroid cartilage**
Oblique left lateral view. The hyaline thyroid cartilage consists of two quadrilateral plates (laminae) that are joined at the anterior midline. The superior portion of this junction is the laryngeal prominence ("Adam's apple"). The posterior ends of the laminae are prolonged forming the superior and inferior horns, which serve as anchors for ligaments.

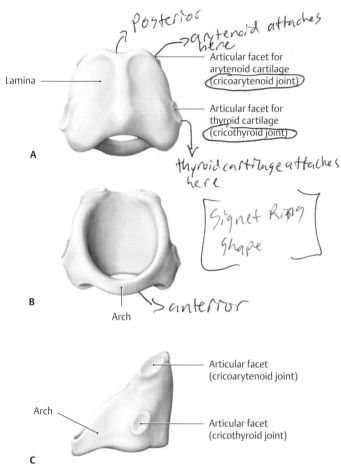

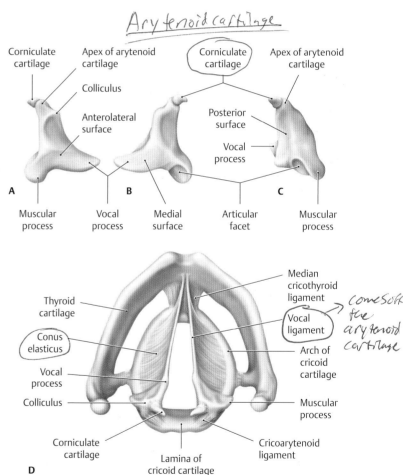

*Fig. 11.6* **Cricoid cartilage**
**A** Posterior view. **B** Anterior view. **C** Left lateral view. The hyaline cricoid cartilage is a ring that is connected inferiorly to the highest tracheal cartilage by the cricotracheal ligament. The cricoid ring is expanded posteriorly to form a lamina. The laminae each have an upper and lower articular facet for the arytenoid cartilage (cricoarytenoid joint) and thyroid cartilage (cricothyroid joint), respectively.

*Fig. 11.7* **Arytenoid and corniculate cartilages**
Right cartilages. **A** Right lateral view. **B** Left lateral (medial) view.
**C** Posterior view. **D** Superior view.
The arytenoid cartilages alter the positions of the vocal cords during phonation. The pyramid-shaped hyaline cartilages have three surfaces (anterolateral, medial, and posterior), an apex, and a base with vocal and muscular processes. The apex articulates with the tiny corniculate cartilages, which are composed of elastic fibrocartilage.

# Laryngeal Muscles

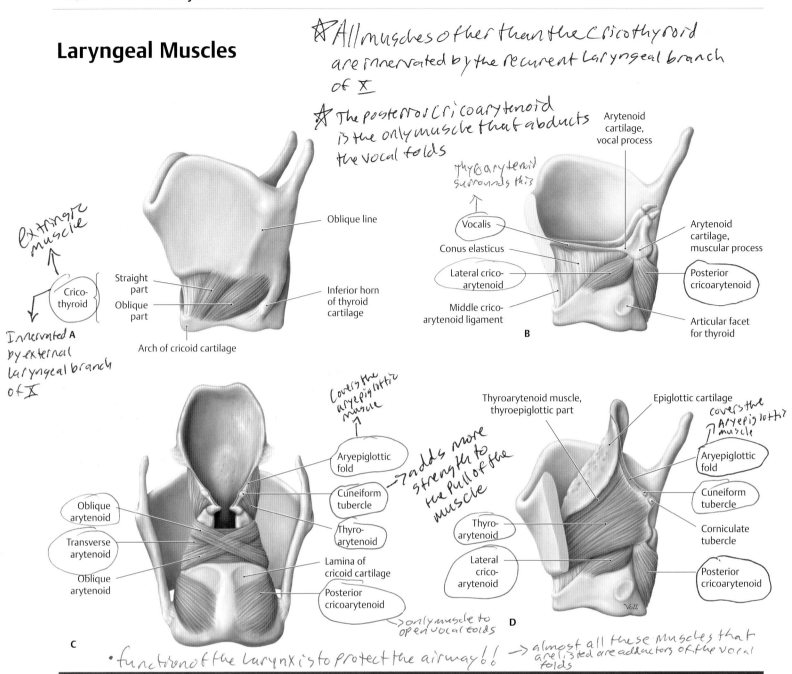

Handwritten notes:

★ All muscles other than the cricothyroid are innervated by the recurrent laryngeal branch of X

★ The posterior cricoarytenoid is the only muscle that abducts the vocal folds

Extrinsic muscle → Crico-thyroid → Innervated by external laryngeal branch of X

**A** — Oblique line, Straight part, Oblique part, Arch of cricoid cartilage, Inferior horn of thyroid cartilage

**B** — Thyroarytenoid surrounds this, Vocalis, Conus elasticus, Lateral crico-arytenoid, Middle crico-arytenoid ligament, Arytenoid cartilage, vocal process, Arytenoid cartilage, muscular process, Posterior cricoarytenoid, Articular facet for thyroid

**C** — covers the aryepiglottic muscle, Aryepiglottic fold, Cuneiform tubercle, Thyro-arytenoid, Oblique arytenoid, Transverse arytenoid, Oblique arytenoid, Lamina of cricoid cartilage, Posterior cricoarytenoid (→ only muscle to open vocal folds), adds more strength to the pull of the muscle

• function of the larynx is to protect the airway!!

**D** — Thyroarytenoid muscle, thyroepiglottic part, Epiglottic cartilage, covers the Aryepiglottic muscle, Aryepiglottic fold, Cuneiform tubercle, Corniculate tubercle, Thyro-arytenoid, Lateral crico-arytenoid, Posterior cricoarytenoid

→ almost all these muscles that are listed are adductors of the vocal folds

## Table 11.1 Laryngeal muscles

The laryngeal muscles move the laryngeal cartilages relative to one another and affect the tension and/or position of the vocal folds. Numerous muscles move the larynx as a whole (infrahyoids, suprahyoids, pharyngeal constrictors, stylopharyngeus, etc.).

| Muscle | Innervation | Action | Vocal folds | Rima glottidis |
|---|---|---|---|---|
| Posterior cricoarytenoid | Recurrent laryngeal n.** | Rotates arytenoid cartilage outward and slightly to the side | Abducts | Opens |
| Lateral cricoarytenoid* | | Rotates arytenoid cartilage inward | Adducts | Closes |
| Transverse arytenoid | | Moves arytenoids toward each other | | |
| Thyroarytenoid | | Rotates arytenoid cartilage inward | Relaxes | Closes |
| Vocalis*** | | Regulates tension of vocal folds | Tightens | None |
| Cricothyroid | External laryngeal n. | Tilts cricoid cartilage posteriorly, acting on the vocalis muscle to increase tension in the vocal folds | | |

*The lateral cricoarytenoid is called the muscle of phonation as it initiates speech production.

**Unilateral loss of the recurrent laryngeal nerve (e.g., due to nodal metastases from a hilar bronchial carcinoma of the left lung) leads to ipsilateral palsy of the posterior cricoarytenoid. This prevents complete abduction of the vocal folds, causing hoarseness. Bilateral nerve loss (e.g., due to thyroid surgery) may cause asphyxiation.

***The vocalis is derived from the inferior fibers of the thyroarytenoid muscle. These fibers connect the arytenoid cartilage with the vocal ligament.

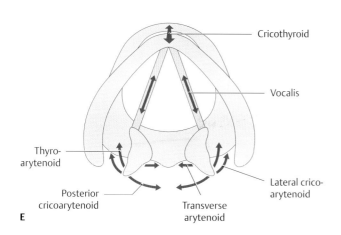

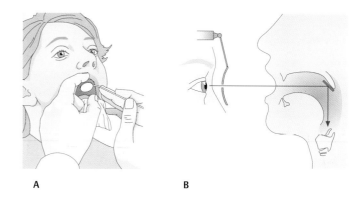

A                              B

## Fig. 11.8 Laryngeal muscles

**A** Left lateral oblique view of extrinsic laryngeal muscles. **B** Left lateral view of intrinsic laryngeal muscles (left thyroid lamina and epiglottis removed). **C** Posterior view. **D** Left lateral view. **E** Actions (arrows indicate directions of pull).

## Fig. 11.9 Indirect laryngoscopy

**A** **Mirror examination of the larynx** from the perspective of the examiner. The larynx is not accessible to direct inspection but can be viewed with the aid of a small mirror. The examiner depresses the tongue with one hand while introducing the laryngeal mirror (or endoscope) with the other hand.

**A** Optical path: The laryngeal mirror is held in front of the uvula, directing light from the examiner's head mirror down toward the larynx. The image seen by the examiner is shown in **Fig. 11.10**.

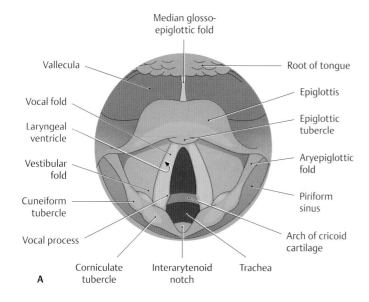

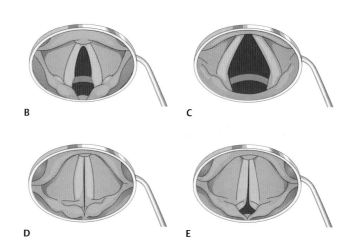

## Fig. 11.10 Indirect laryngoscopy

**A** Laryngoscopic mirror image. **B** Normal respiration. **C** Vigorous respiration. **D** Phonation position (vocal folds completely adducted). **E** Whispered speech (vocal folds slightly abducted).

Indirect laryngoscopy produces a virtual image of the larynx in which the right vocal fold appears on the right side of the mirror image and anterior structures (e.g., tongue base, valleculae, and epiglottis) appear at the top of the image. The vocal folds appear as smooth-edged bands (there are no blood vessels or submucosa below the stratified, nonkeratinized squamous epithelium of the vocal folds). They are therefore markedly lighter than the highly vascularized surrounding mucosa. The glottis can be evaluated in closed (respiratory) and opened (phonation) position by having the patient alternately inhale and sing "hee." The clinician can then determine pathoanatomical changes (e.g., redness, swelling, and ulceration) and functional changes (e.g., to vocal fold position).

# Larynx: Neurovasculature

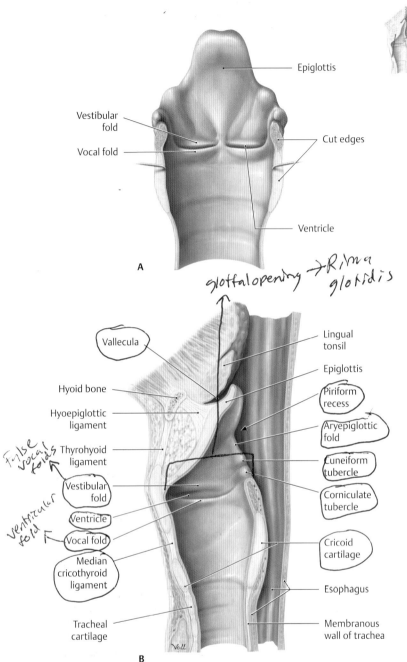

*handwritten:* glottal opening → Rima glotidis

*handwritten labels on figure B (left margin):* False vocal folds; Ventricular fold

**A**

**B**

**Fig. 11.11 Laryngeal mucosa**
**A** Posterior view with pharynx and esophagus cut along the midline and spread open. **B** Left lateral view of midsagittal section. **C** Posterior view with laryngeal levels.
The larynx lies anterior to the laryngopharynx. Air enters through the laryngeal inlet formed by the epiglottis and aryepiglottic folds. Lateral to the aryepiglottic folds are pear-shaped mucosal fossae (piriform recesses), which channel food past the larynx and into the laryngopharynx and on into the esophagus. The interior of the larynx is lined with mucous membrane that is loosely applied to its underlying tissue (except at the vocal folds). The laryngeal cavity can be further subdivided with respect to the vestibular and vocal folds (**Table 11.2**).

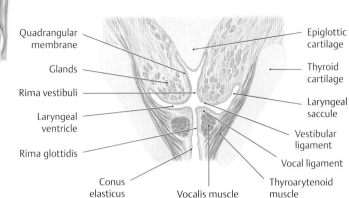

**Fig. 11.12 Vestibular and vocal folds**
Coronal section. The vestibular and vocal folds are the mucosal coverings of underlying ligaments. The vocal folds ("vocal cords") contain the vocal ligament and vocalis muscle. The fissure between the vocal folds is the rima glottidis (glottis). The vestibular folds ("false vocal cords") are superior to the vocal folds. They contain the vestibular ligament, the free inferior end of the quadrangular membrane. The fissure between the vestibular folds is the rima vestibuli, which is broader than the rima glottidis. *Note:* The loose connective tissue of the laryngeal inlet may become markedly swollen (e.g., insect bite, inflammatory process), obstructing the rima vestibuli. This laryngeal edema (often incorrectly called "glottic edema") presents clinically with dyspnea and poses an asphyxiation risk.

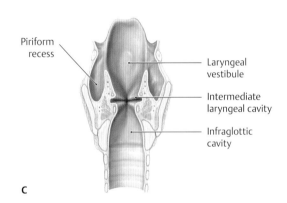

**C**

**Table 11.2 Divisions of the laryngeal cavity**

| Laryngeal level | Boundaries |
| --- | --- |
| I: Laryngeal vestibule (supraglottic space) | Laryngeal inlet (aditus laryngis) to vestibular folds |
| II: Intermediate laryngeal cavity (transglottic space) | Vestibular folds across the laryngeal ventricle (lateral evagination of mucosa) to vocal folds |
| III: Infraglottic cavity (subglottic space) | Vocal folds to inferior border of cricoid cartilage |

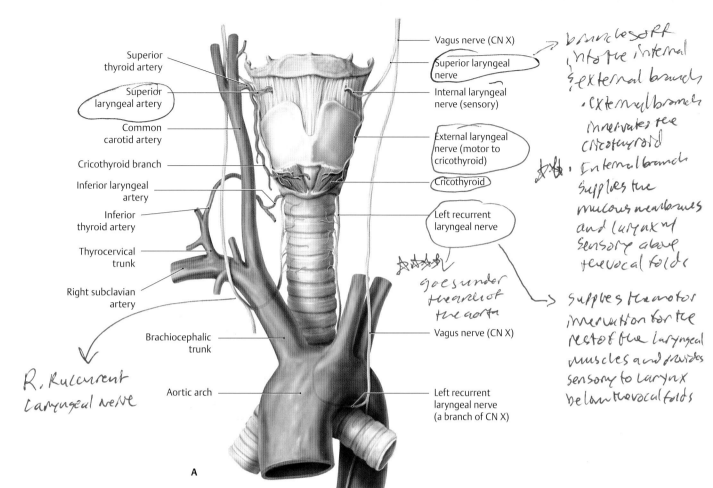

Vagus nerve (CN X)

Superior thyroid artery

Superior laryngeal nerve

Superior laryngeal artery

Internal laryngeal nerve (sensory)

Common carotid artery

External laryngeal nerve (motor to cricothyroid)

Cricothyroid branch

Cricothyroid

Inferior laryngeal artery

Inferior thyroid artery

Left recurrent laryngeal nerve

Thyrocervical trunk

Right subclavian artery

Brachiocephalic trunk

Vagus nerve (CN X)

Aortic arch

Left recurrent laryngeal nerve (a branch of CN X)

**A**

*Handwritten notes:*
- branches off into the internal & external branch
- external branch innervates the cricothyroid
- N.B. Internal branch supplies the mucous membrane and larynx my sensory above the vocal folds
- goes under the arch of the aorta
- supplies the motor innervation for the rest of the laryngeal muscles and provides sensory to larynx below the vocal folds
- R. Recurrent laryngeal nerve

**Fig. 11.13 Laryngeal blood vessels and nerves**

**A** Arteries and nerves, anterior view. **B** Veins, left lateral view.

**Arteries:** The larynx derives its blood supply primarily from the superior and inferior laryngeal arteries. The superior laryngeal artery arises from the superior thyroid artery (a branch of the external carotid artery). The inferior laryngeal artery arises from the inferior thyroid artery (a branch of the thyrocervical trunk).

**Nerves:** The larynx is innervated by the superior laryngeal nerve and the recurrent laryngeal nerve (of the vagus nerve). The superior laryngeal nerve splits into an internal (sensory) and an external (motor) laryngeal nerve. The external laryngeal nerve innervates the cricothyroid. The remaining intrinsic laryngeal muscles receive motor innervation from the recurrent laryngeal nerve, which branches from the vagus nerve below the larynx and ascends. *Note:* The left recurrent laryngeal nerve wraps around the aortic arch, and the right recurrent laryngeal nerve wraps around the subclavian artery. A left-sided aortic aneurysm may cause left recurrent laryngeal nerve palsy, resulting in hoarseness (see p. 263).

**Veins:** The larynx is drained by a superior and an inferior laryngeal vein. The superior laryngeal vein drains to the internal jugular vein (via the superior thyroid vein); the inferior laryngeal vein drains to the left brachiocephalic vein (via the thyroid venous plexus to the inferior thyroid vein).

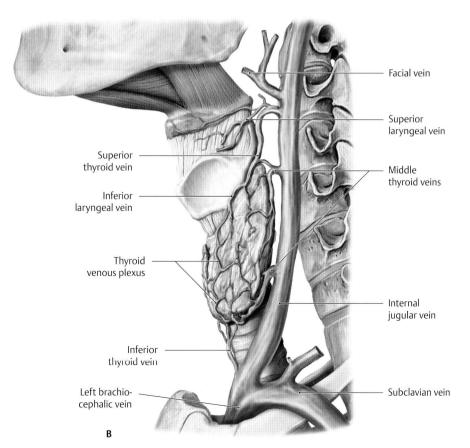

Facial vein

Superior laryngeal vein

Superior thyroid vein

Middle thyroid veins

Inferior laryngeal vein

Thyroid venous plexus

Internal jugular vein

Inferior thyroid vein

Left brachiocephalic vein

Subclavian vein

**B**

# Larynx: Topography

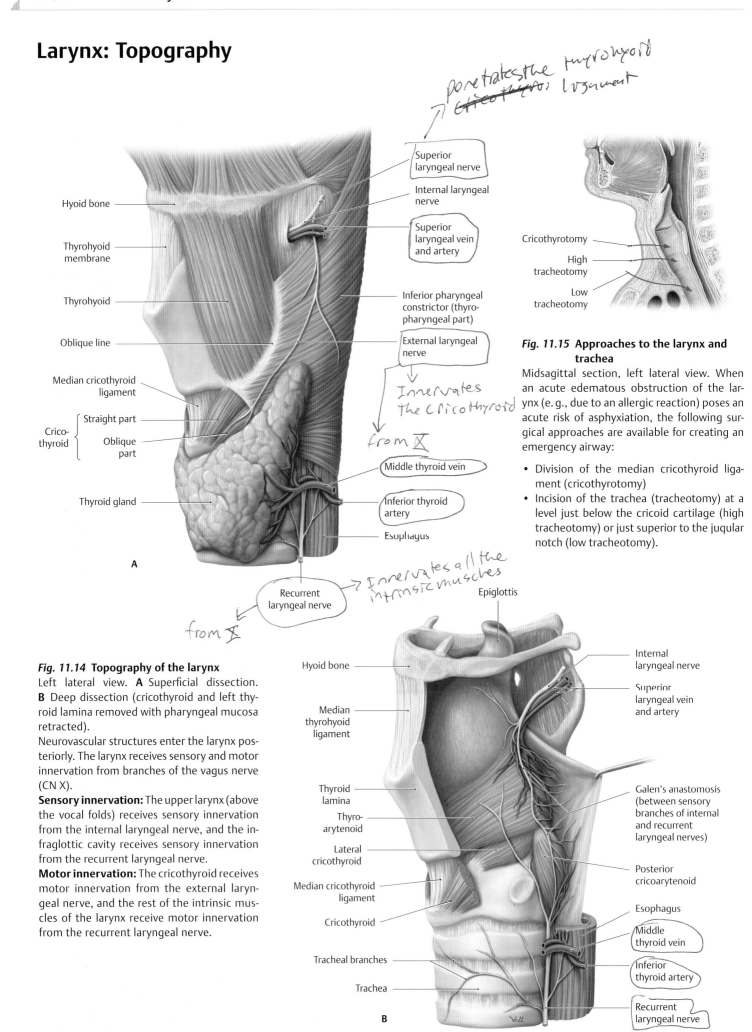

Handwritten notes on figure:
- *penetrates the thyrohyoid / cricothyroid ligament*
- *Innervates the Cricothyroid*
- *from X*
- *from X*
- *Innervates all the intrinsic muscles*

**Fig. 11.14 Topography of the larynx**
Left lateral view. **A** Superficial dissection.
**B** Deep dissection (cricothyroid and left thyroid lamina removed with pharyngeal mucosa retracted).
Neurovascular structures enter the larynx posteriorly. The larynx receives sensory and motor innervation from branches of the vagus nerve (CN X).
**Sensory innervation:** The upper larynx (above the vocal folds) receives sensory innervation from the internal laryngeal nerve, and the infraglottic cavity receives sensory innervation from the recurrent laryngeal nerve.
**Motor innervation:** The cricothyroid receives motor innervation from the external laryngeal nerve, and the rest of the intrinsic muscles of the larynx receive motor innervation from the recurrent laryngeal nerve.

**Fig. 11.15 Approaches to the larynx and trachea**
Midsagittal section, left lateral view. When an acute edematous obstruction of the larynx (e. g., due to an allergic reaction) poses an acute risk of asphyxiation, the following surgical approaches are available for creating an emergency airway:

- Division of the median cricothyroid ligament (cricothyrotomy)
- Incision of the trachea (tracheotomy) at a level just below the cricoid cartilage (high tracheotomy) or just superior to the jugular notch (low tracheotomy).

Labels in figure A: Hyoid bone; Thyrohyoid membrane; Thyrohyoid; Oblique line; Median cricothyroid ligament; Cricothyroid — Straight part, Oblique part; Thyroid gland; Superior laryngeal nerve; Internal laryngeal nerve; Superior laryngeal vein and artery; Inferior pharyngeal constrictor (thyropharyngeal part); External laryngeal nerve; Middle thyroid vein; Inferior thyroid artery; Esophagus; Recurrent laryngeal nerve

Labels in figure 11.15: Cricothyrotomy; High tracheotomy; Low tracheotomy

Labels in figure B: Epiglottis; Hyoid bone; Median thyrohyoid ligament; Thyroid lamina; Thyroarytenoid; Lateral cricothyroid; Median cricothyroid ligament; Cricothyroid; Tracheal branches; Trachea; Internal laryngeal nerve; Superior laryngeal vein and artery; Galen's anastomosis (between sensory branches of internal and recurrent laryngeal nerves); Posterior cricoarytenoid; Esophagus; Middle thyroid vein; Inferior thyroid artery; Recurrent laryngeal nerve

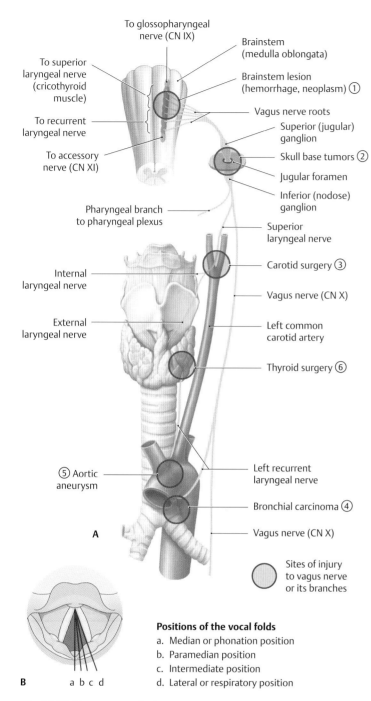

**A**

**B**     a b c d

**Positions of the vocal folds**
a. Median or phonation position
b. Paramedian position
c. Intermediate position
d. Lateral or respiratory position

**Fig. 11.16 Vagus nerve lesions**
The vagus nerve (CN X) provides branchiomotor innervation to the pharyngeal and laryngeal muscles and somatic sensory innervation to the larynx. *Note:* The vagus nerve also conveys parasympathetic motor fibers and visceral sensory fibers to and from the thoracic and abdominal viscera.
**Branchiomotor innervation:** The nucleus ambiguus contains the cell bodies of lower motor neurons whose branchiomotor fibers travel in CN IX, X, and XI. The nuclei of the vagus nerve are located in the middle region of the nucleus ambiguus in the brainstem (the cranial portions of the nucleus send axons via the glossopharyngeal nerve, and the caudal portions send axons via the accessory nerve). Fibers emerge from the middle portion of the nucleus ambiguus as roots and combine into CN X, which passes through the jugular foramen. Branchiomotor fibers are distributed to the pharyngeal plexus via the pharyngeal branch and the cricothyroid muscle via the external laryngeal nerve (a branch of the superior laryngeal nerve). The remaining branchiomotor fibers leave the vagus nerve as the recurrent laryngeal nerves, which ascend along the trachea to reach the larynx.
**Sensory innervation:** General somatic sensory fibers travel from the laryngeal mucosa to the spinal nucleus of the trigeminal nerve via the vagus nerve. The cell bodies of these primary sensory neurons are located in the inferior (nodose) ganglion. *Note:* The superior (jugular) ganglion contains the cell bodies of viscerosensory neurons.

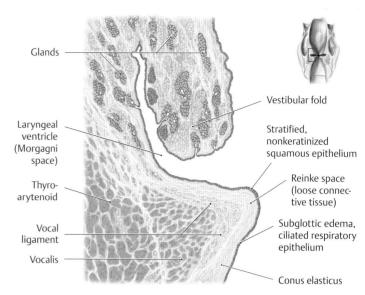

**Fig. 11.17 Vocal folds**
Schematic coronal histologic section, posterior view. The vocal fold, which is exposed to severe mechanical stresses, is covered by nonkeratinized squamous epithelium, unlike the adjacent subglottic space, which is covered by ciliated respiratory epithelium. The mucosa of the vocal folds and subglottic space overlies loose connective tissue. Chronic irritation of the subglottic mucosa (e.g., from cigarette smoke) may cause chronic edema in the subglottic space, resulting in a harsh voice. Degenerative changes in the vocal fold mucosa may lead to thickening, loss of elasticity, and squamous cell carcinoma.

| Table 11.3 Vagus nerve lesions | | |
|---|---|---|
| Lesions of the laryngeal nerves (**Fig. 11.16A**) may cause sensory loss or motor paralysis, which disrupts the position of the vocal folds (**Fig. 11.16B**). | | |
| **Level of nerve lesion and effects on vocal fold position** | | **Sensory loss** |
| ① Central lesion (brainstem or higher) | | |
| E.g., due to tumor or hemorrhage. Spastic paralysis (if nucleus ambiguus is disrupted), flaccid paralysis, and muscle atrophy (if motor neurons or axons are destroyed). | b,c | None |
| ② Skull base lesion* | | |
| E.g., due to nasopharyngeal tumors. Flaccid paralysis of all intrinsic and extrinsic laryngeal muscles on affected side. Glottis cannot be closed, causing severe hoarseness. | b,c | Entire affected side |
| ③ Superior laryngeal nerve lesions* | | |
| E.g., due to carotid surgery. Hypotonicity of the cricothyroid, resulting in mild hoarseness with a weak voice, especially at high frequencies. | d | Above vocal fold |
| Recurrent laryngeal nerve lesions** | | |
| E.g., due to bronchial carcinoma ④, aortic aneurysm ⑤, or thyroid surgery ⑥. Paralysis of all intrinsic laryngeal muscles on affected side. This results in mild hoarseness, poor tonal control, rapid voice fatigue, but not dyspnea. | a,b | Below vocal fold |

*Other motor deficits include drooping of the soft palate and deviation of the uvula toward the affected side, diminished gag and cough reflexes, difficulty swallowing (dysphagia), and hypernasal speech due to deficient closure of the pharyngeal isthmus. Sensory defects include the sensation of a foreign body in the throat.

**Transection of both recurrent laryngeal nerves can cause significant dyspnea and inspiratory stridor (high-pitched noise indicating obstruction), necessitating tracheotomy in acute cases.

# Thyroid & Parathyroid Glands

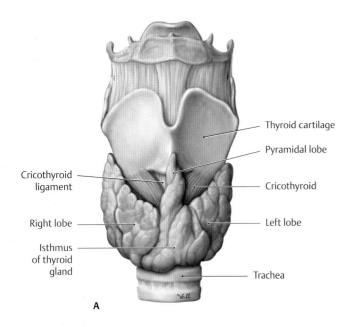

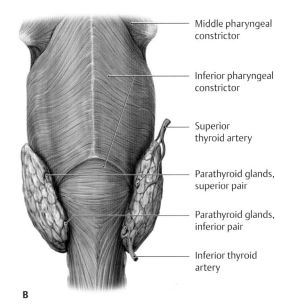

**A**

**B**

**Fig. 11.18 Thyroid and parathyroid glands**
**A** Anterior view. **B** Posterior view.
The thyroid gland consists of two laterally situated lobes and a central narrowing (isthmus). A pyramidal lobe may be found in place of the isthmus; the apex points to the embryonic origin of the thyroid at the base of the tongue (on occasion, a persistent thyroglossal duct may be present, connecting the pyramidal lobe with the foramen cecum of the tongue). The parathyroid glands (generally four in number) show considerable variation in number and location. *Note:* Because the parathyroid glands are usually contained within the thyroid capsule, there is considerable risk of inadvertently removing them during thyroid surgery.

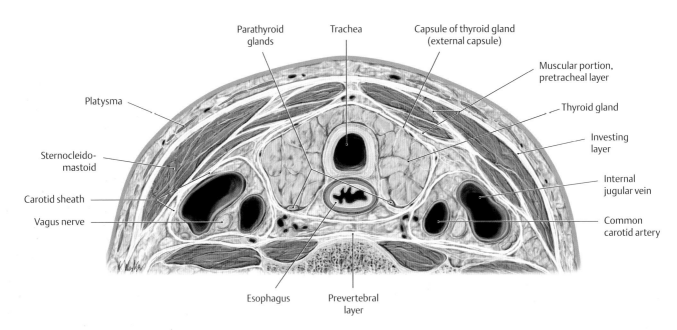

**Fig. 11.19 Topography of the thyroid gland**
Transverse section through the neck at the T 1 level, superior view. The thyroid gland partially surrounds the trachea and is bordered postero-laterally by the carotid sheath. When the thyroid gland is pathologically enlarged (e. g., due to iodine-deficiency goiter), it may gradually compress and narrow the tracheal lumen, causing respiratory distress.
The thyroid gland is surrounded by a fibrous capsule composed of an internal and external layer. The delicate internal layer (*internal capsule*, not shown here) directly invests the thyroid gland and is fused with its glandular parenchyma. Vascularized fibrous slips extend from the internal capsule into the substance of the gland, subdividing it into lobules. The internal capsule is covered by the tough *external capsule*, which is part of the pretracheal layer of the deep cervical fascia. This capsule invests the thyroid gland and parathyroid glands and is also called the "surgical capsule" because it must be opened to gain surgical access to the thyroid gland. Between the external and internal capsules is a potential space that is traversed by vascular branches and is occupied by the parathyroid glands.

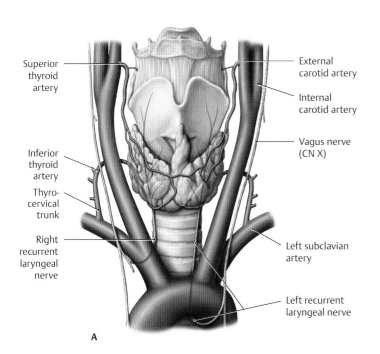

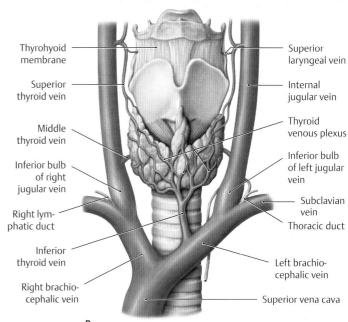

A

B

## Fig. 11.20 Blood supply and innervation of the thyroid gland

Anterior view.

**A Arterial supply:** The thyroid gland derives most of its arterial blood supply from the superior and inferior thyroid arteries. The superior thyroid artery, a branch of the external carotid artery, runs forward and downward to supply the gland. It is supplied from below by the inferior thyroid artery, which branches from the thyrocervical trunk. All of these arteries, which course on the right and left sides of the organ, must be ligated during surgical removal of the thyroid gland. In addition, a rare branch, the thyroidima, may arise from the brachiocephalic trunk or right common carotid artery to supply the gland from below.

*Note:* Operations on the thyroid gland carry a risk of injury to the recurrent laryngeal nerve, which is closely related to the posterior surface of the gland. Because it supplies important laryngeal muscles, unilateral injury to the nerve will cause postoperative hoarseness; bilateral injury may additionally result in dyspnea (difficulty in breathing). Prior to thyroid surgery, therefore, an otolaryngologist should confirm the integrity of the nerve supply to the laryngeal muscles and exclude any preexisting nerve lesion.

**B Venous drainage:** The thyroid gland is drained anteroinferiorly by a well-developed *thyroid venous plexus*, which usually drains through the inferior thyroid vein to the left brachiocephalic vein. Blood from the thyroid gland also drains to the internal jugular vein via the superior and middle thyroid veins.

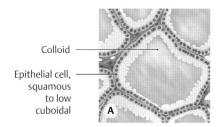

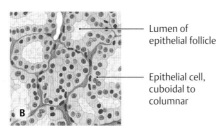

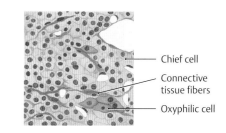

## Fig. 11.21 Histology of the thyroid gland

The thyroid gland absorbs iodide from the blood and uses it to make the thyroid hormones, thyroxine (T4, tetraiodothyronine) and triiodothyronine (T3). These hormones are stored at extracellular sites in the gland, bound to protein, and when needed they are mobilized from the thyroid follicles and secreted into the bloodstream. A special feature of the thyroid gland is the appearance of its epithelium, which varies depending on whether it is storing hormones or releasing them into the blood. The epithelial cells are flattened or squamous when in their resting or "storage state" (**A**), but they are columnar when in their active or "secretory state" (**B**). The epithelial morphology thus indicates the current functional state of the cells. Iodine deficiency causes an enlargement of the colloidal follicular lumen, which eventually results in a gross increase in the size of the thyroid (goiter). With prolonged iodine deficiency, there is a reduction in body metabolism and concomitant lethargy, fatigue, and mental depression. Conversely, hyperactivity of the thyroid, as in Graves' disease (an autoimmune disorder), causes a generalized metabolic acceleration, with irritability and weight loss. In the midst of the thyroid follicles are parafollicular cells (C cells), which secrete calcitonin. Calcitonin inhibits bone resorption and reduces the calcium concentration in the blood.

## Fig. 11.22 Histology of the parathyroid gland

The principal cell type in the parathyroid gland is the *chief cell*, which responds directly to low blood calcium levels by secreting parathyroid hormone (PTH, parathormone). Parathyroid hormone increases calcium concentration in the blood by various means, including the stimulation of bone resorption by osteoclasts and the renal tubular reabsorption of calcium. Parathyroid hormone thus acts antagonistically against calcitonin produced by the thyroid's C cells. Inadvertent removal of the parathyroid glands during thyroid surgery can cause a dramatic fall in serum calcium, with catastrophic consequences. Such a *hypocalcemic* condition causes neuromuscular irritability and, potentially, generalized fatal seizures involving respiratory muscles. Conversely, pathological hyperactivity of the parathyroid can lead to chronic *hypercalcemia*, often associated with bone loss (osteoporosis) and abnormal calcium deposition in the circulatory and urinary systems. Chronic hyperparathyroidism with hypertrophy of chief cells and elevated serum calcium is a common consequence of end-stage renal failure, by a mechanism not clearly established.

# Arteries & Veins of the Neck

## Fig. 12.1 Arteries of the neck

Left lateral view. The structures of the neck are supplied by branches of the external carotid artery and the subclavian artery (the internal carotid artery gives off no branches in the neck). The common carotid artery is enclosed in a fascial sheath (carotid sheath) along with the jugular vein and vagus nerve. The vertebral artery ascends through the transverse foramina of the cervical vertebrae.

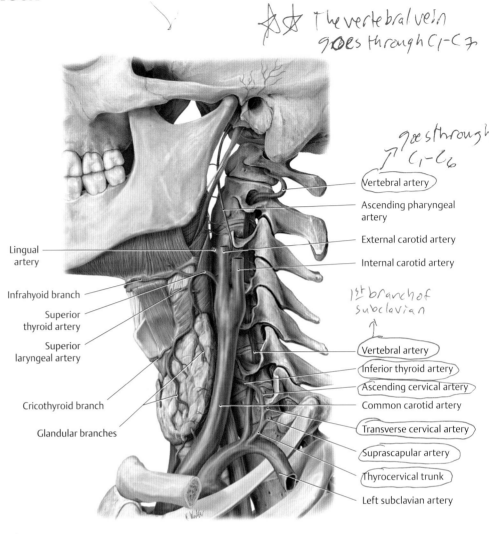

*Handwritten annotations:*
☆☆ The vertebral vein goes through C1-C7

goes through C1-C6 — Vertebral artery

1st branch of subclavian

*Labels:* Vertebral artery; Ascending pharyngeal artery; External carotid artery; Internal carotid artery; Lingual artery; Infrahyoid branch; Superior thyroid artery; Superior laryngeal artery; Cricothyroid branch; Glandular branches; Vertebral artery; Inferior thyroid artery; Ascending cervical artery; Common carotid artery; Transverse cervical artery; Suprascapular artery; Thyrocervical trunk; Left subclavian artery

## Table 12.1 Arteries of the neck

For a complete treatment of the arteries of the head and neck, see **Chapter 3**.

| Artery | Branches | Secondary branches* | |
|---|---|---|---|
| External carotid a. | Superior thyroid a. | Superior laryngeal, cricothyroid, infrahyoid, and sternocleidomastoid aa. | |
| | Ascending pharyngeal a. | Pharyngeal, palatine, prevertebral, inferior tympanic, and meningeal aa. | |
| | Lingual a. | Suprahyoid, dorsal lingual, deep lingual, and sublingual aa. | |
| | Facial a. | Ascending palatine, tonsillar, glandular, and submental aa. | |
| | Occipital a. | Sternocleidomastoid, descending, mastoid, auricular, and meningeal aa. | |
| | Posterior auricular a. | Stylomastoid and auricular aa. | |
| | Superficial temporal a. | (Branching occurs on the face) | |
| | Maxillary a. | (Branches within the infratemporal fossa are listed in **Table 5.1**, p. 102) | |
| Subclavian a. | Vertebral a. | Spinal aa. and muscular aa. | |
| | Thyrocervical trunk | Inferior thyroid a. | Inferior laryngeal, tracheal, esophageal, and ascending cervical aa. |
| | | Suprascapular a. | |
| | | Transverse cervical a. | Superficial and deep branches |
| | Internal thoracic a. | (Branching occurs within the thorax) | |
| | Descending (dorsal) scapular a. | (When present, it supplies the territory of the deep branch of the transverse cervical a.) | |

*Only branches that arise in the neck are listed here.

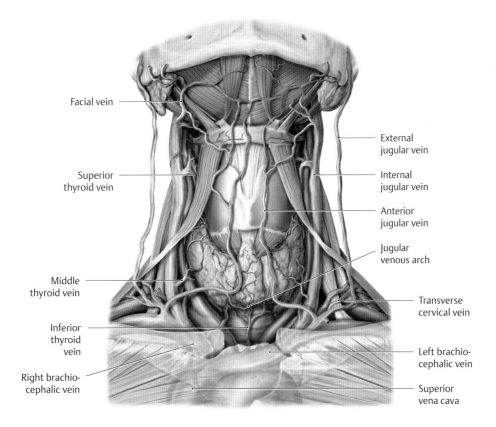

Facial vein

External jugular vein

Superior thyroid vein

Internal jugular vein

Anterior jugular vein

Jugular venous arch

Middle thyroid vein

Inferior thyroid vein

Transverse cervical vein

Right brachiocephalic vein

Left brachiocephalic vein

Superior vena cava

**Fig. 12.2 Veins of the neck**

Anterior view. The veins of the head and neck drain to the superior vena cava via the right and left brachiocephalic veins. The large internal jugular vein combines with the subclavian vein to form the brachiocephalic vein on each side. The internal jugular vein is located within the carotid sheath. It receives blood from the anterior neck and the interior of the skull. The subclavian vein receives blood from the neck via the external and anterior jugular veins, which are located within the superficial cervical fascia. *Note:* The thyroid venous plexus and vertebral veins typically drain directly into the brachiocephalic veins.

| Table 12.2 Veins of the neck | | | |
|---|---|---|---|
| For a complete treatment of the veins of the head and neck, see **Chapter 3**. | | | |
| Right and left brachiocephalic vv.* | Internal jugular v. | Inferior petrosal sinus, pharyngeal vv.; occipital, (common) facial, lingual, and superior and middle thyroid vv. | |
| | Subclavian v. | External jugular v. | Posterior external jugular, anterior jugular, transverse cervical, and suprascapular vv.** |
| | Vertebral v. | Internal and external vertebral venous plexuses; ascending cervical (anterior vertebral) and deep cervical vv. | |
| | Inferior thyroid vv. | Thyroid venous plexus | |

*The brachiocephalic vein is formed by the joining of its two primary tributaries, the internal jugular vein and the subclavian vein. Only tributaries within the neck are listed above.
**The tributaries of the external jugular vein may on occasion drain directly into the subclavian vein.

# Lymphatics of the Neck

A distinction is made between regional lymph nodes, which are associated with a particular organ or region and constitute their primary filtering stations, and collecting lymph nodes, which usually receive lymph from multiple regional lymph node groups. Lymph from the head and neck region, gathered in scattered regional nodes, flows through its system of deep cervical collecting lymph nodes into the right and left jugular trunks, each closely associated with its corresponding internal jugular vein. The jugular trunk on the right side drains into the right lymphatic duct, which terminates at the right jugulosubclavian junction. The jugular trunk on the left side terminates at the thoracic duct, which empties into the left jugulosubclavian junction (see **Fig. 12.6**).

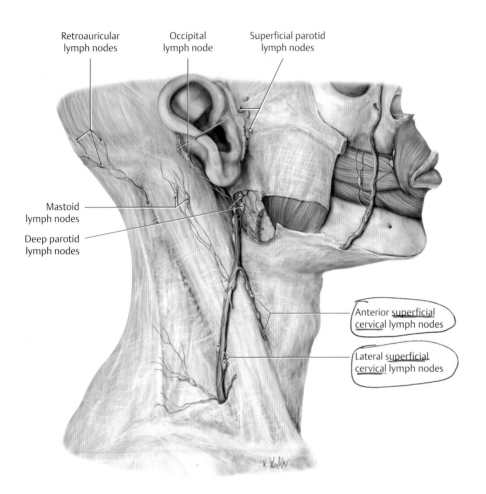

Retroauricular lymph nodes

Occipital lymph node

Superficial parotid lymph nodes

Mastoid lymph nodes

Deep parotid lymph nodes

Anterior superficial cervical lymph nodes

Lateral superficial cervical lymph nodes

**Fig. 12.3 Superficial cervical lymph nodes**
Right lateral view. Enlarged cervical lymph nodes are a common finding at physical examination. The enlargement of cervical lymph nodes may be caused by inflammation (usually a *painful* enlargement) or neoplasia (usually a *painless* enlargement) in the area drained by the nodes. The superficial cervical lymph nodes are primary drainage locations for lymph from adjacent areas or organs.

**Fig. 12.4 Deep cervical lymph nodes**
Right lateral view. The deep lymph nodes in the neck consist mainly of collecting nodes. They have major clinical importance as potential sites of metastasis from head and neck tumors. Affected deep cervical lymph nodes may be surgically removed (neck dissection) or may be treated by regional irradiation. For this purpose, the American Academy of Otolaryngology—Head and Neck Surgery has grouped the deep cervical lymph nodes into six levels (Robbins 1991):

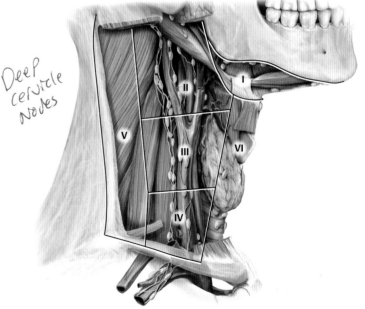

Deep cervicle nodes

I    Submental and submandibular lymph nodes
II–IV Deep cervical lymph nodes along the internal jugular vein (lateral jugular lymph nodes):
   – II   Deep cervical lymph nodes (upper lateral group)
   – III  Deep cervical lymph nodes (middle lateral group)
   – IV   Deep cervical lymph nodes (lower lateral group)
V    Lymph nodes in the posterior cervical triangle
VI   Anterior cervical lymph nodes

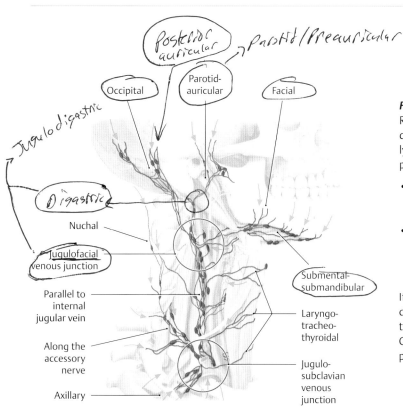

*(handwritten annotations)*
Posterior auricular
Parotid/Preauricular
Jugulodigastric
Occipital
Parotid-auricular
Facial
Digastric
Nuchal
Jugulofacial venous junction
Parallel to internal jugular vein
Along the accessory nerve
Axillary
Submental-submandibular
Laryngo-tracheo-thyroidal
Jugulo-subclavian venous junction

*(handwritten notes top right)*
※ A granulomatous Lymph Node
is a dying Lymph Node
※ Cancerous Lymph Node is hard, doesnt move,
& isnt tender.

**Fig. 12.5 Directions of lymphatic drainage in the neck**
Right lateral view. Understanding this pattern of lymphatic flow is critical to identifying the location of a potential cause of enlarged cervical lymph nodes. There are two main sites in the neck where the lymphatic pathways intersect:

- Jugulofacial venous junction: Lymphatics from the head pass obliquely downward to this site, where the lymph is redirected vertically downward in the neck.
- Jugulosubclavian venous junction: The main lymphatic trunk, the thoracic duct, terminates at this central location, where lymph collected from the left side of the head and neck region is combined with lymph draining from the rest of the body.

If only peripheral nodal groups are affected, this suggests a localized disease process. If the central groups (e.g., those at the venous junctions) are affected, this usually signifies an extensive disease process. Central lymph nodes can be obtained for diagnostic evaluation by prescalene biopsy.

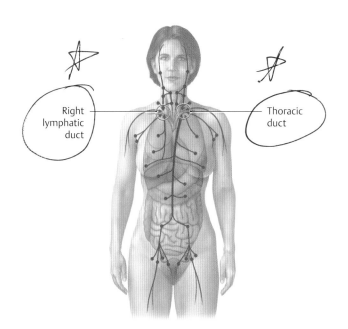

Right lymphatic duct
Thoracic duct

**Fig. 12.6 Relationship of the cervical nodes to the systemic lymphatic circulation**
Anterior view. The cervical lymph nodes may be involved by diseases that are not primary to the head and neck region, because lymph from the entire body is channeled to the left and right jugulosubclavian junctions (red circles). This can lead to retrograde involvement of the cervical nodes. The *right lymphatic duct* terminates at the right jugulosubclavian junction, the *thoracic duct* at the left jugulosubclavian junction. Besides cranial and cervical tributaries, the lymph from thoracic lymph nodes (mediastinal and tracheobronchial) and from abdominal and caudal lymph nodes may reach the cervical nodes by way of the thoracic duct. As a result, diseases in those organs may lead to cervical lymph node enlargement.

For example, gastric carcinoma may metastasize to the left supraclavicular group of lymph nodes, producing an enlarged *sentinel node* that suggests an abdominal tumor. Systemic lymphomas may also spread to the cervical lymph nodes by this pathway.

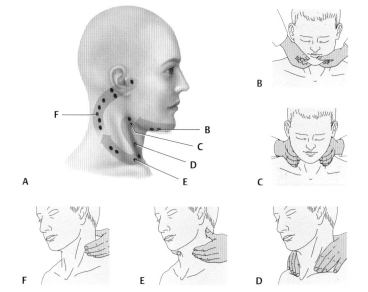

A B C D E F

**Fig. 12.7 Systematic palpation of the cervical lymph nodes**
The cervical lymph nodes are systematically palpated during the physical examination to ensure the detection of any enlarged nodes.
Panel **A** shows the sequence in which the various nodal groups are successively palpated. The examiner usually palpates the submental-submandibular group first (**B**), including the mandibular angle (**C**), then proceeds along the anterior border of the sternocleidomastoid muscle (**D**). The supraclavicular lymph nodes are palpated next (**E**), followed by the lymph nodes along the accessory nerve and the nuchal group of nodes (**F**).

# Cervical Plexus

The neck receives innervation from the cervical spinal nerves as well as three cranial nerves: glossopharyngeal (CN IX), vagus (CN X), and accessory (CN XI). CN IX and X innervate the pharynx and larynx; CN XI provides motor innervation to the trapezius and sternocleido-mastoid. The course and distribution of the cranial nerves are described in **Chapter 4**.

### Fig. 12.8 Cervical spinal nerves

Like all spinal nerves, the cervical spinal nerves emerge from the spinal cord as a dorsal (sensory) root and a ventral (motor) root. The roots combine to form the mixed spinal nerve, which then gives off a dorsal and a ventral ramus.

**Dorsal rami:** Supply motor innervation to the intrinsic back muscles (epiaxial muscle) (**Table 12.3**).

**Ventral rami:** Supply motor innervation to the anterolateral muscles of the neck derived from the hypaxial muscle. The ventral rami of C1–C4 supply motor innervation to the deep neck muscles (scalenes, rectii capitis anterioris) via direct branches. The ventral rami also combine to form the cervical plexus, which supplies the skin and musculature of the anterior and lateral neck.

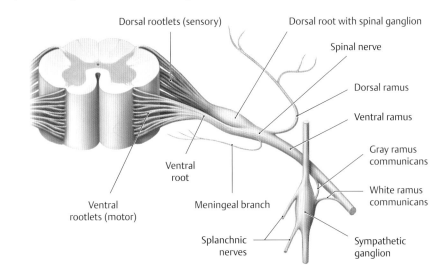

### Table 12.3 Dorsal rami of C1–C3

| Dorsal ramus | | Motor | Sensory |
|---|---|---|---|
| C1 (Suboccipital n.)* | | Nuchal muscles (e.g., superior oblique, inferior oblique, rectus capitis posterior major, rectus capitis posterior minor, semispinalis capitis) | Meninges |
| C2 | Greater occipital n.* (medial branch of C2) | – | C2 dermatome (posterior neck and scalp) |
| | Lateral branch of C2 | Semispinalis capitis, splenius capitis, longissimus capitis | – |
| C3 | Least occipital n.* (medial branch of C3) | – | C3 dermatome (posterior neck) |
| | Lateral branch of C3 | Semispinalis capitis, splenius capitis, longissimus capitis | – |

*The suboccipital nerve is primarily a motor nerve, whereas the greater occipital and least occipital nerves are sensory branches of C2 and C3, respectively.

### Fig. 12.9 Cervical plexus

The ventral rami of spinal nerves C1–C4 emerge from the intervertebral foramina along the transverse processes of the cervical vertebrae. They emerge between the anterior and posterior scalenes and give off short direct branches to the scalenes and rectii capitis anterioris before coursing anteriorly to form the cervical plexus.

**Motor fibers:** Motor fibers from C1 course with the hypoglossal nerve (CN XII). Certain fibers continue with the nerve to innervate the thyrohyoid and geniohyoid. The remainder leave CN XII to form the superior root of the ansa cervicalis. The inferior root is formed by motor fibers from C2 and C3. The ansa cervicalis innervates the omohyoid, sternothyroid, and sternohyoid. Most motor fibers from C4 descend as the phrenic nerve, which innervates the diaphragm.

**Sensory fibers:** The sensory fibers of C2–C4 emerge from the cervical plexus as peripheral nerves. (*Note:* The sensory fibers of C1 go to the meninges.) These peripheral sensory nerves emerge from Erb's point and provide sensory innervation to the anterolateral neck.

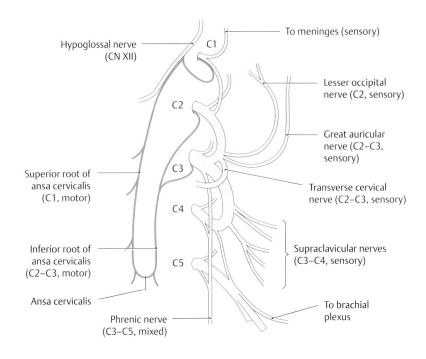

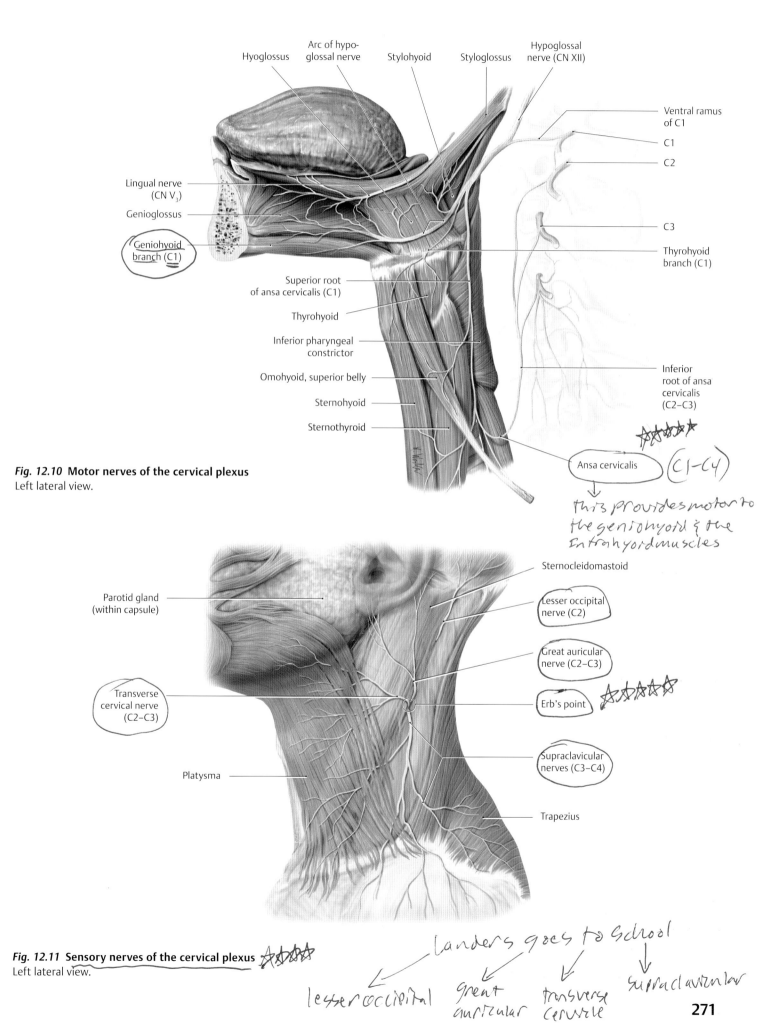

**Fig. 12.10 Motor nerves of the cervical plexus**
Left lateral view.

Hyoglossus

Arc of hypo-glossal nerve

Stylohyoid

Styloglossus

Hypoglossal nerve (CN XII)

Ventral ramus of C1

C1

C2

C3

Thyrohyoid branch (C1)

Lingual nerve (CN V₃)

Genioglossus

Geniohyoid branch (C1)

Superior root of ansa cervicalis (C1)

Thyrohyoid

Inferior pharyngeal constrictor

Omohyoid, superior belly

Sternohyoid

Sternothyroid

Inferior root of ansa cervicalis (C2–C3)

Ansa cervicalis (C1–C4)

this provides motor to the geniohyoid & the Intrahyoid muscles

**Fig. 12.11 Sensory nerves of the cervical plexus**
Left lateral view.

Parotid gland (within capsule)

Transverse cervical nerve (C2–C3)

Platysma

Sternocleidomastoid

Lesser occipital nerve (C2)

Great auricular nerve (C2–C3)

Erb's point

Supraclavicular nerves (C3–C4)

Trapezius

Landers goes to School

lesser occipital    great auricular    transverse cervical    supraclavicular

271

# Cervical Regions (Triangles)

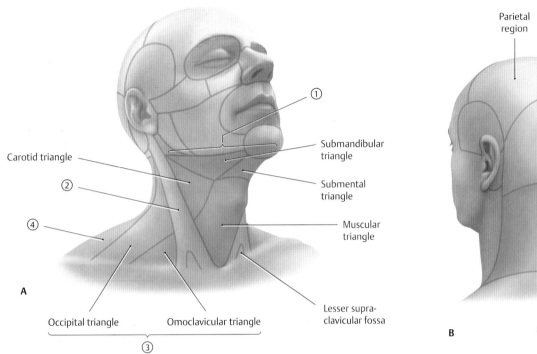

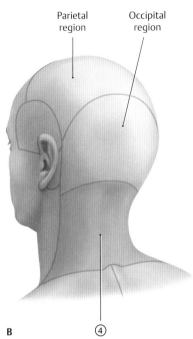

**Fig. 12.12 Cervical regions**
**A** Right lateral oblique view. **B** Right posterior oblique view.
For descriptive purposes, the anterolateral neck is divided into an anterior and a posterior cervical triangle, separated by the sternocleidomastoid. The posterior portion of the neck is referred to as the nuchal region.

| Table 12.4 Cervical regions | |
| --- | --- |
| **Region** | **Subdivision** |
| ① Anterior cervical region (anterior cervical triangle): Bounded by the midline, mandible, and sternocleidomastoid. | Submandibular (digastric) triangle: Bounded by the mandible and the bellies of the digastric muscle. |
| | Carotid triangle: Bounded by the sternocleidomastoid, superior belly of the omohyoid, and posterior belly of the digastric. |
| | Muscular triangle: Bounded by the sternocleidomastoid, superior omohyoid, and sternohyoid. |
| | Submental triangle: Bounded by the anterior bellies of the diagastric, the hyoid bone, and the mandible. |
| ② Sternocleidomastoid region: The region lying under the sternocleidomastoid muscle. | |
| ③ Lateral cervical region (posterior cervical triangle): Bounded by the sternocleidomastoid, trapezius, and clavicle. | Omoclavicular (subclavian) triangle: Bounded by the inferior belly of the omohyoid, the clavicle, and the sternocleidomastoid. |
| | Occipital triangle: Bounded by the inferior belly of the omohyoid, the trapezius, and the clavicle. |
| ④ Posterior cervical Region (nuchal region): Region lying under the trapezius muscle inferior to its insertion at the superior nuchal line and superior to the vertebra prominens (C7). | |

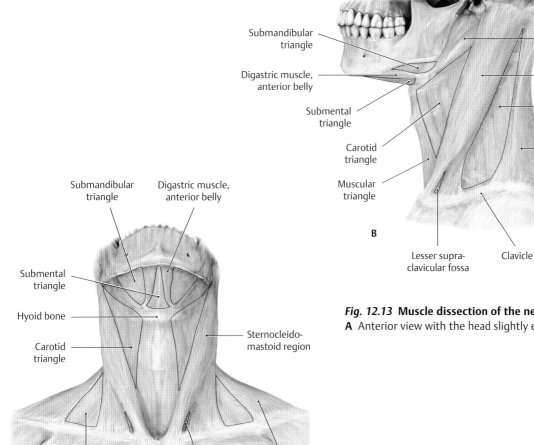

**Fig. 12.13 Muscle dissection of the neck**
**A** Anterior view with the head slightly extended. **B** Left lateral view.

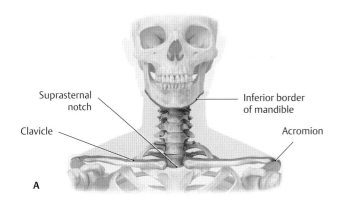

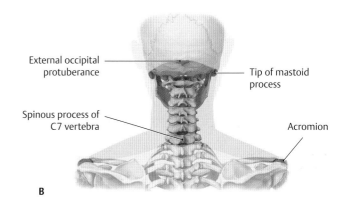

**Fig. 12.14 Palpable bony prominences in the neck**
**A** Anterior view. **B** Posterior view. Certain palpable structures define the boundaries of the neck. The superior boundaries of the neck are the

inferior border of the mandible, tip of the mastoid process, and external occipital protuberance. The inferior boundaries are the suprasternal notch, clavicle, acromion, and spinous process of the C7 vertebra.

# Cervical Fasciae

*See page 286 also* [handwritten]

### Fig. 12.15 Cervical fasciae

The structures of the neck are enclosed by multiple layers of cervical fasciae, sheets of connective tissue that subdivide the neck into compartments. The fascial layers are separated by interfascial spaces. There are four major fascial spaces in the neck: pretracheal, retrovisceral/retropharyngeal, prevertebral, and carotid. These spaces are not prominent under normal conditions (the fasciae lie flat against each other). However, the spaces may provide routes for the spread of inflammatory processes (e.g., tonsillar infections in the infratemporal fossa) to spread from regions of the head and neck into the mediastinum.

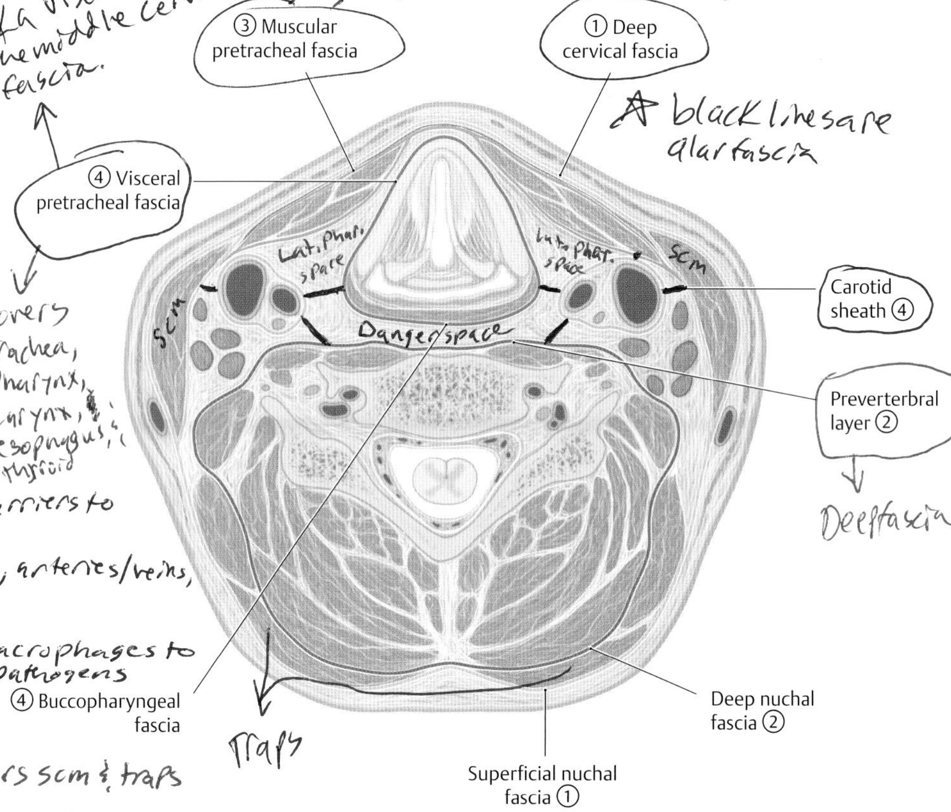

[Handwritten annotations around figure:]
- *aka visceral layer of the middle cervicle fascia*
- *muscular layer of the middle cervicle fascia → covers infrahyoid muscles*
- *Investing layer*
- ③ Muscular pretracheal fascia
- ① Deep cervical fascia
- *black lines are alar fascia*
- ④ Visceral pretracheal fascia
- *covers Trachea, Pharynx, Larynx, & esophagus, & thyroid*
- Lat. Phar. space
- Int. Phar. space
- SCM
- Danger space
- Carotid sheath ④
- Prevertebral layer ②
- *Deep fascia*
- ④ Buccopharyngeal fascia
- *Traps*
- Superficial nuchal fascia ①
- Deep nuchal fascia ②

[Handwritten notes on left:]
- ★ Superficial fascia → Contains fat & are barriers to infection
- ★ Deep fascia → No fat & covers Muscles, arteries/veins, and holds things together
- ★ Both have histiocytes → fixed macrophages to combat pathogens

*Deep fascia has 3 layers*
1) Superficial – Investing layer → Covers scm & traps
2) middle layer
   • muscular portion – covers infrahyoid muscles
   • Visceral layer – covers thyroid, trachea, larynx, & pharynx
3) Deep layer – prevertebral layer

---

### Table 12.5 Cervical fasciae and fascial spaces

Despite generally being continuous, many of the fascial layers bear different names in different regions of the neck relative to the structures they enclose.

| Fascial layer | Description | Contents |
|---|---|---|
| Superficial cervical fascia (not shown) | Subcutaneous tissue that lies deep to the skin and contains the platysma anterolaterally. | Platysma |
| ① Investing layer (yellow) = Deep cervical fascia + Superficial nuchal fascia | Envelops the entire neck and is continuous with the nuchal ligament posteriorly. | Trapezius and (splits around the) sternocleidomastoid |
| ② Prevertebral layer (purple) = Prevertebral fascia + Deep nuchal fascia | Attaches superiorly to the skull base and continues inferiorly into the superior mediastinum, merging with the anterior longitudinal ligament. Continues along the subclavian artery and brachial plexus, becoming continuous with the axillary sheath.<br>• The prevertebral fascia splits into an alar and a prevertebral layer (the "danger space" is located between these layers). | Intrinsic back muscles and prevertebral muscles |
| Pretracheal fascia (green) | ③ Muscular portion (light green) | Infrahyoid muscles |
| | ④ Visceral portion (dark green): Attaches to the cricoid cartilage and is continuous posteriorly with the buccopharyngeal fascia. Continues inferiorly into the superior mediastinum, eventually merging with the fibrous pericardium. | Thyroid gland, trachea, esophagus, and pharynx |
| Carotid sheath (blue) | Consisting of loose areolar tissue, the sheath extends from the base of the skull (from the external opening of the carotid canal) to the aortic arch. | Common and internal carotid arteries, internal jugular vein, and vagus nerve (CN X); in addition, CN IX, CN XI, and CN XII briefly pass through the most superior part of the carotid sheath. |

*✱ Deep fascia covers the temporalis & masseter*
*✱ Superficial fascia covers the muscles of facial expression*

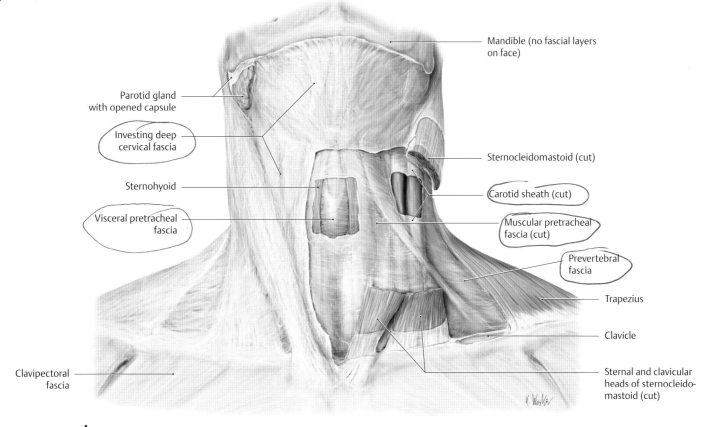

Mandible (no fascial layers on face)

Parotid gland with opened capsule

Investing deep cervical fascia

Sternohyoid

Visceral pretracheal fascia

Clavipectoral fascia

Sternocleidomastoid (cut)

Carotid sheath (cut)

Muscular pretracheal fascia (cut)

Prevertebral fascia

Trapezius

Clavicle

Sternal and clavicular heads of sternocleido-mastoid (cut)

**A**

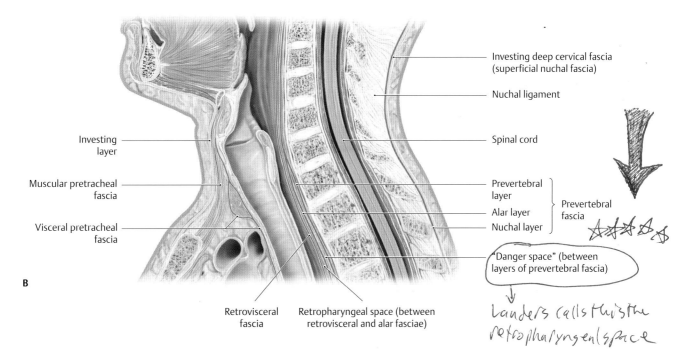

Investing layer

Muscular pretracheal fascia

Visceral pretracheal fascia

Investing deep cervical fascia (superficial nuchal fascia)

Nuchal ligament

Spinal cord

Prevertebral layer

Alar layer

Nuchal layer

Prevertebral fascia

"Danger space" (between layers of prevertebral fascia)

*Landers calls this the retropharyngeal space*

**B**

Retrovisceral fascia

Retropharyngeal space (between retrovisceral and alar fasciae)

**Fig. 12.16 Fascial relationships in the neck**
**A** Anterior view with skin, superficial cervical fascia, and platysma removed. **B** Left lateral view of midsagittal section.
The superficial cervical fascia (not shown) lies just deep to the skin and contains the cutaneous muscle of the neck (platysma). The investing layer of deep cervical fascia contains the remainder of the structures in the neck. It attaches to the inferior border of the mandible and is continuous inferiorly with the clavipectoral fascia (anteriorly) and the thoracolumbar fascia (posteriorly). The deep cervical fascia splits to enclose the parotid gland in a capsule (**A**, swelling of the parotid gland results in pain due to constriction by the capsule). It also splits to enclose the sternocleidomastoid. In the anterior neck, the pretracheal layer lies just deep to the investing layer. It consists of a muscular portion and a visceral portion, which collectively enclose the structures of the anterior neck, including the pharynx, trachea, and esophagus. The portion of the pretracheal fascia posterior to the esophagus is known as the retrovisceral fascia (**B**). It is separated from the prevertebral fascia by the retropharyngeal space. Inferior to the laryngeal inlet, the prevertebral fascia splits into an anterior (alar) and a posterior (prevertebral) layer, which are separated by the "danger space" — a potential route for the spread of infection from the pharynx into the superior mediastinum. With tuberculous osteomyelitis of the cervical spine, a retropharyngeal abscess may develop in the "danger space" along the prevertebral fascia. Both prevertebral layers are continuous posteriorly with the deep nuchal fascia. *Note:* The laterally located carotid sheath (**A**) does not appear in the midsagittal section.

**275**

# Posterior Neck

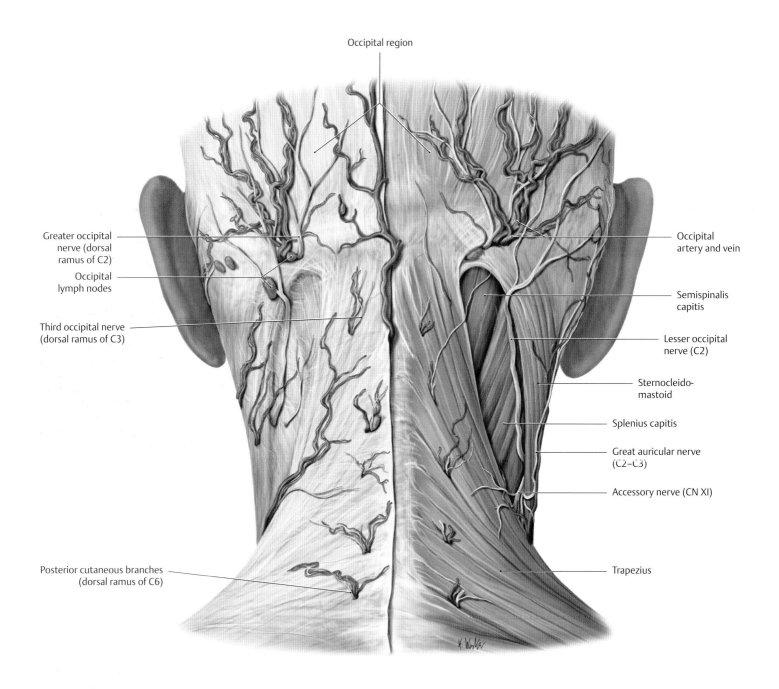

Occipital region

Greater occipital nerve (dorsal ramus of C2)

Occipital lymph nodes

Third occipital nerve (dorsal ramus of C3)

Posterior cutaneous branches (dorsal ramus of C6)

Occipital artery and vein

Semispinalis capitis

Lesser occipital nerve (C2)

Sternocleido-mastoid

Splenius capitis

Great auricular nerve (C2–C3)

Accessory nerve (CN XI)

Trapezius

**Fig. 12.17 Posterior cervical (nuchal) region**
Posterior view. Left side: Subcutaneous layer of superficial nuchal fascia. Right side: All fascia removed (superficial cervical fascia, investing layer, prevertebral layer).
The posterior cervical region is bounded superiorly by the superior nuchal line (the attachment of the trapezius and sternocleidomastoid to the occipital bone) and inferiorly by the palpable spinous process of the last cervical vertebra, the vertebra prominens (C7). The posterior cervical region, like the rest of the neck, is completely enveloped in superficial fascia (left side). The investing layer of deep cervical fascia envelops the trapezius and splits to enclose the sternocleidomastoid.

Both muscles are innervated by the accessory nerve (CN XI). The deep nuchal fascia (the posterior continuation of the prevertebral fascia) lies deep to the trapezius and sternocleidomastoid and encloses the intrinsic back muscles (here: semispinalis and splenius capitis). The intrinsic back muscles receive motor and sensory innervation from the dorsal rami of the spinal nerves (see **Fig. 12.20**). The great auricular and lesser occipital nerves are also visible in this dissection. They are sensory nerves arising from the cervical plexus (formed by the ventral rami of C1–C4). The major artery of the occipital region is the occipital artery, a posterior branch of the external carotid artery.

*(handwritten)* ✕ Suboccipital triangle

*(handwritten)* 8 cervical spinal nerves
7 cervical vertebrae

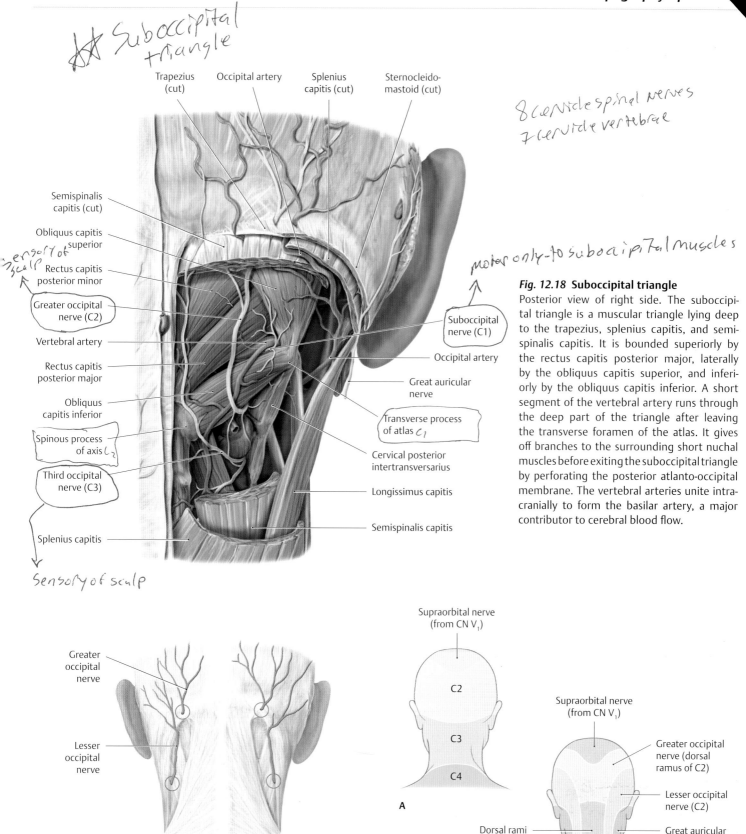

*(handwritten)* Sensory of scalp

*(handwritten)* motor only - to suboccipital muscles

**Fig. 12.18 Suboccipital triangle**
Posterior view of right side. The suboccipital triangle is a muscular triangle lying deep to the trapezius, splenius capitis, and semispinalis capitis. It is bounded superiorly by the rectus capitis posterior major, laterally by the obliquus capitis superior, and inferiorly by the obliquus capitis inferior. A short segment of the vertebral artery runs through the deep part of the triangle after leaving the transverse foramen of the atlas. It gives off branches to the surrounding short nuchal muscles before exiting the suboccipital triangle by perforating the posterior atlanto-occipital membrane. The vertebral arteries unite intracranially to form the basilar artery, a major contributor to cerebral blood flow.

**Fig. 12.19 Sites of emergence of the occipital nerves**
Posterior view. The sites where the lesser and greater occipital nerves emerge from the fascia into the subcutaneous connective tissue are clinically important because they are tender to palpation in certain diseases (e.g., meningitis). The examiner tests the sensation of these nerves by pressing lightly on the circled points with the thumb. If these points (but not their surroundings) are painful, the clinician should suspect meningitis.

**Fig. 12.20 Cutaneous innervation of the posterior neck**
Posterior view. **A** Segmental innervation (dermatomes). **B** Peripheral cutaneous nerves.
The occiput and nuchal regions derive most of their segmental innervation from the C2 and C3 spinal nerves. Of the specific cutaneous nerves, the greater occipital nerve is a dorsal ramus; the lesser occipital, great auricular, and supraclavicular nerves are branches of the cervical plexus (formed from the ventral rami of C1–C4). See p. 65 for segmental versus peripheral cutaneous innervation.

# Lateral Neck

### Fig. 12.21 Lateral neck

Right lateral view. *Removed:* Superficial cervical fascia, platysma, and parotid capsule (investing layer). The investing layer of deep cervical fascia encloses all the structures of the neck with the exception of the platysma. (*Note:* The face does not have fascial layers.) It splits to enclose the parotid gland in a capsule. The capsule has been opened to show the emergence of the cervical branch of the facial nerve (CN VII) from the parotid plexus. The cervical branch provides motor innervation to the platysma. The sensory nerves of the anterolateral neck (lesser occipital, great auricular, transverse cervical, and supraclavicular) arise from the cervical plexus, formed by the ventral rami of C1–C4. They pierce the investing layer at or near the punctum nervosum (Erb's point), midway down the posterior border of the sternocleidomastoid. *Note:* The transverse cervical nerve (sensory) courses deep to the external jugular vein and forms a mixed anastomosis with the cervical branch (motor) of CN VII.

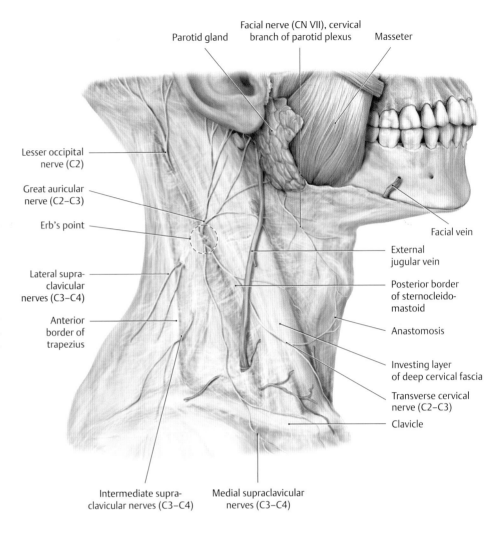

### Fig. 12.22 Posterior cervical triangle

Right lateral view. **A** Investing fascia removed. **B** Pretracheal fascia removed. **C** Prevertebral fascia removed.

The investing layer of deep cervical fascia splits into a superficial and a deep lamina to enclose the sternocleidomastoid and trapezius, both of which are innervated by the accessory nerve (CN XI). (*Note:* The accessory nerve may be injured during lymph node biopsy.) Removing the investing layer between the sternocleidomastoid and trapezius reveals the posterior cervical triangle (bounded inferiorly by the clavicle). This exposes the prevertebral fascia, which encloses the intrinsic and deep muscles of the neck. The prevertebral fascia is fused to the pretracheal fascia, which envelops the omohyoid (**B**). Removing the prevertebral fascia exposes the phrenic nerve (**C**), which arises from the cervical plexus and descends to innervate the diaphragm. The brachial plexus (**C**) is also visible at its point of emergence between the anterior and middle scalenes.

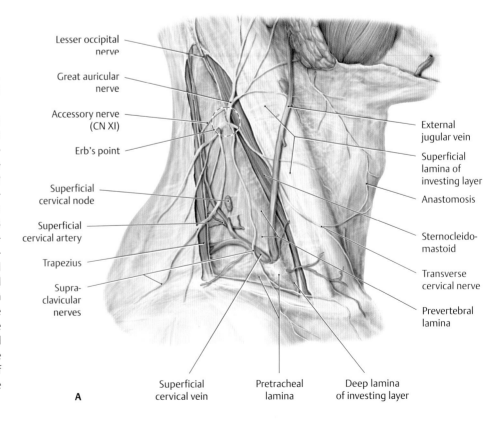

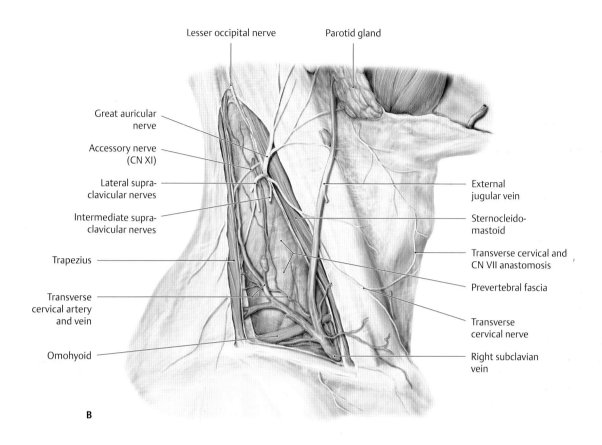

Lesser occipital nerve

Parotid gland

Great auricular nerve

Accessory nerve (CN XI)

Lateral supra-clavicular nerves

Intermediate supra-clavicular nerves

Trapezius

Transverse cervical artery and vein

Omohyoid

External jugular vein

Sternocleido-mastoid

Transverse cervical and CN VII anastomosis

Prevertebral fascia

Transverse cervical nerve

Right subclavian vein

**B**

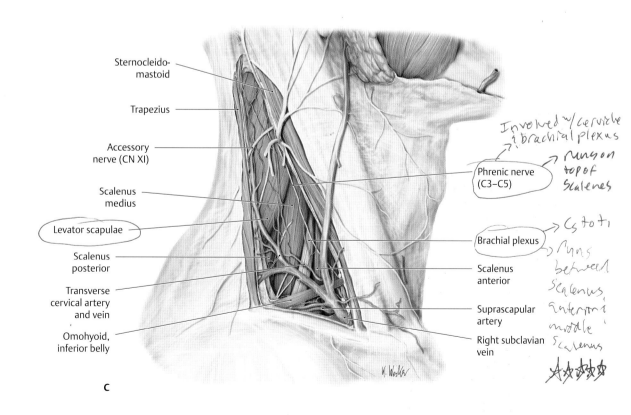

Sternocleido-mastoid

Trapezius

Accessory nerve (CN XI)

Scalenus medius

Levator scapulae

Scalenus posterior

Transverse cervical artery and vein

Omohyoid, inferior belly

Phrenic nerve (C3–C5)

Brachial plexus

Scalenus anterior

Suprascapular artery

Right subclavian vein

*K. Wesker*

**C**

**279**

# Anterior Neck

### Fig. 12.23 Anterior neck

Anterior view. Left neck: Superficial cervical fascia removed to expose platysma. Right neck: Platysma removed to expose investing layer. The investing layer of deep cervical fascia lies just deep to the cutaneous platysma muscle, which is innervated by the cervical branch of the facial nerve (CN VII). It attaches to the inferior border of the mandible and is continuous inferiorly with the clavipectoral fascia. The investing layer splits to form a capsule around the parotid gland. Inflammation of the parotid gland (e.g., mumps) causes conspicuous facial swelling and deformity in this region ("hamster cheeks" with prominent earlobes). The investing layer also divides into a deep and a superficial lamina to enclose the sternocleidomastoid. The investing layer has been cut around the midline to expose the pretracheal layer of deep cervical fascia, which encloses the infrahyoid muscles and the viscera of the anterior neck.

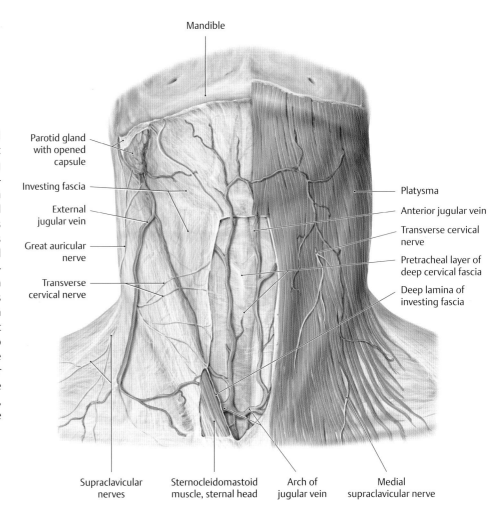

### Fig. 12.24 Anterior cervical triangle

Anterior view. The pretracheal fascia has been removed to expose the anterior cervical triangle, bounded by the mandible and the anterior borders of the sternocleidomastoid muscles. The infrahyoid muscles are enclosed by the muscular pretracheal fascia (removed). The thyroid gland and larynx are enclosed by the visceral pretracheal fascia (removed). The anterior cervical triangle contains neurovasculature of the larynx and thyroid gland, including the first branch of the external carotid artery (the superior thyroid artery). The internal and external laryngeal nerves (from the superior laryngeal branch of CN X) are visible. C1 motor fibers run with the hypoglossal nerve (CN XII) to the thyrohyoid and geniohyoid (not shown). Certain C1 motor fibers leave CN XII to form the superior root of the ansa cervicalis. The inferior root is formed by motor fibers from C2 and C3. The ansa cervicalis innervates the omohyoid, sternothyroid, and sternohyoid.

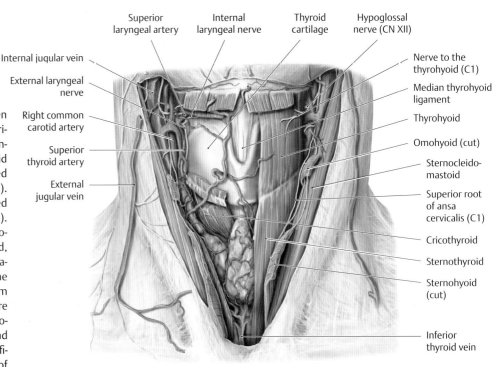

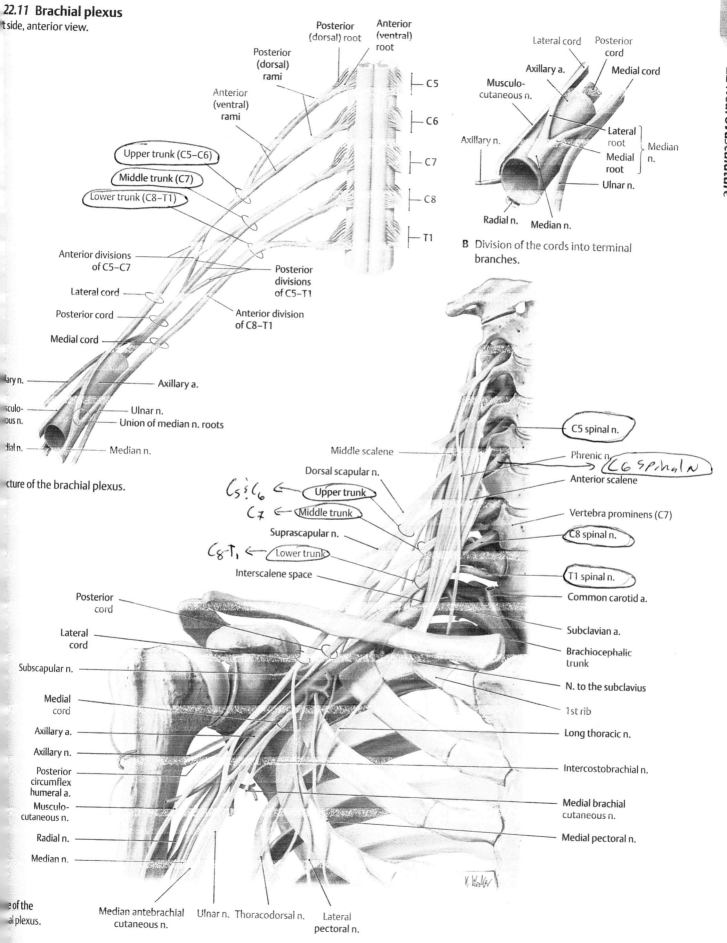

## 22.11 Brachial plexus

t side, anterior view.

Posterior (dorsal) root
Anterior (ventral) root

Posterior (dorsal) rami
Anterior (ventral) rami

Lateral cord    Posterior cord
Axillary a.    Medial cord
Musculo-cutaneous n.
Axillary n.
Lateral root ⎫
Medial root ⎬ Median n.
Ulnar n.
Radial n.    Median n.

C5
C6
C7
C8
T1

**B** Division of the cords into terminal branches.

Upper trunk (C5–C6)
Middle trunk (C7)
Lower trunk (C8–T1)

Anterior divisions of C5–C7
Lateral cord
Posterior cord
Medial cord

Posterior divisions of C5–T1
Anterior division of C8–T1

…ary n.    Axillary a.
…sculo-ous n.    Ulnar n.
Union of median n. roots
…ial n.    Median n.

…cture of the brachial plexus.

Middle scalene
Dorsal scapular n.
Upper trunk
Middle trunk
Suprascapular n.
Lower trunk
Interscalene space

C5 spinal n.
Phrenic n. → C6 spinal N
Anterior scalene
Vertebra prominens (C7)
C8 spinal n.
T1 spinal n.
Common carotid a.
Subclavian a.
Brachiocephalic trunk
N. to the subclavius
1st rib
Long thoracic n.
Intercostobrachial n.
Medial brachial cutaneous n.
Medial pectoral n.

C5 & C6
C7
C8–T1

Posterior cord
Lateral cord
Subscapular n.
Medial cord
Axillary a.
Axillary n.
Posterior circumflex humeral a.
Musculo-cutaneous n.
Radial n.
Median n.

e of the
…al plexus.

Median antebrachial cutaneous n.    Ulnar n.    Thoracodorsal n.    Lateral pectoral n.

321

22 Neurovasculature

*[Handwritten annotations:]*

✗✗✗✗✗ Carotid sheath has...
· Internal Jugular
· common carotid
· Vagus Nerve

Rami form trunks
trunks form plexus'

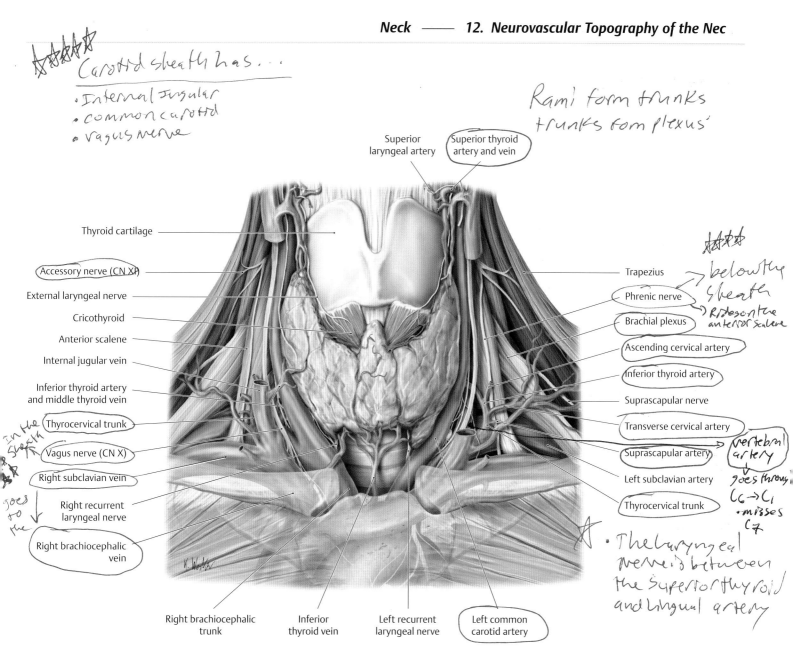

Superior laryngeal artery

Superior thyroid artery and vein

Thyroid cartilage

Accessory nerve (CN XI)

External laryngeal nerve

Cricothyroid

Anterior scalene

Internal jugular vein

Inferior thyroid artery and middle thyroid vein

Thyrocervical trunk

Vagus nerve (CN X)

Right subclavian vein

Right recurrent laryngeal nerve

Right brachiocephalic vein

Right brachiocephalic trunk

Inferior thyroid vein

Left recurrent laryngeal nerve

Left common carotid artery

Trapezius

Phrenic nerve

Brachial plexus

Ascending cervical artery

Inferior thyroid artery

Suprascapular nerve

Transverse cervical artery

Suprascapular artery

Left subclavian artery

Thyrocervical trunk

*[Handwritten annotations:]*

✗✗✗✗
below the sheath
→ Rides on the anterior scalene

In the sheath ✗✗✗

Goes to the

vertebral artery
goes through
C6 → C1
· misses C7

✗ · The laryngeal nerve is between the superior thyroid and lingual artery

K. Wesker

**Fig. 12.25 Root of the neck (thoracic inlet)**
Anterior view. The root of the neck contains numerous structures, including the common carotid artery, subclavian artery, subclavian vein, internal jugular vein, inferior thyroid vein, vagus nerve, phrenic nerve, and recurrent laryngeal nerve. A retrosternal goiter enlarging the inferior pole of the thyroid gland can easily compress neurovascular structures at the thoracic inlet.

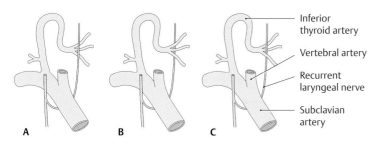

Inferior thyroid artery

Vertebral artery

Recurrent laryngeal nerve

Subclavian artery

A    B    C

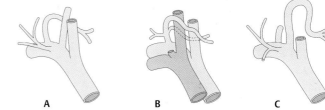

A    B    C

**Fig. 12.26 Course of the right recurrent laryngeal nerve**
    (after von Lanz and Wachsmuth)
Anterior view. The recurrent laryngeal nerve is a somatomotor and sensory branch of the vagus nerve, which innervates all the muscles of the larynx except the cricothyroid muscle. Unilateral damage to this nerve supply results in hoarseness, and bilateral damage leads to a closed glottis with severe dyspnea. The right recurrent laryngeal nerve may pass in front of (**A**), behind (**B**), or between (**C**), the branches of the inferior thyroid artery. Its course should be noted during operations on the thyroid gland due to its close relationship to the posterior surface of the gland. *Note:* The left recurrent laryngeal nerve passes around the aortic arch in proximity to the ligamentum arteriosum.

**Fig. 12.27 Variations in the branching pattern of the right inferior thyroid artery** (after Platzer)
The course of the inferior thyroid artery is highly variable. It may run medially behind the vertebral artery (**A**), divide immediately after arising from the thyrocervical trunk (**B**), or arise as the first branch of the subclavian artery (**C**).

# Deep Anterolateral Neck

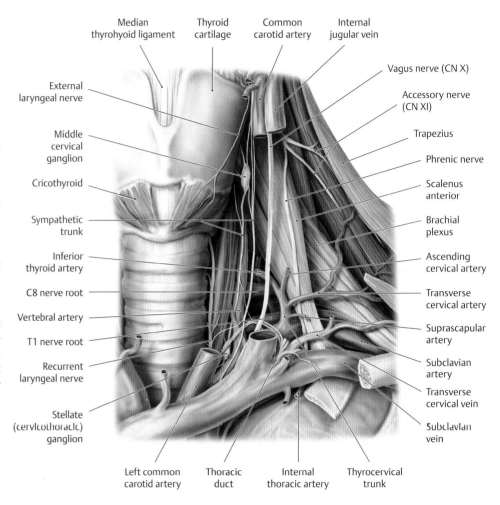

**Fig. 12.28 Root of the neck**

Anterior view of left neck. *Removed:* Clavicle (sternal end), first rib, manubrium sterni, and thyroid gland. The left common carotid artery has been cut to expose sympathetic ganglia and the ascent of the left recurrent laryngeal nerve from the aortic arch (where it arises from CN X). The brachial plexus can be seen emerging from the interscalene space between the anterior and middle scalenes. It courses with the subclavian artery and vein into the axilla. The phrenic nerve descends on the anterior scalene into the mediastinum, where it innervates the diaphragm. The left thoracic duct terminates at the jugulosubclavian venous junction. It receives lymph from the entire body with the exception of the right upper quadrant, which drains to the right lymphatic duct.

Labels (top): Median thyrohyoid ligament — Thyroid cartilage — Common carotid artery — Internal jugular vein

Labels (right): Vagus nerve (CN X) — Accessory nerve (CN XI) — Trapezius — Phrenic nerve — Scalenus anterior — Brachial plexus — Ascending cervical artery — Transverse cervical artery — Suprascapular artery — Subclavian artery — Transverse cervical vein — Subclavian vein

Labels (left): External laryngeal nerve — Middle cervical ganglion — Cricothyroid — Sympathetic trunk — Inferior thyroid artery — C8 nerve root — Vertebral artery — T1 nerve root — Recurrent laryngeal nerve — Stellate (cervicothoracic) ganglion

Labels (bottom): Left common carotid artery — Thoracic duct — Internal thoracic artery — Thyrocervical trunk

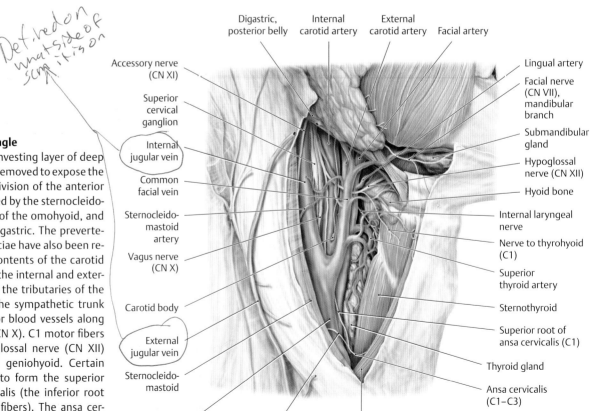

**Fig. 12.29 Carotid triangle**

Right lateral view. The investing layer of deep cervical fascia has been removed to expose the carotid triangle, a subdivision of the anterior cervical triangle bounded by the sternocleidomastoid, superior belly of the omohyoid, and posterior belly of the digastric. The prevertebral and pretracheal fasciae have also been removed to expose the contents of the carotid triangle, which include the internal and external carotid arteries and the tributaries of the internal jugular vein. The sympathetic trunk runs between the major blood vessels along with the vagus nerve (CN X). C1 motor fibers course with the hypoglossal nerve (CN XII) to the thyrohyoid and geniohyoid. Certain C1 motor fibers leave to form the superior root of the ansa cervicalis (the inferior root is formed from C2–C3 fibers). The ansa cervicalis innervates the omohyoid, sternohyoid, and sternothyroid.

Labels (top): Digastric, posterior belly — Internal carotid artery — External carotid artery — Facial artery

Labels (left): Accessory nerve (CN XI) — Superior cervical ganglion — Internal jugular vein — Common facial vein — Sternocleidomastoid artery — Vagus nerve (CN X) — Carotid body — External jugular vein — Sternocleidomastoid

Labels (right): Lingual artery — Facial nerve (CN VII), mandibular branch — Submandibular gland — Hypoglossal nerve (CN XII) — Hyoid bone — Internal laryngeal nerve — Nerve to thyrohyoid (C1) — Superior thyroid artery — Sternothyroid — Superior root of ansa cervicalis (C1) — Thyroid gland — Ansa cervicalis (C1–C3)

Labels (bottom): Internal jugular vein — Inferior root of ansa cervicalis (C2–C3) — Omohyoid

*[handwritten note]: Def. red on what side of SCM it is on*

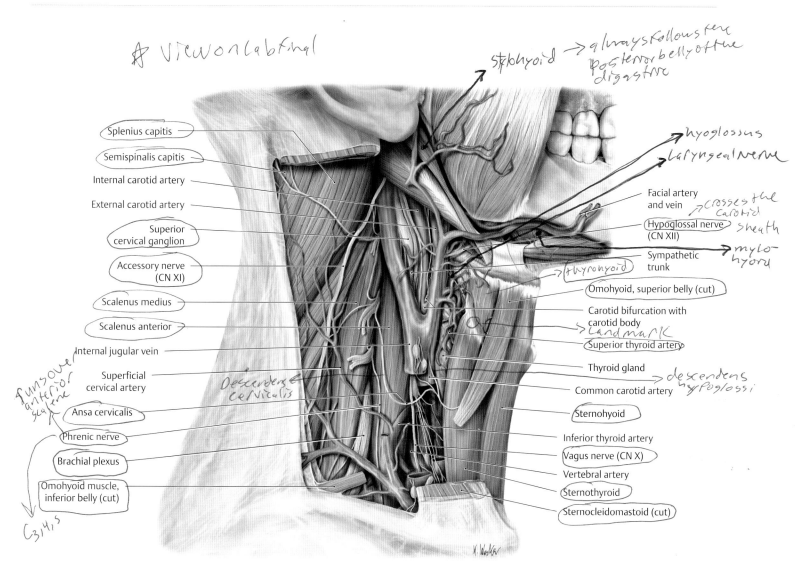

*handwritten annotations:*
★ View on Lab Final

stylohyoid → always follows the posterior belly of the digastric

hyoglossus
laryngeal nerve

crosses the carotid sheath

mylohyoid

thyrohyoid

Descendens cervicalis

descendens hypoglossi

Landmark

funsover anterior scale

C 3,4,5

**Fig. 12.30 Deep lateral cervical region**
Right lateral view. The sternocleidomastoid region and carotid triangle have been dissected along with adjacent portions of the posterior and anterior cervical triangles. The carotid sheath has been removed in this dissection along with the cervical fasciae and omohyoid muscle to demonstrate important neurovascular structures in the neck:

- Common carotid artery with internal and external carotid arteries
- Superior and inferior thyroid arteries
- Internal jugular vein
- Deep cervical lymph nodes along the internal jugular vein
- Sympathetic trunk, including ganglia

- Vagus nerve (CN X)
- Accessory nerve (CN XI)
- Hypoglossal nerve (CN XII)
- Brachial plexus
- Phrenic nerve

The phrenic nerve (C3–C5) originates from the cervical plexus and the brachial plexus. The muscular landmark for locating the phrenic nerve is the scalenus anterior, along which the nerve descends in the neck. The (posterior) interscalene space is located between the scalenus anterior and medius and the first rib and is traversed by the brachial plexus and subclavian artery. The subclavian vein passes the scalenus anterior.

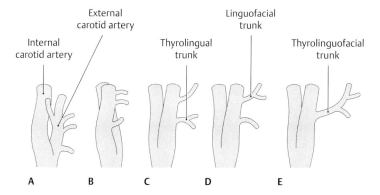

**Fig. 12.31 Variants of the carotid arteries** (after Faller and Poisel-Golth)
The internal carotid artery may arise from the common carotid artery posterolateral (49%, **A**) or anteromedial (9%, **B**) to the external carotid artery, or at other intermediate sites.
The external carotid artery may give origin to a thyrolingual trunk (4%, **C**), linguofacial trunk (23%, **D**), or thyrolinguofacial trunk (0.6%, **E**).

283

# Parapharyngeal Space (I)

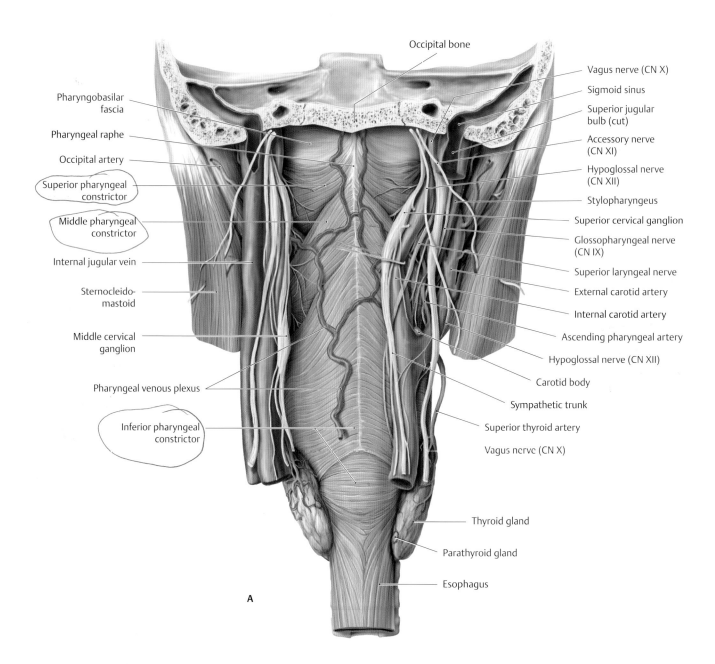

Occipital bone

Vagus nerve (CN X)

Sigmoid sinus

Superior jugular bulb (cut)

Accessory nerve (CN XI)

Hypoglossal nerve (CN XII)

Stylopharyngeus

Superior cervical ganglion

Glossopharyngeal nerve (CN IX)

Superior laryngeal nerve

External carotid artery

Internal carotid artery

Ascending pharyngeal artery

Hypoglossal nerve (CN XII)

Carotid body

Sympathetic trunk

Superior thyroid artery

Vagus nerve (CN X)

Thyroid gland

Parathyroid gland

Esophagus

Pharyngobasilar fascia

Pharyngeal raphe

Occipital artery

Superior pharyngeal constrictor

Middle pharyngeal constrictor

Internal jugular vein

Sternocleido-mastoid

Middle cervical ganglion

Pharyngeal venous plexus

Inferior pharyngeal constrictor

A

**Fig. 12.32 Parapharyngeal space**
Posterior view. **A** *Removed:* Fascial layers and contents of the prevertebral fascia. **B** Pharynx opened along pharyngeal raphe. The common and internal carotid arteries travel with the jugular vein and vagus nerve within the carotid sheath, which attaches to the skull base. The pharynx, thyroid gland, and anterior viscera are enclosed within the pretracheal fascia (the posterior portion, the buccopharyngeal fascia, lies anterior to the prevertebral fascia).

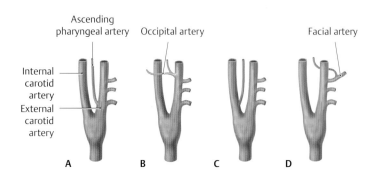

Ascending pharyngeal artery

Occipital artery

Facial artery

Internal carotid artery

External carotid artery

A      B      C      D

**Fig. 12.33 Ascending pharyngeal artery: variants** (after Tillmann, Lippert, and Pabst)
Left lateral view. The main arterial vessel supplying the upper and middle pharynx is the ascending pharyngeal artery. In 70% of cases (**A**) it arises from the posteroinferior surface of the external carotid artery. In approximately 20% of cases it arises from the occipital artery (**B**). Occasionally (8%) it originates from the internal carotid artery or carotid bifurcation (**C**), and in 2% of cases it arises from the facial artery (**D**).

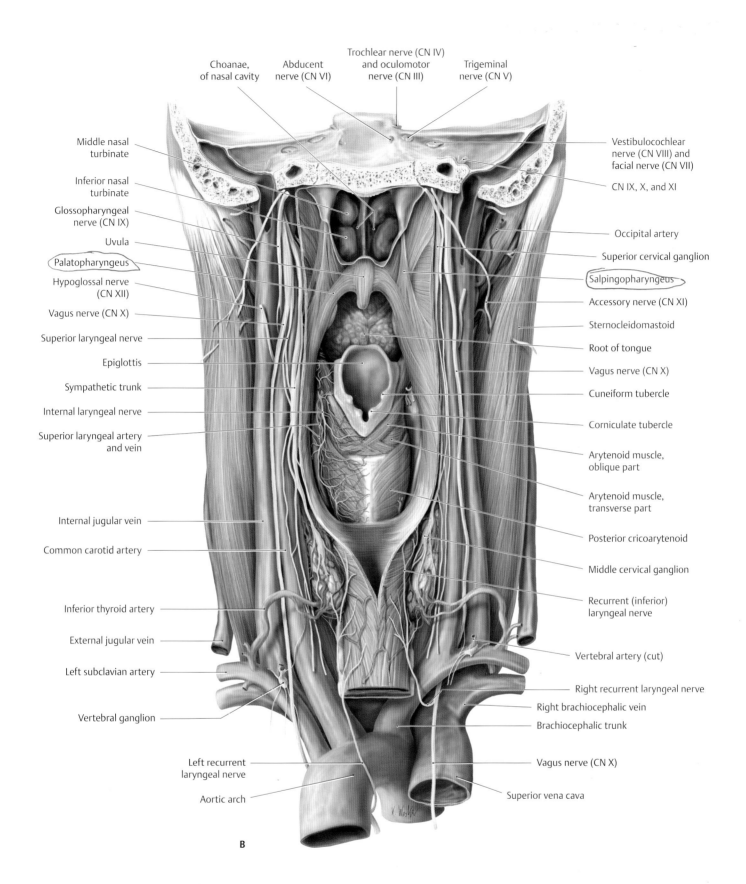

Choanae, of nasal cavity

Abducent nerve (CN VI)

Trochlear nerve (CN IV) and oculomotor nerve (CN III)

Trigeminal nerve (CN V)

Middle nasal turbinate

Inferior nasal turbinate

Glossopharyngeal nerve (CN IX)

Uvula

Palatopharyngeus

Hypoglossal nerve (CN XII)

Vagus nerve (CN X)

Superior laryngeal nerve

Epiglottis

Sympathetic trunk

Internal laryngeal nerve

Superior laryngeal artery and vein

Internal jugular vein

Common carotid artery

Inferior thyroid artery

External jugular vein

Left subclavian artery

Vertebral ganglion

Left recurrent laryngeal nerve

Aortic arch

Vestibulocochlear nerve (CN VIII) and facial nerve (CN VII)

CN IX, X, and XI

Occipital artery

Superior cervical ganglion

Salpingopharyngeus

Accessory nerve (CN XI)

Sternocleidomastoid

Root of tongue

Vagus nerve (CN X)

Cuneiform tubercle

Corniculate tubercle

Arytenoid muscle, oblique part

Arytenoid muscle, transverse part

Posterior cricoarytenoid

Middle cervical ganglion

Recurrent (inferior) laryngeal nerve

Vertebral artery (cut)

Right recurrent laryngeal nerve

Right brachiocephalic vein

Brachiocephalic trunk

Vagus nerve (CN X)

Superior vena cava

**B**

3 pharyngeal elevators

- Stylopharyngeus — IX
- Palatopharyngeus — X
- Salpingopharyngeus — X ⇒ attaches to torus tubarus

# Parapharyngeal Space (II)

*[Handwritten notes:]*
*☆ Infections spread between fascial layers, muscles, & periosthium & bone*
*☆ The parapharyngeal space is broken into the retropharyngeal & lateropharyngeal space*

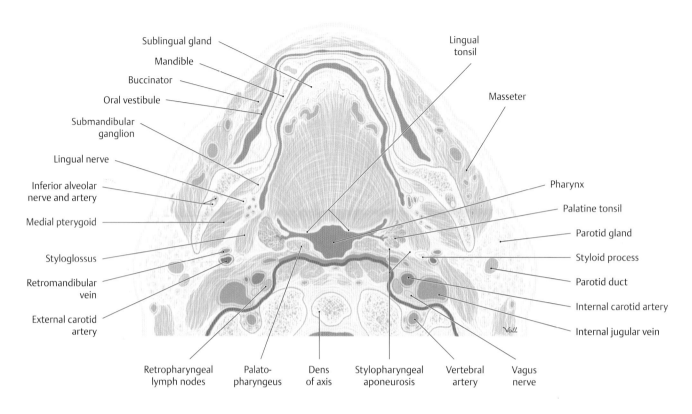

Sublingual gland
Mandible
Buccinator
Oral vestibule
Submandibular ganglion
Lingual nerve
Inferior alveolar nerve and artery
Medial pterygoid
Styloglossus
Retromandibular vein
External carotid artery

Lingual tonsil
Masseter
Pharynx
Palatine tonsil
Parotid gland
Styloid process
Parotid duct
Internal carotid artery
Internal jugular vein

Retropharyngeal lymph nodes
Palato-pharyngeus
Dens of axis
Stylopharyngeal aponeurosis
Vertebral artery
Vagus nerve

### Fig. 12.34  Spaces in the neck

Transverse section, superior view. The pharynx is enclosed by the pretracheal fascia along with the larynx and thyroid gland. The posterior portion of the pretracheal fascia that is in direct contact with the pharynx is called the buccopharyngeal fascia. The fascial space surrounding the pharynx (parapharyngeal space) is divided into a posterior (retropharyngeal) space and a lateral (lateropharyngeal) space. The retropharyngeal space (green) lies between the anterior alar layer of the prevertebral fascia (red) and the buccopharyngeal fascia, the posterior portion of the pretracheal fascia. The lateropharyngeal space is divided by the stylopharyngeal aponeurosis into an anterior and a posterior part. The anterior part (yellow) is contained within the pretracheal fascia in the neck (this section is through the oral cavity). The posterior part (orange) is contained within the carotid sheath.

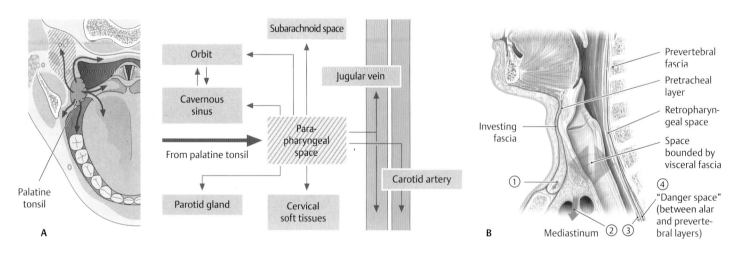

Palatine tonsil

Subarachnoid space
Orbit
Cavernous sinus
Jugular vein
Para-pharyngeal space
From palatine tonsil
Parotid gland
Cervical soft tissues
Carotid artery

A

Investing fascia

Prevertebral fascia
Pretracheal layer
Retropharyngeal space
Space bounded by visceral fascia

① ④ "Danger space" (between alar and prevertebral layers)

Mediastinum ② ③

B

### Fig. 12.35  Clinical significance of the parapharyngeal space
(after Becker, Naumann, and Pfaltz)

Bacteria and inflammatory processes from the oral and nasal cavities (e.g., tonsillitis, dental infections) may invade the parapharyngeal space. From there, they may spread in various directions (**A**). Invasion of the jugular vein may lead to bacteremia and sepsis. Invasion of the subarachnoid space poses a risk of meningitis. Inflammatory processes may also track downward into the mediastinum (gravitation abscess), causing mediastinitus (**B**). These may spread anteriorly in the spaces between the investing and muscular pretracheal layers ① or in the space within the pretracheal fascia ②. They may also spread posteriorly in the retropharyngeal space ③ between the buccopharyngeal prevertebral fascia and the alar prevertebral fascia. Infections that enter the "danger space" ④ between the alar and prevertebral layers of the prevertebral fascia may spread directly into the mediastinum.

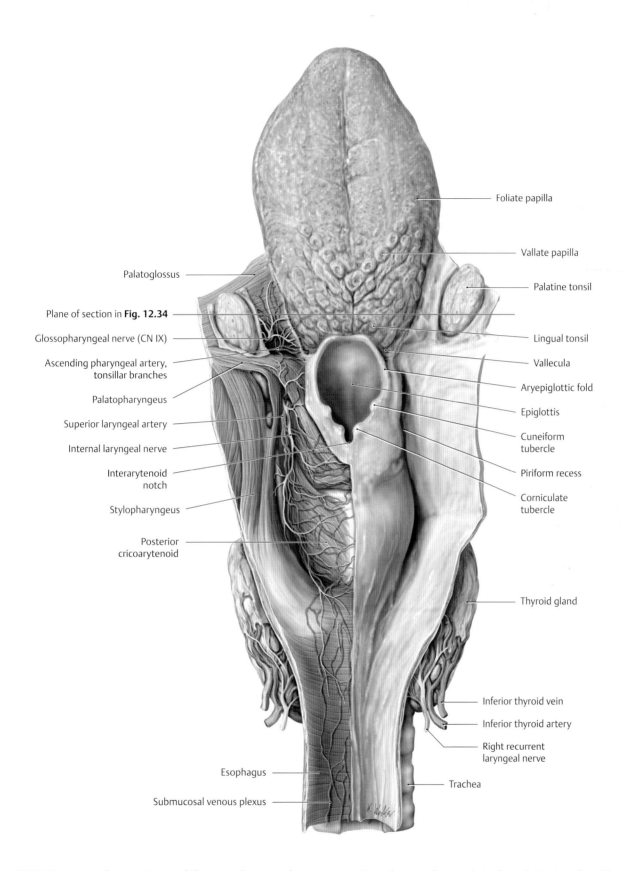

**Fig. 12.36 Neurovascular structures of the parapharyngeal space**
Posterior view of an en bloc specimen composed of the tongue, larynx, esophagus, and thyroid gland, as it would be resected at autopsy for pathologic evaluation of the neck. This dissection clearly demonstrates the branching pattern of the neurovascular structures that occupy the plane between the pharyngeal muscles.

Note the vascular supply to the palatine tonsil and its proximity to the neurovascular bundle, which creates a risk of hemorrhage during tonsillectomy.

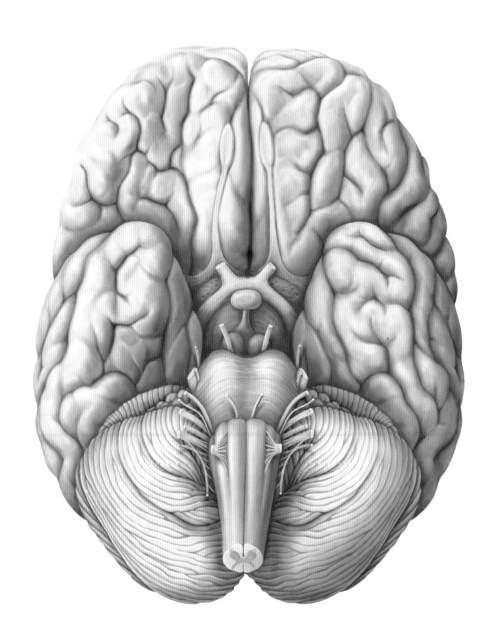

# Neuroanatomy

# Nervous System

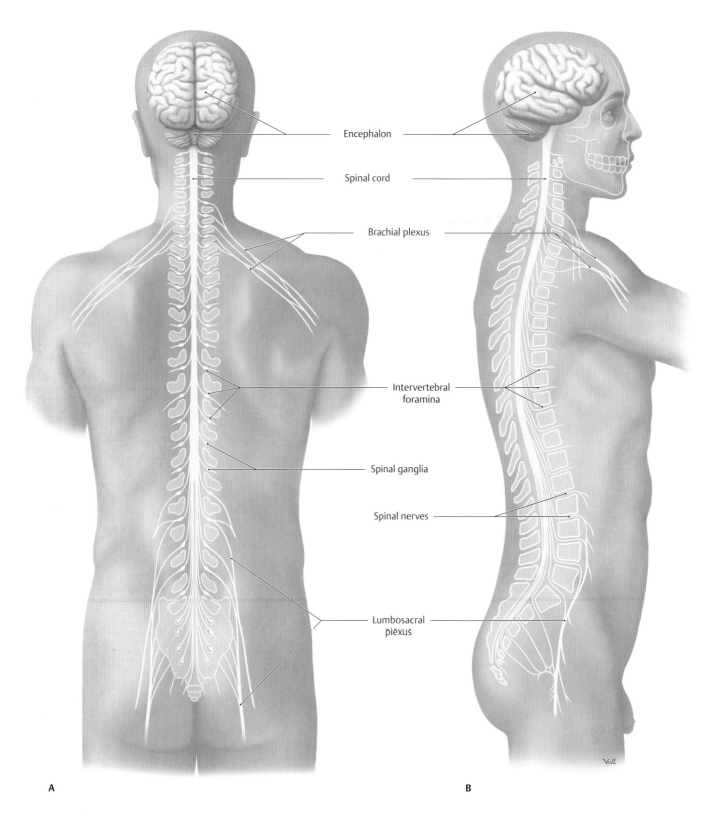

Encephalon

Spinal cord

Brachial plexus

Intervertebral
foramina

Spinal ganglia

Spinal nerves

Lumbosacral
plexus

A

B

**Fig. 13.1 Topography of the nervous system**
**A** Posterior view. **B** Right lateral view.

The *central nervous system* (CNS), consisting of the brain (encephalon) and spinal cord, is shown in pink. The *peripheral nervous system* (PNS), consisting of nerves synd ganglia, is shown in yellow. The nerves arising from the spinal cord leave their bony canal through the *intervertebral foramina* and are distributed to their target structures. The *spinal nerves* are formed in the foramina by the union of their dorsal (poste-

rior) roots and ventral (anterior) roots (see p. 292). The small *spinal ganglion* in the intervertebral foramen appears as a slight swelling of the dorsal root (visible only in the posterior view; its function is described on p. 292).

In the limbs, the ventral rami of the spinal nerves come together to form plexuses. These plexuses then give rise to the peripheral nerves that supply the limbs.

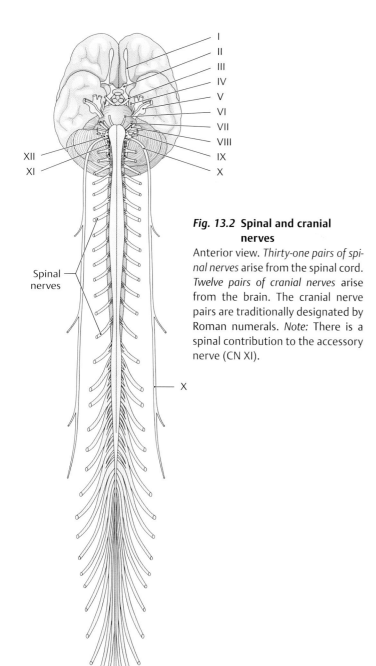

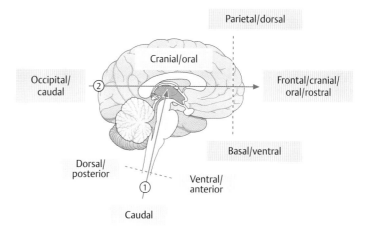

**Fig. 13.2 Spinal and cranial nerves**

Anterior view. *Thirty-one pairs of spinal nerves* arise from the spinal cord. *Twelve pairs of cranial nerves* arise from the brain. The cranial nerve pairs are traditionally designated by Roman numerals. *Note:* There is a spinal contribution to the accessory nerve (CN XI).

**Fig. 13.3 Terms of location and direction in the CNS**

Midsagittal section, right lateral view.
Note two important axes:

① The almost vertical brainstem axis (corresponds approximately to the body axis).
② The horizontal axis through the diencephalon and telencephalon.

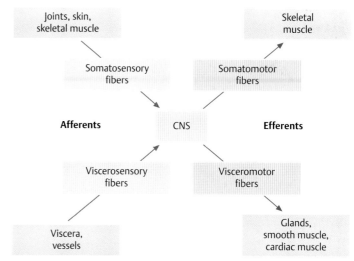

**Fig. 13.4 Information flow in the nervous system**

The information encoded in nerve fibers is transmitted either *to the CNS* (brain and spinal cord) or *from the CNS* to the periphery (PNS, including the peripheral parts of the autonomic nervous system). Fibers that carry information to the CNS are called afferent fibers or *afferents* for short; fibers that carry signals away from the CNS are called efferent fibers or *efferents*.

**291**

# Spinal Cord: Organization

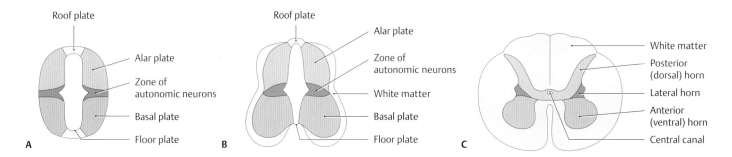

**Fig. 13.5 Development of the spinal cord**

Transverse section, superior view. **A** Early neural tube. **B** Intermediate stage. **C** Adult spinal cord. The spinal cord consists of white matter that encloses gray matter columns arranged about the central canal. The gray matter primarily contains the cell bodies of neurons, and the white matter primarily consists of nerve fibers (axons). Axons with the same function are collected into bundles. Within the spinal cord, these bundles are called tracts (in the periphery they are called nerves). Ascending (afferent or sensory) tracts terminate in the brain. Descending (efferent or motor) tracts pass from the brain into the spinal cord.

The spinal cord develops from the neural tube. *Note:* Neurons do not develop from the roof or floor plates.

- Posterior (dorsal) horn: Develops from basal plate (posterior neural tube, pink). It contains afferent (sensory) neurons.
- Anterior (ventral) horn: Develops from the alar plate (anterior neural tube, blue). It contains efferent (motor) neurons.
- Lateral horn: Develops from the intervening zone. It contains autonomic sympathetic neurons. *Note:* The lateral horn is present in the thoracic and upper lumbar regions of the spinal cord.

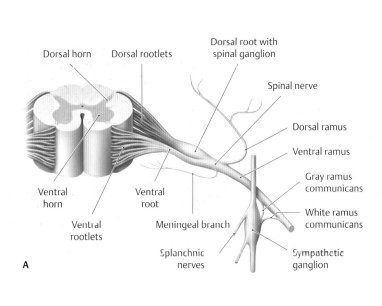

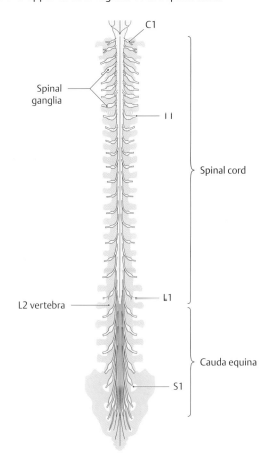

**Fig. 13.6 Organization of spinal cord segments**

**A** Transverse section, superior view. **B** Longitudinal section, posterior view with laminar (neural) arches of vertebral bodies removed. There are two main organizational principles in the spinal cord:

1. Functional organization within segments (**A**). In each spinal cord segment, afferent dorsal rootlets enter the cord posteriorly, and efferent ventral rootlets emerge anteriorly. The rootlets combine to form the dorsal (posterior) and ventral (anterior) roots. The dorsal and ventral roots of each spinal cord segment fuse to form a mixed spinal nerve, which carries both sensory and motor fibers. Shortly

after the fusion of its two roots, the spinal nerve divides into various branches.

2. Topographical organization of segments (**B**). The spinal cord consists of a vertical series of 31 segments. Each segment innervates a specific area. Most spinal nerves emerge inferior to their corresponding vertebra (see **Fig. 13.7**). The spinal cord level does not, however, correspond to the level of the vertebra. The lower end of the adult spinal cord extends only to the first lumbar vertebral body (L1). Below L1, the spinal nerve roots descend to the intervertebral foramina as the cauda equina ("horse's tail"). At the intervertebral foramina, they join to form the spinal nerves.

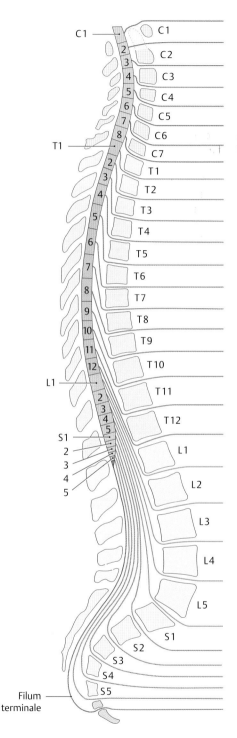

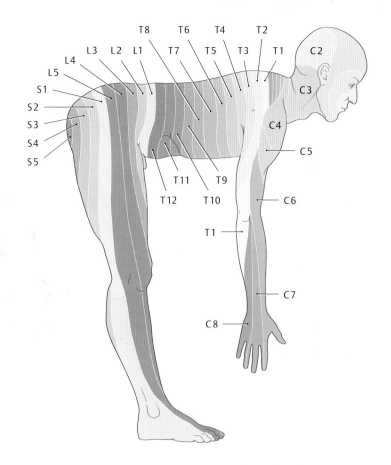

**Fig. 13.8 Dermatomes**
Sensory innervation of the skin correlates with the sensory roots of the spinal nerves. Every spinal cord segment (except for C1) innervates a particular skin area (= dermatome). From a clinical standpoint, it is important to know the precise correlation of dermatomes with spinal cord segments so that the level of a spinal cord lesion can be determined based on the location of the affected dermatome. For example, a lesion of the C8 spinal nerve root is characterized by a loss of sensation on the ulnar (small-finger) side of the hand.

| Table 13.1 Levels of spinal cord segments | | |
|---|---|---|
| **Spinal cord segment** | **Nearest vertebral body** | **Nearest spinous process** |
| C8 | C6 (inferior margin) and C7 (superior margin) | C6 |
| T6 | T5 | T4 |
| T12 | T10 | T9 |
| L3 | T11 | |
| S1 | T12 | |

*Note:* These are only approximations and may differ among individuals.

**Fig. 13.7 Spinal cord segments**
Midsagittal section, viewed from the right side. The spinal cord is divided into five major regions: the cervical cord (C, pink), thoracic cord (T, blue), lumbar cord (L, green), sacral cord (S, yellow), and coccygeal cord (gray). The adult spinal cord generally extends to the level of the L1 vertebral body. The region below, known as the cauda equina (see **Fig. 13.6B**), provides relatively safe access for introducing a spinal needle to sample CSF (lumbar puncture).

**Numbering of spinal cord segments.** The spinal cord segments are numbered according to the exit point of their associated spinal nerve. In most cases, the spinal nerve emerges inferior to its associated vertebra (exceptions: C1–C8*). The emergence point does not necessarily correlate with the nearest skeletal element (see **Table 13.1**). Progressively greater "mismatch" between segments and associated vertebrae occurs at more caudal levels. The relationship between the spinal cord segments and vertebrae can be used to assess injuries to the vertebral column (e.g., spinal fracture or cord lesions).

* *Note:* There are only seven cervical vertebrae but eight pairs of cervical spinal nerves (C1–C8).

**293**

# Brain: Organization

### *Fig. 13.9* Gross anatomy of the brain

**A** Left lateral view with dura mater removed.
**B** Basal (inferior) view with cervical spinal cord sectioned. The central nervous system consists of the brain and spinal cord. The brain is divided into four major parts (**Fig. 13.10**): telencephalon (cerebrum), diencephalon, brainstem, and cerebellum. The telencephalon (cerebrum) is the large outer portion of the brain, consisting of two hemispheres separated by a longitudinal cerebral fissure (**B**). The telencephalon (cerebrum) is divided macroscopically into five lobes: frontal, parietal, temporal, occipital, and central (insular). *Note:* The central (insular) lobe cannot be seen unless the temporal or parietal lobe is retracted at the lateral sulcus. The surface contours of the cerebrum are defined by convolutions (gyri) and depressions (sulci). The central sulcus, an important reference point on the cerebrum, separates the precentral gyrus from the postcentral gyrus. The precentral gyrus mediates voluntary motor activity, and the postcentral gyrus mediates the conscious perception of body sensation. Gyri vary considerably between individuals and may even vary between hemispheres. Sulci may be narrowed and compressed in brain edema (excessive fluid accumulation in the brain). They are enlarged in brain atrophy (e.g., Alzheimer disease), due to tissue loss from the gyri.

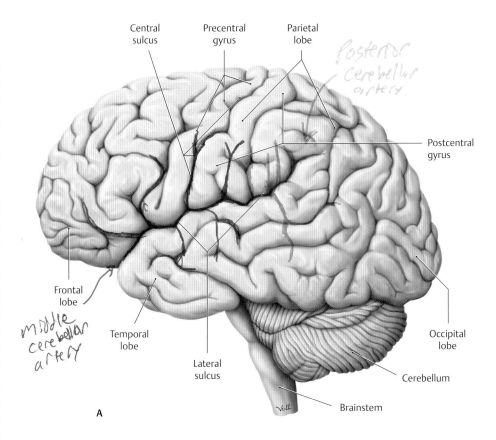

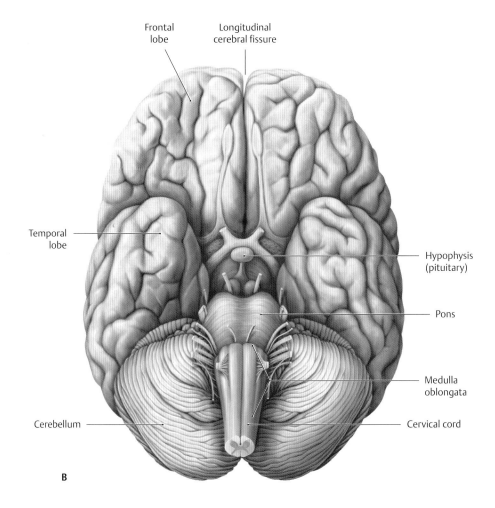

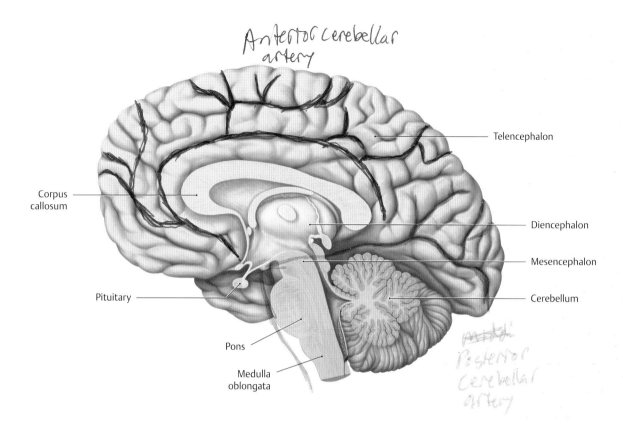

**Fig. 13.10 Developmental organization of the brain**
Midsagittal section of brain (along longitudinal cerebral fissure). Medial view of right hemisphere. The brain is divided developmentally into six major parts: telencephalon (cerebrum), diencephalon, mesencephalon, pons, medulla oblongata, and cerebellum. The mesencephalon, pons, and medulla oblongata are collectively referred to as the brainstem. The medulla oblongata, the caudal portion of the brainstem, is continuous inferiorly with the spinal cord. There is no definite anatomical boundary between them, as the brain and spinal cord are a functional unit (the central nervous system).

| Table 13.2 Development of the brain | | | |
|---|---|---|---|
| **Primary vesicle** | | **Region** | **Structure** |
| Neural tube | Prosencephalon (forebrain) | Telencephalon | Cerebral cortex, white matter, and basal ganglia |
| | | Diencephalon | Epithalamus (pineal), dorsal thalamus, subthalamus, and hypothalamus |
| | Mesencephalon (midbrain)* | | Tectum, tegmentum, and cerebral peduncles |
| | Rhombencephalon (hindbrain) | Metencephalon — Cerebellum | Cerebellar cortex, nuclei, and peduncles |
| | | Pons* | Nuclei and fiber tracts |
| | | Myelencephalon — Medulla oblongata* | |

*The mesencephalon, pons, and medulla oblongata are collectively known as the brainstem.

# Brain & Meninges

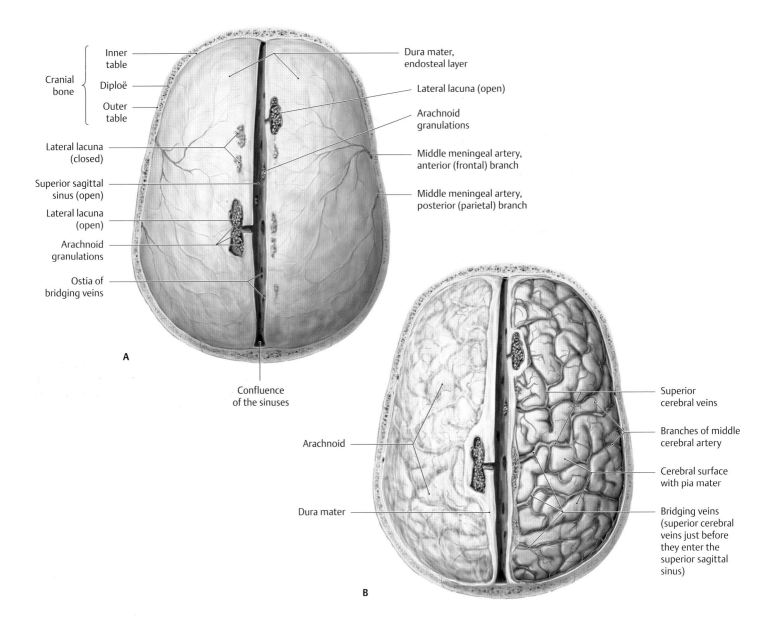

**Fig. 13.11 Brain and meninges in situ**

Superior view. **A** The calvaria has been removed, and the superior sagittal sinus and its lateral lacunae have been opened. **B** The dura mater has been removed from the left hemisphere, and the dura and arachnoid have been removed from the right hemisphere.

The brain and spinal cord are covered by membranes called meninges, which form a sac filled with cerebrospinal fluid (CSF). The meninges are composed of the following three layers:

- Outer layer: The *dura mater* (often shortened to "dura") is a tough layer of collagenous connective tissue. It consists of two layers, an inner meningeal layer and an outer endosteal layer. The periosteal layer adheres firmly to the periosteum of the calvaria within the cranial cavity, but it is easy to separate the inner layer from the bone in this region, leaving it on the cerebrum, as illustrated here (**A**).
- Middle layer: The *arachnoid* (arachnoid membrane) is a translucent membrane through which the cerebrum and the blood vessels in the subarachnoid space can be seen (**B**).

- Inner layer: The *pia mater* directly invests the cerebrum and lines its fissures (**B**).

The arachnoid and pia are collectively called the *leptomeninges*. The space between them, called the subarachnoid space, is filled with CSF and envelops the brain. It contains the major cerebral arteries and the superficial cerebral veins, which drain chiefly through "bridging veins" into the superior sagittal sinus. The dura mater in the midline forms a double fold between the periosteal and meningeal layers that encloses the endothelium-lined superior sagittal sinus, which has been opened in the illustration. Inspection of the opened sinus reveals the arachnoid granulations (pacchionian granulations, arachnoid villi). These protrusions of the arachnoid are sites for the reabsorption of CSF. Arachnoid granulations are particularly abundant in the lateral lacunae of the superior sagittal sinus. The dissection in **A** shows how the middle meningeal artery is situated between the dura and calvaria. Rupture of this vessel causes blood to accumulate between the bone and dura, forming an epidural hematoma.

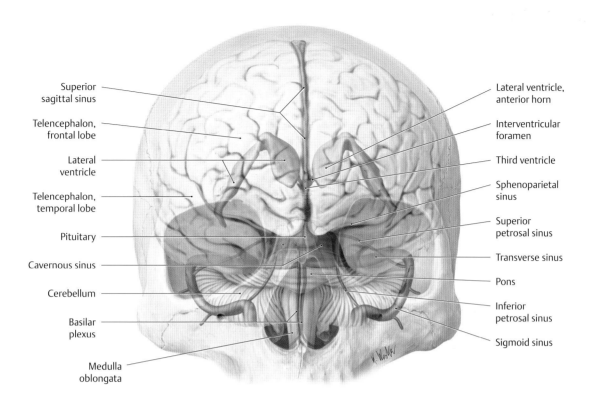

Superior sagittal sinus

Telencephalon, frontal lobe

Lateral ventricle

Telencephalon, temporal lobe

Pituitary

Cavernous sinus

Cerebellum

Basilar plexus

Medulla oblongata

Lateral ventricle, anterior horn

Interventricular foramen

Third ventricle

Sphenoparietal sinus

Superior petrosal sinus

Transverse sinus

Pons

Inferior petrosal sinus

Sigmoid sinus

**Fig. 13.12 Projection of important brain structures**
Anterior view. The largest structures of the cerebrum (telencephalon) are the frontal and temporal lobes. The falx cerebri separates the two cerebral hemispheres in the midline (not visible here). In the brainstem, we can identify the pons and medulla oblongata on both sides of the midline below the telencephalon. The superior sagittal sinus and the paired sigmoid sinuses can also be seen. The anterior horns of the two lateral ventricles are projected onto the forehead.

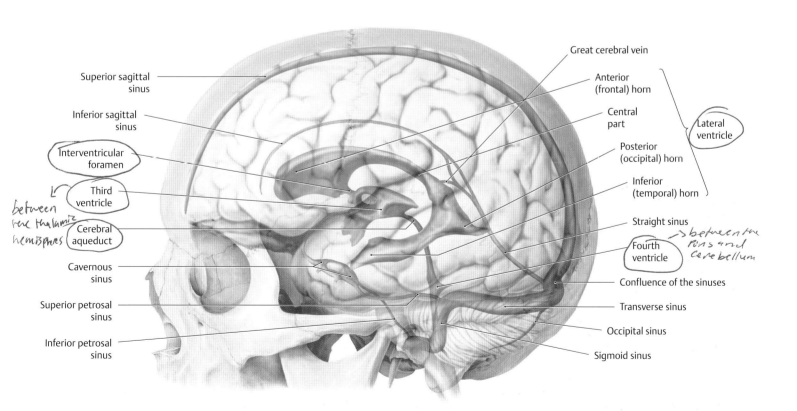

Superior sagittal sinus

Inferior sagittal sinus

Interventricular foramen

Third ventricle

Cerebral aqueduct

Cavernous sinus

Superior petrosal sinus

Inferior petrosal sinus

Great cerebral vein

Anterior (frontal) horn

Central part

Posterior (occipital) horn

Inferior (temporal) horn

Lateral ventricle

Straight sinus

Fourth ventricle

Confluence of the sinuses

Transverse sinus

Occipital sinus

Sigmoid sinus

*(handwritten annotations:)* between the thalamic hemispheres; between the pons and cerebellum

**Fig. 13.13 Projection of important brain structures**
Left lateral view. The relationship of specific lobes of the cerebrum to the cranial fossae can be appreciated in this view. The frontal lobe lies in the anterior cranial fossa, the temporal lobe in the middle cranial fossa, and the cerebellum in the posterior cranial fossa. The following dural venous sinuses can be identified: the superior and inferior sagittal sinus, straight sinus, transverse sinus, sigmoid sinus, cavernous sinus, superior and inferior petrosal sinus, and occipital sinus.

# Spinal Cord & Meninges

### Fig. 13.14  Spinal cord in the vertebral canal

Transverse section at the level of the C4 vertebra, viewed from above. The spinal cord occupies the center of the vertebral foramen and is anchored within the subarachnoid space to the spinal dura mater by the denticulate ligament. The root sleeve, an outpouching of the dura mater in the intravertebral foramen, contains the spinal ganglion and the dorsal and ventral roots of the spinal nerve. The spinal dura mater is bounded externally by the epidural space, which contains venous plexuses, fat, and connective tissue. The epidural space extends upward as far as the foramen magnum, where the dura becomes fused to the cranial periosteum.

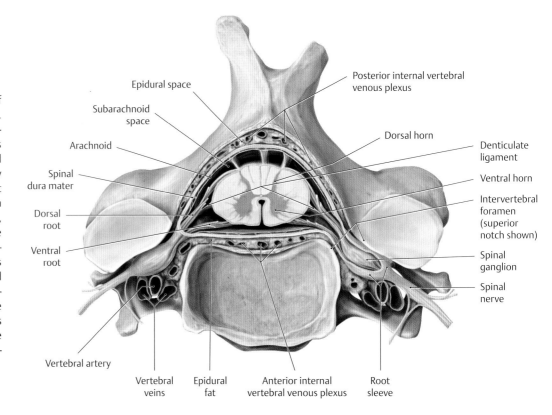

### Fig. 13.15  Cauda equina in the vertebral canal

Transverse section at the level of the L2 vertebra, viewed from below. The spinal cord usually ends at the level of the first lumbar vertebra (L1). The space below the lower end of the spinal cord is occupied by the cauda equina and filum terminale in the dural sac, which ends at the level of the S2 vertebra. The epidural space expands at that level and contains extensive venous plexuses and fatty tissue.

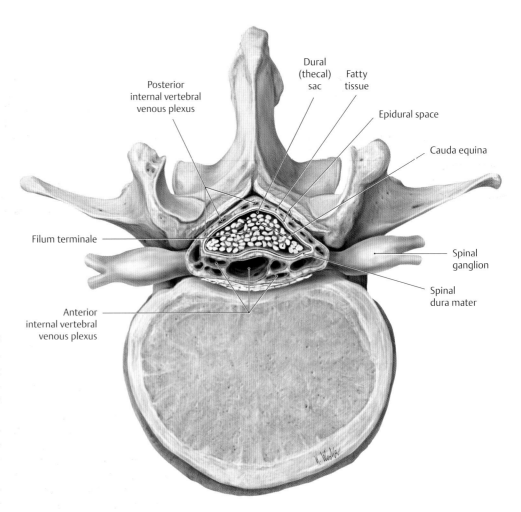

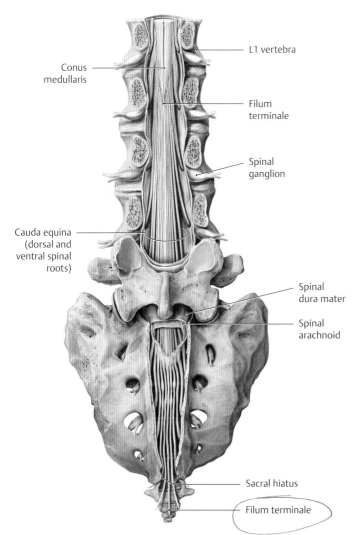

Conus medullaris

L1 vertebra

Filum terminale

Spinal ganglion

Cauda equina (dorsal and ventral spinal roots)

Spinal dura mater

Spinal arachnoid

Sacral hiatus

Filum terminale

**Fig. 13.16 Cauda equina in the vertebral canal**
Posterior view. The laminae and the dorsal surface of the sacrum have been partially removed. The spinal cord in the adult terminates at approximately the level of the first lumbar vertebra (L1). The dorsal and ventral spinal nerve roots extending from the lower end of the spinal cord (conus medullaris) are known collectively as the cauda equina. During lumbar puncture at this level, a needle introduced into the subarachnoid space (lumbar cistern) normally slips past the spinal nerve roots without injuring them.

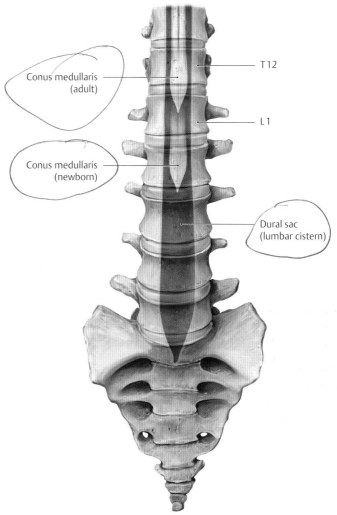

Conus medullaris (adult)

T12

L1

Conus medullaris (newborn)

Dural sac (lumbar cistern)

**Fig. 13.17 Age-related changes of spinal cord levels**
Anterior view. As an individual grows, the longitudinal growth of the spinal cord increasingly lags behind that of the vertebral column. At birth the distal end of the spinal cord, the conus medullaris, is at the level of the L3 vertebral body (where lumbar puncture is contraindicated). The spinal cord of a tall adult ends at the T12/L1 level, whereas that of a short adult extends to the L2/L3 level. The dural sac always extends into the upper sacrum. It is important to consider these anatomical relationships during lumbar puncture. It is best to introduce the needle at the L3/L4 interspace (see **Fig. 13.18**).

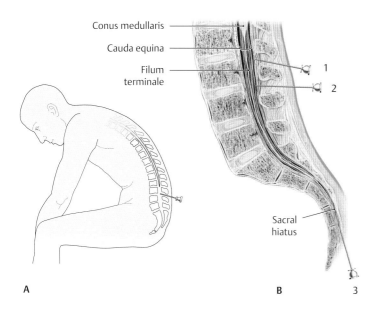

Conus medullaris

Cauda equina

Filum terminale

1

2

Sacral hiatus

A     B     3

**Fig. 13.18 Lumbar puncture, epidural anesthesia, and lumbar anesthesia**
In preparation for a **lumbar puncture**, the patient bends far forward to separate the spinous processes of the lumbar spine. The spinal needle is usually introduced between the spinous processes of the L3 and L4 vertebrae. It is advanced through the skin and into the dural sac (lumbar cistern, see **Fig. 13.17**) to obtain a CSF sample. This procedure has numerous applications, including the diagnosis of meningitis. For **epidural anesthesia**, a catheter is placed in the epidural space without penetrating the dural sac (1). **Lumbar anesthesia** is induced by injecting a local anesthetic solution into the dural sac (2). Another option is to pass the needle into the epidural space through the sacral hiatus (3).

**299**

# Cerebrospinal Fluid (CSF) Spaces

*[handwritten annotations:]*
*★★ One way value back into venous circulation*
*• when impaired this leads to CSF build up →*
*hydrocephalus syndrome*

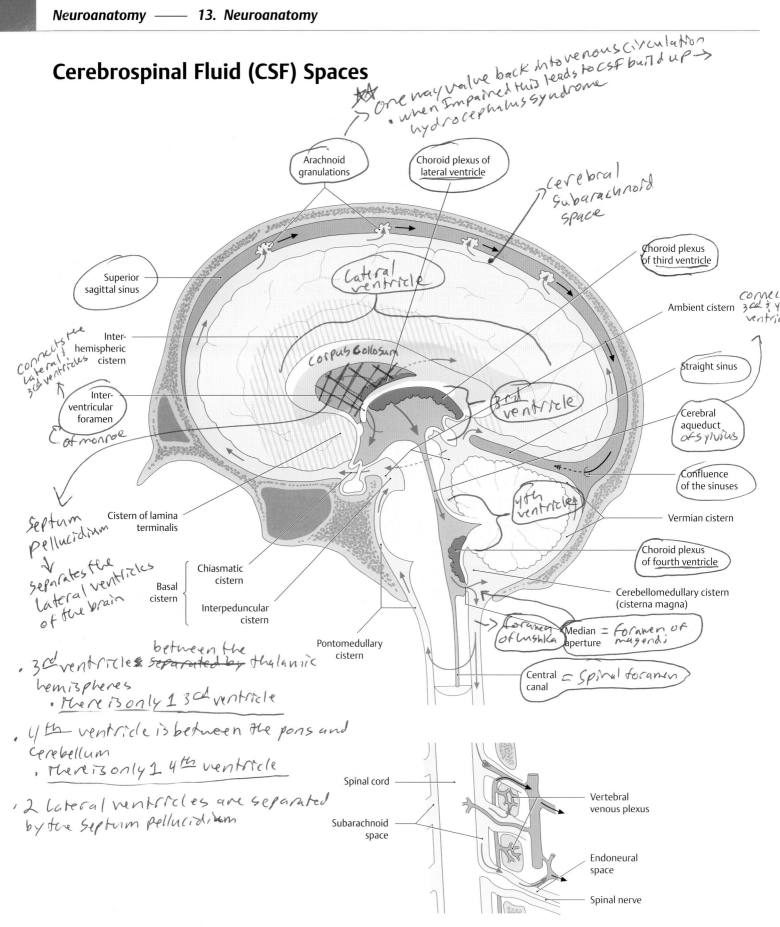

*[handwritten labels on figure:]*
Cerebral subarachnoid space
Lateral ventricle
Corpus collosum
3rd ventricle
4th ventricle
Connects the lateral & 3rd ventricles
...of monroe
Septum pellucidium ↓ separates the lateral ventricles of the brain
Cerebral aqueduct of sylvius
Correl: 3rd & 4th ventricle
Foramen of Lushka
Median = foramen of magendi
Central canal = spinal foramen

*[handwritten notes at bottom:]*
• 3rd ventricles separated by thalanic hemispheres
   • There is only 1 3rd ventricle
• 4th ventricle is between the pons and cerebellum
   • There is only 1 4th ventricle
• 2 lateral ventricles are separated by the septum pellucidium

*[printed figure labels:]*
Arachnoid granulations
Choroid plexus of lateral ventricle
Choroid plexus of third ventricle
Superior sagittal sinus
Ambient cistern
Inter-hemispheric cistern
Straight sinus
Inter-ventricular foramen
Choroid plexus of fourth ventricle
Confluence of the sinuses
Cistern of lamina terminalis
Vermian cistern
Chiasmatic cistern
Basal cistern
Interpeduncular cistern
Cerebellomedullary cistern (cisterna magna)
Median aperture
Pontomedullary cistern
Central canal
Spinal cord
Vertebral venous plexus
Subarachnoid space
Endoneural space
Spinal nerve

**Fig. 13.19 CSF spaces**
Schematized midsagittal section. Medial view of right hemisphere. The brain and spinal cord are suspended in CSF. CSF is located in the subarachnoid space enclosed by the meningeal layers surrounding the brain and spinal cord. The cerebral ventricles and subarachnoid space have a combined capacity of approximately 150 mL of CSF (80% in subarachnoid space, 20% in ventricles). This volume is completely replaced two to four times daily. CSF is produced in the choroid plexus (red), present in each of the four cerebral ventricles (see **Fig. 13.13**). It flows from the ventricles through the median and lateral apertures (not shown) into the subarachnoid space. Most CSF drains from the subarachnoid space through the arachnoid granulations (see **Fig. 13.11**) and the dural sinuses. Smaller amounts drain along the proximal portions of the spinal nerves into venous plexuses or lymphatic pathways. Obstruction of CSF drainage will cause a rapid rise in intracranial pressure due to the high rate of CSF turnover.

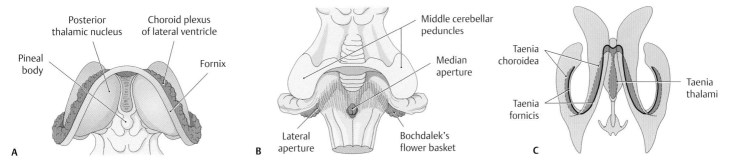

**Fig. 13.20 Choroid plexus**
**A** Lateral ventricles. Rear view of thalamus. **B** Fourth ventricle. Posterior view of partially opened rhomboid fossa (cerebellum removed). **C** Cerebral ventricles, superior view.
The choroid plexus is formed by the ingrowth of vascular loops into the ependyma. The ependyma is firmly attached to the walls of the associated ventricles. Its lines of attachment, the taeniae, are revealed when the plexus tissue is removed with forceps (**C**). As the choroid plexus is adherent to the ventricular wall at only one site, it can float freely in the ventricular system. Free ends of the choroid plexus may extend through the lateral aperture into the subarachnoid space ("Bochdalek's flower basket").

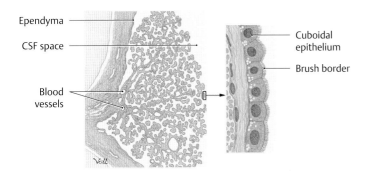

**Fig. 13.21 Histological section of the choroid plexus** (after Kahle)
The choroid plexus is a protrusion of the ventricular wall. It is often likened to a cauliflower because of its extensive surface folds. The epithelium of the choroid plexus consists of a single layer of cuboidal cells and has a brush border on its apical surface (to increase the surface area further).

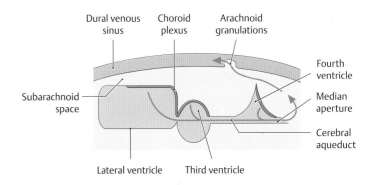

**Fig. 13.22 CSF circulation**
The choroid plexus is present to some extent in each of the four cerebral ventricles. It produces CSF, which flows through the two lateral apertures (not shown) and median aperture into the subarachnoid space. From there, most of the CSF drains through the arachnoid granulations into the dural venous sinuses.

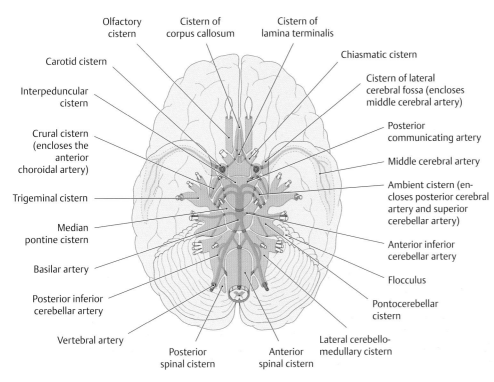

**Fig. 13.23 Subarachnoid cisterns**
(after Rauber and Kopsch)
Basal view. The cisterns are CSF-filled expansions of the subarachnoid space. They contain the proximal portions of some cranial nerves and basal cerebral arteries (veins are not shown). When arterial bleeding occurs (as from a ruptured aneurysm), blood will seep into the subarachnoid space and enter the CSF. A ruptured intracranial aneurysm is a frequent cause of blood in the CSF.

**301**

# Dural Sinuses

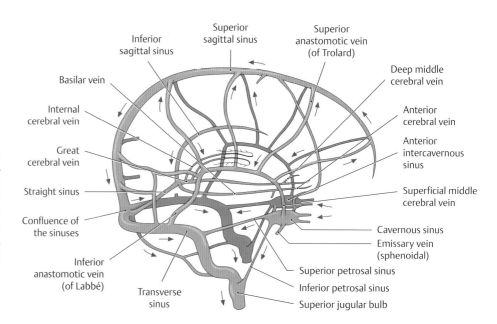

**Fig. 13.24 Dural sinus tributaries from the cerebral veins** (after Rauber and Kopsch)
Right lateral view. Venous blood collected deep within the brain drains to the dural sinuses through superficial and deep cerebral veins. The red arrows in the diagram show the principal directions of venous blood flow in the major sinuses. Because of the numerous anastomoses, the isolated occlusion of a complete sinus segment may produce no clinical symptoms.

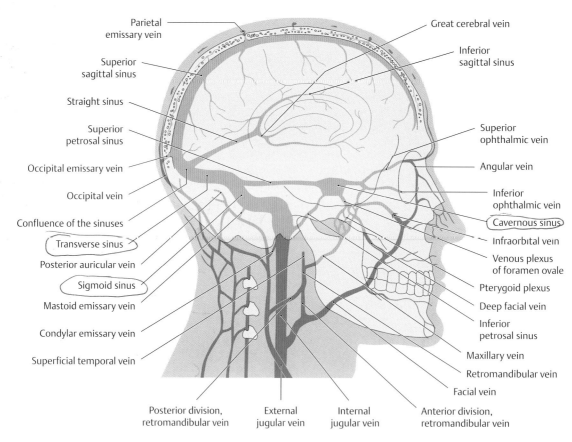

**Fig. 13.25 Accessory drainage pathways of the dural sinuses**
Right lateral view. The dural sinuses have many accessory drainage pathways besides their principal drainage into the two internal jugular veins. The connections between the dural sinuses and extracranial veins mainly serve to equalize pressure and regulate temperature. These anastomoses are of clinical interest because their normal direction of blood flow may reverse (general absence of functional valves in the head and neck), allowing blood from extracranial veins to reflux into the dural sinuses. This mechanism may give rise to sinus infections that lead, in turn, to vascular occlusion (*venous*

*sinus thrombosis*). The most important accessory drainage vessels include the following:

- Emissary veins (diploic and superior scalp veins)
- Superior ophthalmic vein (angular and facial veins)
- Venous plexus of foramen ovale (pterygoid plexus, retromandibular vein)
- Marginal sinus and basilar plexus (internal and external vertebral venous plexus)

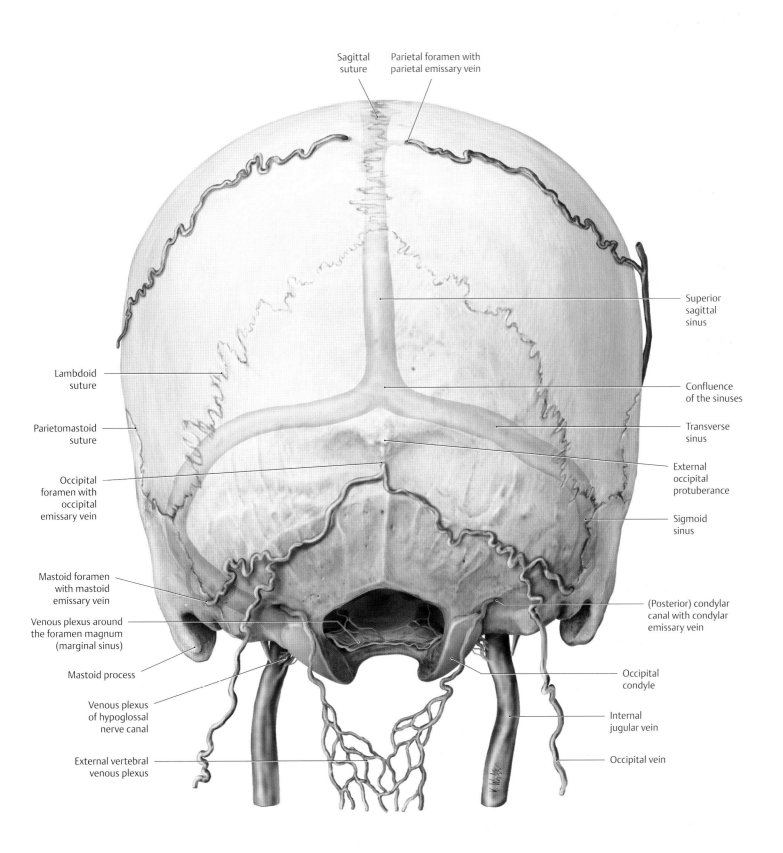

**Fig. 13.26 Emissary veins**

Posterior view of occiput. Emissary veins establish a direct connection between the intracranial dural sinuses and extracranial veins. They run through small cranial openings such as the parietal and mastoid foramina. Emissary veins are of clinical interest because they create a potential route by which bacteria from the scalp may spread to the dura mater and incite a purulent meningitis. Only the posterior emissary veins are shown here.

# Arteries of the Brain

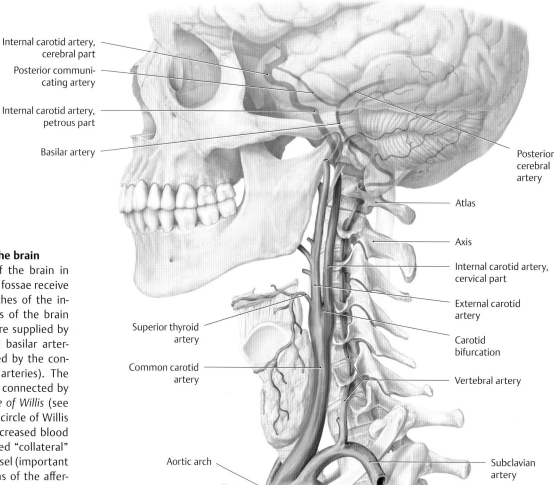

**Fig. 13.27 Arterial supply to the brain**
Left lateral view. The parts of the brain in the anterior and middle cranial fossae receive their blood supply from branches of the internal carotid artery; the parts of the brain in the posterior cranial fossa are supplied by branches of the vertebral and basilar arteries (the basilar artery is formed by the confluence of the two vertebral arteries). The carotid and basilar arteries are connected by a vascular ring called the *circle of Willis* (see **Fig. 13.29**). In many cases the circle of Willis allows for compensation of decreased blood flow in one vessel with increased "collateral" blood flow through another vessel (important in patients with stenotic lesions of the afferent arteries, see **Fig. 13.31**).

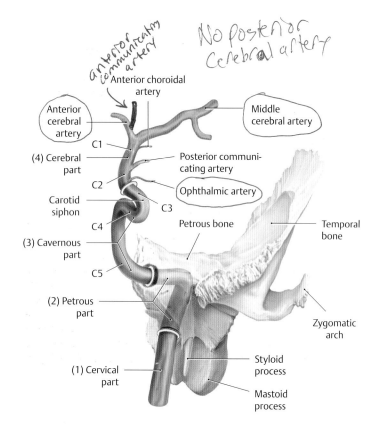

**Fig. 13.28 Anatomical divisions of the internal carotid artery**
Anterior view of the left internal carotid artery. The internal carotid artery consists of four topographically distinct parts between the carotid bifurcation and the point where it divides into the anterior and middle cerebral arteries. The parts (separated in the figure by white disks) are:

(1) Cervical part (red): Located in the lateral pharyngeal space.
(2) Petrous part (yellow): Located in the carotid canal of the petrous bone.
(3) Cavernous part (green): Follows an S-shaped curve in the cavernous sinus.
(4) Cerebral part (purple): Located in the chiasmatic cistern of the subarachnoid space.

Except for the cervical part, which generally does not give off branches, all the other parts of the internal carotid artery give off numerous branches. The *intracranial* parts of the internal carotid artery are subdivided into five segments (C1–C5) based on clinical criteria:

• C1–C2: Supraclinoid segments, located within the cerebral part. C1 and C2 lie above the anterior clinoid process of the lesser wing of the sphenoid bone.
• C3–C5: Infraclinoid segments, located within the cavernous sinus.

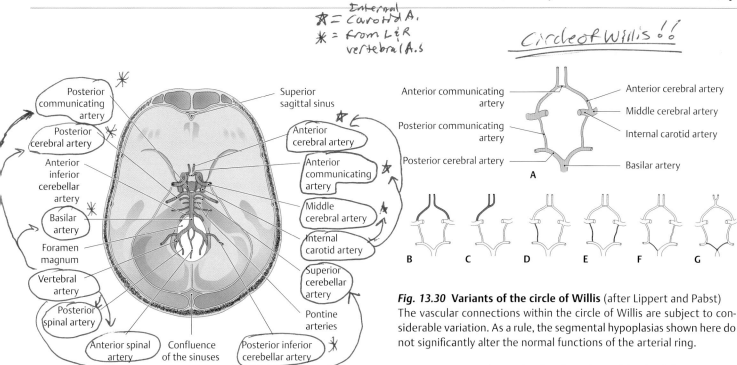

Handwritten notes:
☆ = Internal Carotid A.
✳ = from L & R vertebral A.s

*Circle of Willis!!*

**Fig. 13.29 Circle of Willis**
Superior view. The two vertebral arteries enter the skull through the foramen magnum and unite behind the clivus to form the unpaired basilar artery. This vessel then divides into the two posterior cerebral arteries (additional vessels that normally contribute to the circle of Willis are shown in **Fig. 13.30**).
*Note:* Each middle cerebral artery (MCA) is the direct continuation of the internal carotid artery on that side. Clots ejected by the left heart will frequently embolize to the MCA territory.

**Fig. 13.30 Variants of the circle of Willis** (after Lippert and Pabst)
The vascular connections within the circle of Willis are subject to considerable variation. As a rule, the segmental hypoplasias shown here do not significantly alter the normal functions of the arterial ring.

**A** In most cases, the circle of Willis is formed by the following arteries: the anterior, middle, and posterior cerebral arteries; the anterior and posterior communicating arteries; the internal carotid arteries; and the basilar artery.
**B** Occasionally, the anterior communicating artery is absent.
**C** Both anterior cerebral arteries may arise from one internal carotid artery (10% of cases).
**D** The posterior communicating artery may be absent or hypoplastic on one side (10% of cases).
**E** Both posterior communicating arteries may be absent or hypoplastic (10% of cases).
**F** The posterior cerebral artery may be absent or hypoplastic on one side.
**G** Both posterior cerebral arteries may be absent or hypoplastic. In addition, the anterior cerebral arteries may arise from a common trunk.

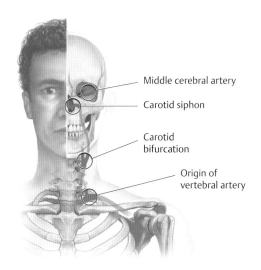

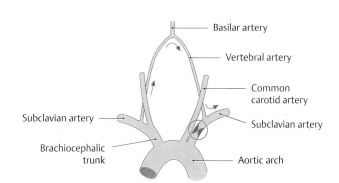

**Fig. 13.31 Stenoses and occlusions of arteries supplying the brain**
Atherosclerotic lesions in older patients may cause the narrowing (stenosis) or complete obstruction (occlusion) of arteries that supply the brain. Stenoses most commonly occur at arterial bifurcations. The sites of predilection are shown with circles. Isolated stenoses that develop gradually may be compensated for by collateral vessels. When stenoses occur simultaneously at multiple sites, the circle of Willis cannot compensate for the diminished blood supply, and cerebral blood flow becomes impaired (varying degrees of cerebral ischemia).
*Note:* The damage is manifested clinically in the brain, but the cause is located in the vessels that supply the brain. Because stenoses are treatable, their diagnosis has major therapeutic implications.

**Fig. 13.32 Anatomical basis of subclavian steal syndrome**
"Subclavian steal" usually results from stenosis of the left subclavian artery (red circle) located proximal to the origin of the vertebral artery. This syndrome involves a stealing of blood from the *vertebral artery* by the subclavian artery. When the left arm is exercised, as during yard work, insufficient blood may be supplied to the arm to accommodate the increased muscular effort (the patient complains of muscle weakness). As a result, blood is "stolen" from the vertebral artery circulation, and there is a reversal of blood flow in the vertebral artery on the *affected* side (arrows). This leads to deficient blood flow in the basilar artery and may deprive the brain of blood, producing a feeling of lightheadedness.

**305**

# Neurons

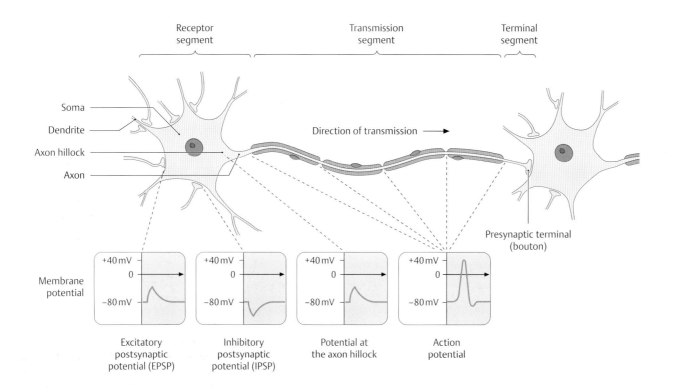

**Fig. 13.33 Neurons (nerve cells)**
Neurons are the smallest functional units of the nervous system. Each neuron is composed of a cell body (soma or perikaryon) and two types of processes: dendrites and axons. The function of the neuron is reflected in the number and type of processes arising from the cell body (see **Fig. 13.35**).

- Dendrite (receptor segment): Conducts impulses from synapse to the cell body. Depending on its function, a neuron may have multiple dendrites. Dendrites may undergo complex arborization to increase their surface area.
- Axon (projecting segment): Conducts impulses to other neurons or cells (e.g., skeletal muscle). Neurons have only one axon. In the CNS, axons are generally myelinated (covered with myelin cells). The cell membranes of myelin cells are predominantly lipid (this gives white matter its fatty appearance). Myelination electrically insulates axons, increasing the speed of impulse conduction.

Neurons communicate at synapses, the junction between the axon of one neuron and the dendrite or cell body of the other (see **Fig. 13.37**). Nerve impulses are propagated through waves of depolarization across cell membranes. Resting nerve cells have a membrane potential of −80 mV (higher concentration of positive ions outside the nerve cell than inside). In response to a nerve impulse, neurotransmitters are released into the synapse. These neurotransmitters bind ion channels that allow positive ions to rush into the cytoplasm. This initiates other channels to open, causing the cell membrane to become massively depolarized (+40 mV). This initiates an action potential at the axon hillock, the origin of the axon on the cell body. The action potential travels along the axon and induces the release of neurotransmitters from the presynaptic terminal at the next synapse. The action potential is therefore propagated rapidly across multiple cells, which are repolarized through the action of ion pumps. *Note:* Neurotransmitters may be either excitatory or inhibitory (create either an excitatory or inhibitory postsynaptic potential at the target neuron).

**Fig. 13.34 Electron microscopy of the neuron**
The organelles of neurons can be resolved with an electron microscope. Neurons are rich in rough endoplasmic reticulum (protein synthesis, active metabolism). This endoplasmic reticulum (called *Nissl substance* under a light microscope) is easily demonstrated by light microscopy when it is stained with cationic dyes (which bind to the anionic mRNA and nRNA of the ribosomes). The distribution pattern of the Nissl substance is used in neuropathology to evaluate the functional integrity of neurons. The neurotubules and neurofilaments that are visible by electron microscopy are referred to collectively in *light microscopy* as neurofibrils, as they are too fine to be resolved as separate structures under the light microscope. Neurofibrils can be demonstrated in light microscopy by impregnating the nerve tissue with silver salts. This is important in neuropathology, for example, because the clumping of neurofibrils is an important histological feature of Alzheimer disease.

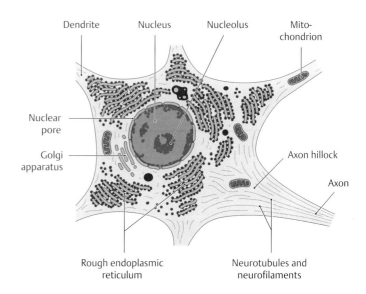

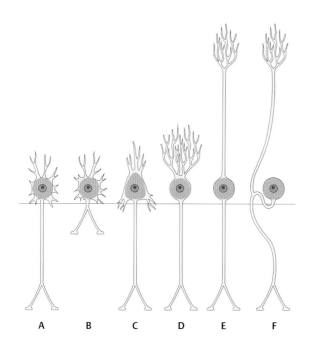

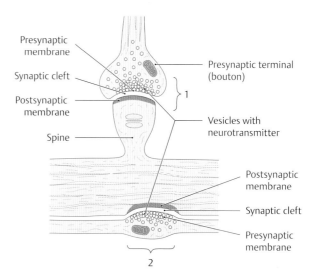

## Fig. 13.35 Basic neuron forms

Neurons consist of a cell body, an axon, and one or more dendrites. The function of the neuron is reflected in its structure. Neurons **A–D** are efferent (motor) neurons, which convey impulses from the CNS to the periphery. Neurons **E** and **F** are afferent (sensory) neurons, which convey impulses to the CNS.

**A, B** Multipolar neurons: Multiple dendrites with either a long (**A**) or short (**B**) axon. Alpha motor neurons of the spinal cord are the long-axon form. Interneurons in the gray matter of the brain and spinal cord are the short-axon form.

**C** Pyramidal cell: Long axon with multiple dendrites only at the apex and base of the triangular cell body (e.g., efferent neurons of cerebral motor cortex).

**D** Purkinje cell: Long axon with elaborately branched dendritic tree from one site on the cell body. Purkinje cells are found within the cerebellum.

**E** Bipolar neuron: Long axon and long dendrite that arborizes in the periphery (e.g., retinal cells).

**F** Pseudounipolar neuron: Long axon and long arborized dendrite that are not separated by the cell body. This is the traditional form of primary afferent (sensory) neurons in spinal nerves. The cell bodies of these neurons form the spinal (dorsal root) ganglion.

## Fig. 13.36 Synapses in the CNS

Synapses are the functional connection between two neurons. They consist of a presynaptic membrane, a synaptic cleft, and a postsynaptic membrane. In a "spine synapse" (1), the presynaptic terminal (bouton) is in contact with a specialized protuberance (spine) of the target neuron. The side-by-side synapse of an axon with the flat surface of a target neuron is called a parallel contact or *bouton en passage* (2). The vesicles in the presynaptic expansions contain the neurotransmitters that are released into the synaptic cleft by exocytosis when the axon fires. From there the neurotransmitters diffuse to the postsynaptic membrane, where their receptors are located. A variety of drugs and toxins act upon synaptic transmission (antidepressants, muscle relaxants, nerve gases, botulinum toxin).

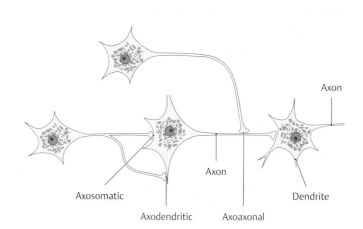

## Fig. 13.37 Synaptic patterns

Axons may terminate at various sites on the target neuron and form synapses there. The synaptic patterns are described as axodendritic, axosomatic, or axoaxonal. Axodendritic synapses are the most common. The cerebral cortex consists of many small groups of neurons that are collected into functional units called columns.

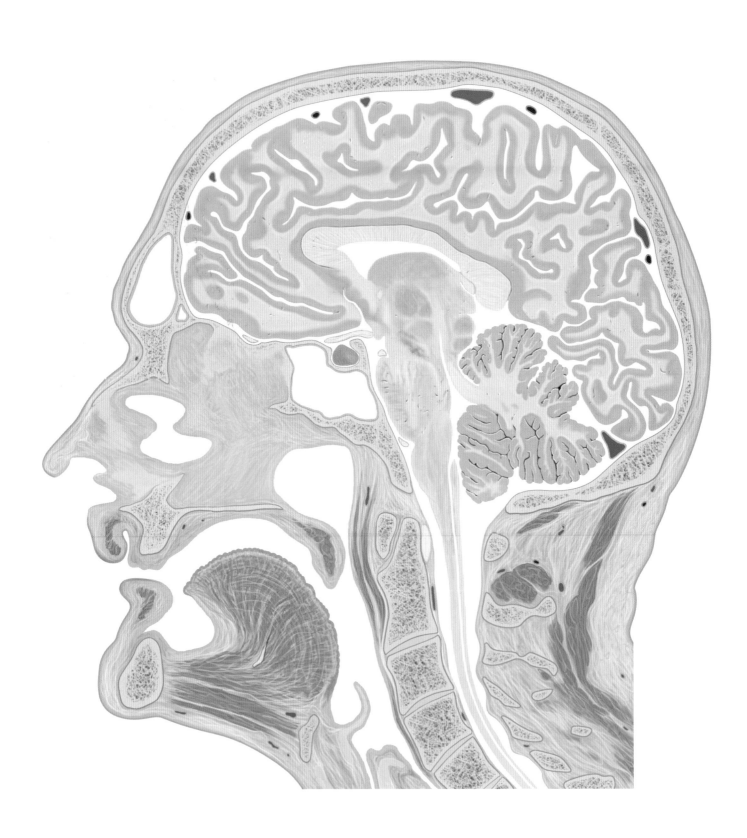

# Sectional Anatomy

# Coronal Sections of the Head (I): Anterior

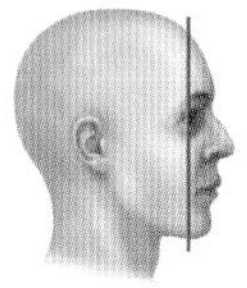

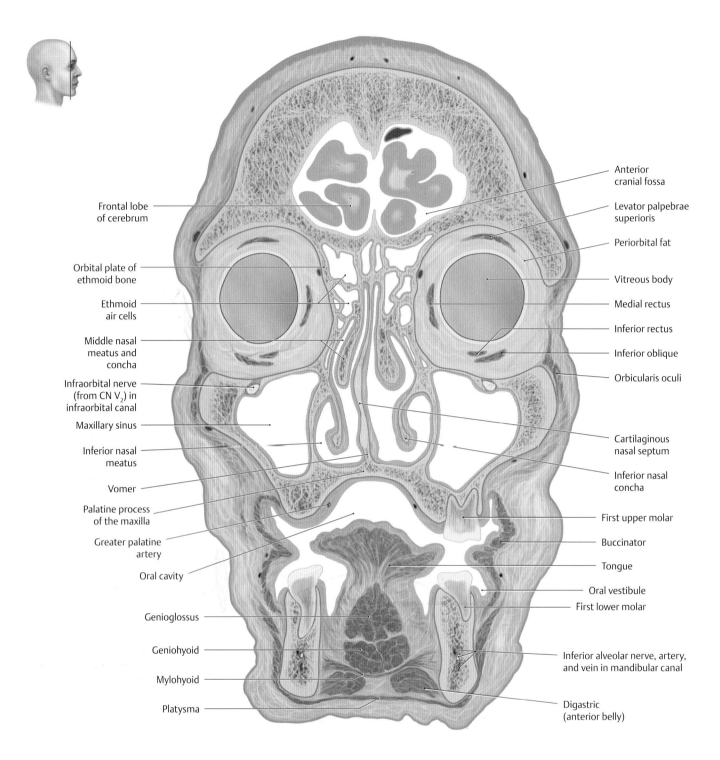

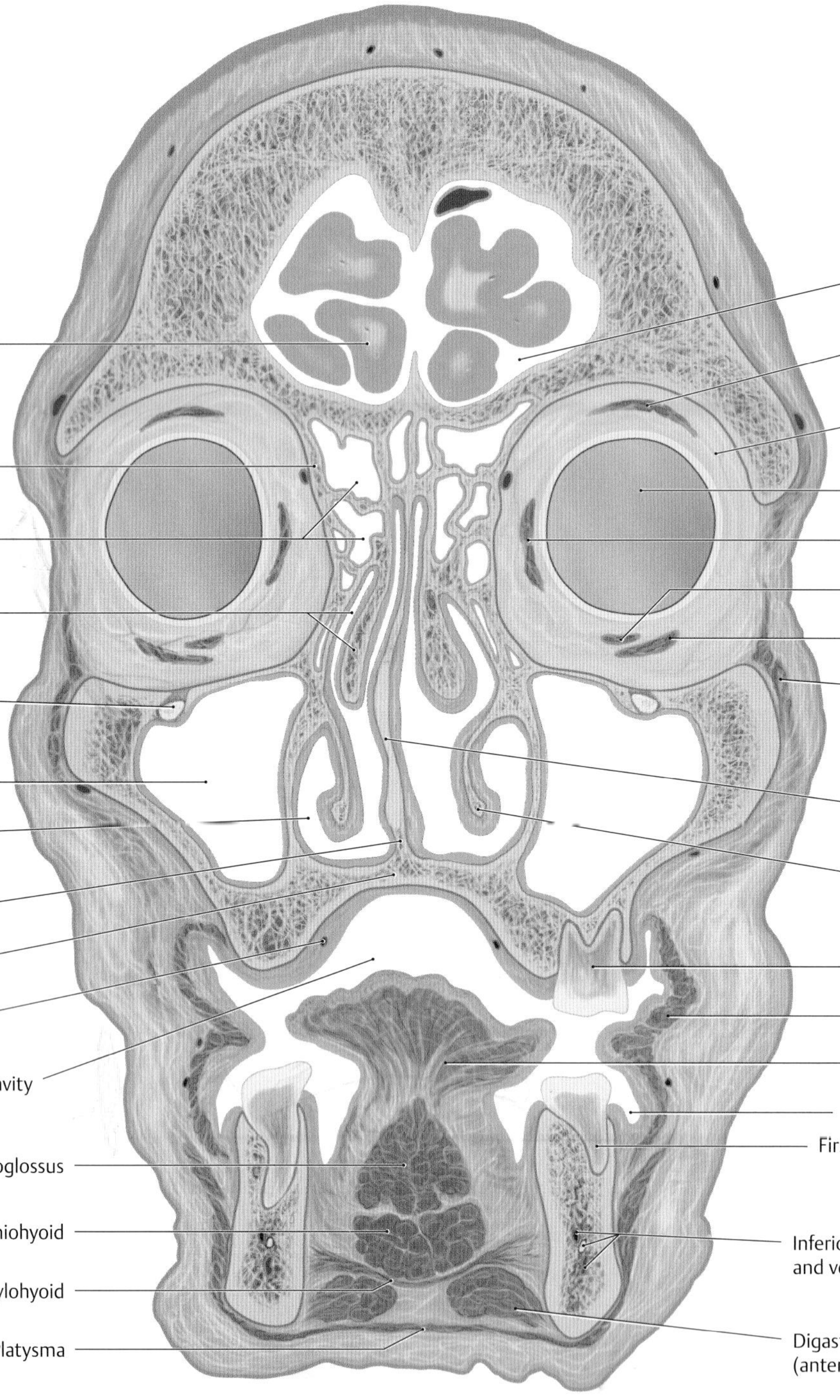
Frontal lobe of cerebrum
Orbital plate of ethmoid bone
Ethmoid air cells
Middle nasal meatus and concha
Infraorbital nerve (from CN V2) in infraorbital canal
Maxillary sinus
Inferior nasal meatus
Vomer
Palatine process of the maxilla
Greater palatine artery
Oral cavity
Genioglossus
Geniohyoid
Mylohyoid
Platysma
Anterior cranial fossa
Levator palpebrae superioris
Periorbital fat
Vitreous body
Medial rectus
Inferior rectus
Inferior oblique
Orbicularis oculi
Cartilaginous nasal septum
Inferior nasal concha
First upper molar
Buccinator
Tongue
Oral vestibule
First lower molar
Inferior alveolar nerve, artery, and vein in mandibular canal
Digastric (anterior belly)

***Fig. 14.1*** **Coronal section through the anterior orbital margin**
Anterior view. This section of the skull can be roughly subdivided into four regions: the oral cavity, the nasal cavity and sinus, the orbit, and the anterior cranial fossa. Inspecting the region in and around the **oral cavity**, we observe the muscles of the oral floor, the apex of the tongue, the neurovascular structures in the mandibular canal, and the first molar. The hard palate separates the oral cavity from the **nasal cavity**, which is divided into left and right halves by the nasal septum. The inferior and middle nasal conchae can be identified along with the laterally situated maxillary sinus. The structure bulging down into the roof of the sinus is the infraorbital canal, which transmits the infraorbital nerve (branch of the maxillary division of the trigeminal nerve, CN $V_2$).

The plane of section is so far anterior that it does not cut the lateral bony walls of the **orbits** because of the lateral curvature of the skull. The section passes through the transparent vitreous body and three of the six extraocular muscles, which can be identified in the periorbital fat. Two additional muscles can be seen in the next deeper plane of section (**Fig. 14.2**). The space between the two orbits is occupied by the ethmoid cells. *Note:* The bony orbital plate is very thin (lamina papyracea) and may be penetrated by infection, trauma, and neoplasms.
In the **anterior cranial fossa**, the section passes through both frontal lobes of the brain in the most anterior portions of the cerebral gray matter. Very little white matter is visible at this level.

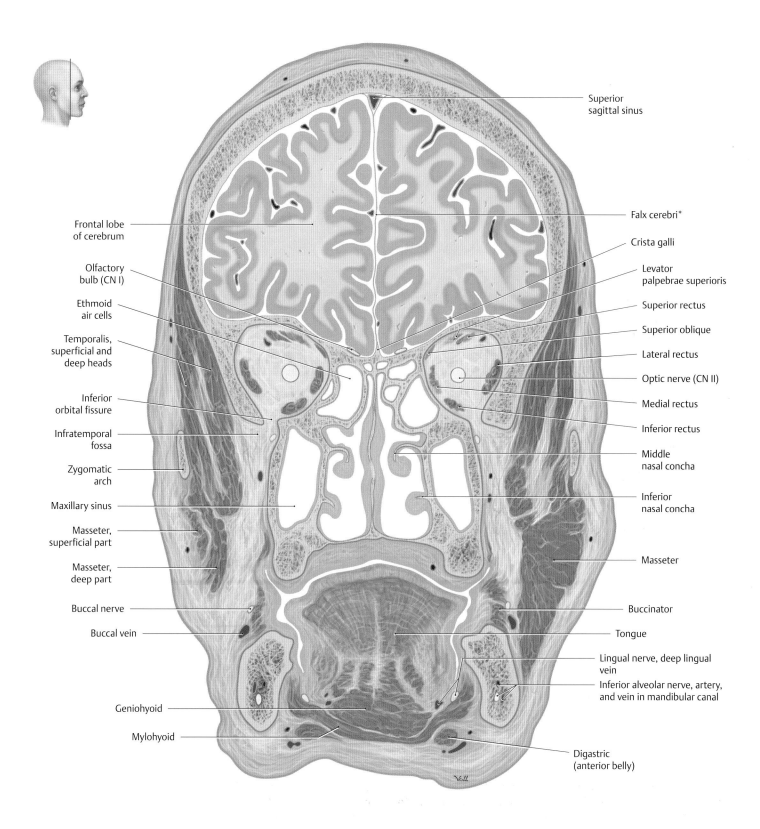

Frontal lobe
of cerebrum

Olfactory
bulb (CN I)

Ethmoid
air cells

Temporalis,
superficial and
deep heads

Inferior
orbital fissure

Infratemporal
fossa

Zygomatic
arch

Maxillary sinus

Masseter,
superficial part

Masseter,
deep part

Buccal nerve

Buccal vein

Geniohyoid

Mylohyoid

Superior
sagittal sinus

Falx cerebri*

Crista galli

Levator
palpebrae superioris

Superior rectus

Superior oblique

Lateral rectus

Optic nerve (CN II)

Medial rectus

Inferior rectus

Middle
nasal concha

Inferior
nasal concha

Masseter

Buccinator

Tongue

Lingual nerve, deep lingual
vein

Inferior alveolar nerve, artery,
and vein in mandibular canal

Digastric
(anterior belly)

**Fig. 14.2 Coronal section through the retrobulbar space**
Anterior view. Here, the tongue is cut at a more posterior level than in
**Fig. 14.1** and therefore appears broader. In addition to the oral floor
muscles, we see the muscles of mastication on the sides of the skull. In
the orbital region we can identify the retrobulbar space with its fatty
tissue, the extraocular muscles, and the optic nerve. The orbit communicates laterally with the infratemporal fossa through the inferior

orbital fissure. This section cuts through both olfactory bulbs in the anterior cranial fossa, and the superior sagittal sinus can be recognized
in the midline.

*Note: More posteriorly, the falx cerebri does not separate the cerebral
hemispheres. Its inferior margin is nonattached, superior to the corpus
callosum.

# Coronal Sections of the Head (II): Posterior

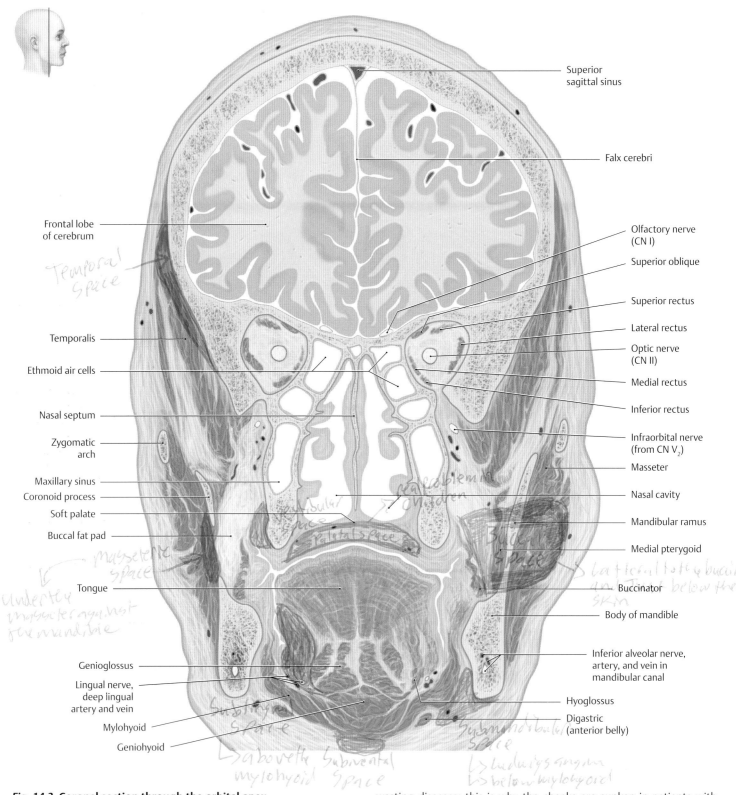

Superior sagittal sinus

Falx cerebri

Frontal lobe of cerebrum

Olfactory nerve (CN I)

Superior oblique

Superior rectus

Temporalis

Lateral rectus

Ethmoid air cells

Optic nerve (CN II)

Medial rectus

Inferior rectus

Nasal septum

Infraorbital nerve (from CN V₂)

Zygomatic arch

Masseter

Maxillary sinus

Nasal cavity

Coronoid process

Mandibular ramus

Soft palate

Medial pterygoid

Buccal fat pad

Tongue

Buccinator

Body of mandible

Inferior alveolar nerve, artery, and vein in mandibular canal

Genioglossus

Lingual nerve, deep lingual artery and vein

Hyoglossus

Mylohyoid

Digastric (anterior belly)

Geniohyoid

**Fig. 14.3 Coronal section through the orbital apex**
Anterior view. The soft palate replaces the hard palate in this plane of section, and the nasal septum becomes osseous at this level. The buccal fat pad is also visible in this plane. The buccal pad is attenuated in wasting diseases; this is why the cheeks are sunken in patients with end-stage cancer. This coronal section is slightly angled, producing an apparent discontinuity in the mandibular ramus on the left side of the figure (compare with the continuous ramus on the right side).

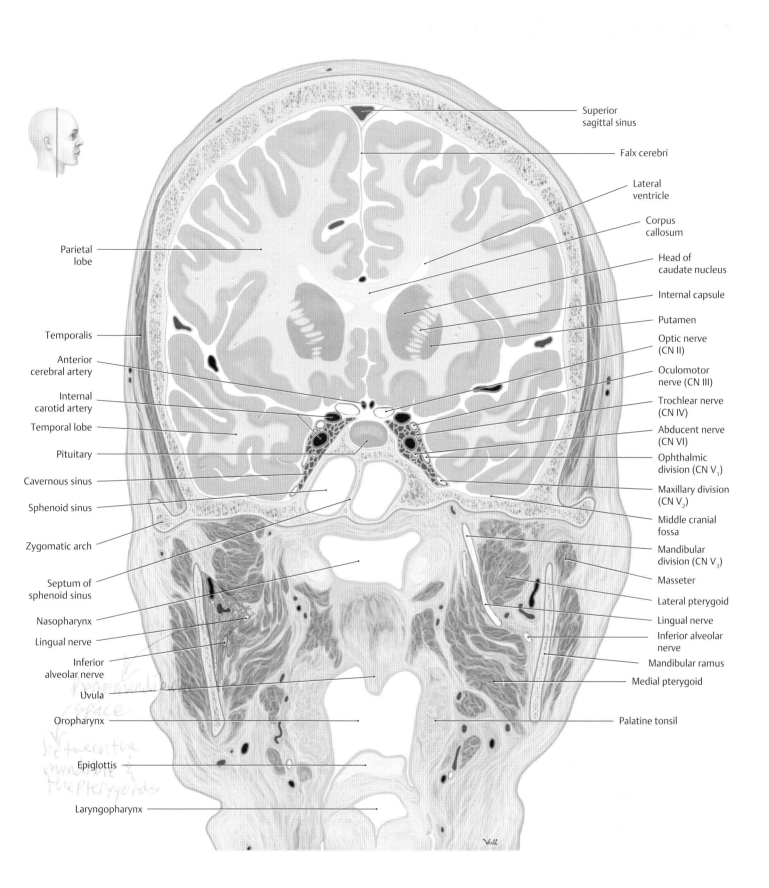

**Superior sagittal sinus**
**Falx cerebri**
**Lateral ventricle**
**Corpus callosum**
**Head of caudate nucleus**
**Internal capsule**
**Putamen**
**Optic nerve (CN II)**
**Oculomotor nerve (CN III)**
**Trochlear nerve (CN IV)**
**Abducent nerve (CN VI)**
**Ophthalmic division (CN V₁)**
**Maxillary division (CN V₂)**
**Middle cranial fossa**
**Mandibular division (CN V₃)**
**Masseter**
**Lateral pterygoid**
**Lingual nerve**
**Inferior alveolar nerve**
**Mandibular ramus**
**Medial pterygoid**
**Palatine tonsil**

**Parietal lobe**
**Temporalis**
**Anterior cerebral artery**
**Internal carotid artery**
**Temporal lobe**
**Pituitary**
**Cavernous sinus**
**Sphenoid sinus**
**Zygomatic arch**
**Septum of sphenoid sinus**
**Nasopharynx**
**Lingual nerve**
**Inferior alveolar nerve**
**Uvula**
**Oropharynx**
**Epiglottis**
**Laryngopharynx**

**Fig. 14.4 Coronal section through the pituitary**
Anterior view. The nasopharynx, oropharynx, and laryngopharynx can now be identified. This section cuts the epiglottis, below which is the supraglottic space. The plane cuts the mandibular ramus on both sides, and a relatively long segment of the mandibular division (CN V₃) can be identified on the left side. Above the roof of the sphenoid sinuses is the pituitary (hypophysis), which lies in the hypophyseal fossa. In the cranial cavity, the plane of section passes through the middle cranial fossa.

Due to the presence of the carotid siphon (a 180-degree bend in the cavernous part of the internal carotid artery), the section cuts the internal carotid artery twice on each side. Cranial nerves can be seen passing through the cavernous sinus on their way from the middle cranial fossa to the orbit. The superior sagittal sinus appears in cross section at the attachment of the falx cerebri. At the level of the cerebrum, the plane of section passes through the parietal and temporal lobes.

**313**

# Coronal MRIs of the Head

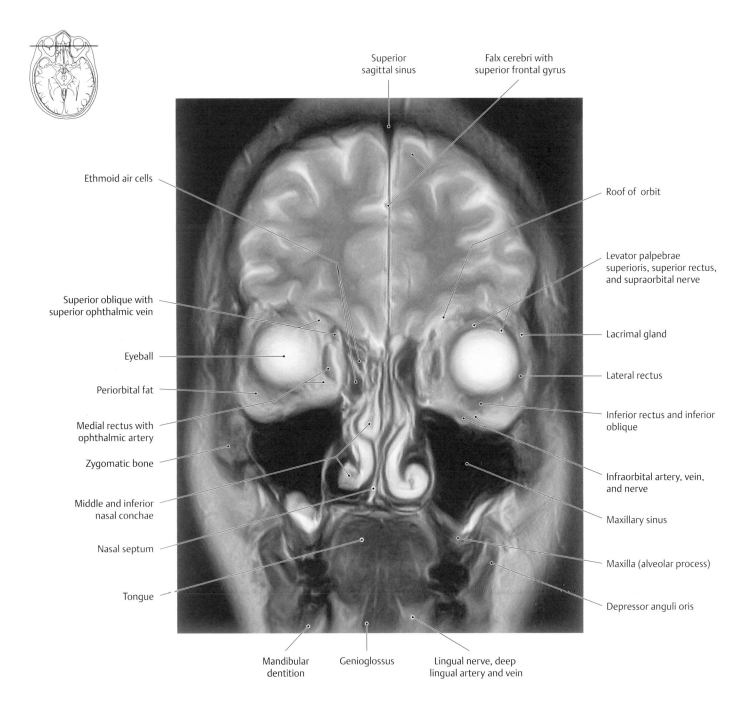

Superior sagittal sinus

Falx cerebri with superior frontal gyrus

Ethmoid air cells

Roof of orbit

Levator palpebrae superioris, superior rectus, and supraorbital nerve

Superior oblique with superior ophthalmic vein

Lacrimal gland

Eyeball

Lateral rectus

Periorbital fat

Inferior rectus and inferior oblique

Medial rectus with ophthalmic artery

Zygomatic bone

Infraorbital artery, vein, and nerve

Middle and inferior nasal conchae

Maxillary sinus

Nasal septum

Maxilla (alveolar process)

Tongue

Depressor anguli oris

Mandibular dentition

Genioglossus

Lingual nerve, deep lingual artery and vein

**Fig. 14.5 Coronal MRI through the eyeball**
Anterior view. In this plane of section, the falx cerebri completely divides the cerebral hemispheres. The extraocular muscles can be used to find the orbital neurovasculature: the supraorbital nerve runs superior to the levator palpebrae superioris and superior rectus, the superior ophthalmic vein runs medial and superior to the superior oblique, and the oph- thalmic artery runs inferior to the medial rectus. The infraorbital canal (containing the infraorbital artery, vein, and nerve) runs inferior to the inferior rectus and oblique. The region medial to the mandibular den- tition and lateral to the genioglossus contains the sublingual gland as well as the lingual nerve, deep lingual artery and vein, hypoglossal nerve (CN XII), and submandibular duct.

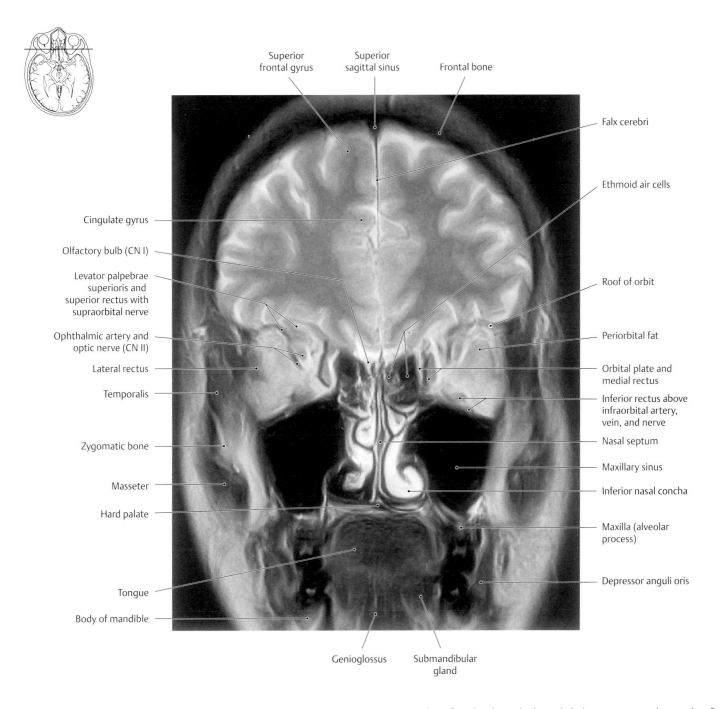

**Fig. 14.6 Coronal MRI through the posterior orbit**

Anterior view. The inferior margin of the falx cerebri is now superior to the cingulate gyrus. In the orbit, the supraorbital nerve runs with the levator palpebrae superioris and superior rectus, and the oculomotor nerve (CN III) runs lateral to the inferior rectus, which in turn runs superior to the infraorbital canal. The ophthalmic artery can be used to find the more medially located optic nerve (CN II), both of which emerge from the optic canal. Note the asymmetrical nature of the nasal cavities. The submandibular gland is more prominent in this section between the genioglossus and the body of the mandible.

# Coronal MRIs of the Neck (I): Anterior

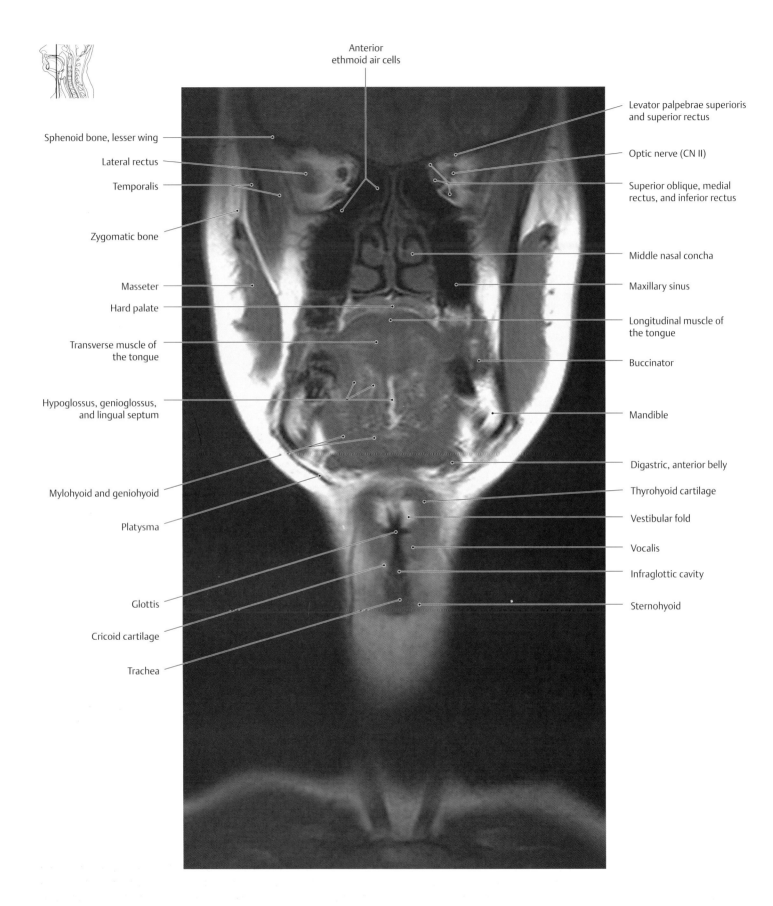

Anterior ethmoid air cells

Sphenoid bone, lesser wing

Lateral rectus

Temporalis

Zygomatic bone

Masseter

Hard palate

Transverse muscle of the tongue

Hypoglossus, genioglossus, and lingual septum

Mylohyoid and geniohyoid

Platysma

Glottis

Cricoid cartilage

Trachea

Levator palpebrae superioris and superior rectus

Optic nerve (CN II)

Superior oblique, medial rectus, and inferior rectus

Middle nasal concha

Maxillary sinus

Longitudinal muscle of the tongue

Buccinator

Mandible

Digastric, anterior belly

Thyrohyoid cartilage

Vestibular fold

Vocalis

Infraglottic cavity

Sternohyoid

**Fig. 14.7 Coronal MRI of the lingual muscles**
Anterior view. This plane of section lies just posterior to the previous one and transects the extrinsic (genioglossus and hypoglossus) and intrinsic (longitudinal and transverse) lingual muscles. The muscles of mastication (temporalis and masseter) are visible, as are the buccinator, mylohyoid, and geniohyoid. This section cuts the larynx and trachea, revealing the vestibular fold, vocalis muscle, and cricoid cartilage.

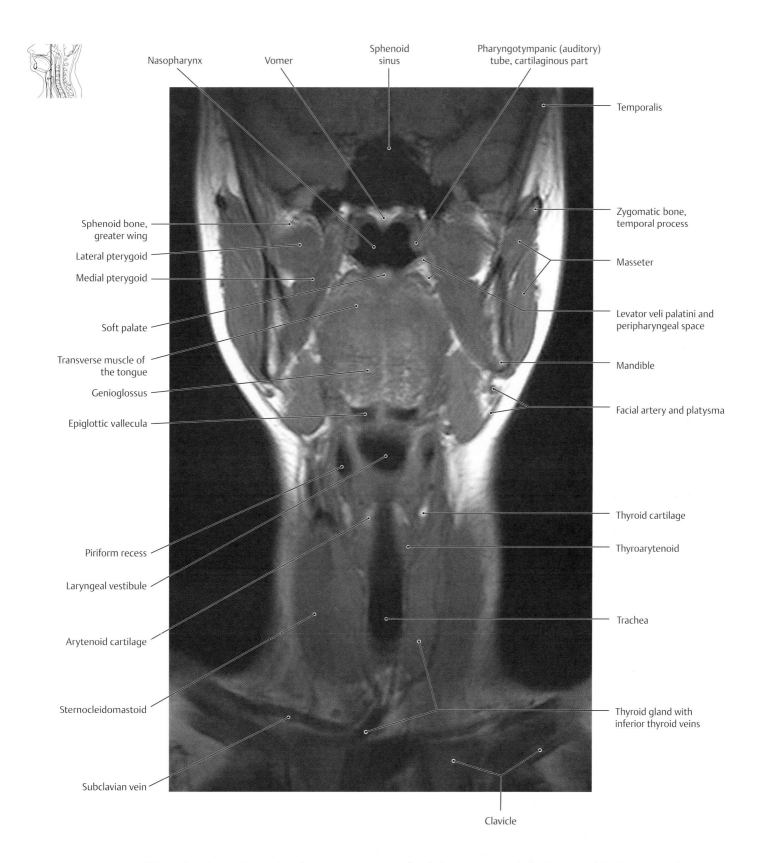

**Fig. 14.8 Coronal MRI of the soft palate and muscles of mastication** Anterior view. This section illustrates the convergence of the air- and foodways in the pharynx. The nasopharynx lies inferior to the sphenoid sinus and superior to the soft palate. It converges with the foodway in the oropharynx, located posterior to the uvula (not shown). The oropharynx continues inferiorly to the epiglottis (the epiglottis vallecula lies anterior to this). The air- and foodways then diverge into the larynx and laryngopharynx, respectively. The laryngeal vestibule is the superior portion of the larynx, above the vocal folds. This section reveals the thyroid and arytenoid cartilage of the larynx. Compare this image to **Fig. 14.9**.

**317**

# Coronal MRIs of the Neck (II)

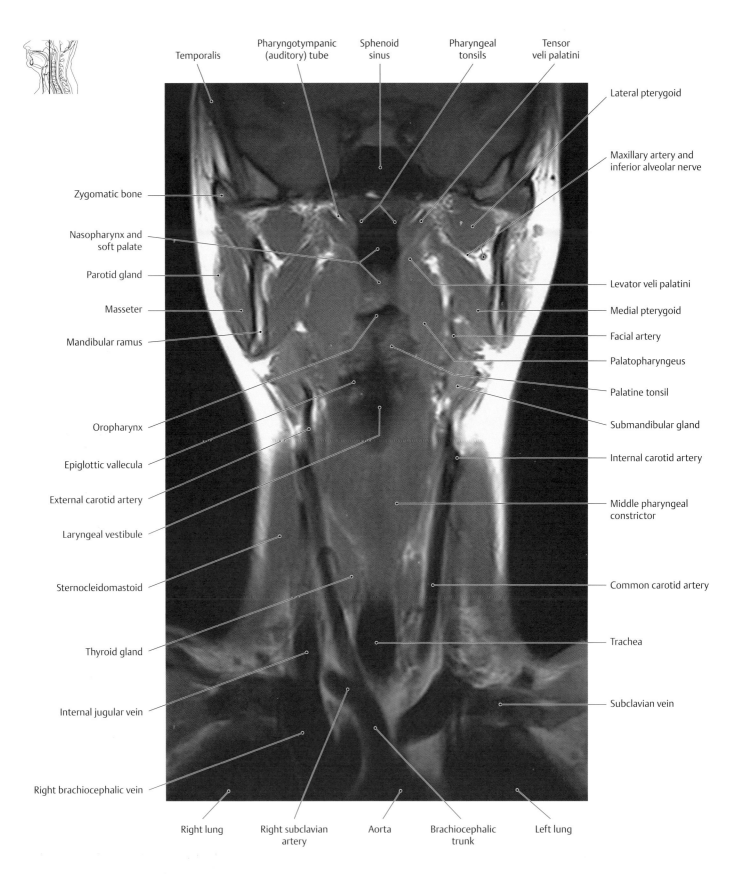

**Fig. 14.9 Coronal MRI of the great vessels**

Anterior view. This image clearly demonstrates the course of the great vessels in the neck. This image is also an excellent demonstration of the structures of the oral cavity. Note the position of the pharyngeal tonsils on the roof of the nasopharynx and the extent of the palatine tonsils in the oropharynx.

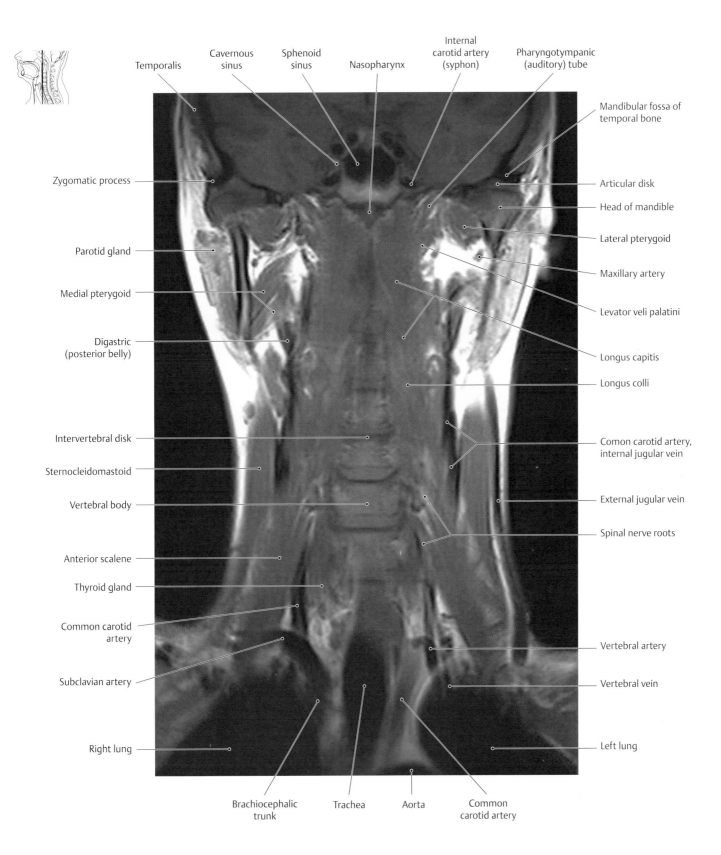

Temporalis
Cavernous sinus
Sphenoid sinus
Nasopharynx
Internal carotid artery (syphon)
Pharyngotympanic (auditory) tube

Zygomatic process

Parotid gland

Medial pterygoid

Digastric (posterior belly)

Intervertebral disk

Sternocleidomastoid

Vertebral body

Anterior scalene

Thyroid gland

Common carotid artery

Subclavian artery

Right lung

Mandibular fossa of temporal bone

Articular disk

Head of mandible

Lateral pterygoid

Maxillary artery

Levator veli palatini

Longus capitis

Longus colli

Comon carotid artery, internal jugular vein

External jugular vein

Spinal nerve roots

Vertebral artery

Vertebral vein

Left lung

Brachiocephalic trunk
Trachea
Aorta
Common carotid artery

**Fig. 14.10 Coronal MRI through the temporomandibular joint (TMJ)**
Anterior view. This image clearly demonstrates the structures of the TMJ, in particular the articular disk and mandibular head. The ramus of the mandible is seen medial to the parotid gland. This image shows the cervical vertebrae with intervertebral disks.

# Coronal MRIs of the Neck (III): Posterior

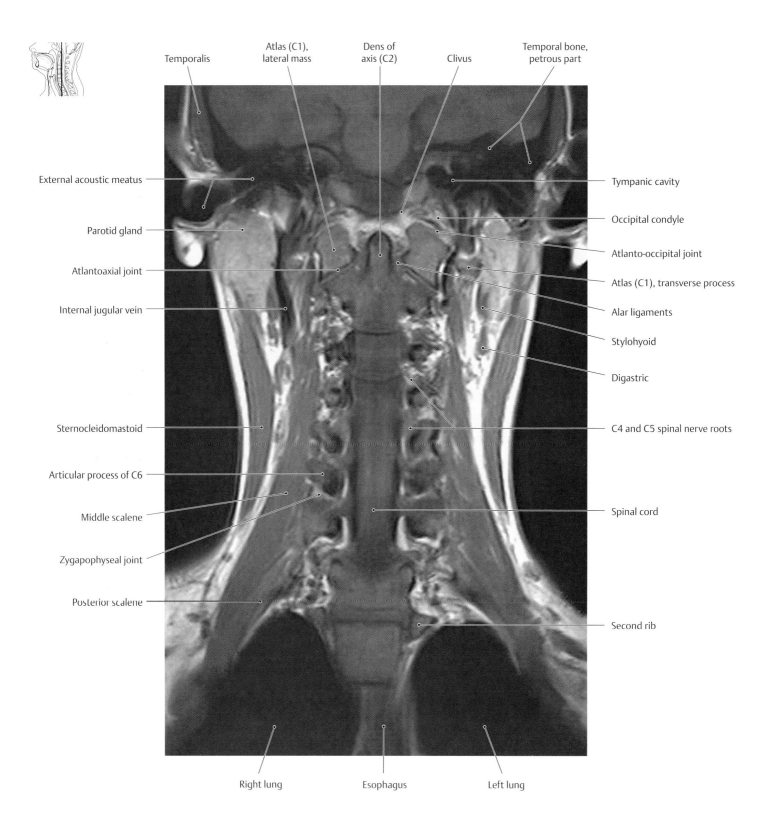

**Fig. 14.11 Coronal MRI through the cervical vertebrae and spinal nerves**

Anterior view. This image clearly shows the C1 through T2 vertebrae. The lateral masses of the atlas (C1) can be seen flanking the dens of the axis (C2). The more inferior vertebrae can be counted using the articular processes of the cervical vertebrae. The spinal nerve roots emerge between the articular processes (note for counting purposes: the C3 root emerges inferior to C2 and superior to the articular processes of C3).

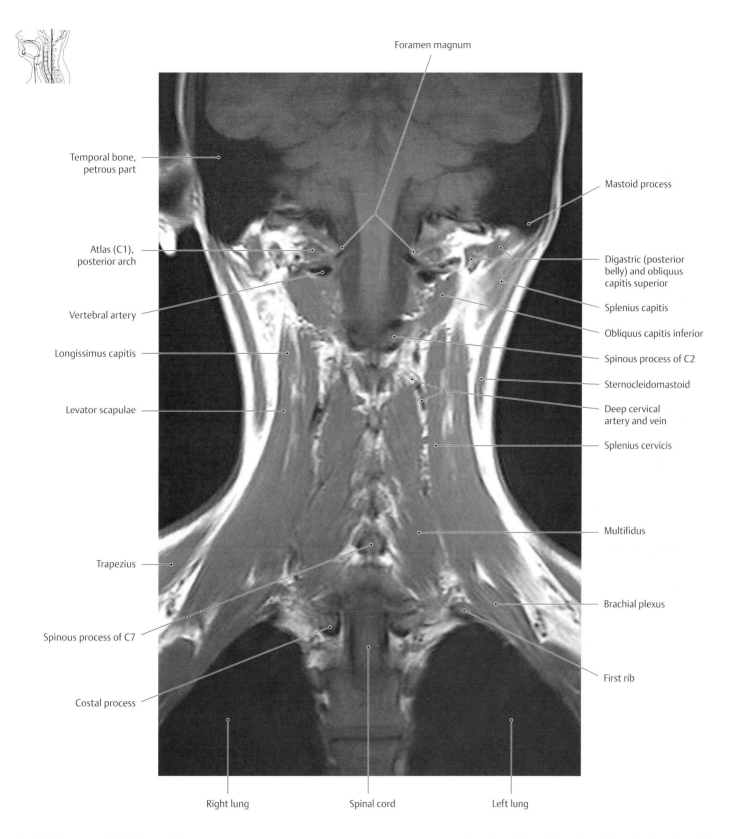

Foramen magnum

Temporal bone, petrous part

Atlas (C1), posterior arch

Vertebral artery

Longissimus capitis

Levator scapulae

Trapezius

Spinous process of C7

Costal process

Right lung

Spinal cord

Left lung

Mastoid process

Digastric (posterior belly) and obliquus capitis superior

Splenius capitis

Obliquus capitis inferior

Spinous process of C2

Sternocleidomastoid

Deep cervical artery and vein

Splenius cervicis

Multifidus

Brachial plexus

First rib

**Fig. 14.12 Coronal MRI through the nuchal muscles**
Anterior view. This image clearly shows the relations of the muscles in the neck. *Note:* The elongated spinous process of the C7 vertebra (ver-tebra prominens) is still visible in this section. The spinal cord is visible both during its passage through the foramen magnum and more cau-dally, posterior to the T1 vertebral body.

**321**

# Transverse Sections of the Head (I): Cranial

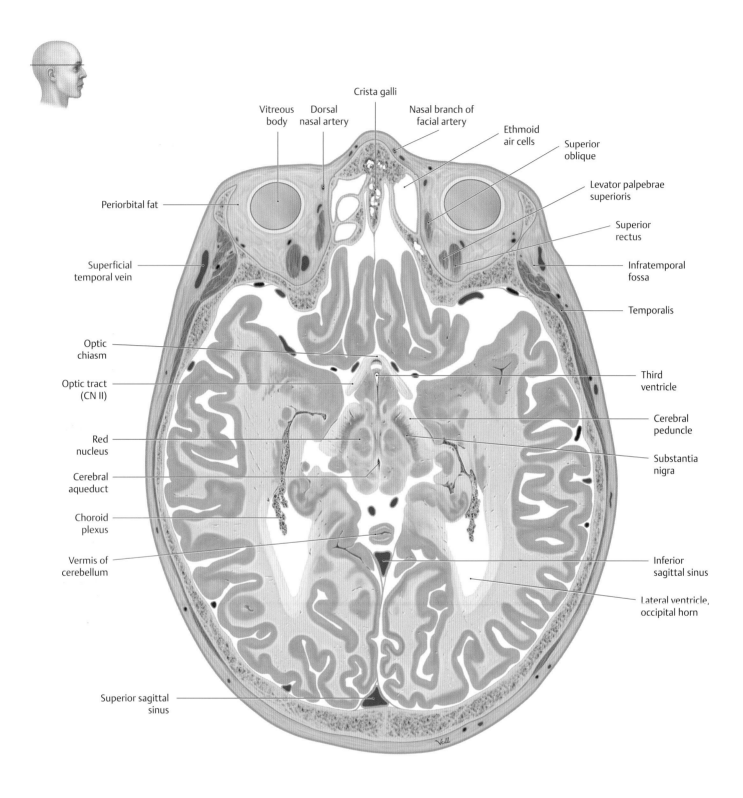

**Fig. 14.13 Transverse section through the upper level of the orbits**
Superior view. The highest section in this series displays the muscles in the upper level of the orbit (the orbital levels are described on p. 116). The section cuts the bony crista galli in the anterior cranial fossa, flanked on each side by cells of the ethmoid sinus. The sections of the optic chiasm and adjacent optic tract are parts of the diencephalon, which surrounds the third ventricle at the center of the section. The red nucleus and substantia nigra are visible in the mesencephalon. The pyramidal tract descends in the cerebral peduncles. The section passes through the posterior (occipital) horns of the lateral ventricles and barely cuts the vermis of the cerebellum in the midline.

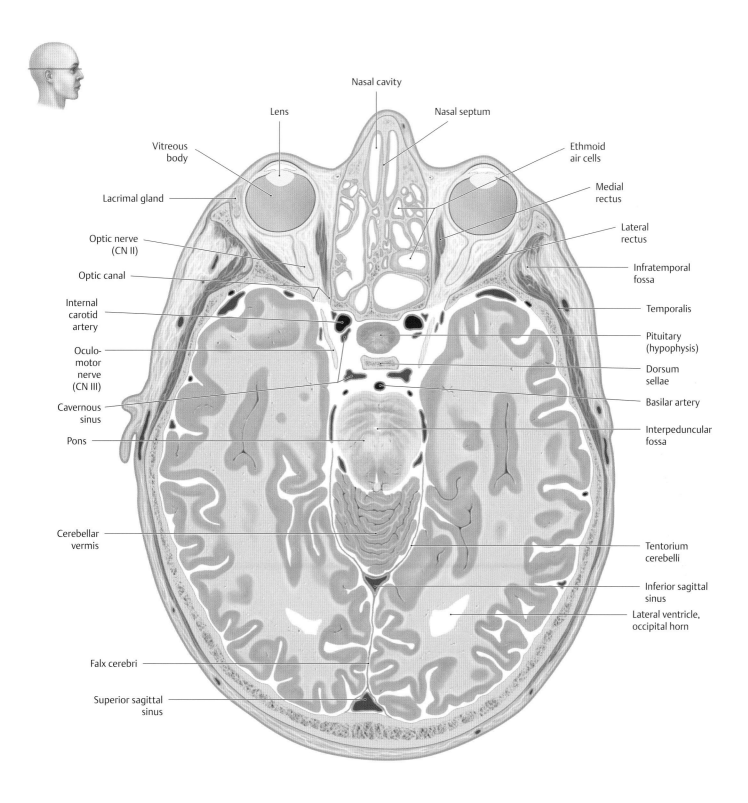

**Fig. 14.14 Transverse section through the optic nerve and pituitary**
Superior view. The optic nerve is seen just before its entry into the optic canal, indicating that the plane of section passes through the middle level of the orbit. Because the nerve completely fills the canal, growth disturbances of the bone at this level may cause pressure injury to the nerve. This plane cuts the ocular lenses and the cells of the ethmoid labyrinth. The internal carotid artery can be identified in the middle cranial fossa, embedded in the cavernous sinus. The section cuts the oculomotor nerve on either side, which courses in the lateral wall of the cavernous sinus. The pons and cerebellar vermis are also seen. The falx cerebri and tentorium cerebelli appear as thin lines that come together at the straight sinus.

# Transverse Sections of the Head (II)

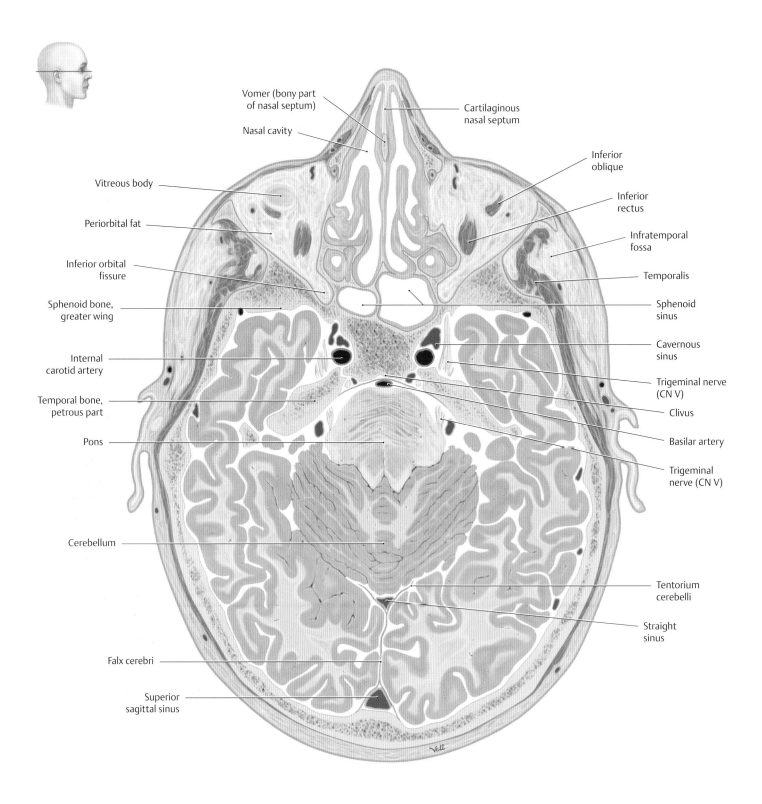

**Fig. 14.15 Transverse section through the sphenoid sinus**
Superior view. This section cuts the infratemporal fossa on the lateral aspect of the skull and the temporalis muscle that lies within it. The plane passes through the lower level of the orbit, which is continuous posteriorly with the inferior orbital fissure. This section displays the anterior extension of the two greater wings of the sphenoid bone and the posterior extension of the two petrous parts of the temporal bones, which mark the boundary between the middle and posterior cranial fossae. The clivus is part of the posterior cranial fossa and lies in contact with the basilar artery. The pontine origin of the trigeminal nerve is visible. *Note:* The trigeminal nerve passes superior to the petrous portion of the temporal bone to enter the middle cranial fossa.

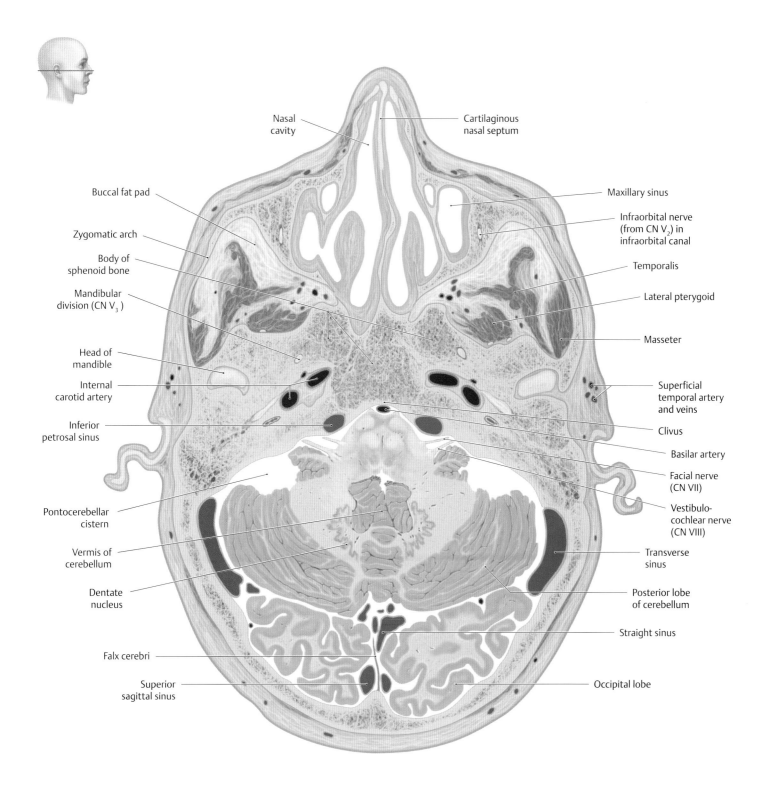

**Fig. 14.16 Transverse section through the middle nasal concha**
Superior view. This section below the orbit passes through the infra-orbital nerve and canal. Medial to the infraorbital nerve is the roof of the maxillary sinus. The zygomatic arch is visible in its entirety, with portions of the muscles of mastication (masseter, temporalis, and lateral pterygoid) and the upper part of the head of the mandible. The mandibular division (CN V$_3$) appears in cross section in its bony canal, the foramen ovale. The body of the sphenoid bone forms the bony center of the base of the skull. The facial and vestibulocochlear nerves emerge from the brainstem and enter the internal acoustic meatus. The dentate nucleus lies within the white matter of the cerebellum. The space around the anterior part of the cerebellum, the pontocerebellar cistern, is filled with cerebrospinal fluid in the living individual. The transverse sinus is prominent among the dural sinuses of the brain.

**325**

# Transverse Sections of the Head (III): Caudal

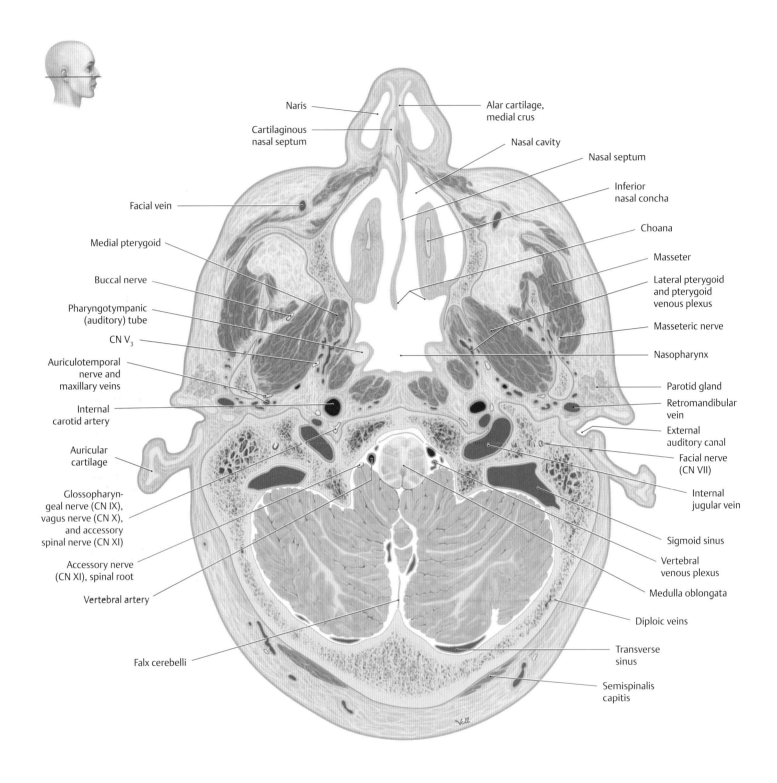

**Fig. 14.17 Transverse section through the nasopharynx**
Superior view. This section passes through the external nose and portions of the cartilaginous nasal skeleton. The nasal cavities communicate with the nasopharynx through the choanae. Cartilaginous portions of the pharyngotympanic tube project into the nasopharynx. The internal jugular vein travels with the vagus nerve (CN X) and common carotid artery as a neurovascular bundle within the carotid sheath, a fascial covering that extends from the base of the skull to the arch of the aorta. Cranial nerves IX, XI, and XII also pierce the upper portion of the carotid sheath. However, these neurovascular structures do not all enter and exit the skull base together. The jugular foramen consists of a neural and a venous portion. The neural portion conducts the glossopharyngeal (CN IX), vagus (CN X), and accessory spinal (CN XI) nerves, and the venous portion contains the jugular bulb, which receives blood from the sigmoid sinus. (*Note:* The internal jugular vein begins at the inferior portion of the jugular foramen.) The internal carotid artery enters the carotid canal, and the hypoglossal (CN XII) nerve enters the hypoglossal canal.

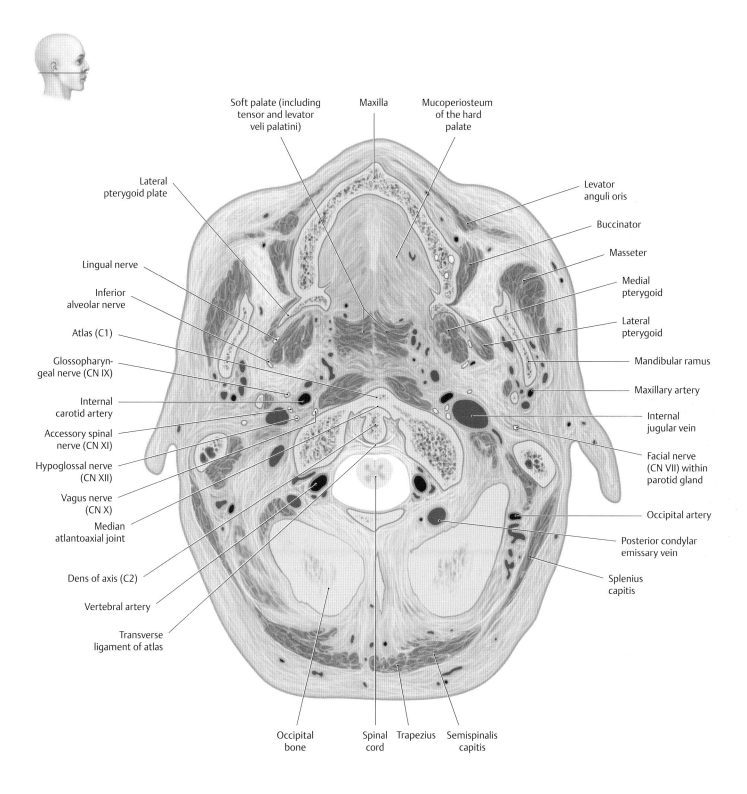

Soft palate (including tensor and levator veli palatini)

Maxilla

Mucoperiosteum of the hard palate

Lateral pterygoid plate

Levator anguli oris

Buccinator

Masseter

Lingual nerve

Medial pterygoid

Inferior alveolar nerve

Lateral pterygoid

Atlas (C1)

Mandibular ramus

Glossopharyngeal nerve (CN IX)

Maxillary artery

Internal carotid artery

Internal jugular vein

Accessory spinal nerve (CN XI)

Facial nerve (CN VII) within parotid gland

Hypoglossal nerve (CN XII)

Vagus nerve (CN X)

Occipital artery

Median atlantoaxial joint

Posterior condylar emissary vein

Dens of axis (C2)

Splenius capitis

Vertebral artery

Transverse ligament of atlas

Occipital bone

Spinal cord

Trapezius

Semispinalis capitis

**Fig. 14.18 Transverse section through the median atlantoaxial joint**
Superior view. The section at this level passes through the connective tissue sheet that stretches over the bone of the hard palate. Portions of the upper pharyngeal muscles are sectioned close to their origin. The neurovascular structures in the carotid sheath are also well displayed. The dens of the axis articulates in the median atlantoaxial joint with the facet for the dens on the posterior surface of the anterior arch of the atlas. The transverse ligament of the atlas that helps to stabilize this joint can also be identified. The vertebral artery and its accompanying veins are displayed in cross section, as is the spinal cord. In the occipital region, the section passes through the upper portion of the posterior neck muscles.

# Transverse Sections of the Neck (I): Cranial

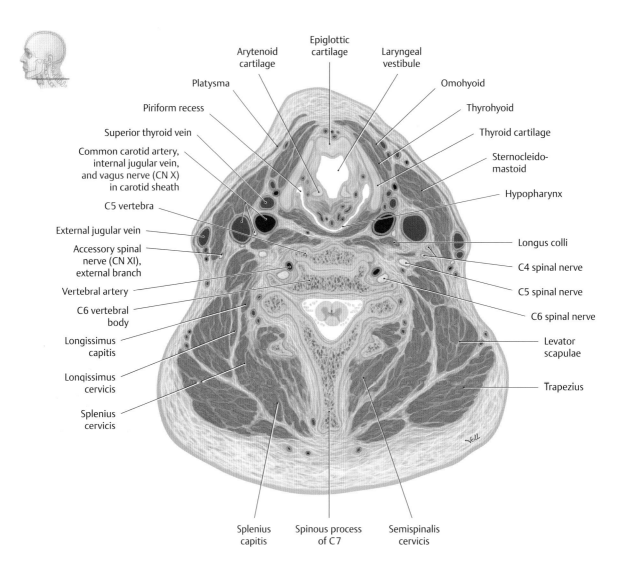

**Fig. 14.19 Transverse section at the level of the C5 vertebral body**
Inferior view. The internal jugular vein travels with the common carotid artery and vagus nerve in the carotid sheath. The accessory spinal nerve (CN XI) is medial to the sternocleidomastoid; more proximal to the skull base it will pierce the carotid sheath to enter the jugular foramen with the internal jugular vein, as well as CN IX and X. The elongated spinous process of the C7 vertebra (vertebra prominens) is visible at this level, owing to the lordotic curvature of the neck. Note that the triangular shape of the arytenoid cartilage is clearly demonstrated in the laryngeal cross section.

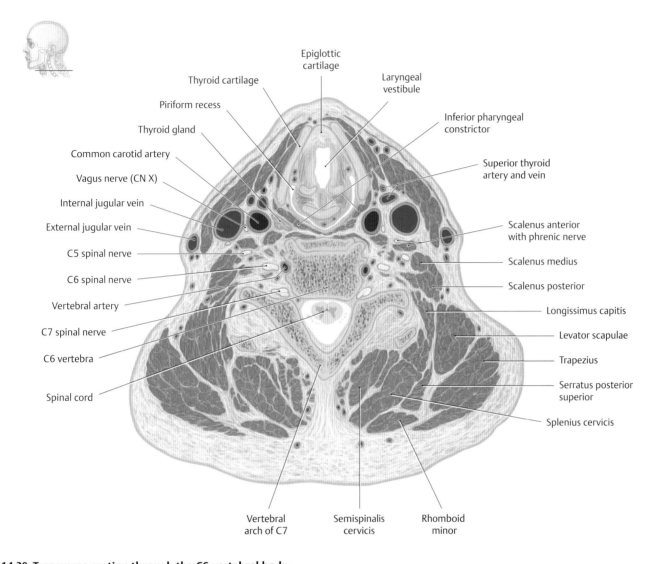

Epiglottic
cartilage

Thyroid cartilage

Laryngeal
vestibule

Piriform recess

Inferior pharyngeal
constrictor

Thyroid gland

Common carotid artery

Superior thyroid
artery and vein

Vagus nerve (CN X)

Internal jugular vein

External jugular vein

Scalenus anterior
with phrenic nerve

C5 spinal nerve

Scalenus medius

C6 spinal nerve

Scalenus posterior

Vertebral artery

Longissimus capitis

C7 spinal nerve

Levator scapulae

C6 vertebra

Trapezius

Spinal cord

Serratus posterior
superior

Splenius cervicis

Vertebral
arch of C7

Semispinalis
cervicis

Rhomboid
minor

*Fig. 14.20* **Transverse section through the C6 vertebral body**
Inferior view. The piriform recess can be identified at this level, and
the vertebral artery is visible in its course along the vertebral body.
The vagus nerve (CN X) lies in a posterior angle between the common
carotid artery and internal jugular vein within the carotid sheath. The
phrenic nerve, which arises from the ventral rami of cervical spinal
nerves C3–C5, lies on the scalenus anterior muscle on the left side.

# Transverse Sections of the Neck (II): Caudal

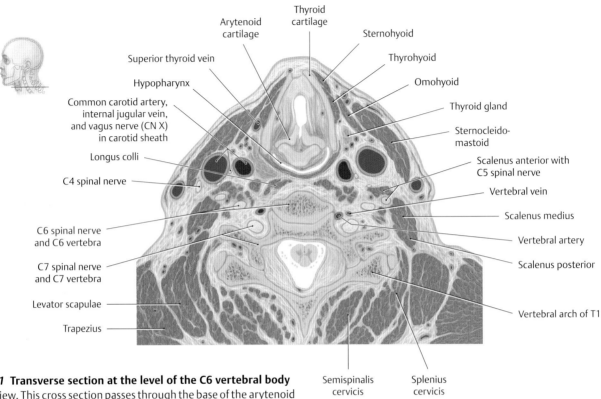

**Fig. 14.21 Transverse section at the level of the C6 vertebral body**
Inferior view. This cross section passes through the base of the arytenoid cartilage in the larynx. The hypopharynx appears as a narrow transverse cleft behind the larynx.

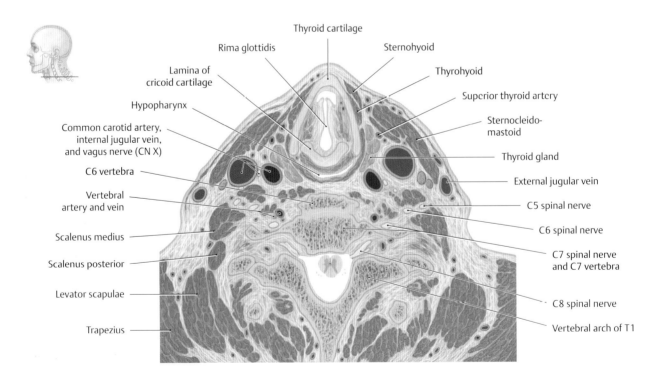

**Fig. 14.22 Transverse section at the level of the C6/C7 vertebral junction**
Inferior view. This cross section passes through the larynx at the level of the vocal folds. The thyroid gland appears considerably smaller at this level than in subsequent views.

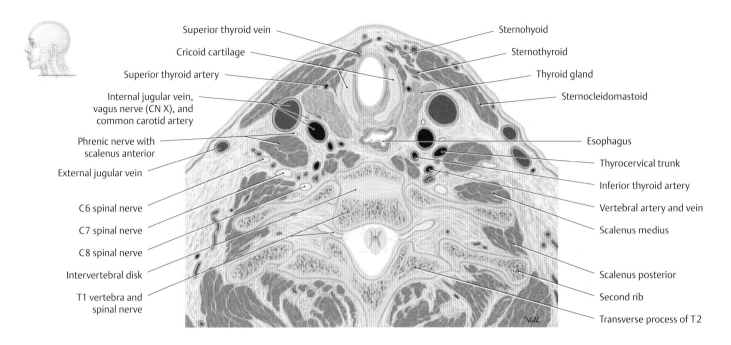

**Fig. 14.23 Transverse section at the level of the C7/T1 vertebral junction**
Inferior view. This cross section clearly displays the scalenus anterior and medius muscles and the interval between them, which is traversed by the C6–C8 roots of the brachial plexus. Note the neurovascular structures (common carotid artery, internal jugular vein, vagus nerve) that lie within the carotid sheath between the sternocleidomastoid, anterior scalene, and thyroid gland.

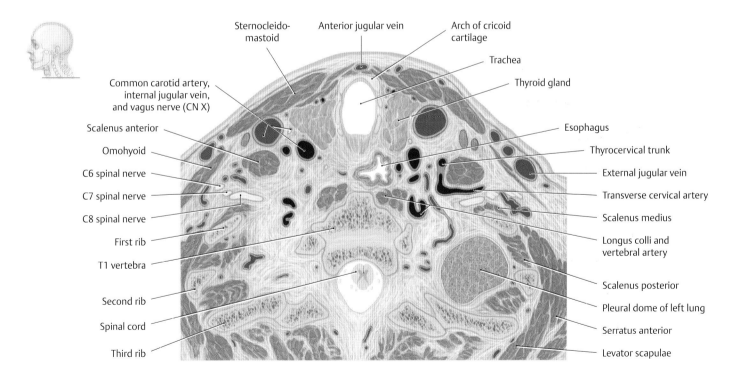

**Fig. 14.24 Transverse section at the level of the T1/T2 vertebral junction**
Inferior view. Due to the curvature of the neck in this specimen, the section also cuts the intervertebral disk between T1 and T2. This section includes the C6–C8 nerve roots of the brachial plexus and a small section of the left pleural dome. The proximity of the pulmonary apex to the brachial plexus shows why the growth of an apical lung tumor may damage the brachial plexus roots. Note also the thyroid gland and its proximity to the trachea and neurovascular bundle in the carotid sheath.

**331**

# Transverse MRIs of the Head

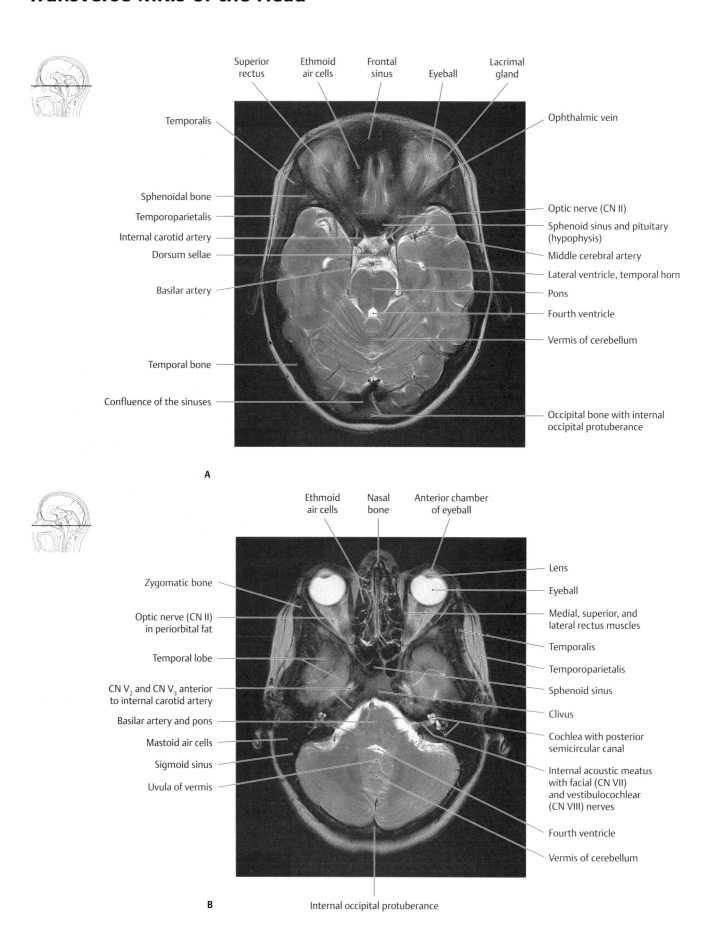

**Fig. 14.25 Transverse MRIs through the orbit and ethmoid air cells**
Inferior view. **A** Superior orbit. This section demonstrates the relationship of the frontal and sphenoid sinuses to the orbit and nasal cavity. **B** Section through optic nerve (CN II). The divisions of the eye can be clearly seen along with the extraocular muscles located in the peri-orbital fat. The sigmoid sinus is located posterior to the mastoid air cells and lateral to the cerebellum. This section clearly displays the internal acoustic meatus, which conducts the facial (CN VII) and vestibulocochlear (CN VIII) nerves.

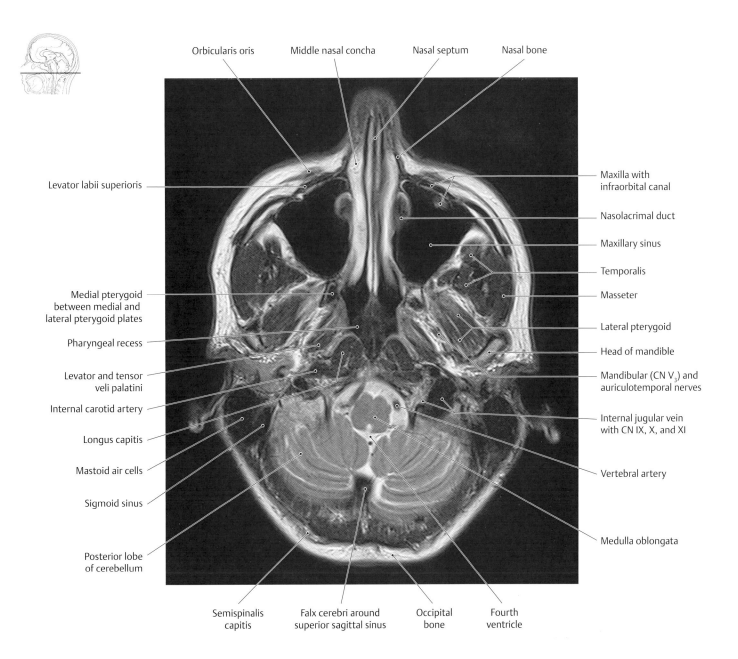

Orbicularis oris    Middle nasal concha    Nasal septum    Nasal bone

Levator labii superioris

Medial pterygoid between medial and lateral pterygoid plates

Pharyngeal recess

Levator and tensor veli palatini

Internal carotid artery

Longus capitis

Mastoid air cells

Sigmoid sinus

Posterior lobe of cerebellum

Maxilla with infraorbital canal

Nasolacrimal duct

Maxillary sinus

Temporalis

Masseter

Lateral pterygoid

Head of mandible

Mandibular (CN V₃) and auriculotemporal nerves

Internal jugular vein with CN IX, X, and XI

Vertebral artery

Medulla oblongata

Semispinalis capitis    Falx cerebri around superior sagittal sinus    Occipital bone    Fourth ventricle

**Fig. 14.26 Transverse MRI through the orbit and nasolacrimal duct**
Inferior view. This section clearly demonstrates the relationships of the infraorbital canal and nasolacrimal duct to the maxillary sinus. The medial and lateral pterygoid plates can be seen flanking the medial pterygoid. The pharyngeal recess is visible, anterior to the longus capitis. The mandibular division of the trigeminal nerve (CN V₃) is lateral to the levator and tensor veli palatini and medial to the lateral pterygoid. Cranial nerves IX, X, and XI run just anteromedial to the internal jugular vein.

**333**

# Transverse MRIs of the Oral Cavity

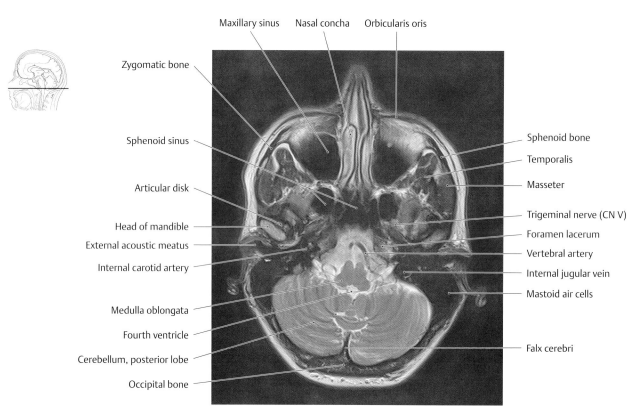

**Fig. 14.27 Transverse MRI through the TMJ**
Inferior view. *Note:* The plane of this section is slightly higher than **Fig. 14.26**. It has been included here in order to show the articular disk of the TMJ and the full extent of the mandible.

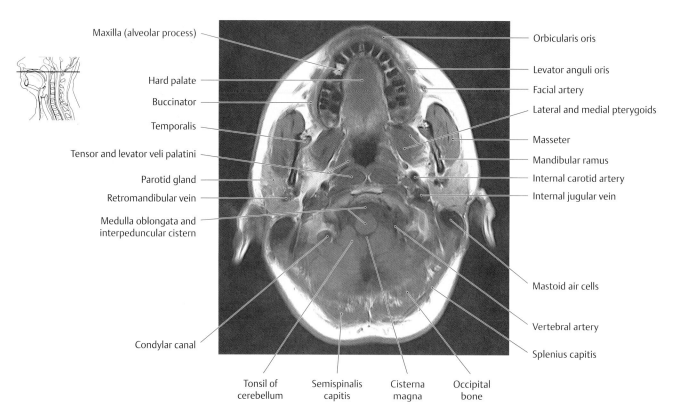

**Fig. 14.28 Transverse MRI through the hard and soft palates**
Inferior view. This section demonstrates the relation of the mandibular ramus to the muscles of mastication in the infratemporal fossa.

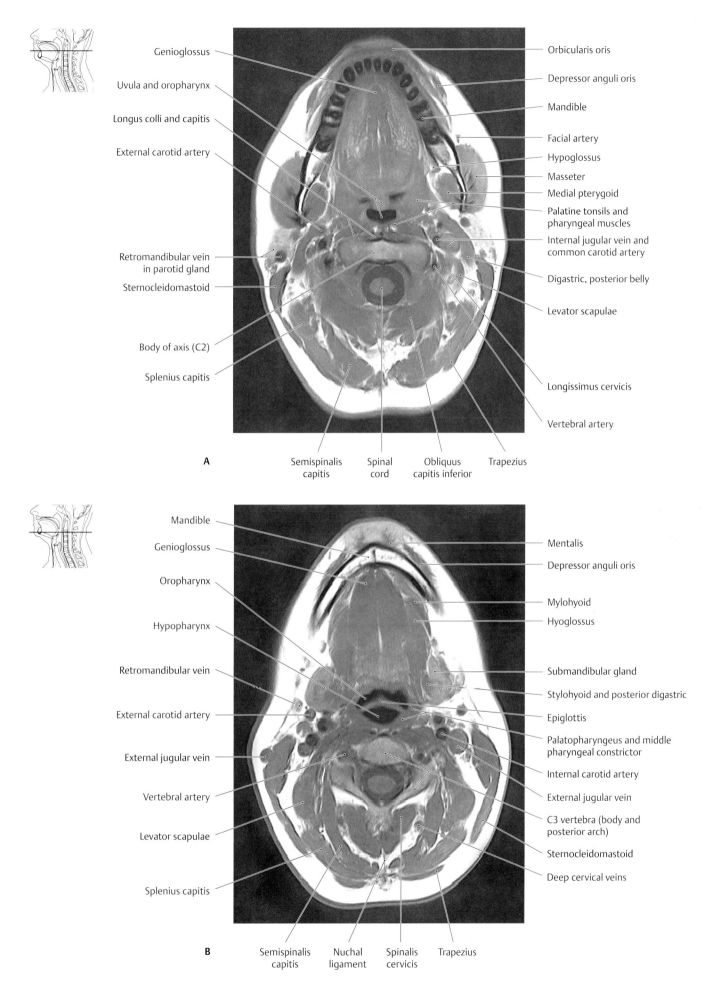

Genioglossus

Uvula and oropharynx

Longus colli and capitis

External carotid artery

Retromandibular vein in parotid gland

Sternocleidomastoid

Body of axis (C2)

Splenius capitis

Orbicularis oris

Depressor anguli oris

Mandible

Facial artery

Hypoglossus

Masseter

Medial pterygoid

Palatine tonsils and pharyngeal muscles

Internal jugular vein and common carotid artery

Digastric, posterior belly

Levator scapulae

Longissimus cervicis

Vertebral artery

**A**   Semispinalis capitis   Spinal cord   Obliquus capitis inferior   Trapezius

Mandible

Genioglossus

Oropharynx

Hypopharynx

Retromandibular vein

External carotid artery

External jugular vein

Vertebral artery

Levator scapulae

Splenius capitis

Mentalis

Depressor anguli oris

Mylohyoid

Hyoglossus

Submandibular gland

Stylohyoid and posterior digastric

Epiglottis

Palatopharyngeus and middle pharyngeal constrictor

Internal carotid artery

External jugular vein

C3 vertebra (body and posterior arch)

Sternocleidomastoid

Deep cervical veins

**B**   Semispinalis capitis   Nuchal ligament   Spinalis cervicis   Trapezius

***Fig. 14.29* Transverse MRIs through the mandible**

Inferior view. **A** Section through mandibular arch. This section demonstrates the relationship of the oropharynx to the soft palate (uvula) and prevertebral muscles (longus colli and capitis). The vessels of the carotid sheath are clearly visible, along with the retromandibular vein in the parotid gland. **B** Section through body of mandible and hypophyarynx.

**335**

# Transverse MRIs of the Neck

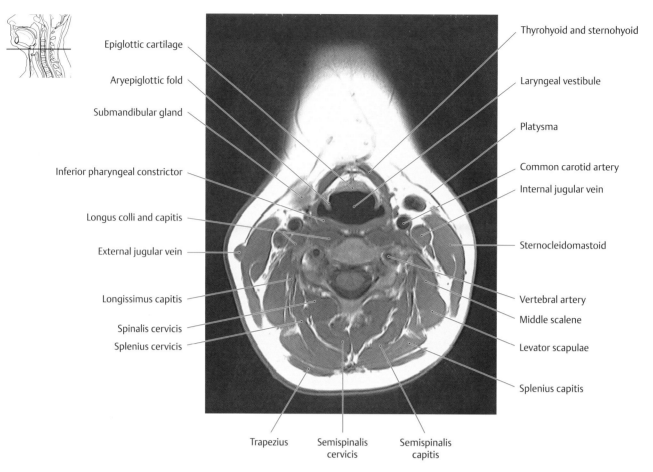

Epiglottic cartilage

Aryepiglottic fold

Submandibular gland

Inferior pharyngeal constrictor

Longus colli and capitis

External jugular vein

Longissimus capitis

Spinalis cervicis

Splenius cervicis

Thyrohyoid and sternohyoid

Laryngeal vestibule

Platysma

Common carotid artery

Internal jugular vein

Sternocleidomastoid

Vertebral artery

Middle scalene

Levator scapulae

Splenius capitis

Trapezius   Semispinalis   Semispinalis
cervicis        capitis

**Fig. 14.30 Transverse MRI through the C4 vertebral body**
Inferior view. This section demonstrates the aryepiglottic fold in the
laryngeal vestibule. Note the proximity of the prevertebral muscles to
the pharyngeal constrictors.

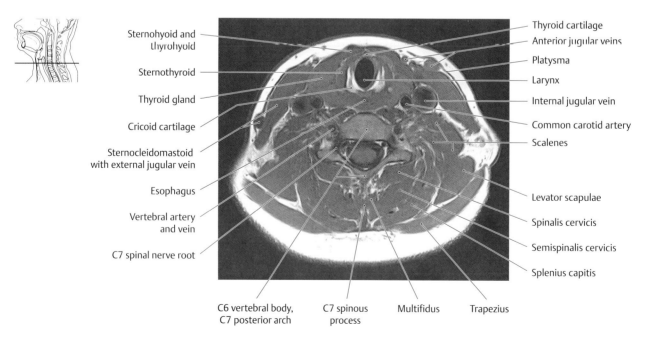

Sternohyoid and
thyrohyoid

Sternothyroid

Thyroid gland

Cricoid cartilage

Sternocleidomastoid
with external jugular vein

Esophagus

Vertebral artery
and vein

C7 spinal nerve root

Thyroid cartilage

Anterior jugular veins

Platysma

Larynx

Internal jugular vein

Common carotid artery

Scalenes

Levator scapulae

Spinalis cervicis

Semispinalis cervicis

Splenius capitis

C6 vertebral body,   C7 spinous   Multifidus   Trapezius
C7 posterior arch      process

**Fig. 14.31 Transverse MRI through the C6 vertebral body**
Inferior view. This section demonstrates the cricoid and thyroid cartilage of the larynx (note the change in shape of the larynx). Due to lordosis of the cervical spine, this section includes the C6 vertebral body
and the C7 spinous process with posterior arch.

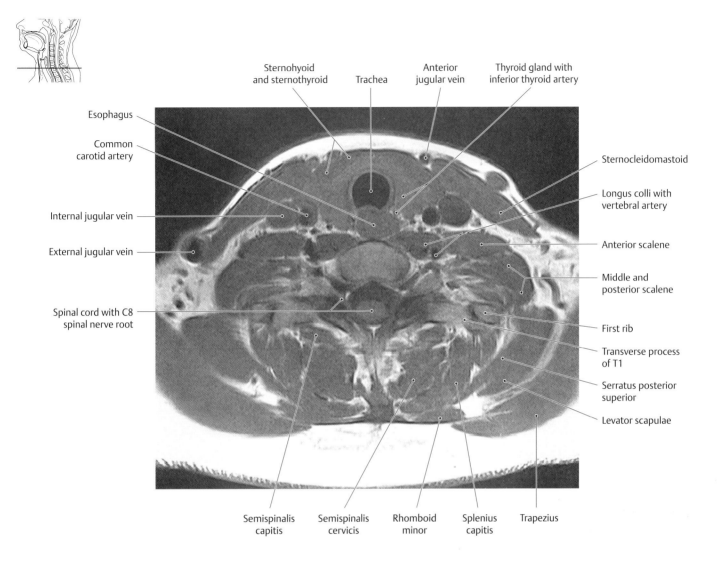

Esophagus

Common carotid artery

Internal jugular vein

External jugular vein

Spinal cord with C8 spinal nerve root

Sternohyoid and sternothyroid    Trachea    Anterior jugular vein    Thyroid gland with inferior thyroid artery

Sternocleidomastoid

Longus colli with vertebral artery

Anterior scalene

Middle and posterior scalene

First rib

Transverse process of T1

Serratus posterior superior

Levator scapulae

Semispinalis capitis    Semispinalis cervicis    Rhomboid minor    Splenius capitis    Trapezius

**Fig. 14.32 Transverse MRI through the C7 vertebra**
Inferior view. This section demonstrates the relationship of the trachea to the esophagus. Note the position of the carotid sheath (containing the common carotid artery, internal jugular vein, and vagus nerve) with respect to the thyroid gland. The C8 spinal nerve root can be seen emerging from the spinal cord. Note the first rib and transverse process of the thoracic vertebra.

# Sagittal Sections of the Head (I): Medial

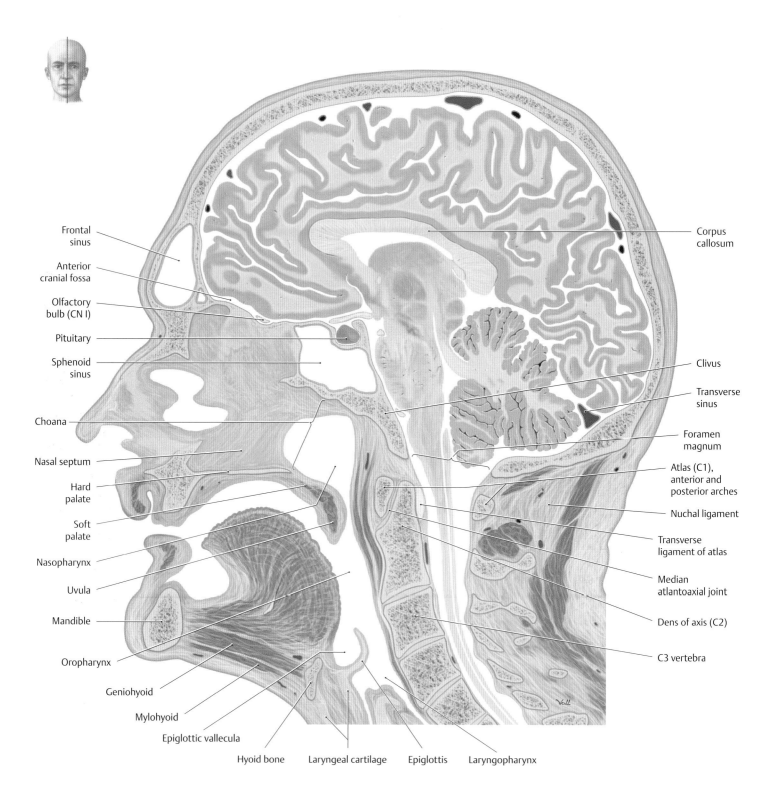

Frontal sinus

Anterior cranial fossa

Olfactory bulb (CN I)

Pituitary

Sphenoid sinus

Choana

Nasal septum

Hard palate

Soft palate

Nasopharynx

Uvula

Mandible

Oropharynx

Geniohyoid

Mylohyoid

Epiglottic vallecula

Hyoid bone          Laryngeal cartilage          Epiglottis          Laryngopharynx

Corpus callosum

Clivus

Transverse sinus

Foramen magnum

Atlas (C1), anterior and posterior arches

Nuchal ligament

Transverse ligament of atlas

Median atlantoaxial joint

Dens of axis (C2)

C3 vertebra

**Fig. 14.33 Midsagittal section through the nasal septum**
Left lateral view. The anatomical structures at this level can be roughly assigned to the **facial skeleton** or neurocranium (cranial vault). The lowest level of the facial skeleton is formed by the oral floor muscles between the hyoid bone and mandible and the overlying skin. This section also passes through the epiglottis and the larynx below it, which are considered part of the cervical viscera. *Note:* The epiglottic vallecula, located in the oropharynx, is bounded by the root of the tongue and the epiglottis. The hard and soft palate with the uvula define the boundary between the oral and nasal cavities. Posterior to the uvula is the oropharynx. The section includes the nasal septum, which divides the nasal cavity into two cavities (sectioned above and in front of the septum) that communicate with the nasopharynx through the choanae. Posterior to the frontal sinus is the anterior cranial fossa, which is part of the **neurocranium**. This section passes through the medial surface of the brain (the falx cerebri has been removed). The cut edge of the corpus callosum, the olfactory bulb, and the pituitary are also shown.

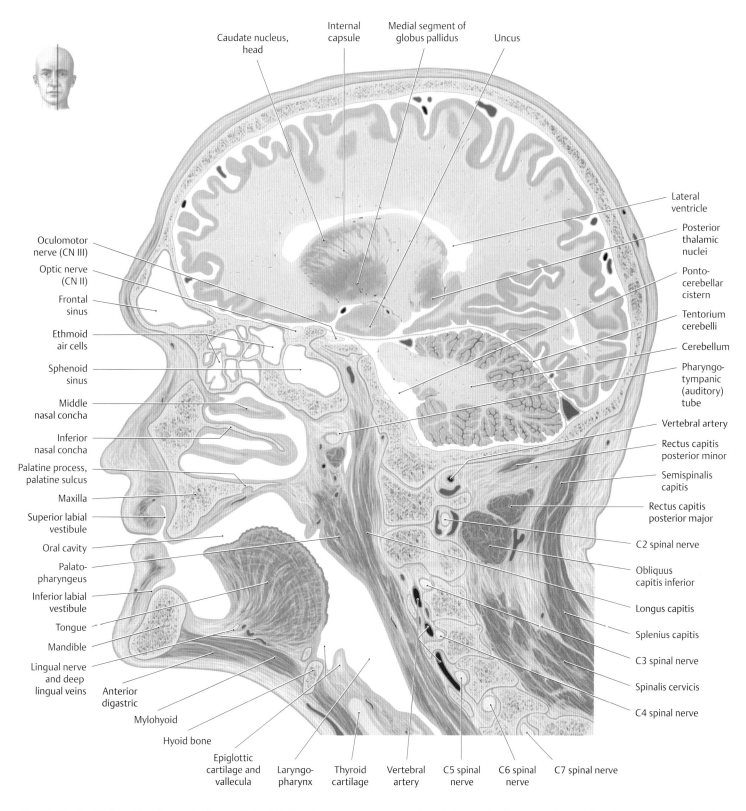

Caudate nucleus, head

Internal capsule

Medial segment of globus pallidus

Uncus

Oculomotor nerve (CN III)

Optic nerve (CN II)

Frontal sinus

Ethmoid air cells

Sphenoid sinus

Middle nasal concha

Inferior nasal concha

Palatine process, palatine sulcus

Maxilla

Superior labial vestibule

Oral cavity

Palato-pharyngeus

Inferior labial vestibule

Tongue

Mandible

Lingual nerve and deep lingual veins

Anterior digastric

Mylohyoid

Hyoid bone

Epiglottic cartilage and vallecula

Laryngo-pharynx

Thyroid cartilage

Vertebral artery

C5 spinal nerve

C6 spinal nerve

C7 spinal nerve

Lateral ventricle

Posterior thalamic nuclei

Ponto-cerebellar cistern

Tentorium cerebelli

Cerebellum

Pharyngo-tympanic (auditory) tube

Vertebral artery

Rectus capitis posterior minor

Semispinalis capitis

Rectus capitis posterior major

C2 spinal nerve

Obliquus capitis inferior

Longus capitis

Splenius capitis

C3 spinal nerve

Spinalis cervicis

C4 spinal nerve

**Fig. 14.34 Sagittal section through the medial orbital wall**
Left lateral view. This section passes through the inferior and middle nasal conchae within the nasal cavity. Above the middle nasal concha are the ethmoid air cells. The only parts of the nasopharynx visible in this section are a small luminal area and the lateral wall, which bears a section of the cartilaginous portion of the pharyngotympanic tube. The sphenoid sinus is also displayed. In the region of the cervical spine, the section cuts the vertebral artery at multiple levels. The lateral sites where the spinal nerves emerge from the intervertebral foramina are clearly displayed. *Note:* This section is lateral to the geniohyoid.

# Sagittal Sections of the Head (II): Lateral

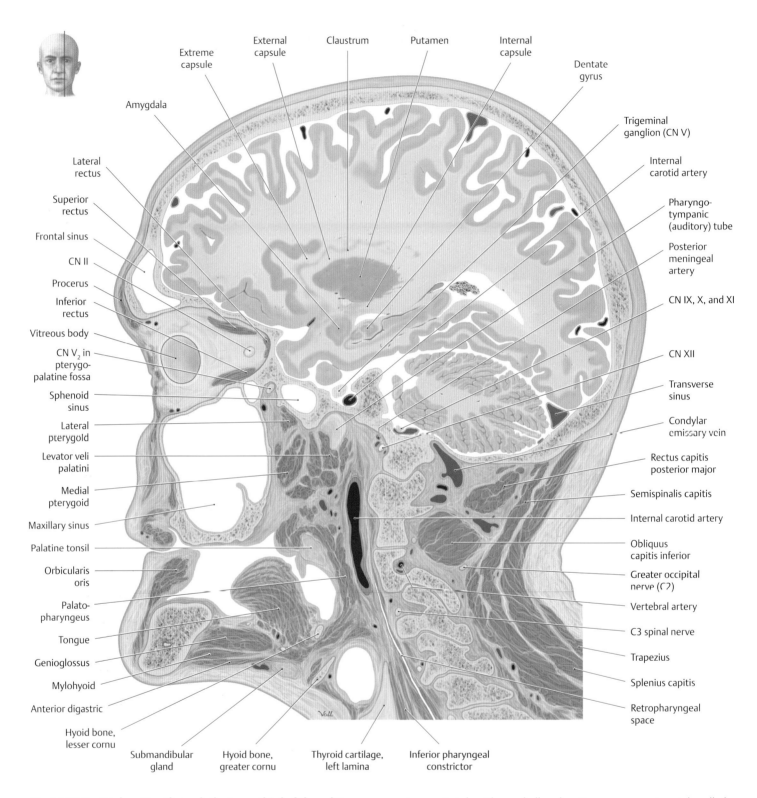

**Fig. 14.35 Sagittal section through the inner third of the orbit**
Left lateral view. This section passes through the maxillary and frontal sinuses while displaying one ethmoid air cell and the peripheral part of the sphenoid sinus. It passes through the medial portion of the internal carotid artery and submandibular gland. The pharyngeal and masticatory muscles are grouped about the cartilaginous part of the pharyn-gotympanic tube. The eyeball and optic nerve are cut peripherally by the section, which displays relatively long segments of the superior and inferior rectus muscles. Sectioned brain structures include the external and internal capsules and the intervening putamen. The amygdala can be identified near the base of the brain. A section of the trigeminal ganglion appears below the cerebrum.

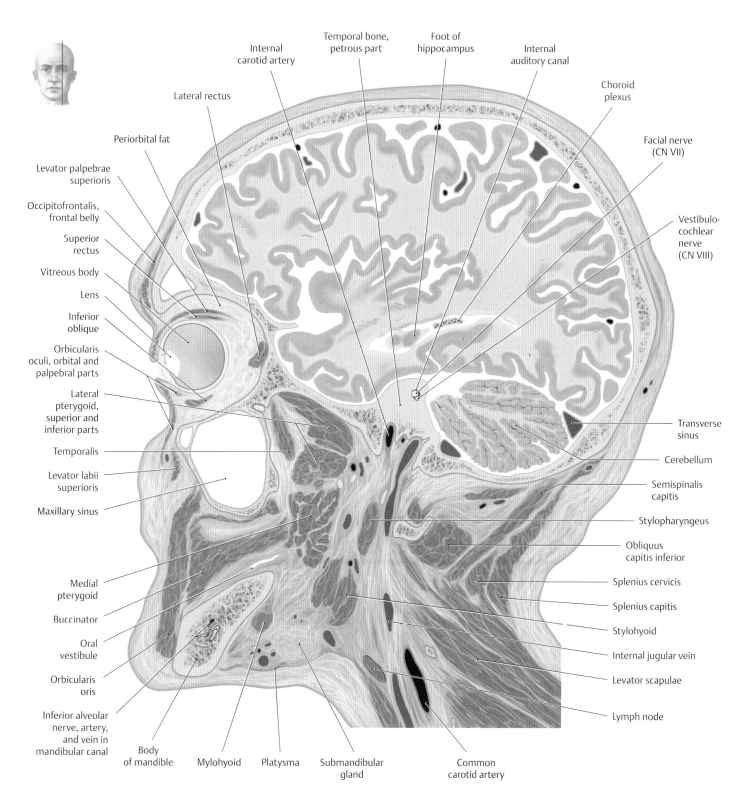

**Fig. 14.36 Sagittal section through the approximate center of the orbit**

Left lateral view. Due to the obliquity of this section, the dominant structure in the oral floor region is the mandible, whereas the oral vestibule appears as a narrow slit. The buccal and masticatory muscles are prominently displayed. Much of the orbit is occupied by the eyeball, which appears in longitudinal section. Aside from a few sections of the extraocular muscles, the orbit in this plane is filled with periorbital fat. Both the internal carotid artery and the internal jugular vein are demonstrated. Except for the foot of the hippocampus, the only visible cerebral structures are the white matter and cortex. The facial nerve and vestibulocochlear nerve can be identified in the internal auditory canal.

**341**

# Sagittal MRIs of the Head

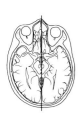

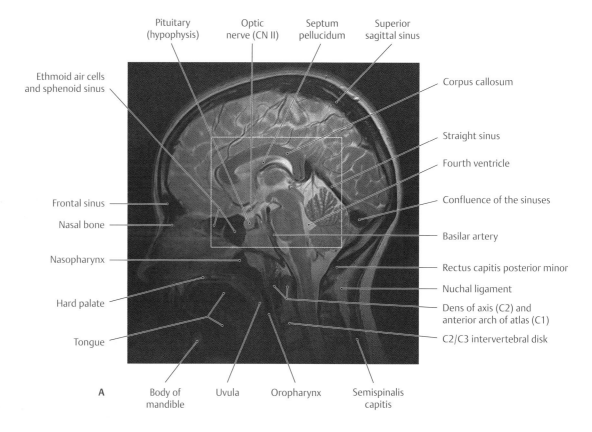

Pituitary (hypophysis)

Optic nerve (CN II)

Septum pellucidum

Superior sagittal sinus

Ethmoid air cells and sphenoid sinus

Corpus callosum

Straight sinus

Fourth ventricle

Frontal sinus

Confluence of the sinuses

Nasal bone

Basilar artery

Nasopharynx

Rectus capitis posterior minor

Hard palate

Nuchal ligament

Dens of axis (C2) and anterior arch of atlas (C1)

Tongue

C2/C3 intervertebral disk

**A**  Body of mandible   Uvula   Oropharynx   Semispinalis capitis

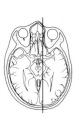

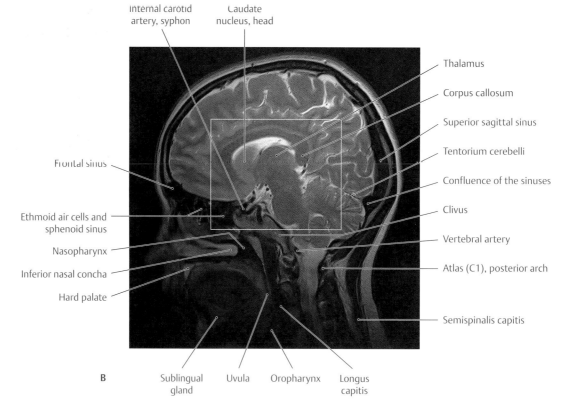

Internal carotid artery, syphon

Caudate nucleus, head

Thalamus

Corpus callosum

Superior sagittal sinus

Frontal sinus

Tentorium cerebelli

Confluence of the sinuses

Ethmoid air cells and sphenoid sinus

Clivus

Nasopharynx

Vertebral artery

Inferior nasal concha

Atlas (C1), posterior arch

Hard palate

Semispinalis capitis

**B**  Sublingual gland   Uvula   Oropharynx   Longus capitis

**Fig. 14.37 Sagittal sections through the nasal cavity**
Left lateral view. **A** Midsagittal section through nasal septum. **B** Sagittal section through inferior and middle nasal conchae. These sections demonstrate the relationship of the nasopharynx to the oropharynx.

The optic nerve (CN II) is visible as the optic chiasm in **A**. The pituitary (hypophysis) can be seen inferior to it, just posterior to the sphenoid sinus. The syphon of the internal carotid artery is beautifully displayed in **B**.

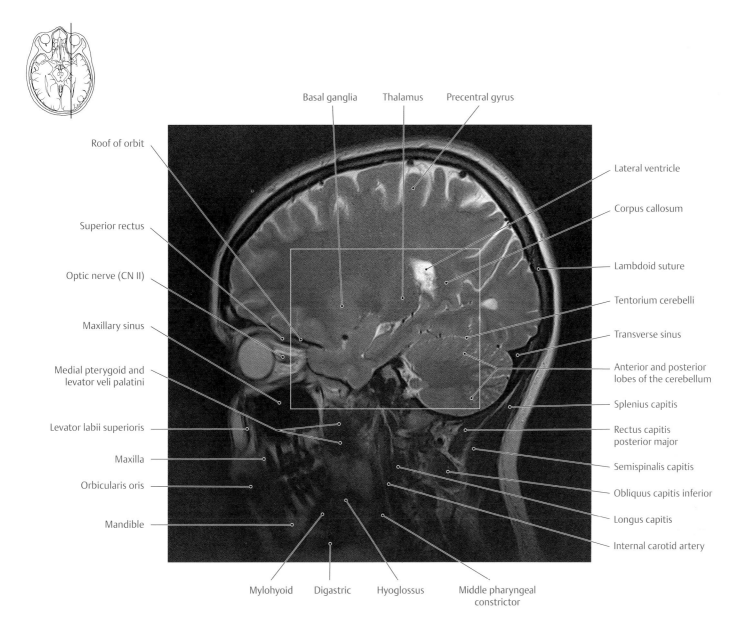

Basal ganglia  Thalamus  Precentral gyrus

Roof of orbit

Superior rectus

Optic nerve (CN II)

Maxillary sinus

Medial pterygoid and
levator veli palatini

Levator labii superioris

Maxilla

Orbicularis oris

Mandible

Lateral ventricle

Corpus callosum

Lambdoid suture

Tentorium cerebelli

Transverse sinus

Anterior and posterior
lobes of the cerebellum

Splenius capitis

Rectus capitis
posterior major

Semispinalis capitis

Obliquus capitis inferior

Longus capitis

Internal carotid artery

Mylohyoid  Digastric  Hyoglossus  Middle pharyngeal
constrictor

*Fig. 14.38* **Sagittal section through the orbit**
Left lateral view. This view exposes the superior and inferior rectus
muscles within the periorbital fat. The course of the optic nerve (CN II)
within the orbit can be seen. Note the proximity of the maxillary dentition to the maxillary sinus. Roots of the maxillary dentition may erupt
into the maxillary sinus. The major forceps of the corpus callosum can
be seen just posterior to the lateral ventricle.

# Sagittal MRIs of the Neck

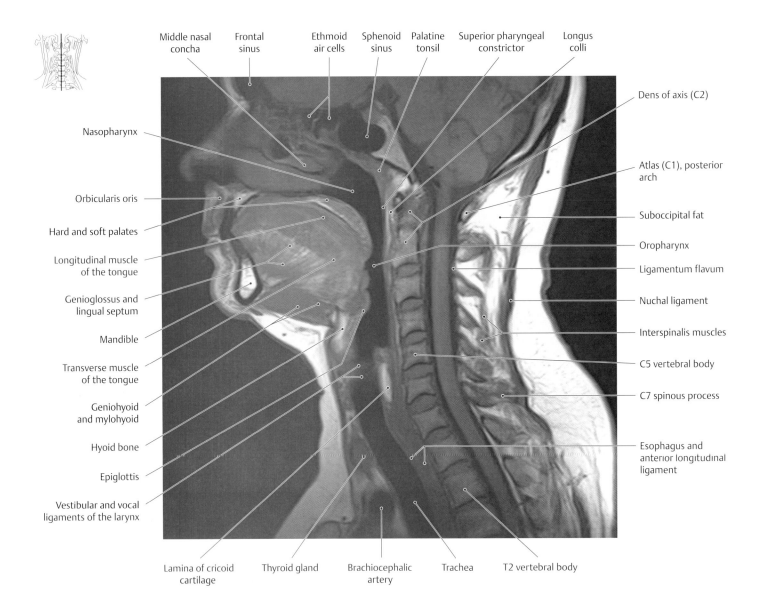

Middle nasal concha — Frontal sinus — Ethmoid air cells — Sphenoid sinus — Palatine tonsil — Superior pharyngeal constrictor — Longus colli

Nasopharynx

Orbicularis oris

Hard and soft palates

Longitudinal muscle of the tongue

Genioglossus and lingual septum

Mandible

Transverse muscle of the tongue

Geniohyoid and mylohyoid

Hyoid bone

Epiglottis

Vestibular and vocal ligaments of the larynx

Dens of axis (C2)

Atlas (C1), posterior arch

Suboccipital fat

Oropharynx

Ligamentum flavum

Nuchal ligament

Interspinalis muscles

C5 vertebral body

C7 spinous process

Esophagus and anterior longitudinal ligament

Lamina of cricoid cartilage — Thyroid gland — Brachiocephalic artery — Trachea — T2 vertebral body

**Fig. 14.39 Midsagittal section**
Left lateral view. This section illustrates the relations between the nasal cavity and ethmoid air cells. The nasal cavity communicates posteriorly (via the choanae) with the nasopharynx, which is separated from the oral cavity by the soft palate and uvula. Inferior to the uvula, the naso-pharynx and oral cavity converge in the oropharynx. Air continues more anteriorly into the laryngopharynx and ultimately the trachea, whereas food passes into the esophagus, posterior to the lamina of the larynx. Note how closely opposed the esophagus is to the anterior sur-face of the vertebral bodies. This section also reveals the cervical verte-brae and ligaments.

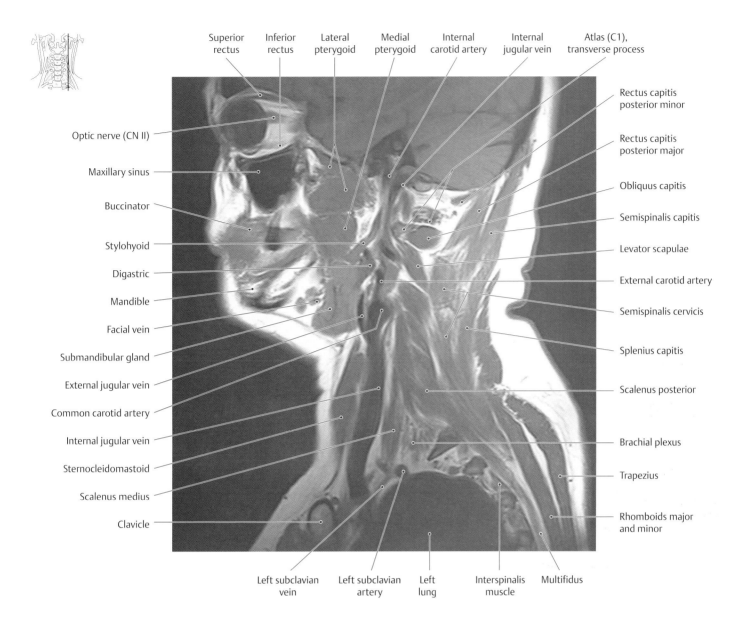

**Fig. 14.40 Sagittal section through carotid bifurcation**
Left lateral view. This section shows the common and external carotid arteries, as well as the internal and external jugular veins. The cranio-vertebral joint muscles are visible along with the nuchal muscles. Note the position of the brachial plexus between the medial and posterior scalenes. The extent of the submandibular gland can be appreciated in this view.

# Appendix

# References

Becker W, Naumann HH, Pfaltz CR. *Otorhinolaryngology* [in German]. 2nd ed. Stuttgart: Thieme; 1983

Faller A, Poisel S, Golth D, Faller A, Schuenke M. *The Human Body* [in German]. 14th ed. Stuttgart: Thieme; 2004

Kahle W, Frotscher M. *Pocket Atlas of Anatomy* [in German]. Vol. 3. 9th ed. Stuttgart: Thieme; 2005

Lippert H, Pabst R. *Arterial Variations in Man.* Munich: Bergmann; 1985

Platzer W. *Pocket Atlas of Anatomy* [in German]. Vol. 1. Stuttgart: Thieme; 1999

Platzer W. *Topographic Anatomy Atlas* [in German]. Stuttgart: Thieme; 1982

Rauber A, Kopsch F. *Human Anatomy* [in German]. Vol. 1–4. Stuttgart: Thieme; Vol. 1, 2: 1997; Vol. 2, 3: 1987; Vol. 4: 1988

Schmidt F. *Innervation of the Temporomandibular Joint* [in German]. Gegenbaurs morphol. Jb. 1067:110;554-573

Tillmann B. *Color Atlas of Anatomy Dental Medicine — Human Medicine* [in German]. Stuttgart: Thieme; 1997

Vahlensieck M, Reiser M. *MRI of the Musculoskeletal System* [in German]. 2nd ed. Stuttgart: Thieme; 2001

Vahlensieck M, Reiser M, eds. *MRI of the Musculoskeletal System* [in German]. 2nd rev. ed. Berlin: Springer; 1959

von Lanz T, Wachsmuth W. *Applied Anatomy* [in German]. Vol. 2, Part 6 (Loeweneck H, Feifel G, eds.), Berlin: Springer; 1993

von Lanz T, Wachsmuth W. *Applied Anatomy* [in German]. Vol. 1, 2: Hals, Berlin: Springer; 1955

# Index

*Note:* Tabular material is indicated by a "t" following the page number.